Inhaled Treatment of Respiratory Infections

Inhaled Treatment of Respiratory Infections

Editors

Philip Chi Lip Kwok
Michael Yee Tak Chow

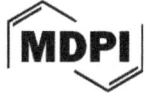 Basel • Beijing • Wuhan • Barcelona • Belgrade • Novi Sad • Cluj • Manchester

Editors

Philip Chi Lip Kwok
Sydney Pharmacy School
The University of Sydney
Camperdown
Australia

Michael Yee Tak Chow
Department of Pharmaceutics,
UCL School of Pharmacy
University College London
London
United Kingdom

Editorial Office
MDPI
St. Alban-Anlage 66
4052 Basel, Switzerland

This is a reprint of articles from the Special Issue published online in the open access journal *Pharmaceutics* (ISSN 1999-4923) (available at: www.mdpi.com/journal/pharmaceutics/special_issues/inhaled_treatment).

For citation purposes, cite each article independently as indicated on the article page online and as indicated below:

Lastname, A.A.; Lastname, B.B. Article Title. *Journal Name* **Year**, *Volume Number*, Page Range.

ISBN 978-3-7258-0392-7 (Hbk)
ISBN 978-3-7258-0391-0 (PDF)
doi.org/10.3390/books978-3-7258-0391-0

Contents

About the Editors

Philip Chi Lip Kwok

Dr Philip Chi Lip Kwok is a Senior Lecturer in Pharmaceutical Sciences in the School of Pharmacy, the University of Sydney. He obtained his Bachelor of Pharmacy degree with First Class Honours in 2002 from this faculty. He became a registered pharmacist after one year of training in a community pharmacy. Dr Kwok then undertook his PhD studies on pharmaceutical aerosol electrostatics in the Faculty of Pharmacy at the University of Sydney and graduated in 2007. He was a research associate in the same group until August 2011 and became an assistant professor in the Department of Pharmacology and Pharmacy at the University of Hong Kong in September 2011. Dr Kwok returned to the University of Sydney as a Lecturer in Pharmaceutical Sciences at the end of July 2017. His research is in pulmonary drug delivery. In particular, he specialises in the engineering, physicochemical characterisation, and electrostatics of pharmaceutical aerosol formulations. He has collaborated with academic and industrial researchers, both locally and internationally, on formulation-focused as well as interdisciplinary projects.

Michael Yee Tak Chow

Dr Michael Yee Tak Chow has been a Postdoctoral Research Fellow in the Department of Pharmaceutics, University College London School of Pharmacy, since February 2023. He obtained his Bachelor of Pharmacy degree with First Class Honours and PhD degree in Pharmacy at the University of Hong Kong in 2012 and 2018, respectively. He became a registered pharmacist under the Hong Kong Pharmacy and Poisons Board in 2013. His PhD project focused on the pharmaceutical formulation development of therapeutic nucleic acids (e.g., RNA) for pulmonary delivery. He worked as a postdoctoral research associate in the Advanced Drug Delivery Group from November 2018 to October 2021 in the Sydney Pharmacy School at the University of Sydney. During this period, he expanded his research area into inhaled bacteriophage formulations to combat respiratory lung infections that are becoming more difficult to treat due to antimicrobial resistance.

Preface

Respiratory infections are conventionally treated with oral or intravenous antimicrobials (antivirals, antibiotics, and antifungals). However, these routes of administration are not ideal because the required drugs are systemically delivered rather than being targeted to the respiratory tract. Higher doses may also be needed to achieve sufficient drug concentrations in the lungs, which may consequently increase the risk of adverse effects. On the other hand, the drugs can be efficiently delivered into the airways as inhaled aerosols. Lower doses can then be used to attain relatively high local concentrations. There are specific challenges to the development of inhaled formulations, such as the optimisation of their physicochemical stability and aerosol performance. In addition, antimicrobial resistance is an urgent global public health issue. Novel strategies are required to overcome these problems.

The papers in this reprint focus on recent advancements in inhaled antimicrobials and vaccines, including those for viral (SARS-CoV-2), bacterial (Mycobacterium tuberculosis, Mycoplasma pneumoniae, Acinetobacter baumanii), and fungal infections (moulds). Tai et al. and D'Angelo et al. studied hydroxychloroquine nebules and an inhalable cyclosporin-A powder for potential COVID-19 treatment, respectively. Sécher et al. reported the physical instability of nebulised immunoglobulin G and the resultant pro-inflammatory and cytotoxic effects. On the other hand, the acute respiratory distress syndrome associated with pulmonary infections such as COVID-19 may be treated with mesh-nebulised plasminogen (Vizzoni et al). Seifelnasr et al. investigated a new method to deliver respiratory vaccines to the posterior nasal area to enhance the mucosal immunisation response. Studies on spray-dried capreomycin (Shao et al), lyophilised isoniazid nanoparticles (Mukhtar et al), and jet-nebulised rifampicin–curcumin micelles for tuberculosis (Galdopórpora et al) are presented. Collins et al. showed that oropharyngeally delivered angiotensin-(1–7) reduced the inflammation and bacterial load in Mycoplasma pneumoniae-infected mice. Yan et al. and Wang et al. characterised inhalable powders containing bacteriophages and ciprofloxacin-polymyxin B, respectively, to combat antimicrobial resistance in Acinetobacter baumannii infections. Son et al. discussed the design and delivery of inhaled high-dose antibiotic powders, whereas the review by Brunet et al. covered a range of inhaled antifungal drugs for invasive pulmonary mould infections.

Philip Chi Lip Kwok and Michael Yee Tak Chow

Editors

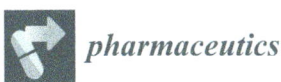

Article

Nebulised Isotonic Hydroxychloroquine Aerosols for Potential Treatment of COVID-19

Waiting Tai [1], Michael Yee Tak Chow [1], Rachel Yoon Kyung Chang [1], Patricia Tang [1], Igor Gonda [2],
Robert B. MacArthur [2], Hak-Kim Chan [1] and Philip Chi Lip Kwok [1,*]

[1]   Advanced Drug Delivery Group, Sydney Pharmacy School, Faculty of Medicine and Health,
      The University of Sydney, Camperdown, NSW 2006, Australia; wtai6746@uni.sydney.edu.au (W.T.);
      yee.chow@sydney.edu.au (M.Y.T.C.); yoon.chang@sydney.edu.au (R.Y.K.C.);
      patricia.tang@sydney.edu.au (P.T.); kim.chan@sydney.edu.au (H.-K.C.)
[2]   Pulmoquine Therapeutics, Inc., 1155 Camino Del Mar Suite 481, Del Mar, CA 92014, USA;
      igonda@pulmoquine.com (I.G.); rmacarthur@rockefeller.edu (R.B.M.)
*   Correspondence: philip.kwok@sydney.edu.au; Tel.: +61-2-8627-6456; Fax: +61-2-9351-4391

Citation: Tai, W.; Chow, M.Y.T.;
Chang, R.Y.K.; Tang, P.; Gonda, I.;
MacArthur, R.B.; Chan, H.-K.;
Kwok, P.C.L. Nebulised Isotonic
Hydroxychloroquine Aerosols for
Potential Treatment of COVID-19.
Pharmaceutics 2021, 13, 1260. https://
doi.org/10.3390/pharmaceutics13081260

Academic Editor: Jason T. McConville

Received: 24 May 2021
Accepted: 12 August 2021
Published: 14 August 2021

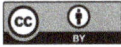
Abstract: The coronavirus disease 2019 (COVID-19) is an unprecedented pandemic that has severely impacted global public health and the economy. Hydroxychloroquine administered orally to COVID-19 patients was ineffective, but its antiviral and anti-inflammatory actions were observed in vitro. The lack of efficacy in vivo could be due to the inefficiency of the oral route in attaining high drug concentration in the lungs. Delivering hydroxychloroquine by inhalation may be a promising alternative for direct targeting with minimal systemic exposure. This paper reports on the characterisation of isotonic, pH-neutral hydroxychloroquine sulphate (HCQS) solutions for nebulisation for COVID-19. They can be prepared, sterilised, and nebulised for testing as an investigational new drug for treating this infection. The 20, 50, and 100 mg/mL HCQS solutions were stable for at least 15 days without refrigeration when stored in darkness. They were atomised from Aerogen Solo Ultra vibrating mesh nebulisers (1 mL of each of the three concentrations and, in addition, 1.5 mL of 100 mg/mL) to form droplets having a median volumetric diameter of 4.3–5.2 μm, with about 50–60% of the aerosol by volume < 5 μm. The aerosol droplet size decreased (from 4.95 to 4.34 μm) with increasing drug concentration (from 20 to 100 mg/mL). As the drug concentration and liquid volume increased, the nebulisation duration increased from 3 to 11 min. The emitted doses ranged from 9.1 to 75.9 mg, depending on the concentration and volume nebulised. The HCQS solutions appear suitable for preclinical and clinical studies for potential COVID-19 treatment.

Keywords: hydroxychloroquine; coronavirus disease 2019 (COVID-19); vibrating mesh nebuliser; inhalation; aerosol; droplet

1. Introduction

Since December 2019, the world has been adversely affected by the coronavirus disease 2019 (COVID-19) pandemic, caused by severe acute respiratory syndrome coronavirus 2 (SARS-CoV-2). As of 17 July 2021, there were 189,482,312 confirmed cases globally, with 4,074,668 deaths [1]. These tolls continue to increase daily at alarming rates. In addition to stressing public health systems, the pandemic has wreaked havoc on the economy and people's livelihoods worldwide. Although various vaccines have been developed and inoculation programmes are progressively being launched in different countries, their effectiveness in achieving general population immunity and reducing viral transmission needs to be yet evaluated [2–4]. Vaccines may not completely restore the present situation to the pre-COVID-19 "norm" [4]. In addition, the long-term safety of the vaccines is yet unclear due to the accelerated development of these products [5]. Public perception of the potential harm from the vaccines versus that from the infection will inevitably influence vaccination rate [6]. Furthermore, various vaccines have been reported to be less effective against SARS-CoV-2 variants, which has prompted questions on how the efficacy of future vaccines can be maintained to tackle incessant viral mutations [7–11]. Therefore, although vaccines are essential, their use alone may not be sufficient to solve the crisis. Drugs for treating the infection are required as a pragmatic strategy. The more effective drugs that are available, the better the health sector is equipped to combat this pandemic.

The course of COVID-19 progresses through two clinical phases. The early phase is predominated by viral replication, whereas the late phase features uncontrolled inflammatory or immune responses to the virus, leading to tissue damage [12]. Thus, the mode of treatment for COVID-19 depends on the stage of the disease, with antiviral and anti-inflammatory therapies being more effective in the early and late phases, respectively. The United States National Institutes of Health advises using anti-SARS-CoV-2 monoclonal antibodies (casirivimab + imdevimab combination or sotrovimab alone) for non-hospitalised patients with mild to moderate COVID-19 at high risk of disease progression [12]. Remdesivir is hitherto the only antiviral drug approved for treating COVID-19 by the United States Food and Drug Administration and European Medicines Agency [13,14]. It is recommended for hospitalised patients on supplemental oxygen and can be used with dexamethasone if oxygen requirement is moderately high [12]. For recently hospitalised patients requiring systemic inflammation using high-flow oxygen or non-invasive ventilation, baricitinib or tocilizumab can be added to dexamethasone with or without remdesivir. Dexamethasone is used alone in the most serious cases, when the patient requires invasive mechanical ventilation or extracorporeal membrane oxygenation [12]. In addition to the drugs mentioned above, the United States Food and Drug Administration has also issued emergency use authorisation for the bamlanivimab + etesevimab combination for mild to moderate COVID-19 [14]. The American Society of Health-System Pharmacists has issued a comprehensive list of approved and experimental drugs for COVID-19 with their clinical evidence that is constantly updated [15]. Some of those drugs (e.g., hydroxychloroquine, azithromycin, lopinavir, ritonavir) have been or are being investigated for repurposing for COVID-19 [16–19]. In particular, hydroxychloroquine is an old 4-aminoquinoline antimalarial chemically similar to, but less toxic than, chloroquine [17,20]. It has been employed for decades for treating autoimmune conditions such as rheumatoid arthritis and lupus erythematosus, due to its immunomodulatory effects [21]. It is administered as hydroxychloroquine sulphate (HCQS) because this salt form is freely soluble in water (aqueous solubility of 1 in 5), with 1 mg of HCQS being equivalent to about 0.775 mg of the base [21,22]. Absorption from the gastrointestinal tract is rapid and extensive [23]. Then, it undergoes hepatic first pass metabolism and results in an oral bioavailability of 79% [24,25].

The proposed use of hydroxychloroquine to prevent and treat COVID-19 is based on its antiviral and immunomodulatory effects reported in the literature. Hydroxychloroquine and chloroquine showed in vitro antiviral activity against SARS-CoV-2 before and after infection in Vero cells, which were derived from the kidney epithelial cells isolated from an African green monkey [26,27]. When the cells were pre-treated with the drugs for 2 h before infection, the half maximal effective concentration (EC_{50}) of hydroxychloroquine and chloroquine for inhibiting viral replication after 48 h of incubation was 5.85 and 18.01 μM, respectively [27]. On the other hand, their EC_{50} was 0.72 and 5.47 μM, respectively, when they were added after infecting with the virus at a multiplicity of infection (MOI) of 0.01. In another study, their EC_{50} on Vero E6 cells (ATCC-1586) at the same MOI was 4.51 and 2.71 μM, respectively [28]. The different EC_{50} for both drugs between the two studies might be due to the different Vero cell lineages used. Nevertheless, those levels were not lethal to the cells because they were significantly lower than the half-maximal cytotoxic concentrations (CC_{50}) on Vero E6 cells (249.50 and 273.20 μM for hydroxychloroquine and chloroquine, respectively) [28]. From these in vitro data, hydroxychloroquine and chloroquine may potentially be used for the prophylaxis and treatment of COVID-19.

Although the antiviral mechanism of these drugs is unclear, they have been shown to prevent the attachment of SARS-CoV-2 to angiotensin-converting enzyme 2 (ACE-2), sialic acid-containing glycoproteins, and gangliosides on the surface of host cells to which the virus needs to bind for entry [29,30]. In addition, the drugs are weak bases so they increase the pH of the normally acidic endosomes and lysosomes in host cells [17,20,29,30]. The alkalinisation alters the homoeostasis of these intracellular organelles and hinders various processes in the viral life cycle that depend on them (e.g., cell entry, replication, release) [29,30].

The initial local airway inflammation in COVID-19 may lead to hypercytokinaemia, or "cytokine storm", the uncontrolled upregulation of multiple pro-inflammatory cytokines such as interleukin (IL)-1β, IL-6, IL-8, tumour necrosis factor-α, and granulocyte-colony stimulating factor [31,32]. Then, the resultant hyperinflammation may cause pulmonary fibrosis, hypoxaemia, damage to other organs, and death. Hydroxychloroquine and chloroquine have long been known to inhibit the production of some of the pro-inflammatory cytokines [33,34]. Therefore, their use in COVID-19 may be beneficial, especially when administered early in the disease to prevent the induction of a cytokine storm and further deterioration of health [25,27,35]. In fact, early treatment of COVID-19 patients with orally administered hydroxychloroquine within one day of hospitalisation (400 mg twice a day on Day 1, followed by 200 mg twice a day on Days 2 to 5) decreased their risk of being transferred to intensive care units by 53%, which is attributed to the anti-inflammatory properties of the drug [36].

Despite the points discussed above suggesting the potential usefulness of hydroxychloroquine in COVID-19, in vivo evidence supporting its clinical application is still lacking. Its benefits were not observed in cynomolgus macaques or human patients infected with SARS-CoV-2 [2,17–19,24,30,37]. This might be due to shortcomings in the route of administration and trial design employed in the clinical studies. The drug was administered orally in all the cases because it is conventionally formulated as tablets. Hydroxychloroquine has a large volume of distribution (5522 L and 44,257 L calculated from blood and plasma data from healthy adults, respectively) and a long terminal elimination half-life of about 40 days as it extensively distributes into and remains in body tissues [38]. Delivering this drug via the oral route is inefficient when the lungs are the primary delivery target site. To achieve a therapeutic drug concentration in the airways, the oral dose needs to be sufficiently high to compensate for the drug loss due to first pass metabolism and distribution into other organs. However, high doses will increase the risk of systemic adverse effects. Indeed, oral hydroxychloroquine has been reported to cause cardiac toxicity including QT prolongation and ventricular arrhythmias in both COVID-19 patients and patients with other illnesses (rheumatoid arthritis, lupus erythematosus, malaria) [21,24,30]. This risk may be further heightened when co-administered with azithromycin [18,24,30]. The lack of robustness of the clinical studies further complicates data interpretation. A number of them were not properly controlled, randomised, or blinded [30]. The patient sample size of some trials was too small for statistical power, while the disease severity amongst certain subject groups varied widely, so it was difficult to interpret the results. Some published studies were not peer-reviewed, especially those from early 2020 as urgent dissemination of medical information on COVID-19 was prioritised [30]. The emergency nature of the pandemic may have imposed limitations on the design and execution of the studies, consequently impacting data quality. Due to its anti-inflammatory properties, inhalation delivery of hydroxychloroquine solutions was tested in sheep for the treatment of asthma [39]. Later research with a soft mist inhaler using an aqueous formulation of HCQS proceeded into humans [40]. The antiviral and anti-inflammatory activities of this drug against rhinoviral infection in human bronchial cells were reported [41].

Robust, controlled clinical trials for hydroxychloroquine utilising a more efficient route of administration are required to better evaluate its efficacy in COVID-19. Since the respiratory tract is the initial site of infection and inflammation, direct inhalation delivery is better targeted than oral administration, as lower doses can be used to achieve high local drug concentrations in the airways to maximise therapeutic action and minimise systemic adverse effects [25,42–44]. Based on the in vitro extracellular concentrations in the activity assays against SARS-CoV-2, direct delivery by inhalation is necessary to achieve adequate HCQS concentration in the upper and central airway target tissues to be effective [45]. Our research group recently characterised jet milled, crystalline HCQS powders deliverable from dry powder inhalers for clinical testing [43]. However, nebulised solutions offer more flexible dose adjustment. Since inhaled dry powders in general and particularly those of HCQS are known to cause coughing [46,47], the use of an isosmotic, pH-neutral formulation was preferable. Nebulisers can be used by patients of all ages, including those who are ventilated. Furthermore, the safety of nebulised HCQS solutions was previously demonstrated in healthy volunteers as well as subjects with pulmonary disease [40,48]. Thus, this paper reports on isotonic HCQS solutions that can be prepared, sterilised, and nebulised for potential treatment of COVID-19.

2. Materials and Methods

2.1. Chemicals

HCQS powder of United States Pharmacopoeia (USP) grade (Lot 1910P031, Batch 033600-192021) was purchased from Sci Pharmtech Inc. (Taoyuan, Taiwan). Chromatographic grade methanol and acetonitrile were bought from RCI Labscan (Bangkok, Thailand) and Honeywell (Morris Plains, NJ, USA), respectively. Deionised water was obtained from a MODULAB® High Flow Water Purification System (Evoqua Water Technologies, Pittsburgh, PA, USA).

2.2. HCQS Nebulised Solutions

Isotonic and pH-neutral solutions containing 20, 50, and 100 mg/mL of HCQS were prepared in volumetric flasks. Then, they were transferred to 50 mL of polypropylene centrifuge tubes (Corning, Corning, NY, USA) and stored in darkness at ambient temperature until use. The osmolality of the solutions was measured with a K-7000 vapor pressure osmometer (Knauer, Berlin, Germany). The cell and head temperatures were set as 60 °C and 62 °C, respectively, and allowed to stabilise for an hour before use. These temperatures followed those recommended in the instrument manual for calibrating and measuring sodium chloride aqueous solutions [49]. The measurement time and gain were 1.5 min and 16, respectively. Approximately 1 mL of each sample solution was drawn into glass microsyringes and inserted into the osmometer. One droplet from each sample was dispensed onto the thermistor for each osmolality measurement. The droplet was replaced by a new one when repeating the measurement. The experiments were conducted in quadruplicate ($n = 4$) for each HCQS solution. The target osmolality range was 260–360 mOsmol/kg H_2O [50,51]. The pH of the solutions was measured with a pH 700 benchtop meter (Oakton, Vernon Hills, IL, USA). The target pH range was 6.8–7.5 [50,51].

2.3. High Performance Liquid Chromatography (HPLC)

HCQS was quantified by a modified reverse phase-HPLC method from the USP [52]. The assay was performed on an automated HPLC system that consisted of a DGU-20A degassing unit, a LC-20AT HPLC pump, a SIL-20A HT autosampler, a CTO-20A column oven, and an SPD-20A UV detector (Shimadzu, Kyoto, Japan). The mobile phase was composed of 10:10:80:0.2 by volume of methanol, acetonitrile, 0.12 g/L sodium 1-pentanesulfonate monohydrate aqueous solution, and orthophosphoric acid. The mobile phase and all other solvents were filtered and degassed before use. The Agilent Zorbax SB-C18 column (5 μm, 4.6 × 250 mm; Agilent, Santa Clara, CA, USA) was kept at 35 °C during the runs. Each sample ran for 15 min at a mobile phase flow rate of 1 mL/min. The injection volume and detection wavelength were 20 μL and 254 nm, respectively. Standard solutions (6.25–1000 μg/mL) were freshly prepared by serially diluting a 100 mg/mL HCQS solution aliquot that had been filtered through a sterile Millex-GP 0.22 μm hydrophilic polyethersulfone membrane syringe filter (Millipore, Burlington, MA, USA) (see below for the method). The diluent for the standard solutions was deionised water and 50:50 *v*/*v* methanol/water, depending on the diluent used for the samples.

2.4. Effect of Filtration on HCQS Solutions

The effect of filtration on the drug concentration, osmolality, and pH was investigated because the HCQS solutions would be sterilised by filtration before nebulisation. Approximately 3 mL of the 20, 50, or 100 mg/mL HCQS solution was drawn into a 3 mL syringe (Terumo, Tokyo, Japan). Then, a sterile Millex-GP 0.22 μm hydrophilic polyethersulfone membrane syringe filter was attached to the syringe. About 1 mL of the solution was ejected through the filter and discarded. The remaining 2 mL in the syringe was filtered and collected into a 2 mL microcentrifuge tube (Quality Scientific Plastics, Petaluma, CA, USA). The drug concentration, osmolality, and pH of the unfiltered and filtered solutions were measured as outlined above. For the HPLC runs, all samples were diluted with deionised water to 500 μg/mL to be within the concentration range of the standard curve.

2.5. Recovery of HCQS from SureGard Filters

SureGard filters (Bird Healthcare, Bayswater, VIC, Australia) were used in the dose output and cascade impaction runs (connected between the impactor and the vacuum pump) to collect the nebulised droplets so the recovery of HCQS from this type of filter was investigated. These filters were spiked with 2 or 75 mg of HCQS by adding 20 or 750 μL of a 100 mg/mL HCQS nebulised solution to a new filter, respectively. The openings of the filter were sealed with Parafilm (Bemis, Oshkosh, WI, USA) after adding 10 mL of deionised water or 50:50 v/v methanol/water. The filters were immediately shook by hand for 5 min or left to stand for 30 min first, followed by 5 min of shaking. The samples were diluted 10-fold with deionised water or 50:50 v/v methanol/water accordingly before HPLC assay.

2.6. Dose Output

The HCQS dose output from three new Aerogen® Solo nebulisers (Mesh numbers C1901059-0822, C1901059-0797, and C1901059-1623; Aerogen, Galway, Ireland) was measured with individualised Aerogen Ultra aerosol chambers. These nebulisers plus aerosol chambers will be referred to in this report as Nebulisers 1, 2, and 3, respectively. The same Aerogen controller was used for all experiments. One SureGard filter was connected to the outlet of the Aerogen Ultra mouthpiece. A filter was also fitted to the exhaust end of the mouthpiece and the exhaust port at the bottom of the Aerogen Ultra (Figure 1). Thus, there were one outlet filter and two exhaust filters. Silicone adaptors were used to connect the mouthpiece to the outlet and one of the exhaust filters (Figure 1). The experiments were conducted under ambient conditions (18–25 °C, 20–65% RH).

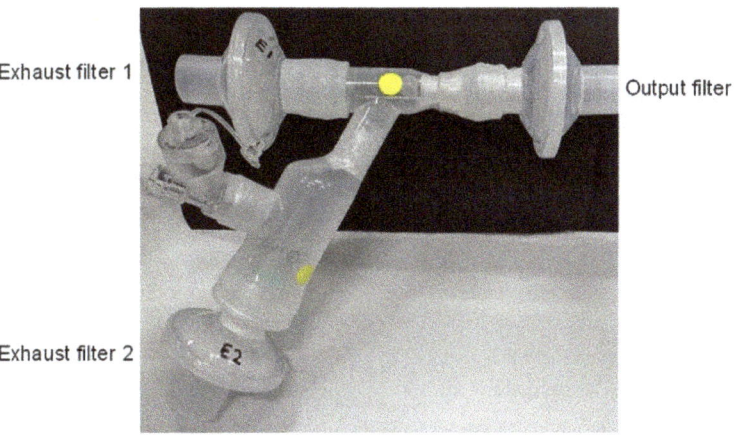

Figure 1. Setup for the dose output runs.

The procedure followed the USP method [52] except that the aerosols were collected from the start to the end of nebulisation instead of collecting them for the first minute using one output filter and then collecting the rest of the aerosols with another output filter. This was to avoid drug loss when changing the filters. It would also simplify the experimental procedure. The output filter was not overloaded by the lengthening of collection duration. The end of nebulisation was determined by visual inspection when no solution remained in the nebuliser.

Nebulised dose output was measured for the following HCQS solutions. The same scheme was adopted for the laser diffraction and cascade impaction experiments (see below).

- 1 mL of 20 mg/mL;
- 1 mL of 50 mg/mL;
- 1 mL of 100 mg/mL;
- 1.5 mL of 100 mg/mL.

HCQS solution was added into the reservoir of the Aerogen Solo by pipetting. The PWG-33 breathing simulator (Piston Medical, Budapest, Hungary) was connected to the output filter. The simulated breathing waveform was sinusoidal at 15 cycles/minute, with an inhalation-to-exhalation ratio of 1:1 and a tidal volume of 500 mL [52]. The outlet and exhaust filters captured droplets exiting the nebulisers during the inhalation and exhalation phases in the breathing cycle, respectively. The nebuliser and breathing simulator were operated from the start to the end of nebulisation, after which the setup was left to stand for 20 min before being removed and assayed. This was to allow the droplets in the Aerogen Ultra to settle by gravitational sedimentation and avoid potential aerosol loss if the setup was disassembled immediately. The runs were conducted in triplicate for each nebuliser.

The openings of the two exhaust filters were sealed with Parafilm after adding in 10 mL of deionised water. Then, the exhaust filters were exhaustively rinsed by shaking for 5 min. The outlet filter was placed into a 600 mL glass beaker. Four hundred millilitres of deionised water, a glass weight, and magnetic stirrer were added into that beaker afterwards. The glass weight was to weigh down the filter to ensure its complete immersion in the water. The mixture was magnetically stirred for 5 min, followed by shaking for another 5 min. The liquid reservoir and outlet of the Aerogen Solo were exhaustively washed with 10 mL of deionised water and 6 min of shaking in total. The same was performed on the two silicone adaptors. The washings were collected into a 100 mL volumetric flask. The openings of the Aerogen Ultra were sealed with Parafilm after adding in about 10 mL of deionised water. The whole chamber was exhaustively rinsed in the same manner as described for Aerogen Solo. All washings were pooled into the same volumetric flask. The volume was made up to 100 mL with deionised water. All samples were assayed by HPLC.

2.7. Laser Diffraction

The nebulised droplets were sized by laser diffraction using Spraytec (Malvern Panalytical, Malvern, UK) with an inhalation cell and at an acquisition frequency of 2.5 kHz. The outlet of the Aerogen Ultra mouthpiece was positioned 1 cm from the laser measurement zone to minimise evaporation during measurement. A vacuum pump connected to the other end of the inhalation cell with entrained dilution air was used to remove the aerosols continuously to (1) prevent droplet re-entrainment of droplets into the laser measurement zone; and (2) maintain the laser signal transmission >70% to minimise multiple scattering. The Aerogen Ultra mouthpiece was not sealed to the inhalation cell, so the airflow through the Aerogen Ultra was unknown. Signals from Detectors 1–10 were excluded to account for beam steering effects. The real and imaginary refractive indices for the droplets were taken to be the same as those for water, which were 1.33 and 0.00, respectively. The refractive index for air was 1.00. These values were deemed appropriate because all measurements showed low residual values (<0.5%). The droplets were sized when the signal transmission was <99%. The duration of nebulisation was the time that aerosols were seen by eye to traverse continuously through the laser measurement zone. The raw data of each run were processed to yield an averaged volumetric diameter distribution, from which the volumetric median diameter (VMD) and geometric standard deviation (GSD) were derived. The percentage of aerosol sample by volume under 1, 2, 3, 5, and 10 μm were also calculated.

2.8. Cascade Impaction

The aerosol performance of the three Aerogen Solo nebulisers coupled to their respective Aerogen Ultra aerosol chambers was measured by the USP method using a Next Generation Impactor (NGI; USP Apparatus 5; Copley, Nottingham, UK) without a preseparator [52]. The same Aerogen controller was used for all the experiments. The NGI and throat were chilled at 5 °C for at least 90 min beforehand. After chilling, a SureGard filter was connected to the NGI after the micro-orifice collector (MOC) to capture any drug that passed beyond the lowest impactor stage. The sealing of the apparatus was verified before each run by a vacuum leak test, after which the airflow rate was set to 15 L/min. A silicone adaptor was used to connect the mouthpiece to the USP induction port (throat). The experiments were conducted under ambient conditions (18–25 °C, 20–65% RH).

HCQS solution was added into the reservoir of the Aerogen Solo by pipetting. No exhaust filters were required to be connected to the Aerogen Ultra because the airflow was suction only. The nebuliser and vacuum pump were operated from the start to the end of nebulisation. The end of nebulisation was determined by visual inspection when no solution remained in the nebuliser. The setup was left to stand for 20 min before being removed and assayed. The co-solvent used for all NGI samples was 50:50 *v/v* methanol:water. For the 20 mg/mL HCQS runs, the Aerogen Solo, and Aerogen Ultra were exhaustively washed with this co-solvent, collected into a 100 mL volumetric flask, and made up to volume. The post-NGI filter was washed with 10 mL of the co-solvent, as for the dose output exhaust filter. The adaptor, throat, and NGI impactor stages were washed with 4 mL of the co-solvent. The assay for the 100 mg/mL HCQS runs was conducted in the same manner, except that Stages 1–6 were washed with 20 mL instead of 4 mL of the co-solvent.

The loaded dose was the amount of HCQS added into the nebuliser. The emitted dose was the total amount of drug assayed from the adaptor to the post-NGI filter. The recovered dose was the total amount of HCQS assayed on all the parts in the experimental setup, i.e., from the nebuliser to the post-NGI filter. Fine particle doses (FPDs) under 1, 2, 3, 5, and 10 μm were calculated, from which the corresponding fine particle fractions (FPFs) with respect to the loaded, emitted, and recovered doses were then derived. Likewise, the mass median aerodynamic diameter (MMAD) and GSD with respect to the recovered dose and the emitted dose were calculated. The MMAD was the diameter at 50% undersize interpolated from the cumulative recovered and emitted doses. The GSD was calculated by dividing the MMAD by the diameter at 16% undersize, which was in turn interpolated from the cumulative recovered and emitted doses.

2.9. Measurement of the Density of HCQS Solutions

The density of HCQS solutions (20, 50, and 100 mg/mL) was measured by first weighing deionised water in a 10 mL volumetric flask, filled to the mark. After discarding the water and drying the volumetric flask, HCQS solution was added to the mark and weighed. The density of the HCQS solutions was calculated with the following equation.

$$\rho_H = \rho_W \, (m_H/m_w) \tag{1}$$

where ρ_H and ρ_W are the densities of HCQS solution and deionised water, respectively; and m_H and m_W are the masses of HCQS solution and deionised water in the 10 mL volumetric flasks, respectively. The density of deionised water at 24 °C, at which the measurements were conducted, was interpolated from the water density data in the CRC Handbook of Chemistry and Physics [53]. Three volumetric flasks were used to obtain triplicate measurements for each solution. The densities of the HCQS solutions were used to convert the volumetric diameters measured by laser diffraction to a volumetric aerodynamic diameter by the following equation [54].

$$d_a = d_v(\rho_H/\rho_0)^{0.5} \tag{2}$$

where d_a and d_v are aerodynamic and volumetric diameters, respectively; and ρ_0 is unit density (1 g/cm^3). The volumetric aerodynamic diameter was used for comparing the droplet sizes measured by laser diffraction to those by cascade impaction.

2.10. Statistical Analysis

One-way analysis of variance followed by Tukey's post hoc test were performed using the SPSS software (IBM, Armonk, NY, USA). Statistical differences were indicated by $p < 0.05$ and $\alpha < 0.05$.

3. Results

3.1. Effect of Filtration on Drug Concentration, Osmolality, and pH

Two batches of 100 mg/mL solutions were made (Batches A and B). Batch A was used to obtain the 20 mg/mL solution by dilution, while Batch B was used directly for the 100 mg/mL experiments and for making the 50 mg/mL solution. No drug degradation was observed over the 15 days during which all the experiments were performed. The drug concentration, osmolality, and pH of the HCQS solutions before and after filtration are presented in Table 1.

Table 1. Drug concentration, osmolality, and pH of HCQS solutions before and after filtration.

	Batch A		Batch B	
	100 mg/mL	20 mg/mL	100 mg/mL	50 mg/mL
Before filtration				
Concentration (mg/mL)	Not measured	20.3 ± 0.2	100.8 ± 0.8	50.8 ± 0.5
Osmolality (mOsmol/kg H$_2$O)	323.0 ± 6.6	286.5 ± 6.6	323.5 ± 14.2	315.5 ± 3.4
pH	7.19	7.38	7.09	7.15
After filtration				
Concentration (mg/mL)	Not measured	20.0 ± 0.3	99.1 ± 1.1	49.9 ± 0.9
Osmolality (mOsmol/kg H$_2$O)	314.0 ± 4.7	275.3 ± 7.2	321.3 ± 13.4	299.3 ± 5.6
pH	7.16	7.25	7.03	7.11

Osmolality is presented as mean ± standard deviation ($n = 4$). One pH measurement was made for each solution ($n = 1$).

The osmolality and pH of all solutions were within the target ranges, regardless of filtration. The five-fold dilution of the Batch A 100 mg/mL solution to 20 mg/mL reduced the osmolality from 323.0 to 286.5 mOsmol/kg H$_2$O, but it was still within the target range. HCQS concentration was not affected by filtration. On the other hand, osmolality and pH decreased after filtration, but the difference was not significant. Similar trends were observed for the Batch B 100 mg/mL and 50 mg/mL solutions. The osmolality and pH of the 50 mg/mL were between those of the 20 mg/mL and 100 mg/mL solutions.

The retention time of the HCQS peak in the HPLC chromatogram was about 8 min. Table 2 shows the regression equations of the calibration curves with the mean slopes and y-intercept. They were obtained using fresh standard solutions over 11 and 14 days with deionised water and 50:50 v/v methanol/water as the diluent, respectively. The standard curves were similar between the days and were linear ($r^2 \approx 1$) from 6.25 to 1000 µg/mL. The detection and quantitation limits were derived by Equations (3) and (4), respectively [55]. The values of slope featured in these equations were taken to be the mean slopes shown in Table 2.

$$\text{Detection limit} = (3.3 \times \text{Standard deviation of the y-intercepts})/\text{Slope} \tag{3}$$

$$\text{Quantitation limit} = (10 \times \text{Standard deviation of the y-intercepts})/\text{Slope} \qquad (4)$$

Table 2. HPLC calibration curves, detection limit, and quantitation limit for HCQS from 6.25 to 1000 μg/mL.

	Regression Equation	Detection Limit (μg/mL)	Quantitation Limit (μg/mL)
Deionised water	A = 43,294C + 32,746	2.7	8.3
50:50 *v/v* methanol:water	A = 42,848C − 19,037	7.2	21.7

A = Peak area at 254 nm. C = HCQS concentration in μg/mL. The slopes and y-intercepts were the mean of 11 and 14 values for water and the co-solvent, respectively.

The HPLC method was more sensitive with deionised water as the diluent, as shown by the lower detection and quantitation limits (Table 2). This is interesting to note because the USP recommends 50:50 *v/v* methanol/water as the diluent.

3.2. Recovery of HCQS from SureGard Filters

The recovery of HCQS from the spiked SureGard filters using deionised water and 50:50 *v/v* methanol/water is presented in Table 3. Deionised water was more efficient than the co-solvent for extracting HCQS from the filters. It obviated the need for the 30-min standing time to allow the filter to soak before shaking. Drug adsorption to the filter was appreciable at the low spiked drug level, as 4–5% of drug could not be recovered even when water was used. This was even more significant (11–12%) with the co-solvent. Therefore, deionised water was better for assaying the drug from SureGard filters.

Table 3. Recovery of HCQS from spiked SureGard filters.

		Deionised Water	50:50 *v/v* Methanol/Water
2 mg HCQS	Immediate 5 min shaking	95.7%	87.3%
	30 min standing, 5 min shaking	95.3%	88.9%
75 mg HCQS	Immediate 5 min shaking	100.7%	94.4%
	30 min standing, 5 min shaking	100.2%	99.3%

One measurement was performed for each scenario ($n = 1$).

3.3. Dose Output

The nebulisation duration of the 1 mL loaded dose runs is shown in Table 4. The correlation between solute concentration and nebulisation duration was non-linear. The nebulisation times with 1.5 mL of 100 mg/mL were understandably longer than with 1 mL.

Table 4. Nebulisation duration of the dose output experiments.

	Nebuliser 1	Nebuliser 2	Nebuliser 3	All Nebulisers
1 mL, 20 mg/mL	3 min 26 s ± 7 s	4 min 27 s ± 31 s	3 min 41 s ± 18 s	3 min 51 s ± 33 s
1 mL, 50 mg/mL	5 min 4 s ± 13 s	5 min 7 s ± 10 s	5 min 8 s ± 16 s	5 min 6 s ± 11 s
1 mL, 100 mg/mL	6 min 24 s ± 26 s	6 min 25 s ± 35 s	6 min 22 s ± 6 s	6 min 24 s ± 22 s
1.5 mL, 100 mg/mL	10 min 55 s ± 43 s	9 min 31 s ± 36 s	10 min 24 s ± 45 s	10 min 17 s ± 52 s

Data presented as mean ± standard deviation ($n = 3$ for Nebulisers 1, 2, and 3; $n = 9$ for all nebulisers).

The recovered dose for the runs was generally 95–105% of the loaded dose, so drug recovery was satisfactory. The absolute and relative doses with respect to the recovered dose for the various parts of the experimental setup are shown in Figure 2. The absolute dose was the assayed HCQS dose expressed in milligrams, whereas the relative dose was the assayed HCQS dose expressed as a percentage of the recovered dose. The data for the absolute doses showed that the amount of drug reaching the exhaust filters was very low. Most of the drug was shared between the output filter and the Aerogen Solo/Ultra. The output dose was approximately proportional to the loaded dose. This was confirmed by the similar distributions of relative doses on the various parts of the experimental setup between the concentration/volume combinations. The amount of drug that exited the nebuliser setup during the exhalation phase of the breathing cycle (i.e., those collected on the two exhaust filters) was low, with <2% of the recovered dose on each filter. About half of the recovered dose was emitted onto the output filter, which represented the amount of HCQS that a patient would inhale, assuming that the simulated breathing cycle is representative of the patient's breathing; the remainder was retained in the Aerogen Solo/Ultra. The output with respect to the recovered dose from 1 mL of 50 mg/mL was slightly lower than that from 1.5 mL of 100 mg/mL (Figure 2). This is explained by the correspondingly higher drug retention in the Aerogen Solo/Ultra.

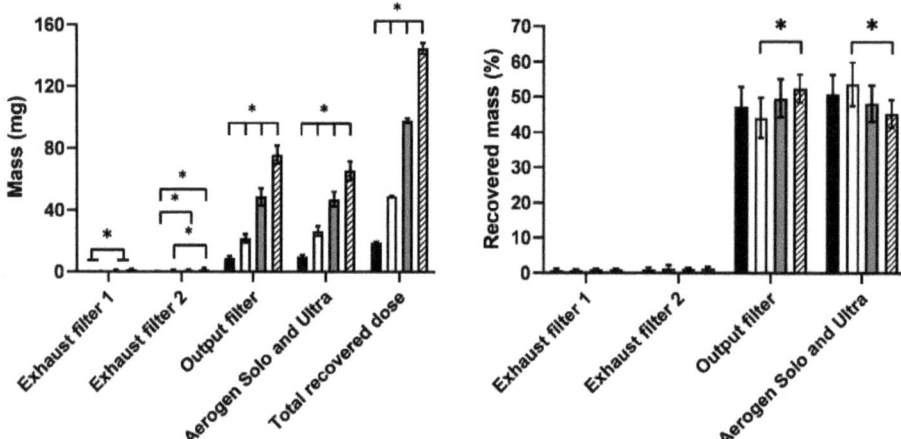

Figure 2. Absolute and relative doses of HCQS on the various parts of the dose output setup. The four bars represent 1 mL of 20 mg/mL (black), 1 mL of 50 mg/mL (white), 1 mL of 100 mg/mL (gray), and 1.5 mL of 100 mg/mL (hatch). Data presented as mean $\pm$ standard deviation ($n = 9$). Statistical difference indicated by * ($p < 0.05$).

3.4. Laser Diffraction

The droplet size distributions measured by laser diffraction were stable over the entire measurement period for each run. The nebulisation duration (Table 5) was longer than the actual measurement time because the aerosol concentrations were low ("thin" aerosols) at the start and end of nebulisation, so the laser signal transmission at these times was higher than the trigger threshold for measurement (99.9%). The measurements generally started a few seconds after aerosols appeared in the measurement zone for all drug concentrations/volumes. The thin aerosol tailing near the end of nebulisation (i.e., thin aerosols in the measurement zone but no sizing was triggered) took about 30 s and was particularly longer (up to 1 min) for 20 mg/mL.

The size distributions were all monomodal and reproducible between the three nebulisers, with the peak at about 5 μm (Figure 3). There was a slight shift in the distribution to the smaller size between 100 mg/mL (both volumes) and the other two HCQS concentrations. This difference was more obvious in the VMD (Figure 4). Although the VMD for all concentrations/volumes was between 4.3 and 5.2 μm, the droplets produced from 100 mg/mL solutions were slightly but significantly ($p < 0.05$) smaller than those from

20 and 50 mg/mL (Figure 4). The GSD was relatively consistent between the four concentrations/volumes, at about 1.8 (Figure 5). However, the GSD from 1.5 mL of 100 mg/mL was also slightly but significantly ($p < 0.05$) lower than that from 1 mL of 20 mg/mL.

Table 5. Nebulisation duration of the laser diffraction experiments.

	Nebuliser 1	Nebuliser 2	Nebuliser 3	All Nebulisers
1 mL, 20 mg/mL	6 min 1 s ± 25 s	5 min 54 s ± 17 s	6 min 7 s ± 15 s	6 min 1 s ± 18 s
1 mL, 50 mg/mL	6 min 24 s ± 22 s	6 min 50 s ± 8 s	6 min 32 s ± 3 s	6 min 35 s ± 16 s
1 mL, 100 mg/mL	7 min 4 s ± 3 s	6 min 51 s ± 13 s	6 min 55 s ± 3 s	6 min 56 s ± 9 s
1.5 mL, 100 mg/mL	11 min 42 s ± 36 s	11 min 23 s ± 31 s	11 min 19 s ± 45 s	11 min 28 s ± 34 s

Data presented as mean ± standard deviation ($n = 3$ for Nebulisers 1, 2, and 3; $n = 9$ for all nebulisers).

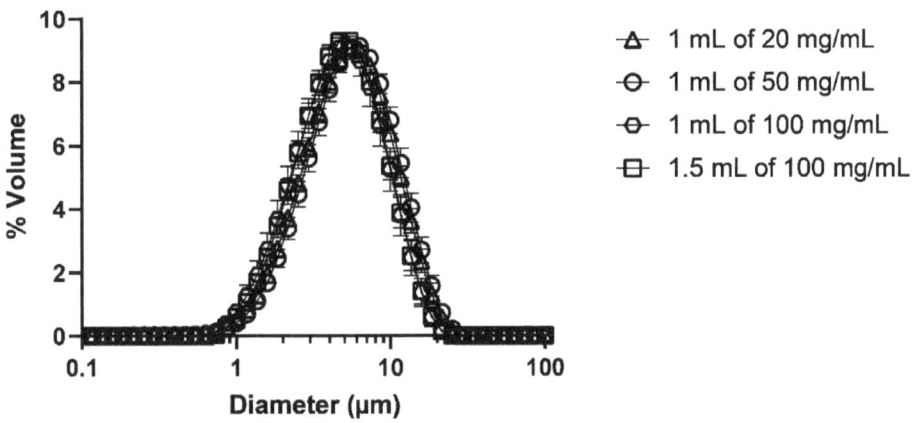

Figure 3. Droplet size distributions measured by laser diffraction. Data presented as mean ± standard deviation ($n = 9$).

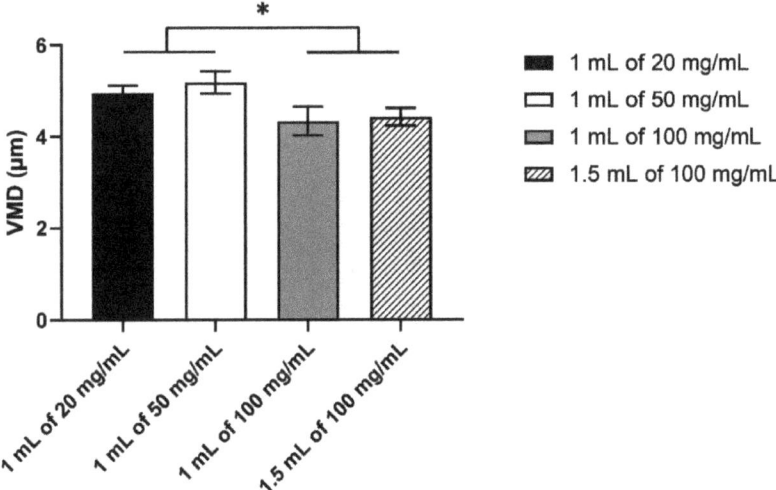

Figure 4. The volumetric median diameter of the droplets measured by laser diffraction. Data presented as mean ± standard deviation ($n = 9$). Statistical difference indicated by * ($p < 0.05$).

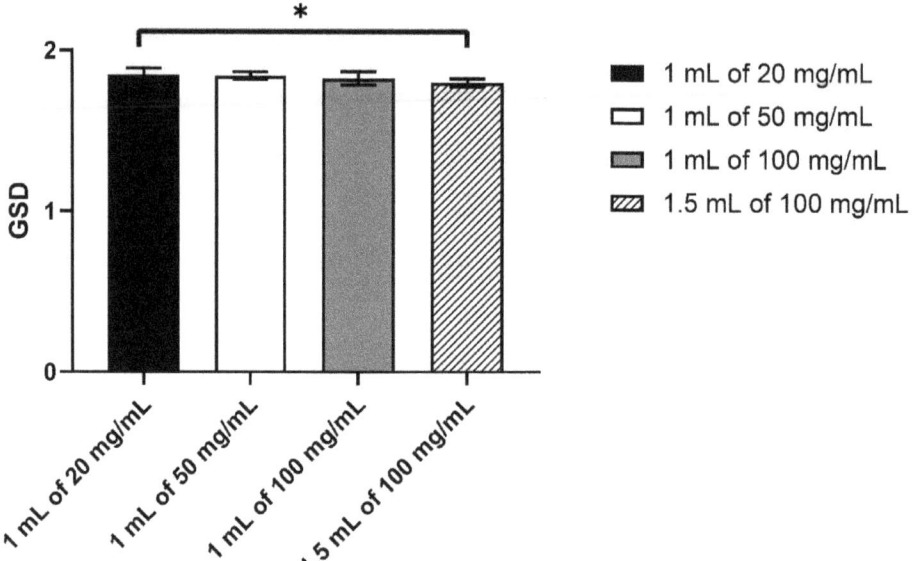

Figure 5. The geometric standard deviation of the droplets measured by laser diffraction. Data presented as mean ± standard deviation (*n* = 9). Statistical difference indicated by * (*p* < 0.05).

The percentage of aerosol sample by volume under 1, 2, 3, 5, and 10 μm is shown in Figure 6. About 50–60% of the aerosols was <5 μm. The nebulisers produced minimal submicron droplets at all concentrations/volumes, but the 100 mg/mL solution consistently produced more droplets by volume than 20 and 50 mg/mL at all cutoff diameters. In other words, the droplets from the 100 mg/mL solution were smaller than those from the other two solutions. No clear dependence between droplet size and relative humidity was observed, so the difference in droplet size was attributed to the solute concentration and the resultant changes in the physicochemical characteristics of the solutions.

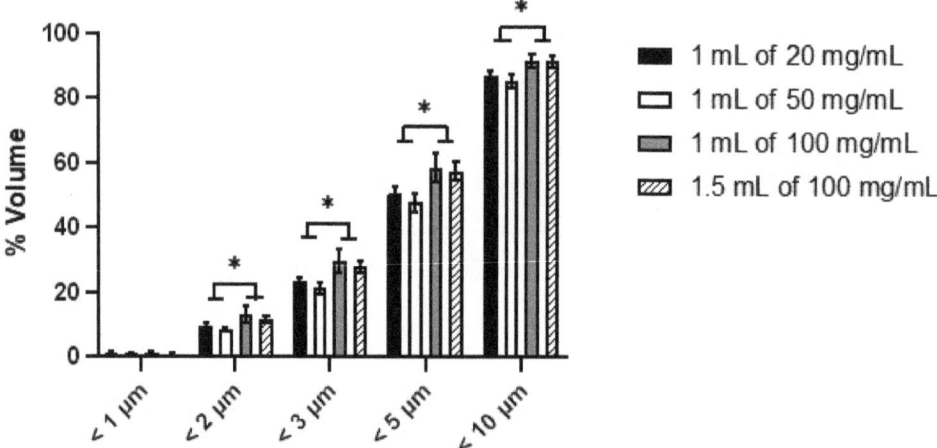

Figure 6. The percentage of aerosol by volume under 1, 2, 3, 5, and 10 μm measured by laser diffraction. Data presented as mean ± standard deviation (*n* = 9). Statistical difference indicated by * (*p* < 0.05).

3.5. Cascade Impaction

The nebulisation durations of the NGI runs (Table 6) were similar to those for the dose output runs (Table 4). The recovered dose was close to the loaded dose for all the runs, so drug recovery was satisfactory. The absolute and relative doses (with respect to the recovered dose) for the various parts of the setup are shown in Figure 7. Only a small amount of HCQS (<1%) was collected on the post-NGI filter, so the NGI captured practically all the emitted doses. About 30–40% of the recovered dose remained in the nebulisers after the NGI runs, compared to 50% after the dose output runs (Figures 2 and 7, respectively). This might be due to the vacuum pump continuously removing droplets from the Aerogen Ultra into the NGI rather than blowing them back repeatedly into the aerosol chamber, as in the case of the breath simulator during the exhalation phase employed in the delivered dose experiments. The overall aerosol performance profiles were similar between the concentrations/volumes, with minimal throat deposition (Figure 7). However, 1.5 mL of 100 mg/mL showed more drug on Stages 4 and 5, so there was a higher proportion of fine droplets.

Table 6. Nebulisation duration of the cascade impaction experiments.

	Nebuliser 1	Nebuliser 2	Nebuliser 3	All Nebulisers
1 mL, 20 mg/mL	3 min 48 s ± 7 s	3 min 50 s ± 44 s	3 min 32 s ± 22 s	3 min 44 s ± 26 s
1 mL, 50 mg/mL	5 min 43 s ± 9 s	5 min 15 s ± 19 s	5 min 35 s ± 10 s	5 min 31 s ± 17 s
1 mL, 100 mg/mL	6 min 41 s ± 42 s	6 min 26 s ± 33 s	6 min 18 s ± 21 s	6 min 28 s ± 30 s
1.5 mL, 100 mg/mL	10 min 48 s ± 20 s	9 min 53 s ± 48 s	9 min 6 s ± 26 s	9 min 56 s ± 53 s

Data presented as mean ± standard deviation (*n* = 3 for Nebulisers 1, 2, and 3; *n* = 9 for all nebulisers).

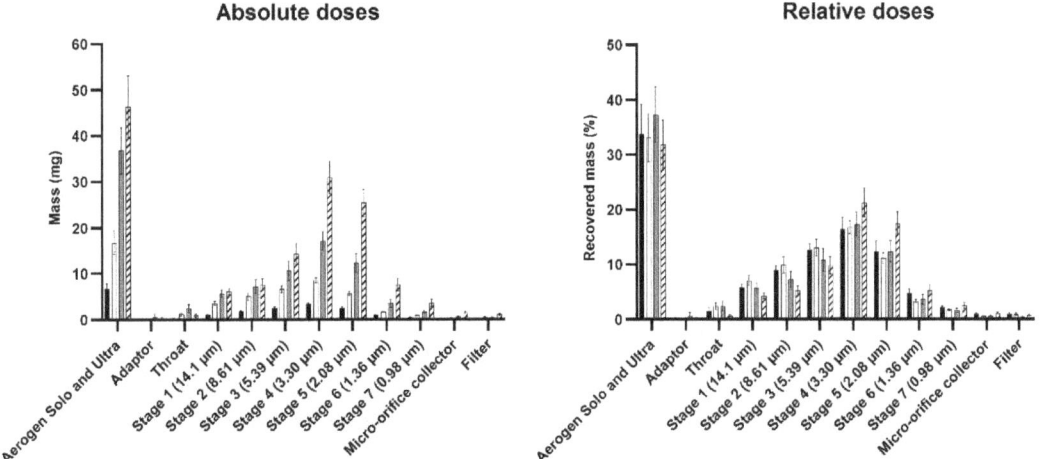

Figure 7. Absolute and relative doses of HCQS on the various parts of the NGI setup. The four bars represent 1 mL of 20 mg/mL (black), 1 mL of 50 mg/mL (white), 1 mL of 100 mg/mL (gray), and 1.5 mL of 100 mg/mL (hatch). Data presented as mean ± standard deviation (*n* = 3).

The emitted dose, FPD, FPF < 5 μm loaded, FPF < 5 μm emitted, MMAD emitted, and GSD emitted derived from the NGI data are summarised in Table 7, together with other key parameters measured in the dose output and laser diffraction experiments for comparison. The overall dose output rate was calculated by dividing the dose of HCQS collected in the output filter by the duration of nebulisation in the dose output experiments. The higher FPF and MMAD of 1.5 mL of 100 mg/mL also indicate that it produced smaller droplets than the other concentrations/volumes. The GSD gradually decreased with increasing concentration/volume, so the size distribution became narrower. These trends were also observed in the VMD and GSD in the laser diffraction data (Table 7). The doses collected in the output filter in the dose output experiments were consistently lower than the emitted doses in cascade impaction. This was because the vacuum pump in the latter constantly pulled the aerosol out of the nebuliser (continuous "inhalation"), and the breath simulator in the former generated a sinusoidal flow (periodic "inhalation" and "exhalation").

Table 7. Summary of the key parameters measured in the dose output, laser diffraction, and cascade impaction experiments.

	1 mL of 20 mg/mL	1 mL of 50 mg/mL	1 mL of 100 mg/mL	1.5 mL of 100 mg/mL
	Dose output			
Dose collected in output filter (mg)	9.05 ± 0.96	21.67 ± 2.81	48.76 ± 5.57	75.88 ± 5.87
Overall dose output rate (mg/min)	2.38 ± 0.38	4.25 ± 0.57	7.63 ± 0.82	7.42 ± 0.71
	Laser diffraction			
VMD (μm)	4.95 ± 0.17	5.19 ± 0.25	4.34 ± 0.31	4.42 ± 0.19
GSD	1.85 ± 0.04	1.84 ± 0.02	1.83 ± 0.04	1.80 ± 0.02
	Cascade impaction			
Emitted dose (mg)	13.2 ± 1.15	33.8 ± 2.19	61.9 ± 5.28	99.0 ± 5.71
FPD < 5 μm (mg)	9.49 ± 1.13	22.7 ± 1.34	44.2 ± 5.60	81.6 ± 6.93
FPF < 5 μm loaded (%)	47.3 ± 5.64	45.3 ± 2.74	44.2 ± 5.60	54.4 ± 4.57
FPF < 5 μm emitted (%)	71.8 ± 3.44	67.3 ± 3.25	71.3 ± 4.71	82.3 ± 3.02
MMAD emitted (μm)	3.00 ± 0.18	3.27 ± 0.25	2.99 ± 0.27	2.50 ± 0.17
GSD emitted	2.02 ± 0.06	1.94 ± 0.14	1.88 ± 0.05	1.75 ± 0.05

Data presented as mean ± standard deviation ($n = 9$).

3.6. Comparison of Dose Output, Laser Diffraction, and Cascade Impaction Data

Laser diffraction and cascade impaction data were compared to check their correlation because cascade impaction measurements can be affected by droplet evaporation in the entrained dilution air [56,57]. To improve the accuracy of the comparison, the major parameters from laser diffraction (VMD and %V < 1, 2, 3, 5, 10 μm) were converted to their volumetric aerodynamic diameters by Equation (2). The density of the 20, 50, and 100 mg/mL HCQS solutions were measured to be 1.008, 1.019, and 1.033 g/cm^3, respectively, and were used in the calculation. The data are shown in Table 8. Correlation between the two techniques was reflected in the percent ratio of each parameter, which was the quotient of a given parameter measured by cascade impaction and that by laser diffraction. The FPFs measured by cascade impaction for all concentrations/volumes were consistently higher than those by laser diffraction at the corresponding cutoff diameters (Table 8). By the same token, the MMAD with respect to the emitted dose measured by cascade impaction was smaller than the volumetric median aerodynamic diameter (VMAD) by laser diffraction. The smaller particle sizes measured by cascade impaction could be attributed to droplet evaporation in the NGI. Despite this, its width remained relatively constant. The deviation between the corresponding GSDs was 97–110%, indicating that evaporation in the NGI was a monotonous shift to the smaller sizes without changing the width of the distribution. The main trend observed in the FPFs and %V undersize was that the lower the cutoff diameter, the larger the deviation between the two datasets, with relatively close agreement at 10 μm (97–104% deviation), to > 120% deviation at 5 μm, and > 200% deviation at 2 μm. This was most likely due to the faster evaporation rates of small droplets, which increased the FPF to a greater extent at the lower cutoff sizes. In addition, the deviation between the two datasets decreased with increasing HCQS concentration for the 1 mL solutions. This might be due to the reduction in vapour pressure with increasing HCQS concentration, which decreased the evaporation rate.

Table 8. Comparison of cascade impaction and laser diffraction data.

1 mL of 20 mg/mL				
Cascade Impaction Data		Laser Diffraction Data (Aerodynamic Diameter)		Cascade Impaction Data/Laser Diffraction Data (%)
FPF emitted < 1 µm (%)	6.28 ± 0.53	%V < 1 µm	1.17 ± 0.53	638.81 ± 277.78
FPF emitted < 2 µm (%)	29.49 ± 0.95	%V < 2 µm	9.79 ± 0.95	305.00 ± 51.55
FPF emitted < 3 µm (%)	50.18 ± 1.29	%V < 3 µm	23.54 ± 1.29	214.19 ± 24.19
FPF emitted < 5 µm (%)	71.76 ± 1.99	%V < 5 µm	50.69 ± 1.99	141.88 ± 10.90
FPF emitted < 10 µm (%)	90.88 ± 1.78	%V < 10 µm	86.94 ± 1.78	104.60 ± 3.58
MMAD emitted (µm)	3.00 ± 0.17	VMAD (µm)	4.97 ± 0.17	60.45 ± 5.11
GSD emitted	2.02 ± 0.04	GSD	1.85 ± 0.04	109.53 ± 4.91
1 mL of 50 mg/mL				
FPF emitted < 1 µm (%)	4.96 ± 0.30	%V < 1 µm	1.05 ± 0.30	506.31 ± 166.86
FPF emitted < 2 µm (%)	24.48 ± 0.67	%V < 2 µm	8.63 ± 0.67	286.29 ± 46.16
FPF emitted < 3 µm (%)	45.29 ± 1.73	%V < 3 µm	21.46 ± 1.73	212.77 ± 28.92
FPF emitted < 5 µm (%)	67.30 ± 2.83	%V < 5 µm	47.93 ± 2.83	140.96 ± 12.42
FPF emitted < 10 µm (%)	88.34 ± 2.04	%V < 10 µm	84.86 ± 2.04	104.17 ± 3.42
MMAD emitted (µm)	3.27 ± 0.25	VMAD (µm)	5.23 ± 0.25	62.77 ± 6.63
GSD emitted	1.94 ± 0.02	GSD	1.84 ± 0.02	105.51 ± 7.74
1 mL of 100 mg/mL				
FPF emitted < 1 µm (%)	4.68 ± 0.36	%V < 1 µm	1.31 ± 0.36	373.53 ± 95.63
FPF emitted < 2 µm (%)	27.62 ± 2.44	%V < 2 µm	13.28 ± 2.44	214.13 ± 50.89
FPF emitted < 3 µm (%)	50.65 ± 3.80	%V < 3 µm	29.73 ± 3.80	172.71 ± 28.55
FPF emitted < 5 µm (%)	71.34 ± 4.29	%V < 5 µm	57.62 ± 4.29	124.33 ± 11.29
FPF emitted < 10 µm (%)	88.44 ± 2.08	%V < 10 µm	91.18 ± 2.08	97.03 ± 2.54
MMAD emitted (µm)	2.99 ± 0.32	VMAD (µm)	4.39 ± 0.32	68.46 ± 7.29
GSD emitted	1.88 ± 0.04	GSD	1.83 ± 0.04	103.18 ± 4.36
1.5 mL of 100 mg/mL				
FPF emitted < 1 µm (%)	6.58 ± 0.20	%V < 1 µm	0.90 ± 0.20	777.58 ± 273.88
FPF emitted < 2 µm (%)	36.57 ± 1.04	%V < 2 µm	11.87 ± 1.04	309.75 ± 39.07
FPF emitted < 3 µm (%)	62.87 ± 1.91	%V < 3 µm	28.15 ± 1.91	223.94 ± 19.12
FPF emitted < 5 µm (%)	82.28 ± 2.74	%V < 5 µm	56.32 ± 2.74	146.31 ± 7.45
FPF emitted < 10 µm (%)	94.29 ± 1.85	%V < 10 µm	90.76 ± 1.85	103.92 ± 2.10
MMAD emitted (µm)	2.50 ± 0.19	VMAD (µm)	4.50 ± 0.19	55.66 ± 3.90
GSD emitted	1.75 ± 0.02	GSD	1.80 ± 0.02	97.43 ± 2.57

Data presented as mean ± standard deviation (n = 9).

4. Discussion

The ClinicalTrials.gov (accessed on 20 May 2021) database records several clinical studies on inhaled hydroxychloroquine for COVID-19 at various stages of progress, from recently completed to not yet recruiting [58]. There are Phase 1 safety, tolerability, and pharmacokinetic studies on healthy subjects (ClinicalTrials.gov Identifier: NCT04461353, NCT04497519, NCT04697654), as well as efficacy studies on COVID-19 patients (NCT04477083, NCT04731051), but no results from the completed trials were available as of 17 July 2021. The formulations investigated included nebulised solutions (NCT04461353, NCT04731051), nebulised liposomal suspension (NCT04697654), and inhaled dry powders (NCT04497519, NCT04477083).

Inhaled hydroxychloroquine solutions had been tested on humans in the past. HCQS (50 µL of 100 mg/mL) aerosolised from the AERx® Pulmonary Delivery System was studied more than a decade ago in Phase 1 and Phase 2 clinical trials for asthma treatment, owing to its anti-inflammatory properties [40]. Subjects inhaling nebulised 20 mg or 50 mg HCQS experienced only mild adverse effects (altered sense of taste and dizziness), with minimal influence on pulmonary and cardiac functions [48]. Two researchers recently self-tested the effects of inhaled hydroxychloroquine by inhaling a nebulised solution (1 mg in 2 mL of normal saline) twice a day [25]. The dose was increased gradually to 4 mg daily over one week. It was also well-tolerated, with the only notable adverse effect being a bitter aftertaste that remained in the mouth for up to 3 h after inhalation [25]. HCQS is bitter [59], which can affect the palatability of the nebulised solutions as the volume delivered is much larger than that from an AERx system. The consumption of peanut butter and hazelnut chocolate spread immediately after oral administration of a bitter drug such as ritonavir has been shown to decrease the duration and intensity of the aftertaste [60]. This practice may be considered after inhaling nebulised HCQS solutions. Alternatively, taste-masking liposomes loaded with the drug may be used instead, but its formulation and drug release profile are more complex [61]. A liposomal HCQS formulation delivered to Sprague–Dawley rats by intratracheal instillation showed higher dose and longer drug retention in the lungs, as well as lower systemic exposure, compared to intravenous injection of unformulated HCQS [62].

Aerogen Solo is a vibrating mesh nebuliser that can be used directly with a mouth-piece/face mask or integrated into breathing circuits with a ventilator/nasal cannula [63]. The Aerogen Ultra acts as an aerosol holding chamber used in conjunction with the Aerogen Solo. It has a port for external air entrainment and optional supplemental oxygen, where an Exhaust filter 2 was connected (Figure 1). The versatility of the nebuliser setup is an advantage for treating COVID-19 because it can be used in patients with various degrees of breathing ability, depending on the severity of the disease. It is also better than jet and ultrasonic nebulisers because the temperature and solute concentration of the liquid in the reservoir remain constant during nebulisation [64]. Its atomisation mechanism is efficient, as the residual volume at the end of nebulisation is only about 50 μL [64]. This nebuliser had been used to administer HCQS to adult subjects in a recent Phase 1 pharmacokinetic study [48]. Therefore, Aerogen Solo was chosen for nebulising the HCQS solutions in the current study.

SARS-Cov-2 is primarily transmitted by the dispersion of bioaerosols from the patient through breathing, speaking, coughing, or sneezing [65]. There is a widely held concern that patients using nebulisers can increase the spread of respiratory pathogens through exhaling contaminated droplets into the surroundings. Nebulisers were consequently banned in Hong Kong during the SARS outbreak there in 2003 [65]. Jet nebulisers would have been the most common nebulisers used at that time. Normally, nebulisers should not produce virus-laden droplets unless they and/or the nebulised liquid are contaminated. The liquid reservoir of jet nebulisers is open to the inhalation/exhalation pathway, so it can be contaminated by bioaerosols from the patient being blown into it or by the materials from the patient's mouth dripping into the nebuliser bowl, thereby generating infected droplets that may escape into the environment if such aerosol leaves the nebuliser system while the patient is exhaling. Furthermore, not all inhaled nebulised droplets will deposit in the lungs. Some of them may be exhaled after a brief stay in the airways. It is still controversial whether these initially virus-free nebulised droplets can become contaminated while inside the airways before they are exhaled. One view is that if an inhaled droplet deposits onto the mucosal lining of the respiratory tract, then it would coalesce and fuse with the airway surface fluid so it cannot be exhaled [65]. For droplets that entered the airways but have not deposited, they should remain virus-free when they are exhaled because they did not contact the infected airway surface [65]. However, it may also be possible that during transit, those initially clean droplets coalesce with virus-laden droplets that are naturally produced in the airways, without contacting the mucosal surface. Then, these contaminated droplets may be exhaled into the surroundings. Whatever the situation is, precaution should be taken when healthcare workers and patients use nebulisers to prevent contamination of the equipment and environment. Both the exhaled aerosol as well as the aerosol that is generated but not inhaled while the patient is exhaling is filtered out by the exhaust filter on the Aerosol Solo Ultra. Exhaust filters should be placed in the manner adopted in the dose output experiments to capture all exhaled droplets (Figure 1). Their collection efficiency was excellent because drug recovery was near 100%. Additionally, the nebulisers should be disinfected thoroughly before and after use.

Filtration of the HCQS solutions through a 0.22 μm syringe filter did not affect the drug concentration, so this could be a suitable sterilisation method. The osmolality and pH of the solutions were controlled because acidity and non-isotonicity may trigger bronchoconstriction and cough [51,66]. The osmolality of normal saline and physiological plasma are 286 and 288 mOsmol/kg H_2O [67]. The osmolality of the normal saline used for dilution in the current study conformed to this range. The osmolality of inhaled solutions should preferably be <320 mOsmol/kg H_2O [66]. After filtration, the osmolality of the HCQS solutions decreased to near or below this level, so they are suitable (Table 1). The airway surface liquid in conducting airways and the alveolar subphase fluid in alveoli have a pH of 6.9 [68]. However, they become more acidic when the lungs are infected and inflamed, with a pH reduction of at least 0.2 from baseline in pneumonia [69]. Airway surface fluid has substantial buffering capacity so that the deposition of unbuffered aerosols, such as the HCQS solutions, would only induce a transient pH change that can quickly be restored [66]. Since the pH of the filtered HCQS solutions was near-neutral (7.03–7.25) (Table 1), disturbance to the pH in the airways should be minimal.

Since chloroquine binds to glass and plastics [70,71], the potential adsorption of hydroxychloroquine to surfaces of the containers and experimental setup in the study was checked in preliminary experiments. The concentration of the HCQS solutions was unchanged after contacting surfaces in Aerogen Solo and Ultra (data not shown). On the other hand, adsorption was observed in the SureGard filters, especially with the lower level of spiked drug (Table 3). The ability of recovering the drug in the assay was different between deionised water and 50:50 methanol/water. This could be due to a difference in the affinity of HCQS between the filter material and the washing liquid. This is analogous to the situation in a HPLC column between the stationary and mobile phases. HCQS was more easily extracted from SureGard filters by water than the co-solvent. The difference in the extraction power of the liquids was more prominent at low drug concentrations because the liquids had to compete with drug adsorption on the filter. The recovery could be improved by soaking the filters with the liquids for 30 min before shaking (Table 3). However, the absolute amount not recovered from 2 mg was only about 0.1 mg for water and 0.24 mg for the co-solvent. These constitute <1.5% of the loaded dose in the nebulisers for the concentrations/volumes investigated in this project so the resultant error in the total recovery was insignificant. Therefore, the final results of the filters did not require correction. On the other hand, recovery from spiked NGI impactor stages with 50:50 methanol/water was high (data not shown) so drug adsorption on the metallic surfaces was negligible. Therefore, the co-solvent was used for the cascade impaction experiments because it is recommended by the USP. The rationale was to follow the USP HPLC method unless there was a need for minor adjustments. Thus, deionised water was used instead for the dose output experiments to maximise recovery because the droplets were collected by SureGard filters rather than metallic impactor stages.

The nebulisation duration in the laser diffraction experiments (Table 5) were longer than those in the dose output (Table 4) and cascade impaction experiments (Table 6), especially for 20 mg/mL. Although the determination of the end of nebulisation was different between these experiments (the aerosol cloud could be easily observed visually in laser diffraction but it could not be seen clearly in the dose output and cascade impaction experiments), it could not account for the doubling of nebulisation duration for 20 mg/mL. It might be due to an effect of lower airflow through the Aerogen Ultra in the laser diffraction experiments and a potential augmented influence from solute concentration on lengthening nebulisation duration.

The HCQS solutions at all concentrations/volumes could form inhalable droplets, but the droplet sizes measured by cascade impaction were consistently smaller than those by laser diffraction, with smaller MMADs and higher FPFs (Table 8). The USP recommends pre-chilling the NGI to minimise droplet evaporation [52]. However, despite that, evaporation could still occur because the dilution air drawn into the impactor was ambient, which was warmer and non-humidified [57,72–74]. The USP does not require the use of humidified air, nor are the nebulisers clinically used with humidified air. However, air is humidified rapidly as it enters the airways, so inhaled isotonic droplets should not evaporate significantly [75]. Therefore, laser diffraction data would better reflect their true size distribution because the measurement zone was close to the exit of the nebuliser mouthpiece, where there was minimal evaporation [72].

Droplet size was observed to decrease with increasing HCQS concentration, especially between 50 and 100 mg/mL (Tables 7 and 8). This trend has been reported in previous studies on vibrating mesh nebulisers [76–79]. An increase in the concentration of ionic species increased the electrical conductivity of the liquid, which then dissipated the high charges that would otherwise be present between water and the nebuliser mesh. Consequently, fluid adhesion to the mesh was reduced, and droplets could be detached easier, resulting in the production of smaller droplets [76–79]. However, the reduction in droplet size with increasing ionic concentration is sigmoidal [79]. In other words, the droplet size will reach a plateau after the ionic concentration exceeds a threshold. The threshold concentration is dependent on the ionic species and liquid vehicle and beyond which other physicochemical factors (e.g., viscosity and surface tension) may then become dominant in affecting droplet size [76–79]. It has been reported that droplet size from vibrating mesh nebulisers decreases with viscosity [76–78]. It should be noted that any factors that affect droplet size may also affect the aerosol output rate. The electrical conductivity, viscosity, and surface tension of the HCQS solutions were not measured in the current study, but the 100 mg/mL solutions were qualitatively more viscous than the 20 and 50 mg/mL solutions. Thus, it is unknown which of the aforementioned physicochemical factors exerted the most effect on the droplet size in the present study.

The in vivo antiviral and anti-inflammatory concentrations of hydroxychloroquine in the airways is unknown, but its in vitro antiviral EC_{50} is approximately 1–5 μM, as discussed in the Introduction. After inhaling a nominal dose of 50 mg HCQS from an Aerogen nebuliser in a Phase 1 study, the peak respiratory tissue concentration was predicted by pharmacokinetic modelling to reach 500 μM, which was at least 100-fold higher than the in vitro antiviral EC_{50} [48]. It decreased to 10 μM at 24 h post-inhalation but was still at least double the in vitro EC_{50}. This supports the feasibility of treating COVID-19 with nebulised HCQS solutions. High drug levels in the airways can be maintained by multiple daily inhalations. Idkaidek et al. employed a physiologically based pharmacokinetic model to estimate the inhaled dose needed for COVID-19 based on this concentration range [80]. The model featured droplets with a VMD of 5.6 μm. The proportions depositing in the trachea, bronchioles, and alveoli were 10, 13, and 30% by mass, respectively [80]. Their sum (53%) could be interpreted as the proportion of the emitted aerosol < 5 μm because they theoretically deposited in the lungs. It was found that inhaling 25 mg of hydroxychloroquine twice a day could achieve a maximum concentration (C_{max}) ≥ 7 μM in the various parts of the lungs, while the plasma C_{max} was only 0.18 μM [80]. If the inhaled dose was doubled to 50 mg hydroxychloroquine twice a day, then the lung C_{max} reached ≥ 13 μM and plasma C_{max} increased to 0.35 μM. Thus, pulmonary drug concentrations higher than the in vitro antiviral EC_{50} with low systemic absorption are potentially achievable. The plasma hydroxychloroquine concentration for rheumatoid arthritis treatment is typically < 1 μM, while serious toxicity was associated with plasma levels from 2.05 to 18.16 μM [81]. Therefore, systemic adverse effects should be minimal with the low plasma concentrations from the inhalation regimens outlined above. The emitted dose obtained from the dose output experiments was 9.1–75.9 mg (Table 7), depending on the concentration/volume of the HCQS solution. This encompassed the range of 25–50 mg hydroxychloroquine (equivalent to 32.3–64.5 mg HCQS) proposed by Idkaidek et al. The VMD of our droplets were 4.3–5.2 μm, with 50–60% of them < 5 μm (Table 7, Figure 6), so they were slightly smaller than those used in their model. This suggests that if our HCQS aerosols were inhaled twice a day, especially with the two volumes of 100 mg/mL HCQS solutions (dose outputs of 48.8–75.9 mg), they may be able to produce pulmonary drug concentrations above the in vitro antiviral EC_{50}. To put this into perspective, 400–600 mg of HCQS were delivered orally per day in previous COVID-19 clinical trials [30]. This is 5–12-fold higher than the emitted doses from the two volumes of 100 mg/mL HCQS solutions. Yao et al. proposed several oral delivery regimens involving hundreds of milligrams HCQS taken twice to four times daily using physiologically based pharmacokinetic modelling to maintain sufficiently high ratios of free lung tissue trough concentration to the in vitro EC_{50} (R_{LTEC}), in the range of 21–169 [27]. The higher the R_{LTEC}, the more likely in vivo antiviral activity is achieved [45]. However, it was found that the free lung trough concentration used by Yao et al. included the in vivo intracellular drug concentration, which is expected to much higher than the in vivo extracellular drug concentration because HCQS highly accumulates in acidic cellular organelles (e.g., endosomes and lysosomes) [45]. Since the reported in vitro EC_{50} was extracellular, Yao et al. overestimated the R_{LTEC}. The corrected R_{LTEC} was much lower after recalculation with the in vivo extracellular drug concentration, ranging from 0.11 to 0.34 [45], which was deemed too low for in vivo antiviral efficacy. Moreover, the risk of systemic adverse effects from the high oral doses outweighed the low to lack of therapeutic effects observed in clinical studies [17,18,30]. Therefore, inhalation would be more efficient and safer for potential treatment of COVID-19.

As mentioned above, intratracheal liposomal HCQS has been tested on rats [62]. There is also a human clinical trial on a nebulised liposomal HCQS suspension (NCT04697654) [58]. Therefore, formulating the drug as simple, aqueous solutions is not the only approach. Multivalent nanoparticles functionalised with ligands targeting SARS-CoV-2 and/or receptors for cellular infection have been proposed for COVID-19 treatment, owing to their engineering flexibility and versatility [82]. They can be designed to target multiple pathogenic pathways of the disease. Multivalent nanoparticles may be employed to deliver otherwise toxic compounds such as oncology drugs (e.g., erlotinib and sunitinib), which may prevent viral entry into cells by inhibiting AP2-associated protein kinase 1 [82]. Systemic adverse effects are minimised due to the specificity offered by the functional ligands. However, although the number of approved nanoparticle products has been growing, their development takes years to decades, as they have unique technical, safety, and regulatory challenges [83]. Moreover, complex constructs such as multivalent nanoparticles may become damaged by the shear and stress during aerosolisation so they may not be a straightforward formulation option. Given the extremely urgent need to develop readily accessible and affordable therapy for the prophylaxis and treatment of COVID-19 for ambulatory and hospitalised patients, including those who may require ventilators, repurposing a well-established drug with antiviral and anti-inflammatory activities that has been used clinically, such as HCQS, is an attractive path to the rapid development of safe and effective treatments. Indeed, the United States and European Union have abbreviated regulatory pathways for drugs previously approved for human use. In addition, the risk of inhaled aqueous HCQS solutions is very low because of the reports of good safety and tolerability, even in patients with pulmonary disease (see above). Therefore, the translational and clinical barriers are significantly lower. The risk of failure due to safety problems is also much reduced.

5. Conclusions

Inhalable droplets of isotonic and pH-neutral HCQS solutions generated from vibrating mesh nebulisers were characterised. Droplet size decreased with increasing solute concentration. A range of emitted and fine particle doses were obtained with 20–100 mg/mL HCQS, with the 100 mg/mL solution potentially able to achieve sufficiently high drug concentrations in the airways for antiviral effects of COVID-19 with low systemic absorption.

Author Contributions: Conceptualization, I.G., R.B.M. and H.-K.C.; methodology, W.T., M.Y.T.C., I.G., H.-K.C. and P.C.L.K.; validation, W.T., M.Y.T.C. and P.C.L.K.; formal analysis, W.T. and P.C.L.K.; investigation, W.T., M.Y.T.C., R.Y.K.C., P.T. and P.C.L.K.; resources, H.-K.C.; data curation, W.T.; writing—original draft preparation, P.C.L.K.; writing—review and editing, I.G., R.B.M., H.-K.C. and P.C.L.K.; visualisation, W.T. and P.C.L.K.; supervision, I.G., H.-K.C. and P.C.L.K.; project administration, P.T. and P.C.L.K.; funding acquisition, I.G., R.B.M. and H.-K.C. All authors have read and agreed to the published version of the manuscript.

Funding: This research was funded by Pulmoquine Therapeutics, Inc. through a contract research project with The University of Sydney (IRMA Project ID 208309).

Institutional Review Board Statement: Not applicable.

Informed Consent Statement: Not applicable.

Data Availability Statement: Not applicable.

Conflicts of Interest: M.Y.T.C., R.Y.K.C., P.T., H.-K.C. and P.C.L.K. are employees of The University of Sydney. W.T. is a PhD student of The University of Sydney under the supervision of P.C.L.K. and H.-K.C. I.G. is a consultant and shareholder in Pulmoquine Therapeutics, Inc. R.B.M. is a founder, equity holder, and member of the scientific advisory board of Pulmoquine Therapeutics, Inc. The Company had no role in the design of the study; in the collection, analyses, or interpretation of data; in the writing of the manuscript, or in the decision to publish the results.

References

1. Johns Hopkins University. COVID-19 Dashboard by the Center for Systems Science and Engineering (CSSE) at Johns Hopkins University (JHU). Available online: https://coronavirus.jhu.edu/map.html (accessed on 17 July 2021).
2. Izda, V.; Jeffries, M.A.; Sawalha, A.H. COVID-19: A review of therapeutic strategies and vaccine candidates. *Clin. Immunol.* **2021**, *222*, 108634. [CrossRef] [PubMed]
3. Krammer, F. SARS-CoV-2 vaccines in development. *Nature* **2020**, *586*, 516–527. [CrossRef] [PubMed]
4. Peiris, M.; Leung, G.M. What can we expect from first-generation COVID-19 vaccines? *Lancet* **2020**, *396*, 1467–1469. [CrossRef]
5. Kostoff, R.N.; Briggs, M.B.; Porter, A.L.; Spandidos, D.A.; Tsatsakis, A. COVID-19 vaccine safety. *Int. J. Mol. Med.* **2020**, *46*, 1599–1602.
6. Karlsson, L.C.; Soveri, A.; Lewandowsky, S.; Karlsson, L.; Karlsson, H.; Nolvi, S.; Karukivi, M.; Lindfelt, M.; Antfolk, J. Fearing the disease or the vaccine: The case of COVID-19. *Personal. Individ. Differ.* **2021**, *172*, 110590. [CrossRef]
7. Wise, J. Covid-19: The E484K mutation and the risks it poses. *BMJ* **2021**, *372*, n359. [CrossRef]
8. Iacobucci, G. Covid-19: Single vaccine dose is 33% effective against variant from India, data show. *BMJ* **2021**, *373*, n1346. [CrossRef]
9. Abu-Raddad, L.J.; Chemaitelly, H.; Butt, A.A. National Study Group for COVID-19 Vaccination. Effectiveness of the BNT162b2 Covid-19 vaccine against the B.1.1.7 and B.1.351 variants. *N. Engl. J. Med.* **2021**, *385*, 187–189. [CrossRef]
10. Luchsinger, L.L.; Hillyer, C.D. Vaccine efficacy probable against COVID-19 variants. *Science* **2021**, *371*, 1116.
11. Madhi, S.A.; Baillie, V.; Cutland, C.L.; Voysey, M.; Koen, A.L.; Fairlie, L.; Padayachee, S.D.; Dheda, K.; Barnabas, S.L.; Bhorat, Q.E.; et al. Efficacy of the ChAdOx1 nCoV-19 Covid-19 vaccine against the B.1.351 variant. *N. Engl. J. Med.* **2021**, *384*, 1885–1898. [CrossRef]
12. COVID-19 Treatment Guidelines Panel. Coronavirus Disease 2019 (COVID-19) Treatment Guidelines. National Institutes of Health. Available online: https://www.covid19treatmentguidelines.nih.gov/ (accessed on 17 July 2021).
13. European Medicines Agency. Treatments and Vaccines for COVID-19: Authorised Medicines. Available online: https://www.ema.europa.eu/en/human-regulatory/overview/public-health-threats/coronavirus-disease-covid-19/treatments-vaccines/treatments-covid-19/covid-19-treatments-authorised (accessed on 17 July 2021).
14. United States Food & Drug Administration. COVID-19 Frequently Asked Questions. Available online: https://www.fda.gov/emergency-preparedness-and-response/coronavirus-disease-2019-covid-19/covid-19-frequently-asked-questions#drugs (accessed on 17 July 2021).
15. American Society of Health-System Pharmacists. Assessment of Evidence for COVID-19-Related Treatments. Available online: https://www.ashp.org/-/media/assets/pharmacy-practice/resource-centers/Coronavirus/docs/ASHP-COVID-19-Evidence-Table.ashx (accessed on 17 July 2021).
16. Majumder, J.; Minko, T. Recent developments on therapeutic and diagnostic approaches for COVID-19. *AAPS J.* **2021**, *23*, 14. [CrossRef]
17. Siemieniuk, R.A.; Bartoszko, J.J.; Ge, L.; Zeraatkar, D.; Izcovich, A.; Kum, E.; Pardo-Hernandez, H.; Rochwerg, B.; Lamontagne, F.; Han, M.A.; et al. Drug treatments for covid-19: Living systematic review and network meta-analysis. *BMJ* **2020**, *370*, m2980. [CrossRef] [PubMed]
18. Boregowda, U.; Gandhi, D.; Jain, N.; Khanna, K.; Gupta, N. Comprehensive literature review and evidence evaluation of experimental treatment in COVID 19 contagion. *Clin. Med. Insights Circ. Respir. Pulm. Med.* **2020**, *14*, 1–7. [CrossRef]
19. Juul, S.; Nielsen, E.E.; Feinberg, J.; Siddiqui, F.; Jørgensen, C.K.; Barot, E.; Holgersson, J.; Nielsen, N.; Bentzer, P.; Veroniki, A.A.; et al. Interventions for treatment of COVID-19: A living systematic review with meta-analyses and trial sequential analyses (The LIVING Project). *PLoS Med.* **2020**, *17*, e1003293. [CrossRef]
20. Warhurst, D.C.; Steele, J.C.P.; Adagu, I.S.; Craig, J.C.; Cullander, C. Hydroxychloroquine is much less active than chloroquine against chloroquine-resistant *Plasmodium falciparum*, in agreement with its physicochemical properties. *J. Antimicrob. Chemother.* **2003**, *52*, 188–193. [CrossRef]
21. *Martindale: The Complete Drug Reference*; Pharmaceutical Press: London, UK, 2021.

22. Moffat, A.C.; Osselton, M.D.; Widdop, B. *Clarke's Analysis of Drugs and Poisons*; Pharmaceutical Press: London, UK; Chicago, IL, USA, 2003.
23. Tett, S.E.; Cutler, D.J.; Day, R.O.; Brown, K.F. Bioavailability of hydroxychloroquine tablets in healthy volunteers. *Br. J. Clin. Pharmacol.* **1989**, *27*, 771–779. [CrossRef] [PubMed]
24. Kaur, K.; Kaushal, S.; Kaushal, I.G. Therapeutic status of hydroxychloroquine in COVID-19: A review. *J. Anaesthesiol. Clin. Pharmacol.* **2020**, *36*, S160–S165. [PubMed]
25. Klimke, A.; Hefner, G.; Will, B.; Voss, U. Hydroxychloroquine as an aerosol might markedly reduce and even prevent severe clinical symptoms after SARS-CoV-2 infection. *Med. Hypotheses* **2020**, *142*, 109783. [CrossRef]
26. Wang, M.; Cao, R.; Zhang, H.; Yang, X.; Liu, J.; Xu, M.; Shi, Z.; Hu, Z.; Zhong, W.; Xiao, G. Remdesivir and chloroquine effectively inhibit the recently emerged novel coronavirus (2019-nCoV) in vitro. *Cell Res.* **2020**, *30*, 269–271. [CrossRef]
27. Yao, X.; Ye, F.; Zhang, M.; Cui, C.; Huang, B.; Niu, P.; Liu, X.; Zhao, L.; Dong, E.; Song, C.; et al. In vitro antiviral activity and projection of optimized dosing design of hydroxychloroquine for the treatment of severe acute respiratory syndrome coronavirus 2 (SARS-CoV-2). *Clin. Infect. Dis.* **2020**, *71*, 732–739. [CrossRef]
28. Liu, J.; Cao, R.; Xu, M.; Wang, X.; Zhang, H.; Hu, H.; Li, Y.; Hu, Z.; Zhong, W.; Wang, M. Hydroxychloroquine, a less toxic derivative of chloroquine, is effective in inhibiting SARS-CoV-2 infection in vitro. *Cell Discov.* **2020**, *6*, 16. [CrossRef]
29. Fantini, J.; Di Scala, C.; Chahinian, H.; Yahi, N. Structural and molecular modelling studies reveal a new mechanism of action of chloroquine and hydroxychloroquine against SARS-CoV-2 infection. *Int. J. Antimicrob. Agents* **2020**, *55*, 105960. [CrossRef]
30. Pastick, K.A.; Okafor, E.C.; Wang, F.; Lofgren, S.M.; Skipper, C.P.; Nicol, M.R.; Pullen, M.F.; Rajasingham, R.; McDonald, E.G.; Lee, T.C.; et al. Review: Hydroxychloroquine and chloroquine for treatment of SARS-CoV-2 (COVID-19). *Open Forum Infect. Dis.* **2020**, *15*, ofaa130. [CrossRef] [PubMed]
31. Romagnoli, S.; Peris, A.; De Gaudio, A.R.; Geppetti, P. SARS-CoV-2 and COVID-19: From the Bench to the Bedside. *Physiol. Rev.* **2020**, *100*, 1455–1466. [CrossRef]
32. Sun, X.; Wang, T.; Cai, D.; Hu, Z.; Chen, J.; Liao, H.; Zhi, L.; Wei, H.; Zhang, Z.; Qiu, Y.; et al. Cytokine storm intervention in the early stages of COVID-19 pneumonia. *Cytokine Growth Factor Rev.* **2020**, *53*, 38–42. [CrossRef]
33. Sperber, K.; Quraishi, H.; Kalb, T.H.; Panja, A.; Stecher, V.; Mayer, L. Selective regulation of cytokine secretion by hydroxychloroquine: Inhibition of interleukin 1 alpha (IL-1-alpha) and IL-6 in human monocytes and T cells. *J. Rheumatol.* **1993**, *20*, 803–808.
34. Jang, C.-H.; Choi, J.-H.; Byun, M.-S.; Jue, D.-M. Chloroquine inhibits production of TNF-alpha, IL-1beta and IL-6 from lipopolysaccharide-stimulated human monocytes/macrophages by different modes. *Rheumatology* **2006**, *45*, 703–710. [CrossRef] [PubMed]
35. Dauby, N. The unfinished story of hydroxychloroquine in COVID-19: The right anti-inflammatory dose at the right moment? *Int. J. Infect. Dis.* **2021**, *103*, 1–2. [CrossRef] [PubMed]
36. Lammers, A.J.J.; Brohet, R.M.; Theunissen, R.E.P.; Koster, C.; Rood, R.; Verhagen, D.W.M.; Brinkman, K.; Hassing, R.J.; Dofferhoff, A.; el Moussaoui, R.; et al. Early hydroxychloroquine but not chloroquine use reduces ICU admission in COVID-19 patients. *Int. J. Infect. Dis.* **2020**, *101*, 283–289. [CrossRef]
37. Maisonnasse, P.; Guedj, J.; Contreras, V.; Behillil, S.; Solas, C.; Marlin, R.; Naninck, T.; Pizzorno, A.; Lemaitre, J.; Gonçalves, A.; et al. Hydroxychloroquine use against SARS-CoV-2 infection in non-human primates. *Nature* **2020**, *585*, 584–587. [CrossRef]
38. Tett, S.E.; Cutler, D.J.; Day, R.O.; Brown, K.F. A dose-ranging study of the pharmacokinetics of hydroxy-chloroquine following intravenous administration to healthy volunteers. *Br. J. Clin. Pharmacol.* **1988**, *26*, 303–313. [CrossRef]
39. Charous, B.L.; Nemeth, A.A.; Serebriakov, I.; Abraham, W.M. Aerosolized hydroxychloroquine (AHCQ) protects against antigen-induced early (EAR) and late airway responses (LAR) and airway hyperresponsiveness (AHR) in allergic sheep. *Am. J. Respir. Crit. Care Med.* **2001**, *163*, A859.
40. Dayton, F.; Owen, S.G.; Cipolla, D.; Chu, A.; Otulana, B.; Di Sciullo, G.; Charous, B.L. Development of an inhaled hydroxychloroquine sulfate product using the AERx® system to treat asthma. In *Respiratory Drug Delivery 2006*; Dalby, R.N., Byron, P.R., Peart, J., Suman, J.D., Farr, S.J., Eds.; Davis Healthcare International Publishing: River Grove, IL, USA, 2006; Volume 2, pp. 429–432.
41. Finkbeiner, W.E.; Charous, B.L.; Dolganov, G.; Widdicombe, J.H. Hydroxychloroquine (HCQ) inhibits rhinovirus (RV) replication in cultured human tracheal epithelial cells. *J. Allergy Clin. Immunol.* **2004**, *113*, S264. [CrossRef]
42. Fassihi, S.C.; Nabar, N.R.; Fassihi, R. Novel approach for low-dose pulmonary delivery of hydroxychloroquine in COVID-19. *Br. J. Pharmacol.* **2020**, *177*, 4997–4998. [CrossRef] [PubMed]
43. Albariqi, A.H.; Chang, R.Y.K.; Tai, W.; Ke, W.-R.; Chow, M.Y.T.; Tang, P.; Kwok, P.C.L.; Chan, H.-K. Inhalable hydroxychloroquine powders for potential treatment of COVID-19. *J. Aerosol Med. Pulm. Drug Deliv.* **2021**, *34*, 20–31. [CrossRef]
44. Mitchell, J.P.; Berlinski, A.; Canisius, S.; Cipolla, D.; Dolovich, M.B.; Gonda, I.; Hochhaus, G.; Kadrichu, N.; Lyapustina, S.; Mansour, H.M.; et al. Urgent appeal from International Society for Aerosols in Medicine (ISAM) during COVID-19: Clinical decision makers and governmental agencies should consider the inhaled route of administration: A statement from the ISAM Regulatory and Standardization Issues Networking Group. *J. Aerosol. Med. Pulm. Drug Deliv.* **2020**, *33*, 235–238. [PubMed]
45. Fan, J.; Zhang, X.; Liu, J.; Yang, Y.; Zheng, N.; Liu, Q.; Bergman, K.; Reynolds, K.; Huang, S.-M.; Zhu, H.; et al. Connecting hydroxychloroquine in vitro antiviral activity to in vivo concentration for prediction of antiviral effect: A critical step in treating COVID-19 patients. *Clin. Infect. Dis.* **2020**, *71*, 3232–3236. [CrossRef]

46. Chang, R.Y.K.; Kwok, P.C.L.; Ghassabian, S.; Brannan, J.D.; Koskela, H.O.; Chan, H.-K. Cough as an adverse effect on inhalation pharmaceutical products. *Br. J. Pharmacol.* **2020**, *177*, 4096–4112. [CrossRef]
47. de Reus, Y.A.; Hagedoorn, P.; Sturkenboom, M.G.G.; Grasmeijer, F.; Bolhuis, M.S.; Sibum, I.; Kerstjens, H.A.M.; Frijlink, H.W.; Akkerman, O.W. Tolerability and pharmacokinetic evaluation of inhaled dry powder hydroxychloroquine in healthy volunteers. *meDrxiv* **2020**, 12.03.20243162.
48. Bentur, O.; Hutt, R.; Brassil, D.; Bäckman, P.; Gonda, I.; Boushey, H.; Cahrous, B.; Coller, B.; MacArthur, R. Phase 1 randomized placebo-controlled study in healthy adult volunteers to evaluate the safety, tolerability, and pharmacokinetics of orally inhaled aerosolized hydroxychloroquine sulfate—A potential treatment for COVID-19. *J. Allergy Clin. Immunol.* **2021**, *147*, AB237. [CrossRef]
49. *K-7000 Vapor Pressure Osmometer User Manual V7109*; Dr. Ing. Herbert Knauer GmbH: Berlin, Germany, 2007.
50. Weers, J. Inhaled antimicrobial therapy—Barriers to effective treatment. *Adv. Drug Deliv. Rev.* **2015**, *85*, 24–43. [CrossRef] [PubMed]
51. Beasley, R.; Rafferty, P.; Holgate, S.T. Adverse reactions to the non-drug constituents of nebuliser solutions. *Br. J. Clin. Pharmacol.* **1988**, *25*, 283–287. [CrossRef]
52. *United States Pharmacopeia 43—National Formulary 38*; United States Pharmacopeial Convention: Rockville, MD, USA, 2020.
53. Chemical Rubber Company. *CRC Handbook of Chemistry and Physics*; Taylor & Francis: Boca Raton, FL, USA, 2020.
54. Hinds, W.C. *Aerosol Technology: Properties, Behavior, and Measurement of Airborne Particles*; John Wiley & Sons: Hoboken, NJ, USA, 1999.
55. *Guidance for Industry—Q2B Validation of Analytical Procedures: Methodology*; Food and Drug Administration: Silver Spring, MD, USA, 1996.
56. Phipps, P.R.; Gonda, I. Droplets produced by medical nebulizers: Some factors affecting their size and solute concentration. *Chest* **1990**, *97*, 1327–1332. [CrossRef]
57. Phipps, P.R.; Gonda, I. Evaporation of aqueous aerosols produced by jet nebulizers: Effects on particle size and concentration of solution in the droplets. *J. Aerosol Med.* **1994**, *7*, 239–258. [CrossRef]
58. United States National Library of Medicine. ClinicalTrials.gov. Available online: https://www.clinicaltrials.gov/ (accessed on 17 July 2021).
59. Pauli, E.; Joshi, H.; Vasavada, A.; Brackett, J.; Towa, L. Evaluation of an immediate-release formulation of hydroxychloroquine sulfate with an interwoven pediatric taste-masking system. *J. Pharm. Sci.* **2020**, *109*, 1493–1497. [CrossRef]
60. Morris, J.B.; Tisi, D.A.; Tan, D.C.T.; Worthington, J.H. Development and palatability assessment of Norvir® (ritonavir) 100 mg powder for pediatric population. *Int. J. Mol. Sci.* **2019**, *20*, 1718. [CrossRef]
61. Schuster, J.A.; Cipolla, D.C.; Farr, S. Processes for Taste-Masking of Inhaled Formulations. U.S. Patent Application No. 2008/0138397 A1, 12 June 2008.
62. Tai, T.-T.; Wu, T.-J.; Wu, H.-D.; Tsai, Y.-C.; Wang, H.-T.; Wang, A.-M.; Shih, S.-F.; Chen, Y.-C. A strategy to treat COVID-19 disease with targeted delivery of inhalable liposomal hydroxychloroquine: A preclinical pharmacokinetic study. *Clin. Transl. Sci.* **2021**, *14*, 132–136. [CrossRef] [PubMed]
63. Aerogen. *Aerogen®Solo System Instruction Manual*; Aerogen: Galway, Ireland, 2016.
64. Lin, H.-L.; Chen, C.-S.; Fink, J.B.; Lee, G.-H.; Huang, C.-W.; Chen, J.-C.; Chiang, Z.Y. In vitro evaluation of a vibrating-mesh nebulizer repeatedly use over 28 days. *Pharmaceutics* **2020**, *12*, 971. [CrossRef] [PubMed]
65. Fink, J.B.; Ehrmann, S.; Li, J.; Dailey, P.; McKiernan, P.; Darquenne, C.; Martin, A.R.; Rothen-Rutishauser, B.; Kuehl, P.J.; Häussermann, S.; et al. Reducing aerosol-related risk of transmission in the era of COVID-19: An interim guidance endorsed by the International Society of Aerosols in Medicine. *J. Aerosol Med. Pulm. Drug Deliv.* **2020**, *33*, 300–304. [CrossRef]
66. Desager, K.N.; Van Bever, H.P.; Stevens, W.J. Osmolality and pH of anti-asthmatic drug solutions. *Agents Actions* **1990**, *31*, 225–228. [CrossRef]
67. Zander, R. Intrakranieller Druck und hypotone Infusionslösungen (Intracranial pressure and hypotonic infusion solutions). *Anaesthesist* **2009**, *58*, 405–409. [CrossRef] [PubMed]
68. Ng, A.W.; Bidani, A.; Heming, T.A. Innate host defense of the lung: Effects of lung-lining fluid pH. *Lung* **2004**, *182*, 297–317. [CrossRef]
69. Karnad, D.R.; Mhaisekar, D.G.; Moralwar, K.V. Respiratory mucus pH in tracheostomized intensive care unit patients: Effects of colonization and pneumonia. *Crit. Care Med.* **1990**, *18*, 699–701. [CrossRef] [PubMed]
70. Yahya, A.M.; McElnay, J.C.; D'Arcy, P.F. Binding of chloroquine to glass. *Int. J. Pharm.* **1985**, *25*, 217–223. [CrossRef]
71. Yahya, A.M.; McElnay, J.C.; D'Arcy, P.F. Investigation of chloroquine binding to plastic materials. *Int. J. Pharm.* **1986**, *34*, 137–143. [CrossRef]
72. Clark, A.R. The use of laser diffraction for the evaluation of the aerosol clouds generated by medical nebulizers. *Int. J. Pharm.* **1995**, *115*, 69–78. [CrossRef]
73. Finlay, W.H.; Stapleton, K.W. Undersizing of droplets from a vented nebulizer caused by aerosol heating during transit through an Andersen impactor. *J. Aerosol Sci.* **1999**, *30*, 105–109. [CrossRef]
74. Kwong, W.T.J.; Ho, S.L.; Coates, A.L. Comparison of nebulized particle size distribution with Malvern laser diffraction analyzer versus Andersen cascade impactor and low-flow Marple personal cascade impactor. *J. Aerosol Med.* **2000**, *13*, 303–314. [CrossRef]
75. Daviskas, E.; Gonda, I.; Anderson, S.D. Mathematical modeling of heat and water transport in human respiratory tract. *J. Appl. Physiol.* **1990**, *69*, 362–372. [CrossRef]

76. Chan, J.G.Y.; Kwok, P.C.L.; Young, P.M.; Chan, H.-K.; Traini, D. Mannitol delivery by vibrating mesh nebulisation for enhancing mucociliary clearance. *J. Pharm. Sci.* **2011**, *100*, 2693–2702. [CrossRef]
77. Ghazanfari, T.; Elhissi, A.M.A.; Dong, Z.; Taylor, K.M.G. The influence of fluid physicochemical properties on vibrating-mesh nebulization. *Int. J. Pharm.* **2007**, *339*, 103–111. [CrossRef]
78. Chan, J.G.Y.; Traini, D.; Chan, H.-K.; Young, P.M.; Kwok, P.C.L. Delivery of high solubility polyols by vibrating mesh nebulizer to enhance mucociliary clearance. *J. Aerosol Med. Pulm. Drug Deliv.* **2012**, *25*, 297–305. [CrossRef] [PubMed]
79. Beck-Broichsitter, M.; Oesterheld, N. Electrolyte type and nozzle composition affect the process of vibrating-membrane nebulization. *Eur. J. Pharm. Biopharm.* **2017**, *119*, 11–16. [CrossRef]
80. Idkaidek, N.; Hawari, F.; Dodin, Y.; Obeidat, N. Development of a physiologically-based pharmacokinetic (PBPK) model of nebulized hydroxychloroquine for pulmonary delivery to COVID-19 patients. *Drug Res.* **2021**, *71*, 250–256.
81. Jordan, P.; Brookes, J.G.; Nikolic, G.; Le Couteur, D.G. Hydroxychloroquine overdose: Toxicokinetics and management. *Clin. Toxicol.* **1999**, *37*, 861–864. [CrossRef]
82. Tabish, T.A.; Hamblin, M.R. Multivalent nanomedicines to treat COVID-19: A slow train coming. *Nano Today* **2020**, *35*, 100962. [CrossRef] [PubMed]
83. Soares, S.; Sousa, J.; Pais, A.; Vitorino, C. Nanomedicine: Principles, properties, and regulatory Issues. *Front. Chem.* **2018**, *6*, 360. [CrossRef] [PubMed]

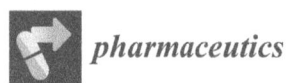

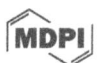

Article

An Enhanced Dissolving Cyclosporin-A Inhalable Powder Efficiently Reduces SARS-CoV-2 Infection In Vitro

Davide D'Angelo [1], Eride Quarta [1], Stefania Glieca [1], Giada Varacca [1], Lisa Flammini [1], Simona Bertoni [1], Martina Brandolini [2,3], Vittorio Sambri [2,3], Laura Grumiro [3], Giulia Gatti [2], Giorgio Dirani [3], Francesca Taddei [3], Annalisa Bianchera [1], Fabio Sonvico [1], Ruggero Bettini [1] and Francesca Buttini [1,*]

[1] Food and Drug Department, University of Parma, Parco Area delle Scienze 27a, 43124 Parma, Italy
[2] Department of Experimental, Diagnostic and Speciality Medicine, University of Bologna, 40138 Bologna, Italy
[3] Microbiology Unit, The Great Romagna Area Hub Laboratory, Piazza della Liberazione 60, Pievesestina, 47522 Cesena, Italy
* Correspondence: francesca.buttini@unipr.it

Abstract: This work illustrates the development of a dry inhalation powder of cyclosporine-A for the prevention of rejection after lung transplantation and for the treatment of COVID-19. The influence of excipients on the spray-dried powder's critical quality attributes was explored. The best-performing powder in terms of dissolution time and respirability was obtained starting from a concentration of ethanol of 45% (v/v) in the feedstock solution and 20% (w/w) of mannitol. This powder showed a faster dissolution profile (Weibull dissolution time of 59.5 min) than the poorly soluble raw material (169.0 min). The powder exhibited a fine particle fraction of 66.5% and an MMAD of 2.97 μm. The inhalable powder, when tested on A549 and THP-1, did not show cytotoxic effects up to a concentration of 10 μg/mL. Furthermore, the CsA inhalation powder showed efficiency in reducing IL-6 when tested on A549/THP-1 co-culture. A reduction in the replication of SARS-CoV-2 on Vero E6 cells was observed when the CsA powder was tested adopting the post-infection or simultaneous treatment. This formulation could represent a therapeutic strategy for the prevention of lung rejection, but is also a viable approach for the inhibition of SARS-CoV-2 replication and the COVID-19 pulmonary inflammatory process.

Keywords: cyclosporine-A; spray-drying; dry powder inhaler; SARS-CoV-2; cytokine storm; transplant rejection

Citation: D'Angelo, D.; Quarta, E.; Glieca, S.; Varacca, G.; Flammini, L.; Bertoni, S.; Brandolini, M.; Sambri, V.; Grumiro, L.; Gatti, G.; et al. An Enhanced Dissolving Cyclosporin-A Inhalable Powder Efficiently Reduces SARS-CoV-2 Infection In Vitro. *Pharmaceutics* **2023**, *15*, 1023. https://doi.org/10.3390/pharmaceutics15031023

Academic Editors: Michael Yee Tak Chow and Philip Chi Lip Kwok

Received: 8 February 2023
Revised: 8 March 2023
Accepted: 18 March 2023
Published: 22 March 2023

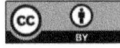

1. Introduction

Cyclosporine-A (CsA) is a cyclic peptide with an immunosuppressive action, administered for the treatment of various pathologies that share uncontrolled activation of the immune system, e.g., atopic dermatitis and psoriasis. Since entering the market in 1983, CsA, a calcineurin inhibitor peptide, has been widely used in the treatment of various autoimmune conditions characterised by the strong activation of the immune system [1]. The success of this molecule is related to its selective and reversible inhibition of the production of pro-inflammatory cytokines by T-lymphocytes [2]. CsA is intravenously and orally (as soft capsules) administered and is currently used for the prevention of allograft rejection in various organ transplantations. Indeed, the continuous activation of T-cells in the transplanted lung is the key factor bringing on bronchiolitis obliterans syndrome (BOS) characterised by extensive fibroproliferation and loss of lung functionality [3]. BOS is considered a marker of chronic rejection and causes 30% of deaths after lung transplantation [4,5].

Despite the efficacy of CsA, severe adverse side effects including nephrotoxicity, hepatotoxicity, hypertension, and neurotoxicity, usually arise during chronic treatment with CsA [6,7]. Moreover, the delivery of a sufficient and reproducible amount of CsA can hardly be achieved by oral administration because of its poor aqueous solubility, its pre-systemic metabolism at the gut level [8,9], and its erratic absorption related to interindividual variability, food intake, and by comorbidities such as diabetes [10,11]. Overall, the oral bioavailability of CsA is around 30%, which entails a dosage range between 5 and 15 mg/kg/day, and the need to carefully monitor the patient's drug plasma concentration over time [12].

For this reason, pulmonary administration would be a promising strategy for the treatment of lung transplant patients, given the possibility of (i) avoiding pre-systemic metabolism and obtaining high drug local concentrations, (ii) having a rapid onset of action, and (iii) administering lower doses than the oral route with limited systemic exposure to the drug. In this regard, the administration of a 100 μg intratracheal dose of CsA to rats, in addition to being effective in reducing lung inflammation, led to a distribution of CsA in the side effect-related organs that were one hundred times lower than that of an oral dose of 10 mg/kg [13]. The pulmonary administration of a dose of just 5 mg of CsA by nebulisation of a propylene glycol solution was able to produce an improvement in lung-transplanted patients' conditions, expressed as forced expiratory volume in one second (FEV1) [14]. This study demonstrated a strong relationship between the administration of CsA directly to the lungs and an increased anti-rejection effect. Further clinical trials have confirmed the benefits of direct pulmonary administration of CsA by nebulisation in patients who underwent single or double lung transplantation [15] or in BOS patients [16].

Besides the effect on the prevention of allograft rejection, CsA has also been widely studied as a potential anti-viral drug [17–19]. In 2011, de Wilde and colleagues first demonstrated the in vitro inhibitory activity of CsA at micromolar concentrations on the replication of different coronavirus genera [20]. The effective inhibition of replication towards SARS-CoV-2 has also recently been demonstrated by Fenizia et al. on the human lung epithelium Calu3 cell line [19]. In addition, CsA anti-inflammatory and immunomodulatory activities would be beneficial in containing the cytokine storm experienced by many COVID-19 patients, leading to airway damage and respiratory loss of function [19,21].

COVID-19 is currently treated using antiviral drugs such as molnupiravir [22], nirmatrelvir [23], ritonavir [24], and remdesivir [25], anti-inflammatory drugs (dexamethasone [26]), immunomodulatory agents such as baricitinib and tocilizumab, an anti-IL-6 antibody [27], and monoclonal antibodies against the receptor binding domain such as sotrovimab [28].

The aim of this work was the development of a highly respirable formulation of CsA obtained by spray drying with excipients already approved for inhalation. A critical parameter for the evaluation of the quality of the produced powders was the Weibull dissolution time obtained from the in vitro release rate profile. The most promising powder was then further analysed in terms of tolerability, reduction of inflammation, and antiviral activity in terms of SARS-CoV-2 reduction of infection in Vero E6 cells.

2. Materials and Methods

CsA (Metapharmaceutical, Barcelona, Spain) was purchased from ACEF (Fiorenzuola d'Arda, Italy). HPMC extra-dry capsules for use in dry powder inhalers, Quali-V®-I size #3, were provided by Qualicaps (Madrid, Spain), while the high-resistance dry powder inhaler RS01 was gifted by Plastiape (Lecco, Italy). Mannitol was purchased from Roquette (Lestrem, France) and glycine was purchased from Sigma Aldrich (Merck, Milano, Italy). All other chemicals used were obtained from commercial suppliers and were at least of analytical grade. The human lung adenocarcinoma cell line A549 (CRM-CCL-185), monocytic cell line THP-1 (TIB-202), and Vero E6 (CRL-1586) were purchased from American Type Culture Collection (ATCC, Manassas, VA, USA).

2.1. Preparation of CsA Spray-Dried Powders

The spray-dried (SD) CsA powders were obtained starting from a solution of water and ethanol 96% with a variable ratio according to the design of experiment (DOE) containing 1% (*w/v*) solids. The effect of different amounts of excipients on the yield of production, respirability, residual solvent, and dissolution rate was assessed. The experiments were designed by means of the Design-Expert 12 software (Stat-Ease, Inc., Minneapolis, MN, USA). A half-fractional factorial design with three factors at two levels and three additional centre points for curvature check was applied, requiring a total of 11 experiments, as detailed in Table 1. The mannitol (10–20% w/w) and glycine (0–5% w/w) content in the dry formulation and ethanol (45–60% v/v) concentration in the feed solution were the three factors investigated, fixed at two levels equally distant from the central point.

Table 1. Composition of powders studied according to the DOE with three factors at two levels and three centre points (*). M = mannitol; G = glycine. Each experimental point was replicated to calculate the experimental error.

Powder (#, Code)	Factor A: Mannitol (% w/w)	Factor B: Glycine (% w/w)	Factor C: Ethanol (% v/v)
1 (CsA_M15) *	15	2.5	52.5
2 (CsA_M10G)	10	5	45
3 (CsA_M20G)	20	5	60
4 (CsA_M10)	10	0	60
5 (CsA_M20)	20	0	45
6 (CsA_M20G)	20	5	60
7 (CsA_M15) *	15	2.5	52.5
8 (CsA_M15) *	15	2.5	52.5
9 (CsA_M20)	20	0	45
10 (CsA_M10G)	10	5	45
11 (CsA_M10)	10	0	60

CsA raw material (CsA_rm) was solubilised in ethanol where the solubility of CsA is more than 100 mg/g [29], while mannitol and glycine were solubilised in water at room temperature. The aqueous solution was added to the CsA solution under magnetic stirring (160 rpm). The CsA remained in solution in all the ranges of water added (from 40 to 55 % v/v) in the hydroalcoholic solution.

To produce the powders, 50 mL solution was spray dried (Mini Spray Dryer B-290, Büchi, Flawill, Switzerland) using the following parameters: inlet temperature 140 °C, drying air flow rate 742 L/h, aspiration 35 m³/h, solution feed rate of 3.5 mL/min, and a nozzle diameter 0.7 mm. Under these conditions, an outlet temperature of 80–87 °C was measured.

An analysis of variance (ANOVA) was performed to investigate the effect of factors on the critical quality attributes (CQAs). In detail, the CQAs selected were the production yield, the percentage of residual solvent, and the Weibull dissolution time obtained from the dissolution profile. The probability value of the model was considered significant when lower than 0.05.

2.2. CsA Quantification by High-Performance Liquid Chromatography (HPLC)

The quantification of CsA in the spray-dried powders was achieved by dissolving 20 mg of powder in 25 mL of water:acetonitrile 40:60. Six samples were prepared and analysed by HPLC. The drug content analysis was conducted after the powder preparation and during the stability study.

CsA was quantified using an HPLC (LC-10, Shimadzu, Kyoto, Japan) equipped with a UV–Vis detector, set at a wavelength of 230 nm and using the column Nova-Pak C18 (3.9 × 150 mm, 4 µm; Waters, Italy). The mobile phase was constituted by a mixture of 65% acetonitrile and 35% ultrapure water, acidified at 0.1% with trifluoroacetic acid. The column temperature was set at 65 °C and the flow rate was fixed at 1.6 mL/min. The injection volume was 10 µL, the run time of was 10 min and the retention time for the CsA was about 5 min. The method linearity was over the range 0.1–2 mg/mL.

2.3. Aerodynamic Performance Characterisation

The screening of the aerodynamic performance of all CsA batches produced was achieved using Fast Screening Impactor (FSI; Copley Scientific, Nottingham, UK), with a 65 L/min insert to provide a 5 μm cut-off size. The FSI was connected to an SCP5 vacuum pump (Copley Scientific, Nottingham, UK) through a critical flow controller (TPK Copley Scientific, Nottingham, UK). A flow rate of 65 L/min, measured with a DFM 2000 Flow Meter (Copley Scientific, UK), was required to activate the RS01 (Plastiape, Lecco, Italy) device at a 4 kPa pressure drop. The TPK actuation time was adjusted so that a volume of 4 L of air was drawn through the inhaler. The content of one capsule, filled with 20 mg of powder, was discharged and each experiment was repeated three times. The amount of CsA present in the formulation was in the range between 15 to 18 mg according to the formulation drug content. CsA was quantified by HPLC using to the method reported in Section 2.2. The emitted fraction (EF) was calculated as the percentage ratio between the total CsA mass recovered in FSI and the CsA loaded in the capsule. The respirable fraction (RF) was calculated as the percentage ratio between the mass of particles with an aerodynamic diameter less than 5 μm and the emitted dose.

The same analysis setup was maintained to further investigate the aerodynamic performance using the Next Generation Impactor (NGI; Copley Scientific, Nottingham, UK). To obtain a more accurate analysis and avoid the eventual particles bouncing, the cups of the impactor were coated using a solution of 2% (w/v) Tween 20 in ethanol. As above, the content of one capsule of 20 mg was aerosolised and the CsA in the NGI was collected and quantified by HPLC.

The metered dose (MD) is the total mass of the drug, quantified by HPLC, recovered in the inhaler and the impactor (induction port, stages 1 to 7, and Micro Orifice Collector (MOC)). The emitted dose (ED) is the amount of drug leaving the device and entering the impactor (induction port, stages 1 to 7, and MOC). The mass median aerodynamic diameter (MMAD) was determined by plotting the cumulative percentage of mass less than the stated aerodynamic diameter for each NGI stage from 1 to 7, on a probability scale versus the aerodynamic diameter of the stage on a logarithmic scale. The fine particle dose (FPD) is defined as the mass of drug with an aerodynamic diameter less than 5 μm (calculated from the log-probability plot equation) and the extra fine particle dose (EFPD) is the mass of the drug with an aerodynamic diameter less than 2 μm. The fine particle fraction (FPF) and the extra fine particle fraction (EFPF) were calculated as the percentage ratio between the FPD or EFPD, respectively, and the ED.

2.4. Thermogravimetric Analysis (TGA)

The analysis was carried out using the TGA/DSC 1 STARe System (Mettler Toledo, Columbus, OH, USA) to determine the loss on drying (LOD), i.e., the percentage of residual humidity and solvents present in the powder at the end of the manufacturing process. For this purpose, approximately 4 mg of powder was placed in a pan of aluminium oxide, and the analysis was carried out in a nitrogen flow at 80 mL/min. The temperature was increased from 25 °C to 150 °C with a rate of 10 °C/min. The LOD was measured in the range 25–125 °C.

2.5. Dissolution Profile of Respirable Particle Fraction

In vitro dissolution tests to compare the dissolution performance of CsA powders were conducted using RespiCell™ [30], an innovative vertical diffusion cell apparatus.

The apparatus comprises a 170 cm³ receiving cell filled with the dissolution media, and the sampling was performed through the side arm. The apparatus constitutes two portions: the upper part acts as a donor chamber and the lower part is a receptor chamber maintained under magnetic stirring at 180 rpm.

The receptor was filled with 170 mL of medium consisting of phosphate-buffered saline (PBS) containing 0.2% of sodium dodecyl sulphate and the cell was connected to a heating thermostat (Lauda eco silver E4, DE) set at 37 ± 0.5 °C. The dissolution was carried out on the RF of the powder, following separation by FSI. In the case of spray-dried CsA, four capsules of 20 mg were aerosolised for each experiment and the analysis was performed in triplicate. In the case of the raw material, the content of ten capsules was aerosolised due to the low respirability of the material. The filter (Type A/E glass filter 7.6 cm diameter, Pall Corp.) containing the mass of powder < 5 μm was then placed on the diffusion area of the RespiCell and 2 mL of PBS containing 0.2% of SDS was added before starting the dissolution to create a thin liquid layer on the powder bed. At fixed intervals, 1 mL of the receiving solution was removed and replaced with 1 mL of fresh buffer to maintain a constant volume inside the receptor chamber.

Finally, at the end of the experiment, the residual undissolved powder was recovered by washing out the filter with 10 mL of ethanol:water (50:50 v/v). The samples were quantified by HPLC according to the method described. The drug dissolved was expressed as a percentage of CsA dissolved relative to the total CsA recovered at the end of the test both on the filter and receptor compartment.

The dissolution profiles were analysed by means of the Weibull equation [31] in order to determine the time parameter, recognised as the time at which the 63.2 per cent of the drug was dissolved.

2.6. Morphological Analysis by SEM

Particle morphology was determined by scanning electron microscopy (SEM, Zeiss AURIGA, Zeiss, Oberkochen, Germany) and was operated under high-vacuum conditions with an accelerating 1.0 kV voltage at a magnification of 5k times. The powders were deposited on adhesive black carbon tabs pre-mounted on aluminium stubs and imaged without undergoing any metallisation process.

2.7. Viability Study on A549 and THP-1

A549 cells (seeding 10^4 cells/well), following overnight culture, and THP-1 cells (seeding 5×10^4 cells/well), immediately after seeding in a 96-well plate at 37 °C, were exposed to the following treatments: vehicle (DMSO 0.5% in PBS), CsA_rm (1, 10 μg/mL), spray-dried powder CsA_M20 (containing 20% w/w of mannitol) (1, 10 μg/mL of CsA), and mannitol 2 μg/mL. Cell viability was quantified using the MTS assay. Briefly, 20 μL of 3-(tributylammonium)-propyl methanethiosulfonate bromide solution (MTS, 1 mg/mL) was added to each well and, following 4 h incubation at 37 °C, the supernatants were collected. The absorbance of each well was measured at 490 nm on a microplate reader (Sunrise™ powered by Magellan™ data analysis software, TECAN, Mannedorf, Switzerland). The impact of the various treatments on cell viability was expressed as the percentage of viability with respect to vehicle-treated cells.

2.8. Co-Culture Assays and Cytokine Determination

For the co-cultures, A549 cells (10^5 cells/well) were seeded at the bottom and THP-1 cells (10^5 cells/well) were plated on the insert (0.4 μm pore polyester filter) of Transwell culture plates (#3470, Corning Inc., Corning, NY, USA), with the two cell cultures being physically separated to avoid direct contact, according to the method described by Li et al. [32]. After 24 h co-culture, the cells were exposed to the following treatments: vehicle (DMSO 0.5% in PBS), CsA_rm 10 μg/mL, CsA_M20 at 10 μg/mL in respect to CsA, mannitol 2 μg/mL in DMSO 0.5% in PBS. After 1 h, LPS 1 μg/mL (*Escherichia coli* O55:B5; cat# L6529; Sigma Aldrich, Merck, Milano, Italy) was added to the culture and maintained for 24 h. Cells incubated with the vehicle and not exposed to LPS were used as the control. The concentration of IL-6 in the conditioned media was subsequently determined using an ELISA kit (Boster Biological Technology, Milano, Italy; cat. no. IL-6, EK0410), according to the manufacturer's protocol and expressed as pg/mL.

2.9. Cell Treatment and Viral Replication Inhibition Assay

The inhibitory effect of CsA_M20, CsA_rm, and mannitol on viral replication on Vero E6 cell cultures was tested against Omicron subvariant BA.1 (lineage B.1.1.529.BA.1).

The viral strain was isolated from a residual clinical specimen conferred to the Unit of Microbiology, Greater Romagna Area Hub Laboratory (Cesena, Italy). The sample underwent an anonymisation procedure in order to adhere to the regulations issued by the local Ethical Board (AVR-PPC P09, rev.2; based on Burnett et al., 2007 [33]). Detailed descriptions of Vero E6 cell culture and propagation, as well as titration and isolation of the virus from biological samples, are reported in the Supplementary Materials.

The day before treatment and infection, Vero E6 cells were seeded at a density of 2×10^6 cells/well in 96-well plates and allowed to attach for 16 to 24 h at 37 °C, 5% CO_2. On the day of infection, each tested compound stock suspension in PBS was freshly diluted in cell culture medium containing 2% FBS. CsA_rm was tested at concentrations of 8, 16, 32, and 64 μM, corresponding to 9.6, 19.2, 38.4, and 76.9 μg/mL; CsA_M20 was diluted to obtain the same CsA concentrations considering the exact CsA content in the powder (determined by HPLC) of about 80% *(w/w)*. The selected CsA concentrations, in the case of powder CsA_M20, involved the presence of dissolved mannitol at concentrations of 2.4, 4.8, 9.6, and 19.2 μg/mL since mannitol represents 20% *(w/w)* of the formulation. These values were then adopted when mannitol was applied to the cells and tested as vehicle alone.

To better determine at which level the viral replication cycle was inhibited, the cells were subjected to different treatment regimens: treatment 1 h before infection (pre-treatment), treatment 2 h after infection (post-infection), and treatment during infection (simultaneous). Each treatment lasted one hour then was removed. Antiviral efficacy was tested against the viral concentration of 0.0005 moi. Infected cultures were incubated for one hour at 37 °C to allow viral adsorption then the supernatant was removed, and cells were washed with PBS. Treated and infected cultures, were incubated with cell medium at 37 °C, 5% CO_2 for 72 h. For each treatment protocol, the cell culture was infected directly with the virus suspension to assess viral replication in the absence of any potential inhibition.

2.10. SARS-CoV-2 Nucleic Acid Quantification

Viral replication in treated and untreated cell cultures was evaluated by qRT-PCR by comparing the cycle threshold (Ct) values of each treated sample (Ct treated) and its corresponding untreated control (Ct control) obtained after 72 h of incubation. For this purpose, the Allplex SARS-CoV-2 Extraction-Free system (Seegene Inc., Seoul, South Korea) was used. It consists of a real-time qRT-PCR multiplex assay based on the use of TaqMan probes. The sample preparation, reaction setup, and analysis were performed according to the manufacturer's instructions and the details are described in the Supplementary Materials. Positive and negative controls were included in each run. Fluorescent signals were acquired after every amplification cycle. By comparing the Ct values referring to the N-gene of each treated sample and its corresponding untreated control obtained at the end of the test, the percentage of infectivity reduction was calculated, as follows:

$$\% \text{ viral infectivity reduction} = \frac{\text{Ct treated} - \text{Ct control}}{\text{Ct}_0 - \text{Ct control}} * 100$$

where Ct_0 represents the cycle threshold at the time of treatment application.

Cells treated with the same treatment protocols, but not infected, were used to assess the effects on cell viability. To quantify cell viability, after the incubation period, the cell monolayers were fixed and stained using 4% formaldehyde solution in crystal violet; absorbance was read at 595 nm. For each tested compound concentration, the percentage of viable cells for each tested concentration was calculated, setting the mean absorbance value of the cell control wells (neither treated nor infected cells) as 100% viability. None of the CsA_M20, CsA, or mannitol concentrations significantly compromised the cell viability.

2.11. Stability Studies

Stability studies were conducted on CsA_M20 spray-dried powder by storing the capsules containing 20 mg of powder at 25 °C and 60% of relative humidity (RH) and 40 °C and 75% of RH. The CsA content and in vitro aerodynamic performance by NGI were studied after 1 and 3 months of storage.

2.12. Statistical Analysis

Statistical analysis was conducted using the analysis of variance (ANOVA test) with a post hoc test using Prism 9 (GraphPad Software, v.9.4.0). Data were considered to be statistically significant when the *p*-value was < 0.05 (* = $p < 0.05$; ** = $p < 0.01$).

3. Results and Discussion

3.1. CsA Dry Powder Development by DOE

CsA is a lipophilic molecule with a logP of 3 and poor water solubility (3.69 mg/L at 37 °C), falling into class II of the Biopharmaceutical Classification System (BCS) among molecules with low water solubility and high permeability [34]. These physico-chemical properties limit the bioavailability of CsA, and many studies have been performed to improve the dissolution profile of CsA including the use of nanoparticles incorporated into microparticles by spray drying or spray freeze drying [13,35,36].

Moreover, the direct deposition of CsA to the lung could be an effective strategy in preventing lung rejection due to the high local drug availability also enhanced by the avoidance of intestinal pre-systemic metabolism.

The low water solubility of CsA represents an issue for the development of an inhalation product both from the point of view of the formulation and the release of the drug on site. In the case of a nebulisation product, a CsA solution using propylene glycol as a solvent [14] or a liposomal formulation has been proposed to increase the pulmonary exposure of the drug. Despite the good performance in clinical trials, the CsA solution for nebulisation did not reach the market, perhaps because of the possible irritant effect of the solvent used [37,38]. Other clinical trials conducted using inhaled liposomal CsA demonstrated the capability of the drug to increase BOS-free survival [39,40].

Compared to a CsA liquid nebulisation, the use of a CsA inhalation powder offers numerous advantages: the powder can be administered by a quick inhalation act and, as a solid-state formulation, the stability of the product is increased. On the other hand, the development of a powder containing CsA requires particular attention to be paid to the choice of excipients and the production technique capable of improving the release of the drug from the solid particles. In this context, some strategies have been proposed to enhance pulmonary release and absorption, such as the construction of CsA particles with pulmonary surfactants or with hydroxypropyl-beta-cyclodextrin and hydrosoluble chitosan [41–43].

In this work, the spray-drying process and water-soluble excipients were chosen to develop physically stable CsA respirable particles with improved dissolution. Mannitol was selected as it is currently approved for pulmonary administration [44] and is widely used in particle engineering. The addition of glycine was investigated to promote powder deaggregation and aerosolisation.

A preliminary study was carried out to identify the most suitable amount of mannitol to add to the formulation and subsequently to keep it as a starting point for a more in-depth investigation by DOE. Figure 1A illustrates the EF and RF of powders containing CsA and mannitol in the two ratios of 80:20 (CsA_M20) and 50:50 (CsA_M50), spray-dried starting from a solution containing 45% (v/v) ethanol in water. Similar EF and RF values were shown by the two CsA–mannitol powders: the EF was around 85% and RF was about 68–70%. On the contrary, CsA_rm, which had a volume median diameter of 7.67 μm, had a large deposition in the induction port of the impactor, which led to a very low RF of 6%.

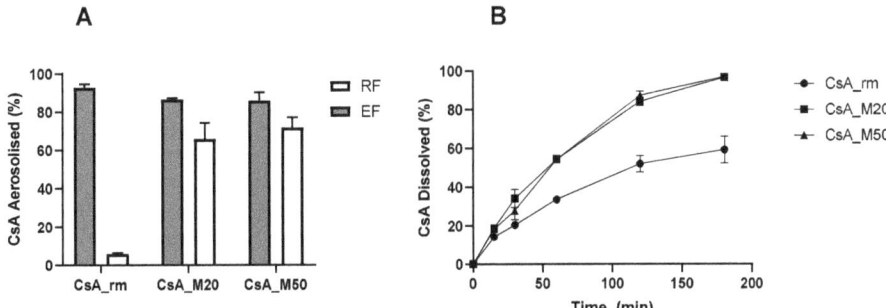

Figure 1. Aerosolisation performance (RF = respirable fraction, EF = emitted fraction) (**A**) and dissolution profiles (**B**) of CsA raw material (CsA_rm), CsA_M20, and CsA_M50. Data presented as n = 3, mean value ± SD.

Both of the CsA spray-dried powders exhibited a faster dissolution rate than the CsA_rm: approximately 87% of the spray-dried powder was dissolved after 3 h of the experiment, while only 50% of the raw material was dissolved (Figure 1B). However, the addition of mannitol in different quantities did not lead to a difference in the release profiles of CsA_M20 and CsA_M50. This preliminary test shows that, when mannitol exceeded 20% (w/w) in the powder composition, it no longer had any positive effect on the formulation for either of the qualitative parameters studied. Hence, with the purpose of limiting the amount of powder to inhale, it was decided that the amount of mannitol in the formulation would remain fixed at 20%.

A screening DoE was set up to investigate the influence of excipients on the quality of the powders. The effect of the ethanol content in the feedstock solution and the addition of glycine along with mannitol on the CQAs of the powders were investigated and are illustrated in Table 2. The yield of the process and the loss on drying (LOD) describe the quality of the spray-drying process, whereas the powder's aerodynamic behaviour (i.e., RF) and the dissolution time are related to the quality of the formulation. The residual solvent in the dried powder could affect not only its chemical stability, but also its respirability over time, as it could modify the powder's properties.

Table 2. Values of the CQAs investigated for the eleven CsA spray-dried powders: yield of the production process, respirable fraction (RF) < 5 μm, loss on drying (LOD), and time parameter of Weibull equation (time for 63.2% of CsA dissolved from composite powders) indicated as WDT. Data presented as n = 3, mean value ± SD.

Batch	Yield	RF (%)	LOD (%)	WDT (min)
1 (CsA_M15) *	55.7 ± 2.6	64.5 ± 6.3	2.85 ± 0.20	89.7 ± 7.4
2 (CsA_M10G)	55.4 ± 4.1	71.6 ± 1.6	3.41 ± 0.31	99.9 ± 4.8
3 (CsA_M20G)	59.1 ± 7.9	72.0 ± 4.1	1.96 ± 0.12	116.2 ± 8.3
4 (CsA_M10)	61.1 ± 3.8	64.5 ± 1.6	1.75 ± 0.33	109.6 ± 5.7
5 (CsA_M20)	59.5 ± 6.5	70.9 ± 0.4	2.04 ± 0.24	61.7 ± 0.2
6 (CsA_M20G)	56.9 ± 3.2	61.7 ± 0.3	1.98 ± 0.14	138.5 ± 6.7
7 (CsA_M15) *	62.6 ± 6.0	65.4 ± 2.4	2.52 ± 0.55	90.8 ± 14.1
8 (CsA_M15) *	65.0 ± 3.2	70.5 ± 8.7	2.45 ± 0.14	89.7 ± 13.7
9 (CsA_M20)	61.6 ± 4.1	59.9 ± 3.1	2.12 ± 0.31	57.7 ± 0.2
10 (CsA_M10G)	61.1 ± 5.1	61.3 ± 4.4	3.06 ± 0.42	110.6 ± 1.5
11 (CsA_M10)	65.3 ± 2.9	56.6 ± 2.9	1.75 ± 0.25	119.3 ± 10.1

* = central points of the DOE.

An ANOVA of the responses for the selected factorial model was performed. The generated model was not significant for the yield of production and for the respirable fraction. In fact, the yield value was similar for all powders, regardless of the composition of the stock solution. In general, the results indicate that the process was efficient in terms of the amount of powder produced and was robust. The yield of the manufacturing process was in the range of 55–65% for all powders. In all cases, the microparticles did not give rise to visible aggregates and the powders were not electrostatic. Not only the process was considered robust with acceptable values, but also, regarding the respirable fraction, the composition of the feed solution did not have a significant impact within the investigated ranges.

Conversely, the ANOVA revealed that the model was significant for the LOD and WDT with probability values of 0.033 and 0.006, respectively (Table 3). Furthermore, the robustness of the relationship between the model and the variables analysed was high, as indicated by the R^2 values. Figure 2 illustrates the perturbation graph of WDT versus the three critical factors and contour plot of LOD and WDT as a function of ethanol and glycine proportion.

Table 3. Probability values for the model terms relating to selected CQAs. RF = respirable fraction; LOD = loss on drying; WDT = Weibull dissolution time. The model was significant at $p < 0.05$ and highlighted in bold.

Term	Yield	RF	LOD	WDT
Model	0.425	0.748	**0.033**	**0.006**
R^2	0.312	0.187	0.944	0.934
Mannitol	0.643	0.580	**0.006**	0.107
Glycine	0.152	0.443	**0.006**	**0.015**
Ethanol	0.568	0.636	**0.0004**	**0.004**

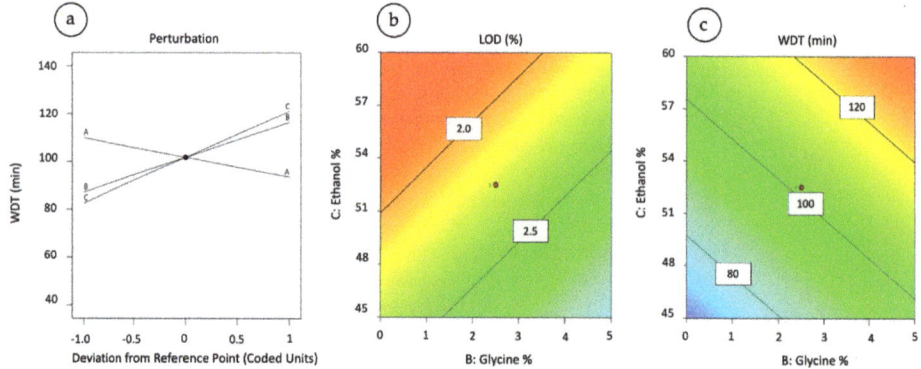

Figure 2. Perturbation graph of Weibull dissolution time (WDT) versus the critical factors plotted as deviation from the reference point (A = mannitol; B = glycine; C = ethanol) (**a**). Contour plot of LOD (**b**) and WDT (**c**) as a function of ethanol and glycine proportion in feed solution at the mannitol concentration of 15% (*w/w*).

Ethanol is the main factor influencing the different degrees of residual solvents in the particles. As the percentage of ethanol increases, the LOD value approaches zero per cent. On the contrary, glycine had a negative effect on the powder LOD: the presence of this excipient increased the amount of residual solvent in the powder; hence, it was not beneficial for the formulation quality aspects. According to this model, the percentage of mannitol also positively influences the LOD; however, this would seem to be a parameter deriving from the combined effect of ethanol and glycine. A low LOD value is important because it usually correlates with improved peptide stability in a solid-state formulation and decreases the possibility of mannitol recrystallisation. The graph in Figure 2b illustrates the trend of the LOD as the ethanol and glycine vary.

The main contribution to the variation in the dissolution time is due to glycine and ethanol, while the effect of mannitol was not significant. Therefore, as the percentage of ethanol and glycine increases, the time to dissolve the 63.2% of the API rises (see Figure 2c). Mannitol did not have a statistically significant effect, although it was indicated as a factor reducing WDT, i.e., leading to a faster dissolution rate (see Figure 2a).

In general, the spray-drying process was always able to produce particles with an enhanced dissolution rate compared to the non-formulated CsA (WDT of 169.0 min). Among all of the formulations, the powder CsA_M20, which was prepared starting from a feed solution containing 45% ethanol and without glycine, had the lowest WDT of approximately 59 min. The drug release profile of CsA_M20 was similar to that obtained by Yamasaki et al. (WDT of approx. 62 min) when CsA was precipitated in nanoparticles and spray-dried into nano-matrix structures with lactose mannitol and lecithin [35]. However, although the dissolution profile of the engineered powders was improved compared to the raw material, it is still a rather slow dissolution rate, which places undissolved particles at risk of removal by mucociliary clearance or phagocytosis. Therefore, in vivo studies will be useful to fully prove the beneficial effect of such formulations.

The observed behaviour indicated that when the particle composition consisted only of mannitol and CsA, this was more favourable for dissolution and in terms of residual solvent content. The reason why the composite CsA particles have a higher dissolution rate than the raw material is because during particle formation, the mannitol precipitates together with the CsA, forming a solid structure where the two materials are intimately dispersed. In contact with an aqueous medium, the mannitol dissolves immediately, leaving the CsA, with a high surface area, free for dissolution. Interestingly, the presence of glycine lowered the release of CsA, although it is a hydrophilic excipient, but less hygroscopic than mannitol.

Given the significance of the data, it will be worthwhile to further investigate the effect of the interactions between the factors and the CQAs using a full factorial DOE.

The ethanol content of the feed solution also influenced the morphology of the microparticles obtained. When the ethanol was 45% (Figure 3A), the particles appeared to be less inflated and more corrugated than the particles produced from a solution containing 60% ethanol (Figure 3B), where a greater number of large, fractured particles were observed. This behaviour is in agreement with what was reported for the production of amikacin spray-drying powders [45]: the particles are much larger or exploded when the evaporation rate is rapid, and therefore the precipitation of the solute occurs early. The evaporation rate increases as the percentage (v/v) of ethanol in the feed solution rise.

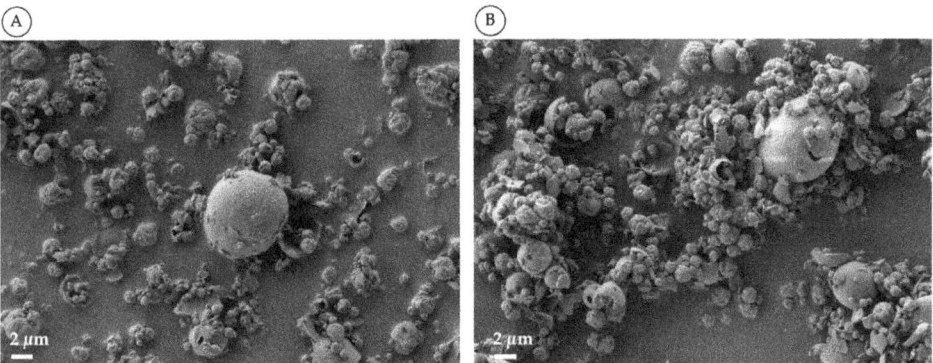

Figure 3. SEM images of CsA spray-dried powders produced with 45% (v/v) (**A**) and 60% (v/v) (**B**) of ethanol in the feedstock solution.

With regard to the solid state of the produced CsA powders, all were amorphous, as evidenced by the typical halo of the X-ray pattern (see Supplementary Materials). The structure of the CsA raw material was also amorphous before spray drying and no crystallinity peaks were observed in the powders after production.

From this first part of the work, CsA_M20 was selected as the best-performing powder and was then further characterised and tested for its tolerability, anti-inflammatory and antiviral activity.

3.2. Full Characterisation of the CsA_M20 Spray-Dried Powder

The CsA drug loading in the CsA_M20 powder after its production was $76.3 \pm 1.4\%$. This value agreed with the theoretical one (80%) considering that the powder had a solvent content, determined by TGA, of about 2%.

The aerodynamic particle size distribution of the powder CsA_M20, assessed by NGI, showed that the formulation had a very high respirability. The emitted amount of powder from the RS01 device was 16 mg (corresponding to 90% of the metered dose) containing 13.2 mg of CsA. The FPD was 8.8 mg of CsA, which corresponds to an FPF of 66.5 % (Table 4). The favourable aerodynamic behaviour can be attributed both to the poor cohesiveness of the particles and their good flowability and to the efficient deaggregation mechanism of the RS01 device.

Table 4. Aerodynamic characterisation of the CsA_M20 powder at time zero and during the stability investigation in standard and accelerated conditions (n = 3, mean value $\pm$ SD).

	Metered Dose (mg)	Emitted Dose (mg)	MMAD (μm)	FPD (mg)	FPF (%)	EFPD (mg)	EFPF (%)
CsA_M20 0 time	14.8 ± 0.1	13.2 ± 0.3	2.97 ± 0.12	8.80 ± 0.18	66.5 ± 2.6	3.61 ± 0.08	27.3 ± 1.2
CsA_M20 1 month 25 °C	14.7 ± 0.3	13.0 ± 0.5	2.58 ± 0.03	9.35 ± 0.46	71.4 ± 0.9	4.24 ± 0.13	32.4 ± 0.2
CsA_M20 1 month 40 °C	15.3 ± 0.3	12.6 ± 0.2	2.38 ± 0.12	8.82 ± 0.41	69.7 ± 4.4	4.38 ± 0.29	34.6 ± 2.8
CsA_M20 3 months 25 °C	14.6 ± 0.3	12.6 ± 0.3	2.61 ± 0.10	9.47 ± 0.22	74.7 ± 0.1	4.11 ± 0.09	32.4 ± 1.5
CsA_M20 3 months 40 °C	15.0 ± 0.3	12.5 ± 0.9	2.58 ± 0.15	8.55 ± 0.85	68.3 ± 2.0	3.75 ± 0.04	30.1 ± 1.8

From Figure 4, illustrating the deposition of the CsA in the NGI, it is possible to observe that most of the particles were collected in stages 2, 3, and 4 and about 4% was collected in the MOC capturing particles with a size lower than 0.5 μm. This led to obtaining an MMAD value of 2.97 μm.

A clinical trial evaluating the CsA anti-inflammatory efficacy in BOS by the nebulisation of 300 mg demonstrated that a deposition of CsA greater than 5 mg in the lung correlates with an improvement in lung functionality, and 12 mg was indicated as an anti-rejection protective dose [14]. In light of these results, it can be considered that the FPD of 8.8 mg, generated by the aerosolisation of 20 mg of CsA_M20, is in the correct therapeutic range for the prevention of BOS.

Regarding the management of the COVID-19 infection, there are no efficacy or pharmacokinetic data upon the delivery of CsA by inhalation. However, COVID-19 patients who received 300 mg of CsA orally showed positive results on survival [46]. At this dose, the amount of CsA available to the lung will have been very low, but still sufficient to dampen the inflammatory reaction of the respiratory tract. Inhalation administration would make it possible to obtain equal or higher efficacy in the face of a reduction in the administered dosage and reduced systemic exposure.

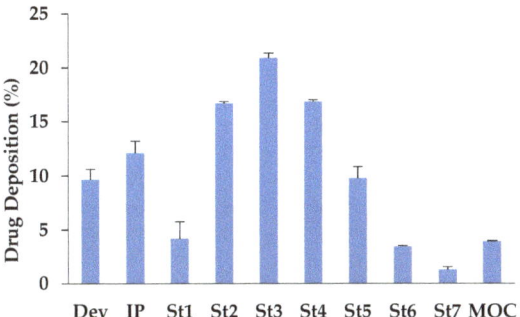

Figure 4. Distribution of CsA_M20 powder on Next Generation Impactor. The loaded amount of powder in the capsule was 20 mg containing 16 mg of CsA, (n = 3, mean value ± SD). Dev = device; IP = induction port; St = stage; MOC = micro-orifice collector.

Stability analyses on the CsA_M20 powder stored in HPMC capsules, conducted at 1 and 3 months in standard and accelerated conditions, provided drug content values in a range between 78 and 82% without being significantly different from the time zero ($p < 0.05$). In the aerodynamic assessment, the CsA ED was around 13 mg and the FPD was in the range of 8–9 mg, independently of the storage conditions and the check time of the analysis (Table 4). These data, albeit preliminary, show that the use of mannitol as a bulking excipient was able to protect the physicochemical stability of the formulation, preserving its initial characteristics. The use of Quali_V®_I capsules in this work, specifically produced for DPI, with optimised puncturing properties and internal lubricant features, certainly contributed to this positive achievement [47]. Finally, the CsA_M20 showed a differential scanning calorimetry profile at three months equal to that at time zero, evidencing that the powder did not undergo solid-state transformations during the observation time (see Supplementary Materials).

3.3. CsA_M20 Cytotoxicity and Anti-Inflammatory Efficiency

The viability of human lung adenocarcinoma cell line A549 and monocytic cell line THP-1 was not affected by the various CsA tested treatments, which were well tolerated by cells, as reported in Figure 5. Indeed, under these conditions, neither CsA_rm nor the spray-dried powder of CsA containing mannitol displayed any cytotoxic effect on the two cell cultures compared to the vehicle (0.5% DMSO in PBS).

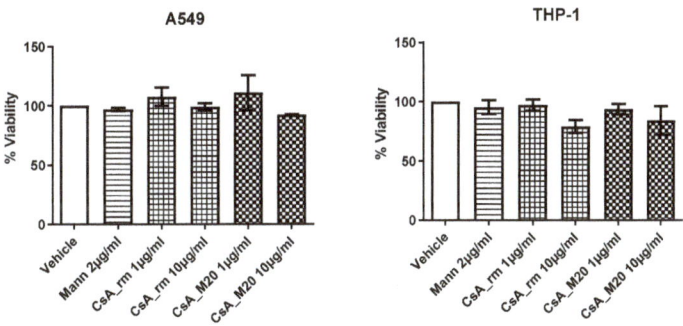

Figure 5. Viability of A549 and THP-1 cell cultures exposed to the vehicle, mannitol (Mann) 2 µg/mL, CsA_rm at 1 and 10 µg/mL, CsA_M20 spray-dried powder at of 1, and 10 µg/mL of CsA. Data are expressed as a percentage with respect to the vehicle.

IL-6 is a pro-inflammatory cytokine involved in numerous cellular processes such as proliferation and survival. Furthermore, the high serum levels of IL-6 in patients who have undergone a lung transplant were a marker for the development of chronic lung allograft dysfunction [48,49]. In parallel, it was observed that COVID-19 infection is accompanied by an aggressive inflammatory response with the release of a large amount of pro-inflammatory serum cytokines in an event known as a "cytokine storm" [50]. In particular, IL-6 was reported to be a potential predictor for the development of severe COVID-19, since elevated levels of this cytokine were associated with critical patient conditions such as acute respiratory distress syndrome and the need for mechanical ventilation [50]. As IL-6 is the most frequently reported cytokine to be increased in COVID-19 patients and as IL-6 elevated levels have been associated with higher mortalities, this cytokine was selected in this work to test the CsA anti-inflammatory effect.

The levels of IL-6 were determined by ELISA test 24 h after the treatment of cell co-cultures exposed to LPS. The levels of the cytokine were significantly reduced either by CsA_rm or by formulated CsA compared to the vehicle (Figure 6). Mannitol, used as an excipient in the formulation, also showed a slight anti-inflammatory effect albeit not statistically significant, as already reported in vivo [51]. The results confirm that through the spray-drying process, it was possible to construct highly respirable particles with improved dissolution rates, preserving the CsA anti-inflammatory effect. An inhaled powder of CsA, therefore, represents a favourable therapeutic strategy to avoid the triggering of a vigorous immune reaction in the lungs. Consequently, this action would limit the production of cytokines and their consequent spillover into the circulatory system, preventing the systemic cytokine storm.

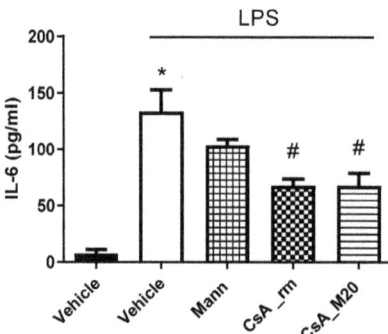

Figure 6. In vitro inhibition of IL-6 production by THP-1/A549 co-culture exposed to LPS in the presence of the vehicle, CsA_rm at 10 µg/mL, CsA_M20 at 10 µg/mL of CsA, or mannitol (Mann) at 2 µg/mL; * $p < 0.05$ vs. vehicle; # $p < 0.05$ vs. vehicle + LPS, ANOVA test followed by Bonferroni's post-test.

3.4. In Vitro Anti-Viral Efficacy against SARS-CoV-2

As mentioned before, CsA has been shown to have a direct inhibitory effect on the replication of different types of coronaviruses, including SARS-CoV-2. For this purpose, orally administered CsA has also been the subject of clinical trials, reporting positive results on the survival of patients affected by COVID-19 [46,52]. Moreover, to date, a further ten clinical trials are ongoing, although the results have not yet become available, indicating the high interest in CsA for the treatment of this disease.

In light of these considerations, the last part of the study explored the inhibition activity of CsA_M20 powder on viral replication in Vero E6 cells in comparison to the CsA_rm. Furthermore, different types of treatment (pre-treatment, post-treatment, or simultaneous regimen) were adopted to assess the more effective one to contain the virus.

The infected cells were treated with CsA_rm, CsA_M20, or mannitol powders applied according to the different treatments. Figure 7 illustrates the virus infectivity reduction in relation to the CsA concentrations applied. The effect of mannitol alone was as well assessed since it is a component of the engineered CsA powder. The range of CsA concentrations investigated was selected according to the one proposed by de Wilde et al. [20]. A 100% viral infectivity reduction corresponds to the maximal reduction in the viral load.

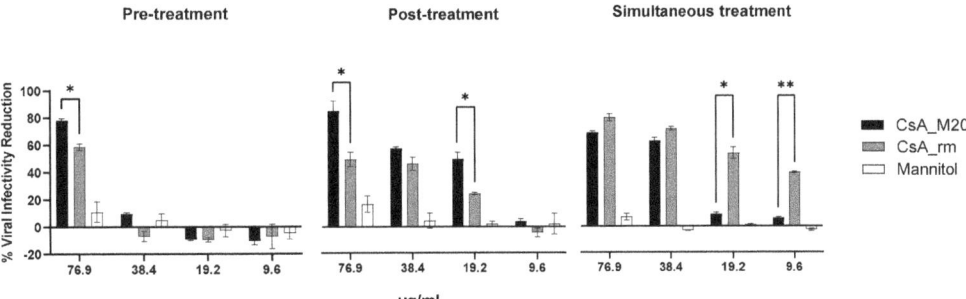

Figure 7. In vitro SARS-CoV-2 Omicron BA.1 infectivity reduction produced by CsA_rm, CsA_M20 or mannitol. Pre-treatment: one hour before infection. Post-treatment: two hours after infection. Simultaneous treatment: cells were infected and treated with the powders at the same time. The mannitol concentrations corresponding to CsA formulation at 76.9, 38.4, 19.2, and 9.6 µg/mL were respectively 15.4, 7.7, 3.8, and 1.9 µg/mL. Data were analysed with two-way analysis of variance (ANOVA) (* $p < 0.05$; ** $p < 0.01$; CsA_M20 vs. CsA_rm).

During the pre-treatment, only the highest CsA concentration applied (76.9 µg/mL) showed an antiviral effect. The reduction of viral infectivity was 78% when the drug was formulated as a spray-dried powder and was statistically superior to the raw material, which reduced the infection by 58%. At lower concentrations, CsA did not have any relevant antiviral effect. Similarly, mannitol did not produce inhibitory effects at any of the tested concentrations. At the lowest concentrations (19.2 and 9.6 µg/mL) of all of the treatments, even greater viral growth was observed in the treated samples compared to the control; this is identified by the negative value of the infectivity percentage. To interpret the data, it should be mentioned that the cell culture medium containing CsA was replaced with fresh medium before applying the virus; therefore, the drug that interacted with the pathogen replication was only the fraction that was internalised by the cell. The fact that CsA_M20 has superior efficacy to CsA_rm could be due to the higher solubility of these composite particles, possibly increasing the host intracellular concentration of the drug where the virus was replicating. These positive inhibition results show that CsA is active not only against SARS-CoV, as shown in 2011 by de Wilde et al. [20], but also on the SARS type CoV-2 responsible for the current sanitary emergency. It was demonstrated that CsA treatment rendered the virus RNA and protein synthesis almost undetectable [20]. In parallel, the reduction of cyclophilins did not interfere with the SARS-CoV replication. Finally, a further blocking mechanism has been recently in silico demonstrated: through molecular docking, CsA was able to bind and block two membrane proteins (TMPRSS2 and CTSL) necessary for SARS-CoV-2 to penetrate the host cell [53].

Differently from the pre-treatment condition, in the post-treatment regimen, the viral inhibitory activity was present for all CsA concentrations tested except for the lowest one. Furthermore, the CsA_M20 powder was always more effective than the CsA_rm, although statistically superior only at the concentration of 19.2 and 76.9 µg/mL. Mannitol, as in the previous case, showed a slight activity of reducing infectivity. With regard to the adopted protocol, in this case, the treatment was applied after the virus had been allowed to absorb and then removed from the culture. Therefore, as in the case of the pre-treatment, the block of the virus infection presumably took place within the host cell, where the viruses remained after washing resided. The engineered CsA powder had, in these conditions, superior efficacy likely due to its enhanced dissolution, leading to a higher amount of the drug entering the host cell where the virus was replicating.

In the simultaneous treatment, the CsA_M20 and CsA_rm powders performed similarly at the two highest concentrations tested where the inhibition reached 75–80%. This trend changed at 19.2 and 9.6 µg/mL, at which only raw CsA showed an antiviral effect of 30% significantly higher than that of CsA_M20 (5%). This was the only experimental protocol in which the cells were exposed to the virus simultaneously with the treatment, therefore the only situation in which the drug–virus interaction took place both in the extracellular compartment and subsequently intracellularly. The inhibition data of the CsA_rm highlight that an interaction may occur between drug suspension and the virus, which does not happen in the case of the more soluble CsA_M20 powder. In fact, the members of the *Coronaviridae* family possess a phospholipid envelope, therefore an interaction between the pure CsA_rm and the viral membrane would be possible. It is known that CsA binds lipid membranes following the classic hydrophobic effect and that CsA affects the membranes in a concentration-dependent manner by the perturbation of the organisation of fatty chains [54]. Hence, it can be hypothesised that in the case of the CsA_rm, the solid particles create a concentration at the particle–virus interface close to saturation, higher than that generated by the CsA_M20 solubilised in the medium. This difference could explain the high ability to interact with the cell membrane of the virus. Furthermore, the presence of solid particles could represent a further obstacle to infection as they act as a physical barrier and reduce the surface area available for virus adsorption. In contrast, CsA_M20, which was successfully dissolved in the medium, could little hinder the interaction between the virus and the host cell membrane. In this regard, the creation of a polymeric barrier is exploited as a system to inhibit virus–cell interaction by numerous commercially available nasal sprays to antagonise the infection.

In summary, the most effective treatment regimens were post-infection or simultaneous infection treatment. In both cases, the infectivity of SARS-CoV-2 was reduced and in the case of post-treatment, more efficiently by the CsA_M20 powder than the raw material. This post-infection approach is also the most plausible considering that pharmacological treatment commonly follows and does not simultaneously accompany the entry of the virus. Moreover, the raw material, although effective, cannot be administered as such due to its low respirability. At variance, the prophylactic treatment, despite the in vitro data, has not been proven to be effective except at the highest concentration tested, probably because in cases of treatment with a lower dosage, an effective drug concentration is not internalised and retained by the cells.

4. Conclusions

The work demonstrated that, through the modulation of mannitol and ethanol, it was possible to achieve an inhalation powder with high respirability (FPF of 66.5%) and improved CsA release (WDT of 59.5 min). This aspect is of crucial importance considering that CsA has a very low oral bioavailability and therefore a rapid lung release would be extremely advantageous to obtain high pulmonary exposure.

Besides the fact that the inhalation powder developed could represent an advantageous strategy in the prevention of lung transplant rejection, the collected findings provide strong in vitro evidence that this therapeutic approach could be efficient in the reduction of SARS-CoV-2 infectivity, especially as a post-infection treatment. CsA_M20 powder, applied to cells one hour after contact with the virus, was able to inhibit its replication by 93%. Finally, the CsA-engineered powder showed an anti-inflammatory effect in terms of IL-6 reduction that could also be useful in containing the COVID-19 cytokine storm in the lungs.

Supplementary Materials: The following supporting information can be downloaded at: https://www.mdpi.com/article/10.3390/pharmaceutics15031023/s1, Figure S1. XRPD scan of spray-dried powders and raw materials; Figure S2. XRPD scan of mannitol raw material (light blue), CsA raw material (green), CsA_M20 powder at time 0 (blue) and after 6 months (red); Figure S3. DSC scan of: CsA raw material (CsA_rm) in black; CsA pure spray dried: (CsA_SD) in red; Figure S4. DSC scan of mannitol spray-dried (red) and mannitol raw material (black); Figure S5. CsA_M20 powder at time 0 after production (red) and CsA_M20 after 6 months at room temperature (black). References [33,55–60] are cited in the supplementary materials.

Author Contributions: Conceptualisation, F.S. and F.B.; formal analysis, D.D.; investigation, D.D., L.F., M.B., L.G., G.G. and F.T.; supervision, S.B., V.S., G.D., A.B., F.S., R.B. and F.B.; writing—original draft, D.D., E.Q., S.G., G.V. and M.B. All authors have read and agreed to the published version of the manuscript.

Funding: This research received no external funding.

Institutional Review Board Statement: Ethical approval or informed consent were not required because the anti-viral efficacy study has been performed using exclusively anonymized, leftover samples deriving from the routine diagnostic procedures. The anonymization was achieved by using the current procedure (AVR-PPC P09, rev.2) checked by the local Ethical Board.

Informed Consent Statement: Not applicable.

Data Availability Statement: The data presented in this study are available on request from the corresponding author.

Acknowledgments: The authors thank Qualicaps and Plastiape for kindly providing the capsules and inhalers, respectively.

Conflicts of Interest: The authors declare no conflict of interest.

References

1. Fahr, A. Cyclosporin Clinical Pharmacokinetics. *Clin. Pharmacokinet.* **1993**, *24*, 472–495. [CrossRef] [PubMed]
2. Forsythe, P.; Paterson, S. Ciclosporin 10 Years on: Indications and Efficacy. *Vet. Rec.* **2014**, *174*, 13–21. [CrossRef] [PubMed]
3. Tissot, A.; Danger, R.; Claustre, J.; Magnan, A.; Brouard, S. Early Identification of Chronic Lung Allograft Dysfunction: The Need of Biomarkers. *Front. Immunol.* **2019**, *10*, 1681. [CrossRef] [PubMed]
4. Barr, M.; Chaparro, C.; Corris, P.; Doyle, R.; Glanville, A.; Klepetko, W.; Mcneil, K.; Orens, J.; Singer, L.; Trulock, E.; et al. Bronchiolitis Obliterans Syndrome 2001: An Update of the Diagnostic. *J. Heart Lung Transplant.* **2001**, *21*, 297–310.
5. Boehler, A.; Estenne, M. Post-Transplant Bronchiolitis Obliterans. *Eur. Respir. J.* **2003**, *22*, 1007–1018. [CrossRef]
6. Chan, C. Side Effects of Systemic Cyclosporine in Patients Not Undergoing Transplantation. *Am. J. Med.* **1984**, *77*, 652–656.
7. Parekh, K.; Trulock, E.; Patterson, G.A. Use of Cyclosporine in Lung Transplantation. *Transplant. Proc.* **2004**, *36*, S318–S322. [CrossRef]
8. Kolars, J.C.; Awni, W.M.; Merion, R.M.; Watkins, P.B. First-Pass Metabolism of Cyclosporin by the Gut. *Lancet* **1991**, *338*, 1488–1490. [CrossRef]
9. Wu, C.Y.; Benet, L.Z.; Hebert, M.F.; Gupta, S.K.; Rowland, M.; Gomez, D.Y.; Wacher, V.J. Differentiation of Absorption and First-Pass Gut and Hepatic Metabolism in Humans: Studies with Cyclosporine. *Clin. Pharmacol. Ther.* **1995**, *58*, 492–497. [CrossRef]
10. Bennani Rtel, M.; Ternant, D.; Büchler, M.; El Hassouni, M.; Khabbal, Y.; Achour, S.; Sqalli, T. Food and Lipid Intake Alters the Pharmacokinetics of Cyclosporine in Kidney Transplants. *Fundam. Clin. Pharmacol.* **2020**, *35*, 446–454. [CrossRef]
11. Mendonza, A.E.; Gohh, R.Y.; Akhlaghi, F. Blood and Plasma Pharmacokinetics of Ciclosporin in Diabetic Kidney Transplant Recipients. *Clin. Pharmacokinet.* **2008**, *47*, 733–742. [CrossRef]
12. Taylor, W.J.; Robinson, J.D.; Burckart, G.J.; Canafax, D.M.; Yee, G.C. Cyclosporine Monitoring. *Ann. Pharmacother.* **2007**, *41*, 1277–1280. [CrossRef] [PubMed]
13. Sato, H.; Suzuki, H.; Yakushiji, K.; Wong, J.; Seto, Y.; Prud'homme, R.K.; Chan, H.K.; Onoue, S. Biopharmaceutical Evaluation of Novel Cyclosporine A Nano-Matrix Particles for Inhalation. *Pharm. Res.* **2016**, *33*, 2107–2116. [CrossRef] [PubMed]
14. Corcoran, T.E.; Smaldone, G.C.; Dauber, J.H.; Smith, D.A.; McCurry, K.R.; Burckart, G.J.; Zeevi, A.; Griffith, B.P.; Iacono, A.T. Preservation of Post-Transplant Lung Function with Aerosol Cyclosporin. *Eur. Respir. J.* **2004**, *23*, 378–383. [CrossRef]
15. Groves, S.; Galazka, M.; Johnson, B.; Corcoran, T.; Verceles, A.; Britt, E.; Todd, N.; Griffith, B.; Smaldone, G.C.; Iacono, A. Inhaled Cyclosporine and Pulmonary Function in Lung Transplant Recipients. *J. Aerosol Med. Pulm. Drug Deliv.* **2010**, *23*, 31–39. [CrossRef]
16. Iacono, A.; Wijesinha, M.; Rajagopal, K.; Murdock, N.; Timofte, I.; Griffith, B.; Terrin, M. A Randomised Single-Centre Trial of Inhaled Liposomal Cyclosporine for Bronchiolitis Obliterans Syndrome Post-Lung Transplantation. *ERJ Open Res.* **2019**, *5*, 1–11. [CrossRef]
17. Nagy, P.D.; Wang, R.Y.; Pogany, J.; Hafren, A.; Makinen, K. Emerging Picture of Host Chaperone and Cyclophilin Roles in RNA Virus Replication. *Virology* **2011**, *411*, 374–382. [CrossRef]
18. Tanaka, Y.; Sato, Y.; Sasaki, T. Suppression of Coronavirus Replication by Cyclophilin Inhibitors. *Viruses* **2013**, *5*, 1250–1260. [CrossRef] [PubMed]

19. Fenizia, C.; Galbiati, S.; Vanetti, C.; Vago, R.; Clerici, M.; Tacchetti, C.; Daniele, T. Cyclosporine A Inhibits Viral Infection and Release as Well as Cytokine Production in Lung Cells by Three SARS-CoV-2 Variants. *Microbiol. Spectr.* **2021**, *10*, 1–16. [CrossRef]
20. de Wilde, A.H.; Zevenhoven-Dobbe, J.C.; van der Meer, Y.; Thiel, V.; Narayanan, K.; Makino, S.; Snijder, E.J.; van Hemert, M.J. Cyclosporin A Inhibits the Replication of Diverse Coronaviruses. *J. Gen. Virol.* **2011**, *92*, 2542–2548. [CrossRef] [PubMed]
21. Molyvdas, A.; Matalon, S. Cyclosporine: An Old Weapon in the Fight against Coronaviruses. *Eur. Respir. J.* **2020**, *56*, 2002484. [CrossRef] [PubMed]
22. Jayk Bernal, A.; Gomes da Silva, M.M.; Musungaie, D.B.; Kovalchuk, E.; Gonzalez, A.; Delos Reyes, V.; Martín-Quirós, A.; Caraco, Y.; Williams-Diaz, A.; Brown, M.L.; et al. Molnupiravir for Oral Treatment of Covid-19 in Nonhospitalized Patients. *N. Engl. J. Med.* **2022**, *386*, 509–520. [CrossRef]
23. Shrestha, N.K.; Burke, P.C.; Nowacki, A.S.; Terpeluk, P.; Gordon, S.M. Molnupiravir and Nirmatrelvir-Ritonavir: Oral COVID Antiviral Drugs Louis. *Clin. Infect. Dis.* **2022**, *76*, 165–171. [CrossRef]
24. Lamb, Y.N. Nirmatrelvir Plus Ritonavir: First Approval. *Drugs* **2022**, *82*, 585–591. [CrossRef]
25. Lin, H.X.J.; Cho, S.; Meyyur Aravamudan, V.; Sanda, H.Y.; Palraj, R.; Molton, J.S.; Venkatachalam, I. Remdesivir in Coronavirus Disease 2019 (COVID-19) Treatment: A Review of Evidence. *Infection* **2021**, *49*, 401–410. [CrossRef] [PubMed]
26. Sinha, S.; Rosin, N.L.; Arora, R.; Labit, E.; Jaffer, A.; Cao, L.; Farias, R.; Nguyen, A.P.; de Almeida, L.G.N.; Dufour, A.; et al. Dexamethasone Modulates Immature Neutrophils and Interferon Programming in Severe COVID-19. *Nat. Med.* **2022**, *28*, 201–211. [CrossRef]
27. Ely, E.W.; Ramanathan, K.; Antognini, D.; Combes, A.; Paden, M.; Zakhary, B.; Ogino, M.; Maclaren, G.; Brodie, D. Efficacy and Safety of Baricitinib plus Standard of Care for the Treatment of Critically Ill Hospitalised Adults with COVID-19 on Invasive Mechanical Ventilation or Extracorporeal Membrane Oxygenation: An Exploratory, Randomised, Placebo-Controlled Trial. *Lancet Respir. Med.* **2020**, *10*, 327–336. [CrossRef]
28. Gupta, A.; Gonzalez-Rojas, Y.; Juarez, E.; Crespo Casal, M.; Moya, J.; Falci, D.R.; Sarkis, E.; Solis, J.; Zheng, H.; Scott, N.; et al. Early Treatment for Covid-19 with SARS-CoV-2 Neutralizing Antibody Sotrovimab. *N. Engl. J. Med.* **2021**, *385*, 1941–1950. [CrossRef]
29. Berton, P.; Mishra, M.K.; Choudhary, H.; Myerson, A.S.; Rogers, R.D. Solubility Studies of Cyclosporine Using Ionic Liquids. *ACS Omega* **2019**, *4*, 7938–7943. [CrossRef]
30. Sonvico, F.; Chierici, V.; Varacca, G.; Quarta, E.; D'Angelo, D.; Forbes, B.; Buttini, F. Respicelltm: An Innovative Dissolution Apparatus for Inhaled Products. *Pharmaceutics* **2021**, *13*, 1541. [CrossRef]
31. Langenbucher, F. Letters to the Editor: Linearization of Dissolution Rate Curves by the Weibull Distribution. *J. Pharm. Pharmacol.* **1972**, *24*, 979–981. [CrossRef] [PubMed]
32. Li, Y.; Su, R.; Chen, J.; Li, Y.; Su, R.; Chen, J. Co-Culture Systems of Drug-Treated Acute Myeloid Leukemia Cells and T Cells for In Vitro and In Vivo Study. *STAR Protoc.* **2020**, *1*, 100097. [CrossRef] [PubMed]
33. Burnett, L.; McQueen, M.J.; Jonsson, J.J.; Torricelli, F. IFCC Position Paper: Report of the IFCC Taskforce on Ethics: Introduction and Framework. *Clin. Chem. Lab. Med.* **2007**, *45*, 1098–1104. [CrossRef] [PubMed]
34. Sato, H.; Kawabata, Y.; Yuminoki, K.; Hashimoto, N.; Yamauchi, Y. Comparative Studies on Physicochemical Stability of Cyclosporine A-Loaded Amorphous Solid Dispersions. *Int. J. Pharm.* **2012**, *426*, 302–306. [CrossRef]
35. Yamasaki, K.; Kwok, P.C.L.; Fukushige, K.; Prud'Homme, R.K.; Chan, H.K. Enhanced Dissolution of Inhalable Cyclosporine Nano-Matrix Particles with Mannitol as Matrix Former. *Int. J. Pharm.* **2011**, *420*, 34–42. [CrossRef]
36. Leung, S.S.Y.; Wong, J.; Guerra, H.V.; Samnick, K.; Prud'homme, R.K.; Chan, H.K. Porous Mannitol Carrier for Pulmonary Delivery of Cyclosporine A Nanoparticles. *AAPS J.* **2017**, *19*, 578–586. [CrossRef]
37. Iacono, A.T.; Johnson, B.A.; Grgurich, W.F.; Youssef, J.G.; Corcoran, T.E.; Seiler, D.A.; Dauber, J.H.; Smaldone, G.C.; Zeevi, A.; Yousem, S.A.; et al. A Randomized Trial of Inhaled Cyclosporine in Lung-Transplant Recipients. *N. Engl. J. Med.* **2006**, *354*, 141–150. [CrossRef]
38. Iacono, A. Capitalizing on the Concept of Local Immune Suppression by Inhalation for Lung Transplant Recipients. *Am. J. Transplant.* **2021**, *22*, 9–11. [CrossRef]
39. Neurohr, C.; Kneidinger, N.; Ghiani, A.; Monforte, V.; Knoop, C.; Jaksch, P.; Parmar, J.; Ussetti, P.; Sole, A.; Quernheim, J.M.-; et al. A Randomized Controlled Trial of Liposomal Cyclosporine A for Inhalation in the Prevention of Bronchiolitis Obliterans Syndrome Following Lung Transplantation. *Am. J. Transplant.* **2022**, *22*, 222–229. [CrossRef]
40. Behr, J.; Zimmermann, G.; Baumgartner, R.; Leuchte, H.; Neurohr, C.; Brand, P.; Herpich, C.; Sommerer, K.; Seitz, J.; Menges, G.; et al. Lung Deposition of a Liposomal Cyclosporine a Inhalation Solution in Patients after Lung Transplantation. *J. Aerosol Med. Pulm. Drug Deliv.* **2009**, *22*, 121–129. [CrossRef]
41. Wu, X.; Zhang, W.; Hayes, D.; Mansour, H.M. Physicochemical Characterization and Aerosol Dispersion Performance of Organic Solution Advanced Spray-Dried Cyclosporine A Multifunctional Particles for Dry Powder Inhalation Aerosol Delivery. *Int. J. Nanomed.* **2013**, *8*, 1269–1283. [CrossRef]
42. Suzuki, H.; Ueno, K.; Mizumoto, T.; Seto, Y.; Sato, H.; Onoue, S. Self-Micellizing Solid Dispersion of Cyclosporine A for Pulmonary Delivery: Physicochemical, Pharmacokinetic and Safety Assessments. *Eur. J. Pharm. Sci.* **2017**, *96*, 107–114. [CrossRef]
43. Yang, T.T.; Wen, B.F.; Liu, K.; Qin, M.; Gao, Y.Y.; Ding, D.J.; Li, W.T.; Zhang, Y.X.; Zhang, W.F. Cyclosporine A/Porous Quaternized Chitosan Microspheres as a Novel Pulmonary Drug Delivery System. *Artif. Cells Nanomed. Biotechnol.* **2018**, *46*, 552–564. [CrossRef] [PubMed]

44. Anderson, S.; Atkins, P.; Bäckman, P.; Cipolla, D.; Clark, A.; Daviskas, E.; Disse, B.; Entcheva-Dimitrov, P.; Fuller, R.; Gonda, I.; et al. Inhaled Medicines: Past, Present, and Future. *Pharmacol. Rev.* **2022**, *74*, 50–118. [CrossRef]
45. Belotti, S.; Rossi, A.; Colombo, P.; Ruggero, B.; Rekkas, D.; Politis, S.; Colombo, G.; Balducci, A.G.; Buttini, F. Spray-dried amikacin sulphate powder for inhalation in cystic fibrosis patients: The role of ethanol in particle formation. *Eur. J. Pharm. Biopharm.* **2015**, *93*, 165–172. [CrossRef] [PubMed]
46. Guisado-Vascoa, P.; Valderas-Ortegab, S.; Carralòn-Gonzalez, M.M.; Roda-Santacruzc, A.; Lucia Gonzalez-CortijoGabriel, G.S.-F.; Roda-santacruz, A.; Gonz, L.; Martí-ballesteros, E.M.; Luque-pinilla, J.M.; Almagro-casado, E.; et al. Clinical Characteristics and Outcomes among Hospitalized Adults with Severe COVID-19 Admitted to a Tertiary Medical Center and Receiving Antiviral, Antimalarials, Glucocorticoids, or Immunomodulation with Tocilizumab or Cyclosporine: A Retrospective O. *EClinicalMedicine* **2020**, *28*, 100591. [CrossRef] [PubMed]
47. Buttini, F.; Quarta, E.; Allegrini, C.; Lavorini, F. Understanding the Importance of Capsules in Dry Powder Inhalers. *Pharmaceutics* **2021**, *13*, 1936. [CrossRef]
48. Wheeler, D.S.; Misumi, K.; Walker, N.M.; Vittal, R.; Combs, M.P.; Aoki, Y.; Braeuer, R.R.; Lama, V.N. Interleukin 6 Trans-Signaling Is a Critical Driver of Lung Allograft Fibrosis. *Am. J. Transplant.* **2021**, *21*, 2360–2371. [CrossRef]
49. Rose-John, S.; Winthrop, K.; Calabrese, L. The Role of IL-6 in Host Defence against Infections: Immunobiology and Clinical Implications. *Nat. Rev. Rheumatol.* **2017**, *13*, 399–409. [CrossRef]
50. Zhou, J.; He, W.; Liang, J.; Wang, L.; Yu, X.; Bao, M.; Liu, H. Association of Interleukin-6 Levels with Morbidity and Mortality in Patients with Coronavirus Disease 2019 (COVID-19). *Jpn. J. Infect. Dis.* **2021**, *74*, 293–298. [CrossRef]
51. Reisi Nassab, P.; Blazsó, G.; Nyári, T.; Falkay, G.; Szabó-Révész, P. In Vitro and In Vivo Investigations on the Binary Meloxicam-Mannitol System. *Pharmazie* **2008**, *63*, 319–320. [CrossRef]
52. Blumberg, E.A.; Noll, J.H.; Tebas, P.; Fraietta, J.A.; Frank, I.; Marshall, A.; Chew, A.; Veloso, E.A.; Carulli, A.; Rogal, W.; et al. A Phase I Trial of Cyclosporine for Hospitalized Patients with COVID-19. *JCI Insight* **2022**, *7*, 155682. [CrossRef] [PubMed]
53. Prasad, K.; Ahamad, S.; Kanipakam, H.; Gupta, D.; Kumar, V. Simultaneous Inhibition of SARS-CoV-2 Entry Pathways by Cyclosporine. *ACS Chem. Neurosci.* **2021**, *12*, 930–944. [CrossRef] [PubMed]
54. Czogalla, A. Oral Cyclosporine A—The Current Picture of Its Liposomal and Other Delivery Systems. *Cell. Mol. Biol. Lett.* **2009**, *14*, 139–152. [CrossRef] [PubMed]
55. Ammerman, N.; Beier-Sexton, M.; Azad, A. Growth and Maintenance of Vero Cell Lines. *Curr. Protoc. Microbiol.* **2009**, *11*, A-4E. [CrossRef]
56. Lei, C.; Yang, J.; Hu, J.; Sun, X. On the Calculation of TCID50 for Quantitation of Virus Infectivity. *Virol. Sin.* **2021**, *36*, 141–144. [CrossRef]
57. Reed, L.J.; Muench, H. A Simple Method of Estimating Fifty per Cent Endpoints. *Am. J. Epidemiol.* **1938**, *27*, 493–497. [CrossRef]
58. Jiang, X.; Zhao, Y.; Guan, Q.; Xiao, S.; Dong, W.; Lian, S.; Zhang, H.; Liu, M.; Wang, Z.; Han, J. Amorphous Solid Dispersions of Cyclosporine A with Improved Bioavailability Prepared via Hot Melt Extrusion: Formulation, Physicochemical Characterization, and in Vivo Evaluation. *Eur. J. Pharm. Sci.* **2022**, *168*, 1–9. [CrossRef] [PubMed]
59. Benetti, A.A.; Bianchera, A.; Buttini, F.; Bertocchi, L.; Bettini, R. Mannitol Polymorphs as Carrier in Dpis Formulations: Isolation Characterization and Performance. *Pharmaceutics* **2021**, *13*, 1113. [CrossRef]
60. Adi, H.; Young, P.M.; Chan, H.K.; Agus, H.; Traini, D. Co-Spray-Dried Mannitol-Ciprofloxacin Dry Powder Inhaler Formulation for Cystic Fibrosis and Chronic Obstructive Pulmonary Disease. *Eur. J. Pharm. Sci.* **2010**, *40*, 239–247. [CrossRef]

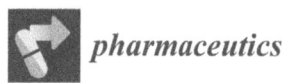

Article

Aggregates Associated with Instability of Antibodies during Aerosolization Induce Adverse Immunological Effects

Thomas Sécher [1,2], Elsa Bodier-Montagutelli [1,2,3,†], Christelle Parent [1,2,†], Laura Bouvart [1,2,4], Mélanie Cortes [1,2], Marion Ferreira [1,2,5], Ronan MacLoughlin [6,7,8], Guy Ilango [1,2], Otmar Schmid [9], Renaud Respaud [1,2,3] and Nathalie Heuzé-Vourc'h [1,2,*]

[1]   INSERM, Centre d'Etude des Pathologies Respiratoires, U1100, F-37032 Tours, France; secher.thomas@gmail.com (T.S.); montage@ch-blois.fr (E.B.-M.); christelle.parent@univ-tours.fr (C.P.); laura.bouvart@gmail.com (L.B.); cortes.melanie@wanadoo.fr (M.C.); marion-ferreira@hotmail.fr (M.F.); guy.ilango@univ-tours.fr (G.I.); renaud.respaud@gmail.com (R.R.)
[2]   Faculté de Médecine, Université de Tours, F-37032 Tours, France
[3]   Service de Pharmacie, Centre Hospitalier Régional Universitaire de Tours, F-37032 Tours, France
[4]   Département de Médecine Pédiatrique, Centre Hospitalier Régional Universitaire de Tours, F-37032 Tours, France
[5]   Département de Pneumologie et d'Exploration Respiratoire Fonctionnelle, Centre Hospitalier Régional Universitaire de Tours, F-37032 Tours, France
[6]   Research and Development, Science and Emerging Technologies, Aerogen Limited, Galway Business Park, H91 HE94 Galway, Ireland; rmacloughlin@aerogen.com
[7]   School of Pharmacy & Biomolecular Sciences, Royal College of Surgeons in Ireland, D02 YN77 Dublin, Ireland
[8]   School of Pharmacy and Pharmaceutical Sciences, Trinity College, D02 PN40 Dublin, Ireland
[9]   Institute of Lung Health and Immunology/Comprehensive Pneumology Center with the CPC-M bioArchive, Helmholtz Zentrum München, Member of the German Center for Lung Research (DZL), 85764 Munich, Germany; otmar.schmid@helmholtz-muenchen.de
*   Correspondence: nathalie.vourch@univ-tours.fr
†   These authors contributed equally to this work.

Citation: Sécher, T.; Bodier-Montagutelli, E.; Parent, C.; Bouvart, L.; Cortes, M.; Ferreira, M.; MacLoughlin, R.; Ilango, G.; Schmid, O.; Respaud, R.; et al. Aggregates Associated with Instability of Antibodies during Aerosolization Induce Adverse Immunological Effects. *Pharmaceutics* 2022, 14, 671. https://doi.org/10.3390/pharmaceutics14030671

Academic Editors: Philip Chi Lip Kwok, Michael Yee Tak Chow and Jesus Perez-Gil

Received: 21 February 2022
Accepted: 16 March 2022
Published: 18 March 2022

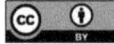
Abstract: Background: Immunogenicity refers to the inherent ability of a molecule to stimulate an immune response. Aggregates are one of the major risk factors for the undesired immunogenicity of therapeutic antibodies (Ab) and may ultimately result in immune-mediated adverse effects. For Ab delivered by inhalation, it is necessary to consider the interaction between aggregates resulting from the instability of the Ab during aerosolization and the lung mucosa. The aim of this study was to determine the impact of aggregates produced during aerosolization of therapeutic Ab on the immune system. Methods: Human and murine immunoglobulin G (IgG) were aerosolized using a clinically-relevant nebulizer and their immunogenic potency was assessed, both in vitro using a standard human monocyte-derived dendritic cell (MoDC) reporter assay and in vivo in immune cells in the airway compartment, lung parenchyma and spleen of healthy C57BL/6 mice after pulmonary administration. Results: IgG aggregates, produced during nebulization, induced a dose-dependent activation of MoDC characterized by the enhanced production of cytokines and expression of co-stimulatory markers. Interestingly, in vivo administration of high amounts of nebulization-mediated IgG aggregates resulted in a profound and sustained local and systemic depletion of immune cells, which was attributable to cell death. This cytotoxic effect was observed when nebulized IgG was administered locally in the airways as compared to a systemic administration but was mitigated by improving IgG stability during nebulization, through the addition of polysorbates to the formulation. Conclusion: Although inhalation delivery represents an attractive alternative route for delivering Ab to treat respiratory infections, our findings indicate that it is critical to prevent IgG aggregation during the nebulization process to avoid pro-inflammatory and cytotoxic effects. The optimization of Ab formulation can mitigate adverse effects induced by nebulization.

Keywords: therapeutic antibody; aerosol; aggregates; immunogenicity

1. Introduction

Therapeutic antibodies (Ab), which mainly consist of monoclonal IgG, represent the fastest growing class of protein therapeutics, accounting for 90% of proteins on the market [1]. As recently highlighted during the COVID-19 pandemic, Ab have a tremendous potential to provide a rapid neutralizing response to emerging viral respiratory pathogens, augmenting vaccines for the control of respiratory infections. Interestingly, both pulmonary and nasal delivery of therapeutic proteins are receiving increasing interest, as the airways are a relevant non-invasive entry portal to the respiratory tract for local-acting protein therapeutics [2–4]. For the treatment of respiratory diseases, several preclinical studies have demonstrated that inhaled protein therapeutics, including Ab, are efficacious and display a better pharmacokinetic profile, as compared to other routes [5–7]. Despite the recent clinical development of oral anti-infective Ab, in the context of the global response to SARS-CoV2 pandemic, the inhalation route remains unexploited for Ab. One of the unknowns is the biological consequence of Ab instability during aerosolization. Inhalation requires transformation of a (bulk) protein formulation in an aerosol, i.e., dispersion of a solution/suspension or a dry-powder into micron-sized particles suspended in a gaseous medium. As with 75% of the inhaled protein therapeutics in clinical development, nebulization of liquid formulations is often the primary technique used for the inhalation of proteins [5]. Nebulization generates a significant air–liquid interface which, combined with the potential for nebulization-induced temperature increase and/or shear forces, can be deleterious for proteins. In response to such stresses, proteins are prone to unfolding, aggregating and, in some cases, being partly inactivated [8,9]. Aggregation is a key marker of instability in full-length Ab during nebulization [10,11] and its extent mainly depends on the type of Ab, the aerosol generator type and the formulation characteristics.

Aggregates are associated with Ab-related adverse immunogenicity [12–14]. Immunogenicity refers to the inherent properties of a molecule to stimulate an immune response. Adverse immunogenicity is due to uncontrolled and protracted immune responses and has major consequences for product safety and pharmacology [15–17]. For instance, adverse immunogenicity is associated with patient's immunization and production of anti-drug antibodies (ADAs) and affects protein therapeutic pharmacokinetics (PK), pharmacodynamics, efficacy and safety, sometimes resulting in extremely harmful side effects [18,19]. To date, many factors have been implicated in adverse immunogenicity [20–23] and they include the content of aggregates and the route of administration, which are important parameters for Ab inhalation.

After inhalation, aggregates from aerosolized Ab will encounter the airways immune system, which has evolved over time to recognize and prevent foreign particles, including aggregates, from penetrating the body. The airway mucosa is sentinelled by a high density of antigen-presenting cells (APC) that quickly and efficiently orchestrate local immune responses against inhaled antigens [24]. In the present study, we analyzed, both in vitro and in vivo, the immunological consequences of Ab aggregates generated during aerosolization and delivered through the airways. First, we screened the potency of IgG aggregates generated by nebulization to activate APC in vitro, using a standard human monocyte-derived dendritic cell (MoDC) assay. Considering the complexity of the immune system and the lung mucosal environment, we evaluated the impact of nebulization-mediated IgG aggregates on immune cells in vivo after pulmonary administration. Our findings show that aggregation attributable to Ab nebulization induced immune cell activation, in a dose-dependent manner and delivering a high-level of aggregates through the pulmonary route had a dramatic effect on immune cell homeostasis, but also that this was avoidable through appropriate formulation approaches.

2. Materials and Methods

Mice

Adult male C57BL/6jrj (B6) mice (5 to 7 weeks old) were obtained from Janvier (France). All mice were housed under specific pathogen-free conditions at the PST Animaleries animal facility (France) and had access to food and water ad libitum. All animal experiments complied with the current European legislative, regulatory and ethical requirements and were approved by the local animal care and use committee (reference: APAFIS No.10200-2017061311352787).

Antibodies

Abs 1, 2 and 3 are full-length IgG1 (named hIgG1-1, hIgG1-2 and hIgG1-3) used in the clinics, supplied in their commercial formulation with endotoxin levels meeting acceptance thresholds (according to their certificate of analysis). To avoid any interference on the aggregation propensity of each Ab, excipients were removed by hydroxyapatite chromatography and subsequent dialysis against phosphate-buffered saline (1X-PBS). Protein concentration was then evaluated for each Ab: hIgG1-1 (1.7 mg/mL), hIgG1-2 (1.9 mg/mL) and hIgG1-3 (2.38 mg/mL)

mAb166 (mIgG2b-1) is a murine monoclonal IgG2b,κ Ab against pcrV, a component of a type three secretion system (T3SS) of *Pseudomonas aeruginosa* [25]. MPC11 (mIgG2b-2) is the control isotype of mAb166. Both were supplied as sterile, pyrogen-free solution in 1X-phosphate-buffered saline (1X-1X-PBS), in accordance with good manufacturing practice, by BioXcell (New Lebanon, NH, USA) with endotoxin level < 1 EU/mL (according to their certificate of analysis). They were supplied as follows: mIgG2b-1 (2.5 mg/mL), mIgG2b-2 (8.5 mg/mL). In some experiments, Ab formulations were supplemented with Polysorbate 80 (PS80; Sigma–Aldrich, Saint-Quentin Fallavier, France) at 0.01% or 0.05% (final volume) prior to nebulization.

Antibody nebulization

For sterility purposes, this procedure was performed under a cell-culture hood. All antibodies were filtered in suspension on a 0.22 μm syringe filter (Millipore, Guyancourt, France). For in vitro assay, all antibodies were diluted in PBS1X to a final concentration of ~1.7 mg/mL before nebulization. For each Ab, 1 mL were nebulized using the clinically-relevant Aeroneb Pro™ vibrating-mesh nebulizer (Aerogen, Ireland), connected with a 13 mL polypropylene tube (Dutscher, Bernolsheim, France) or the VITROCELL Cloud 12 system (VITROCELL Systems, Waldkirch, Germany), which is the commercial version of the Air–Liquid Interface Cell Exposure–Cloud (ALICE-cloud) system, described by Lenz and colleagues [26]. Nebulization duration was measured and lasted ~5 min for each sample (i.e., 0.4 mL/min liquid output rate). For in vitro aerosol-cell exposures, using the VITROCELL Cloud 12 system, the aerosol cloud was allowed to settle for 20 min before removing cells. When necessary, nebulized Ab solutions were filtered on a 0.45 μm syringe filter (Millipore, Guyancourt, France) prior to further use. Nebulizers were washed extensively between each nebulization sessions using 0.22 μm autoclaved water and 1X-PBS. Subsequently, nebulized 1X-PBS was analyzed by flow cell microscopy and the nebulizer was considered cleaned and operating for Ab nebulization when the nebulized 1X-PBS samples contained less than 300 particles/mL. To rule out that cell activation may be attributable to contamination released during nebulization, the activation potency of nebulized 1X-PBS (vehicle solution) was also investigated in vitro. Our analysis revealed that nebulized 1X-PBS had no impact on MoDC activation (data not shown).

Dynamic Light Scattering (DLS) analysis of antibodies

Native and nebulized Ab were analyzed by dynamic light scattering with a Dynapro Nanostar® (Wyatt Technology, Goleta, CA, USA) after appropriate dilution to 100 μg/mL in 1X-PBS in UVette (Eppendorf, Montesson, France). For each sample, the acquisition was performed 10 times for 7 s each, at a temperature of 25 °C with a detection angle of 90°. The particle diameter (nm) and polydispersion index (pdi) were analyzed using DynamicsTM software (Wyatt Technology, Goleta, CA, USA). Samples with less than 70% of successful analyses were considered multimodal and non-analyzable as recommended by the manufacturer (depicted as n/a).

Flow cell microscopy (FCM) of antibodies

Native and nebulized Ab were analyzed by flow cell microscopy with an Occhio® FC200S+ (Occhio, Angleur, Belgium) after appropriate dilution to 100 μg/mL in medium in the flowcell. Briefly, 250 µL of each antibody solution passed continuously in the flow cell, where particles were automatically detected, sized and counted by a camera. Particle counting, size assessment and distribution were analyzed using CallistoTM software (Occhio, Angleur, Belgium).

Monocyte-derived dendritic cells (MoDC) preparation

Human peripheral mononuclear cells (PBMC) were purified from cytapheresis, obtained from naïve donors (Etablissement Français du Sang, Centre Hospitalier Régional Universitaire Bretonneau, Tours, France) by centrifugation on a Ficoll density gradient (Eurobio, Les Ulis, France). MoDC were prepared from PMBC as previously described [27]. Briefly, CD14+ monocytes were isolated using magnetic cell sorting (Miltenyi Biotec, Bergisch Gladbach, Germany) and cultured during 6 days, at 1×10^6 cells/mL in RPMI1640-GlutamaxTM (Gibco, Illkirch, France) supplemented with 10% of FCS (Dutscher, France), 1X-Penicillin/Streptomycin (Gibco, Illkirch, France) in the presence of 25 ng/mL of IL-4 (Miltenyi Biotec, Bergisch Gladbach, Germany) and 100 ng/mL of GM-CSF. On day 6, homogeneity and viability of MoDC population was checked by flow cytometry based on their physical characteristics (forward scatter (FSC) and side scatter (SSC)) and incorporation of vital dye (LiveDead^{TM}, Invitrogen, Illkirch, France). The immature phenotype of MoDC was checked based on their DC-SIGN+, CD80low, CD83low and HLA-DR low phenotype.

MoDC stimulation with antibody preparation

On day 6, immature MoDC were harvested and washed in complete medium (RPMI1640-Glutamax^{TM} supplemented with 10% of FCS (Dutscher, Bernolsheim, France) and 1X-Penicillin/Streptomycin). For experiments using Ab aerosols collected in a 13 mL polypropylene tube, 1×10^5 cells/well were plated in 75 µL in a U-bottom 96-well plate (Falcon, Becton Dickinson, France) for 4 h. A total of 75 µL of nebulized or native Ab was then added to a final concentration of 1, 10, 100 and 200 µg/mL depending on the experiments. For experiments using the VITROCELL Cloud 12 system, 1×10^5 cells/well were plated in 150 µL on a 24-well plate permeable insert (Corning, Hazebrouck, France) for 18 h. The insert was then placed in the VITROCELL Cloud 12 system with 200 µL in the basolateral compartment to prevent cell drying and cells were exposed to Ab aerosol as described above. Inserts were then put back on a companion 24-well plate.

Cells were incubated in 150 µL of complete medium for 18 h at 37 °C with 5% CO_2. Lipopolysaccharide (LPS, from *Escherichia coli* O111:B5, Sigma-Aldrich, France) was used at 1 µg/mL as a positive control. Untreated and nebulized -1X-PBS (Gibco, Illkirch, France) were used as vehicle controls. Each condition was tested in 3–9 replicates.

Analysis of MoDC activation by flow cytometry

After 18 h of stimulation, MoDC were harvested and saturated in -1X-PBS supplemented with 2% of FCS, 2 mM EDTA and 1X-human Fc-Block (Becton Dickinson, France) for 15 min at 4 °C. Cells were washed and stained in FACS buffer (1X-PBS supplemented with 2% FCS and 2 mM EDTA) with antibodies described in Supplementary Table S2, for 20 min at 4 °C in the dark. FMO controls were generated for each parameter analyzed. All antibodies were from Biolegend (London, UK). Data acquisition was conducted on the 8-colors MACSQuant flow cytometer (Miltenyi Biotec, Bergisch Gladbach, Germany) on a minimum of 10,000 living cells. MoDC analysis was performed using VenturiOne software (Applied Cytometry, Sheffield, UK). Analysis was conducted on singlet (FSC-A/FSC-H gating) and CD45+ live cells (negative for LiveDead staining). Costimulatory protein expression was expressed as a ratio of the median fluorescence intensity (MFI) of cells treated with nebulized Ab/MFI of cells treated with native Ab.

Cytokine, chemokine and protein assays

All assays were performed on Immulon^{TM} 96-well plates (ThermoFischer Scientific, Illkirch, France). Concentrations of CXCL8 (IL-8), human IL-6 in cell-free MoDC supernatants and TNF, IL6, IL1b and CXCL1 (KC) were measured using specific ELISAs (Biolegend, London, UK; limit of detection: at 15.6 pg/mL) according to the manufacturer's instructions and were normalized based on the mean concentration of total protein. Total protein concentration was determined using a BCA assay (ThermoFischer Scientific, Illkirch, France), according to the manufacturer's instructions (limit of detection: 15 µg/mL). Protein expression was expressed as a ratio of the protein concentration of cells treated with nebulized Ab/protein concentration of cells treated with native Ab.

Animal experiments

For each experiment, 5 mice per group were used. Animal experiments were performed 2–3 times. Nebulized or native mIgG2b-1 and mIgG2b-2 (100 µg/animal, in 40 µL) were administered orotracheally or through intravenous injection using a restraining tube at days 0, 7, 14, 21 and 28. For orotracheal administration, mice were anesthetized with isofluorane 4% and an operating otoscope fit with intubation specula was introduced both to maintain tongue retraction and to visualize the glottis. A fiber optic wire threaded through a 20 G catheter and connected to torch stylet (Harvard Apparatus, Holliston, MA, USA) was inserted into the mouse trachea. Correct intubation was confirmed using a lung inflation bulb test and 40 µL of the bacterial solution was applied using an ultrafine pipette tip. For the acute treatment assessment, animals were euthanized using a lethal dose of ketamine/xylazine at 4 h, on day 1 and 14 days after a single administration. In the chronic treatment groups, animals were euthanized at day 29.

At the time of necropsy, blood was recovered by intracardiac puncture. Bronchoalveolar lavage fluid (BALF) was then collected by cannulating the trachea and washing the lung twice with 1.2 mL of 1X-PBS at room temperature. The lavage fluid was centrifuged at $400\times g$ for 10 min at 4 °C, and the supernatant was stored at -20 °C until analysis. The cell pellet was resuspended in FACS buffer and counted in a hemocytometer chamber. Peripheral blood was washed out by intracardiac perfusion with 10 mL of 1X-PBS. Lung and spleen homogenates were then prepared in 2 mL of RPMI1640 containing 125 µg/mL of Liberase (Sigma–Aldrich, France) and 100 µg/mL of DnaseI (Sigma–Aldrich, Saint-Quentin Fallavier, France) using a GentleMACS tissue homogenizer (Miltenyi Biotec, Bergisch Gladbach, Germany). Cells were isolated through a 100 µm cell strainer and purified with a 20% Percoll (Sigma–Aldrich, Saint-Quentin Fallavier, France) density gradient. Cell preparation was centrifuged at $400\times g$ for 10 min at 4 °C, and the pellet was resuspended in FACS buffer, and counted in a hemocytometer chamber.

Immune cell phenotyping by flow cytometry

BALF, lung and spleen cells isolated as described above were saturated in 1X-PBS supplemented with 2% of FCS, 2 mM EDTA and 1X- human Fc-Block (Becton Dickinson, France) for 15 min at 4 °C. Cells were washed and stained with antibodies described in Supplementary Table S2 for 20 min at 4 °C in the dark. Data acquisition was made on the 8-colors MACSQuant flow cytometer (Miltenyi Biotec, Bergisch Gladbach, Germany) on a minimum of 100,000 living cells. Analysis was performed using VenturiOne software (Applied Cytometry, Sheffield, UK). Analysis was made on singlet (FSC-A/FSC-H gating) and CD45+ live cells (negative for LiveDead staining). Immune cell phenotypes were determined as described in Supplementary Table S2. Data were normalized based on the mean concentration of respective native Ab conditions or expressed as a number of cells calculated as follows: % of the total CD45+ immune cell population x total number of cells. For Annexin-V/PI staining, data were normalized as follows: % of the positive population for nebulized Ab/% of the positive population for native Ab.

Histology

Lungs were fixed in 10% buffered formalin (Shandon), dehydrated in ethanol and embedded in paraffin. Serial sections (3 mm) were stained with hematoxylin and eosin (HE) or Congo red. Ten HE sections per mouse were randomly evaluated to count the cell nucleus using a machine-learning pixel classification plugin for Image J (https://imagej.net/plugins/tws/, as available on 17 March 2022), as described previously [28].

Statistical analysis

Differences between experimental groups were determined using Kruskal –Wallis or t-test comparing two groups, using one or two-way analysis of variance (ANOVA) followed by Newman–Keuls or Bonferroni post-test (for comparison between more than two groups), after confirmation that the data were normally distributed. All statistical tests were performed with GraphPad Prism software (version 4.03 for Windows, GraphPad Software Inc., San Diego, CA, USA). All data are presented as mean ± standard error of the mean (SEM). The threshold for statistical significance was set to $p < 0.05$.

3. Results

3.1. Aggregation of Antibodies Is Heterogeneous during Nebulization

Nebulization promotes Ab aggregation [10,11]. In this study, mesh nebulization was used since it is less deleterious on Ab and often considered for aerosolization of proteins [5]. Full-length Ab, commercially available or under preclinical development, were reformulated in 1X-PBS and nebulized with the Aeroneb Pro™ vibrating-mesh nebulizer.

Ab aggregation results in a broad range of particles, from dimers (several nanometers) to micron-sized, and even visible particles in some cases [29], requiring the combination of different complementary analytical techniques. The aggregation profiles of Ab were assessed using DLS and FCM to report particles at the submicrometric and micrometric scales, respectively (Figure 1).

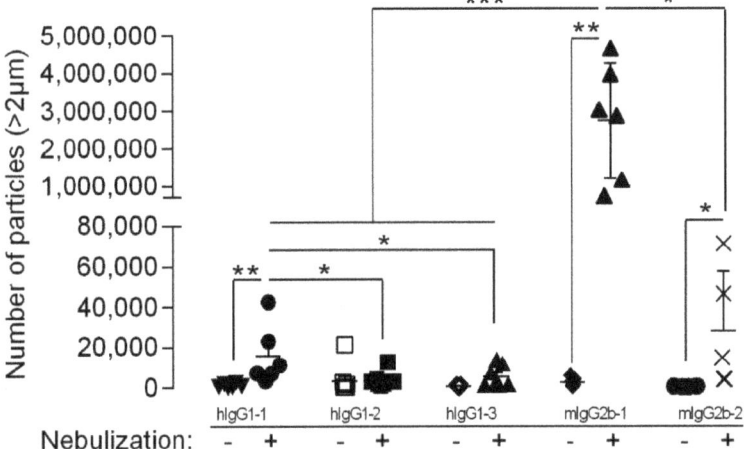

Figure 1. Antibodies were either nebulized using an Aeroneb Pro™ vibrating-mesh nebulizer and collected (Nebulization +) or left untreated (Nebulization −). The total number of particles (with diameter >2 μm) was quantified using a flow microscope. The data are quoted as the mean ± SEM. *, **, ***: $p < 0.05$, $p < 0.01$ and $p < 0.001$, respectively, in a one-way ANOVA with Newman–Keuls correction for multiple comparisons. The results represent three to eight independent nebulizations.

Nebulization led to an increase in the concentration of particles > 2 μm for hIgG1-1, mIgG2b-1 and mIgG2b-2, as compared to their native counterparts. Conversely, no significant increase in particle count was observed for hIgG1-2 and hIgG1-3 (Figure 1). Furthermore, comparing nebulized Ab, we observed that hIgG1-1 and mIgG2b-1 had significantly more particles than the other human and murine Ab, respectively. In addition to differences in total particle concentration, there were also differences in particle size distribution. Nebulized hIgG1-1 and -2 had more than 78% of their particles smaller than 5 μm, while hIgG1-3, mIgG2b-1 and mIgG2b-2 comprised more than 33% of their particles above 5 μm (Table 1). For murine mIgG2b-1 and mIgG2b-2, aggregation was also observed at the submicron scale, most notably for nebulized mIgG2b-1, which could not even be analyzed by DLS due to the large heterogeneity of the particle size distribution (most likely all-sized Ab aggregates), which cannot be clearly structured in defined size modes—a prerequisite for DLS measurements. Nebulized mIgG2b-2 exhibited a significant reduction (7%) in monomeric Ab amount (Supplementary Table S1). Overall, our results highlight the substantial heterogeneity of Ab aggregation during mesh nebulization, most likely depending on Ab sequence/structure.

Table 1. Particle size distribution (%) of nebulized antibodies.

Antibody	2–5 µm	5–25 µm	>25 µm
hIgG1-1	84.3	14.7	1.1
hIgG1-2	78.4	21.1	0.4
hIgG1-3	53.8	45.8	0.4
mIgG2b-1	67	32.3	0.7
mIgG2b-2	57.8	40.7	1.6

3.2. Ab Aggregates, Produced during Mesh Nebulization, Activate Antigen-Presenting Cells

The dramatic consequences of adverse immunogenicity have prompted regulatory authorities to establish a guidance to test the immunogenicity of therapeutic protein products and industry to propose screening approaches [30,31]. They include investigating the ability of protein aggregates to activate immune cells, in vitro.

Here, we incubated human monocyte-derived dendritic cells (MoDC) overnight with native or nebulized Abs (hIgG1-1 to -3) and analyzed both the release of pro-inflammatory cytokines and expression of co-stimulatory proteins involved in the DC-T synapse (CD25, CD83, CD86 and CD80). Neither the native Ab, nor the nebulized buffer without Ab (data not shown) promoted IL-6 or IL-8 production by MoDC (Figure 2A,B) and modulated cell markers as compared to untreated MoDC (Figure 2E–H). Nebulized and aggregated hIgG1-1 induced a significant and dose-dependent increase in cytokine production (Figure 2A–D) whereas the other nebulized Ab solutions had only a minor and inconsistent impact on cytokine level. The nebulized and aggregated hIgG1-1 induced a slight but significant increase in all cell markers, whereas the effect of other nebulized Ab was limited (Figure 2E–H). Interestingly, the filtration of Ab solutions after nebulization, removing micrometric particles (data not shown), resulted in the abrogation of both cytokine release and expression of co-stimulatory markers by MoDC (Figure 2A–H, gray bars). In addition, when comparing nebulized antibodies, our analysis revealed that activation potency of hIgG1-1 was higher than for hIgG1-2 and hIgG1-3. Altogether, our results suggest that activation of APC was attributable to the presence of aggregates and that the extent of this activation was correlated to the number of particles (Figure 1). Since the aerosol collection system may modulate the amount and the size distribution of Ab aggregates after nebulization [11], we determined whether collection might induce a bias in APC activation. We directly exposed MoDC to hIgG1-1 aerosols using the VITROCELL Cloud 12 system [26]. As observed in Supplementary Figure S1, we obtained similar results on MoDC activation independent of whether the cells were directly exposed to hIgG1-1 aerosols (through use of the VITROCELL Cloud 12 system) or exposed to them after collection as a bulk solution, supporting our decision of adopting the latter approach. Collectively, our results showed that nebulized Ab induced MoDC maturation and activation as compared to native Ab and confirmed the involvement of Ab aggregates in this response.

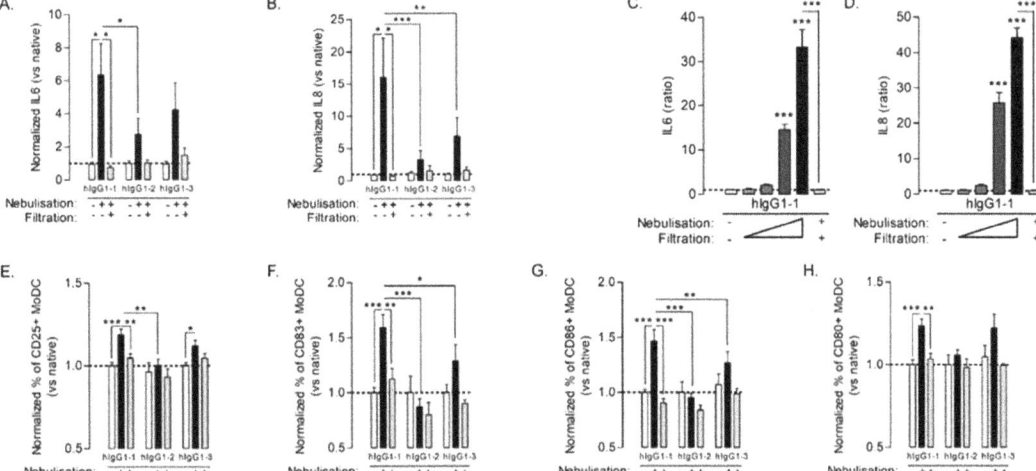

Figure 2. MoDC were stimulated using equal final concentration of Ab at 100 μg/mL, either native (white bars), nebulized (black bars) or nebulized and 0.45 μm-filtered (gray bars) for 18 h. IL6 (**A**) and IL8 (**B**) were quantified in cell-free supernatant. MoDC were stimulated with 1, 10, 100 or 200 μg/mL (gray to black bars) of nebulized hIgG1 or 100 μg/mL of nebulized and 0.45 μm-filtered hIgG1 (last bar) or left untreated (white bars) for 18 h. IL6 (**C**) and IL8 (**D**) were quantified in cell-free supernatant. MoDC were stimulated using equal final concentration of Ab at 100 μg/mL either native (white bars), nebulized (black bars) or nebulized and 0.45 μm-filtered (gray bars) for 18 h. CD25 (**E**), CD83 (**F**), CD86 (**G**) and CD80 (**H**) expression were measured using flow cytometry. The data are quoted as the mean ± SEM. *, **, ***: $p < 0.05$, $p < 0.01$ and $p < 0.001$, respectively, in a one-way ANOVA with Newman–Keuls correction for multiple comparisons. The results are representative of six independent experiments (n = 6–9 technical replicates/experiment).

3.3. High-Level of Nebulization-Mediated Antibody Aggregates Impair Lung Cell Homeostasis after Lung Delivery

Historically, in vitro assays have been widely used to describe the potential immunogenicity of biotherapeutic aggregates [13]. However, they display several limitations: (i) the amount of aggregates inducing a response in vitro may not directly translate into in vivo response and (ii) they may not predict the impact of the pulmonary delivery route. To gain insight into the broad effects of Ab aggregates produced by aerosolization within the lung compartment, we selected two murine IgG2b–mIgG2b-1 and mIgG2b-2-producing different amounts of aggregates during mesh nebulization (Figure 1) which differentially activate MoDC (Supplementary Figure S2). We administered them through the airways in naive mice. Remarkably, the nebulized and aggregated mIgG2b-1 resulted in a dramatic reduction in the total cell number in the airway compartment of mice (BAL), as compared to native antibodies administered by the same route (Figure 3A). Moreover, nebulized mIgG2b-2, producing 10-fold fewer aggregates after mesh nebulization than mIgG2b-1 (Figure 1), showed no statistically significant reduction in BAL cell number (Figure 3G). Of note, the animals that received the native Ab through the airways had similar cell count as sham animals (data not shown), which implies that the orotracheal application itself did not obfuscate our results.

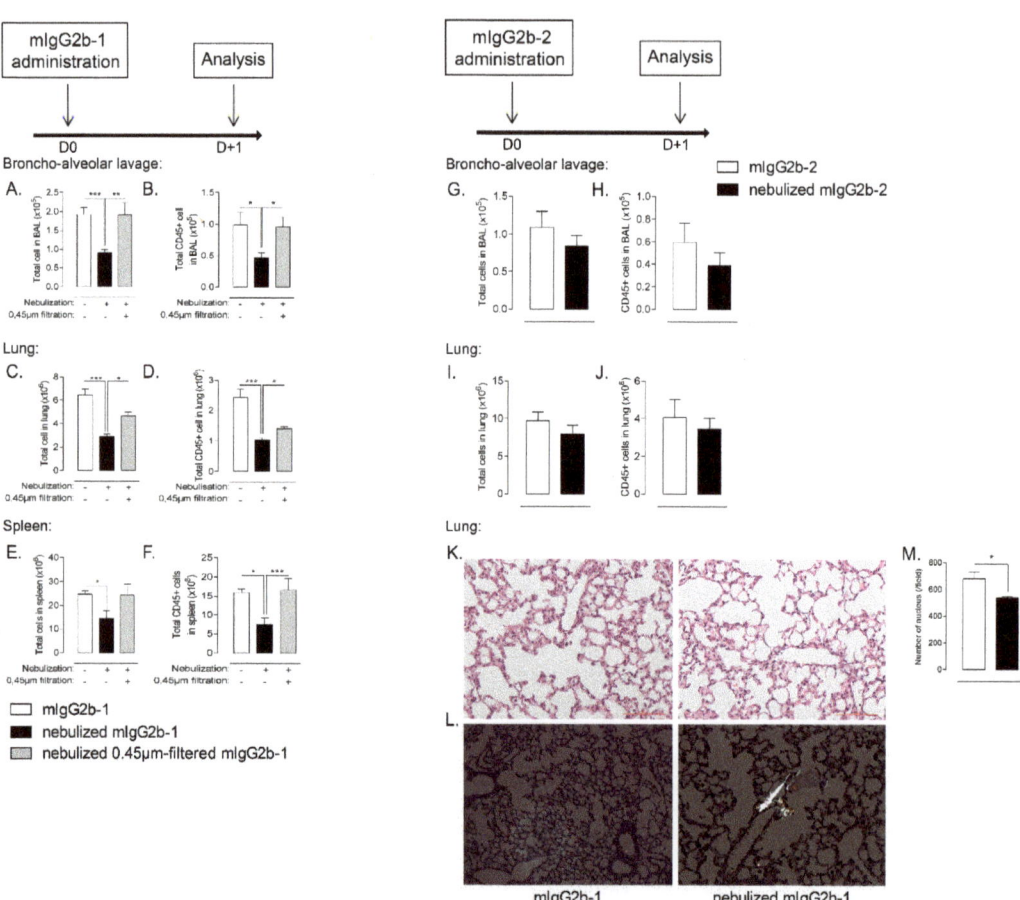

Figure 3. B6 mice received a 40 µL orotracheal instillation of mIgG2b-1 at 100 µg/mL either native (white bars), nebulized (black bars) or nebulized and 0.45 µm-filtered (gray bars). The total number of cells (**A,C,E**) and CD45+ cells (**B,D,F**) were quantified in BAL (**A,B**), in the lungs (**C,D**) and the spleen (**E,F**) using flow cytometry, 18 h after the administration. B6 mice received a 40 µL orotracheal instillation of mIgG2b-2 at 100 µg/mL either native (white bars) or nebulized (black bars). The total number of cells (**G,I**) and CD45+ cells (H and J) were quantified in BAL (**G,H**), in the lungs (**I,J**) using flow cytometry, 18 h after the administration. Lung tissues of mice treated with either native (white bars) or nebulized (black bars) mIgG2b-1 were histologically examined 18 h after the administration. (**K**) Hematoxylin-eosin sections were used to quantify cell nucleus (**M**) by machine-learning (see material and methods section). (**L**) Congo red sections were observed under polarized light. Aggregates are identified as apple-green birefringence artifacts. 10 sections/mouse were observed at ×20 magnification and used for machine-learning quantification. The data are quoted as the mean ± SEM. *, **, ***: $p < 0.05$, $p < 0.01$ and $p < 0.001$, respectively, in a one-way ANOVA with Newman–Keuls correction for multiple comparisons. The results are representative of three independent experiments (n = 5 mice/experiment).

Analysis of the cellular phenotype of the BAL cells revealed an analogous result for immune (CD45+ leukocytes) cells (Figure 3B,H). Further analysis did not reveal any impact on specific lineage as almost all immune cell types were affected after the administration of aggregated Ab (Supplementary Figure S3A–E). In the lung tissue, nebulized mIgG2b-1 caused a 2-fold reduction in total cell and leukocyte counts relative to controls (Figure 3C,D), while nebulization of mIgG2b-2 did not modify leukocyte counts (Figure 3I,J). This decrease affected both myeloid (neutrophils, monocytes/macrophages and dendritic cells) (Supplementary Figure S3F–I) and lymphoid lineages (B, T CD4+/CD8+ cells) (Supplementary Figure S3J–L). The modification of cell homeostasis in the airway compartment was not associated with an alteration of the lung epithelial barrier (Supplementary Figure S4), but was mostly attributable to micron-sized particles as 0.45 μm-filtration of nebulized mIgG2b-1 prevented these adverse effects (Figure 3A–F, gray bars). The filtration step did not significantly modify Ab particle size distribution (Supplementary Tables S4 and S5) or concentration (Supplementary Table S6), as compared to native Ab.

Interestingly, we observed protein aggregates (appearing as apple-green birefringence structures under polarized light) on Congo red stained lung sections from animals treated with nebulized mIgG2b-1 (Figure 3L). Unsupervised machine learning, which was used to quantify the cell nucleus on HE-stained lung section, confirmed that local administration of nebulized mIgG2b-1 was associated with a significant reduction of lung cells after 18 h (Figure 3K,M). Unexpectedly, the number of total and immune cells was also diminished, even though to a lesser extent, in the spleen (Figure 3E,F), indicating that the impairment of cellular homeostasis reached the systemic compartment. Contraction of cell number 18 h after a single airway administration of nebulized Ab primarily occurred in the airways, and then probably extended through the lung tissue and systemically as it was restricted to the airway compartment after 4 h (Figure 4A–F). Moreover, this effect was sustained for at least up to 14 days after Ab administration (Figure 4G,H), or after repeated administrations (Figure 4I–N). For either single or repeated administrations of nebulized mIg2b-1, we did not observe any sign of general toxicity, including body-weight loss (data not shown). Overall, our results suggest that airway administration of aggregated IgG (>0.45 μm) profoundly affected cellular homeostasis, in a time-dependent manner, both locally and systemically.

3.4. Nebulized Aggregated Antibody Induced Immunologically Silent Cell Death after Lung Administration

Next, we investigated the mechanisms accounting for host cell contraction and hypothesized that it was associated with cell death. Cell death occurs in multiple forms and can be divided in accidental cell death (ACD; necrosis) or regulated cell death (RCD; apoptosis) [32]. ACD is characterized by a dramatic and instantaneous collapse of cells and can be triggered in response to different stresses, including chemical, physical or mechanical insults, whereas RCD relies on committed molecular machinery [33]. Using Annexin-V/propidium iodide (PI) staining, which allows the discrimination of early apoptotic cells (Annexin-V+/PI-), late apoptotic cells (Annexin-V+/PI+) and necrotic cells (Annexin-V-/PI+) [34], we quantified the proportion of each cell death phenotypes in both total cells and CD45+ leukocytes population, 18 h after a single administration of mIgG2b-1. We observed that administration of nebulized mIgG2b-1 provoked a significant increase in both late apoptotic and necrotic spleen cells while lung and airway cells were suffering from necrosis as compared to mice treated with native Ab (Figure 5A–F) or with nebulized mIgG2b-2 (Supplementary Figure S5). The type of cell death could also be determined by the analysis of mediators released in the environment. When comparing BALs from animals treated with native and nebulized mIgG2b-1, we did not observe any significant difference in the production of TNF, IL-6, IL-1b or CXCL1 (KC) (Figure 5G–J). These data suggest that the cell contraction occurring after single or multiple airway administration of nebulized and aggregated IgG was associated with an inflammatory silent cell death process.

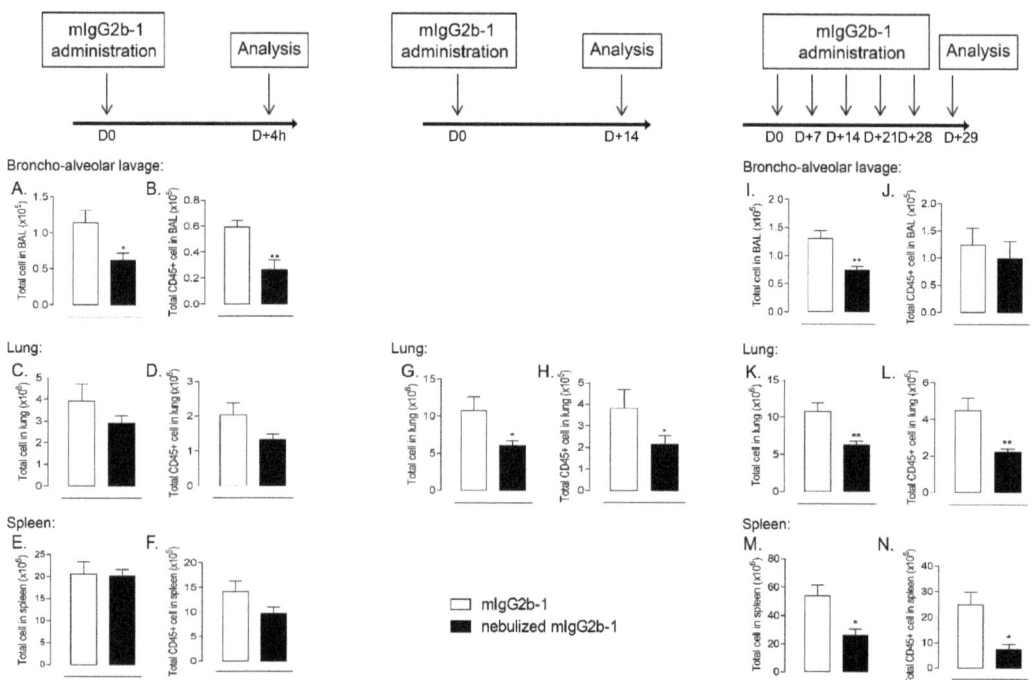

Figure 4. B6 mice received a 40 μL orotracheal instillation of mIg2b-1 at 100 μg/mL either native (white bars) or nebulized (black bars) through the airways at D0, or D + 0, D + 7, D + 14, D + 21 and D + 28. The total number of cells (**A,C,E,G,I,K,M**) and CD45+ cells (**B,D,F,H,J,L,N**) were quantified in BAL (**A,B,I,J**), in the lungs (**C,D,G,H,K,L**) and the spleen (**E,F,M,N**) using flow cytometry, 4 h, 14 days or 29 days after the first administration. The data are quoted as the mean ± SEM. *, **: $p < 0.05$ and $p < 0.01$, respectively, in a t-test. The results are representative of two independent experiments ($n = 5$ mice/experiment).

3.5. The Effect of Nebulization-Mediated Antibody Aggregates on Immune Cell Homeostasis Is Specific of the Pulmonary Route

Immunogenicity of Ab is also dependent on their route of administration [20–22]. Thus, we investigated the effect of native or nebulized-mIgG2b-1 after intravenous injection. In contrast to what was observed after airway administration, there were no significant differences in the BAL or lung cell counts in the animals who received native or nebulized mIgG2b-1 intravenously (Figure 6A–D). Interestingly, these results were substantiated when analyzing cell number after repeated administration of nebulized mIgG2b-1 (Supplementary Figure S6), where no differences were noticed in the airways or lungs of animals treated by repeated intravenous injections as compared to animals, which received the IgG in the lungs. Our data suggest that the route of administration played an important role on the adverse effect of IgG aggregates produced during nebulization on cell homeostasis.

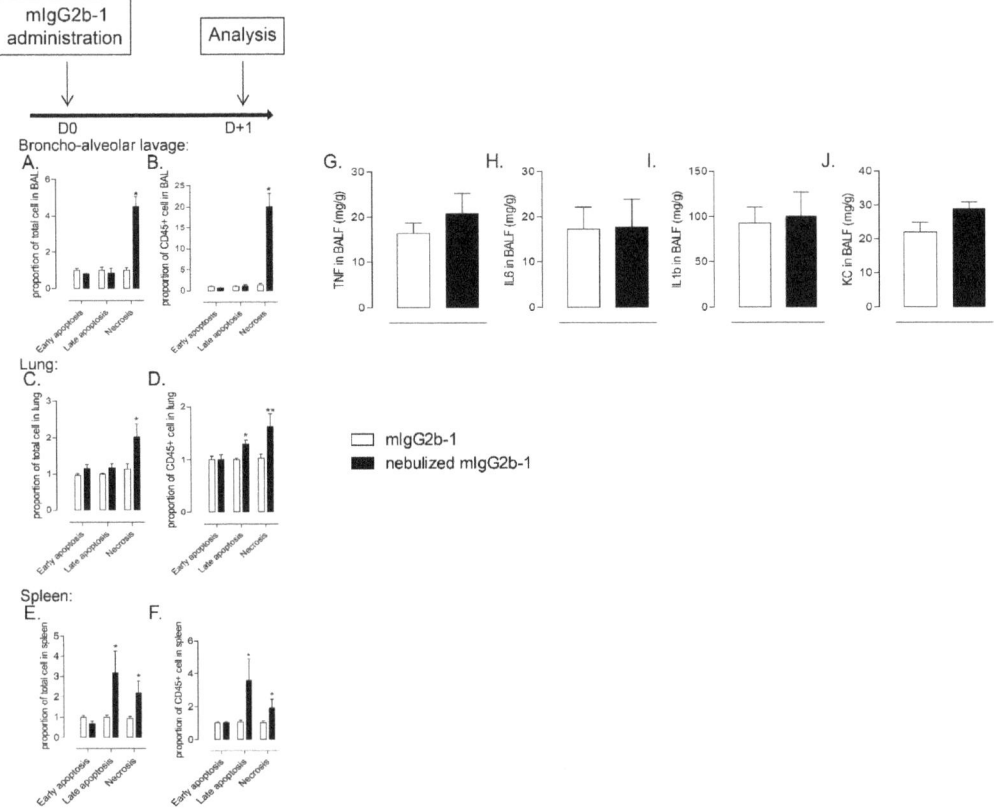

Figure 5. B6 mice received a single 40 µL orotracheal instillation of mIg2b-1 at 100 µg/mL either native (white bars) or nebulized (black bars). The proportion of early apoptotic cells (Annexin-V+/PI-), late apoptotic cells (Annexin-V+/PI+) and necrotic cells (Annexin-V-/PI+) were quantified in total cell (**A,C,E**) or CD45+ cell (**B,D,F**), 18 h after the administration in BAL (**A,B**), lungs (**C,D**) and spleen (**E,F**) relative to mice treated with native Ab using flow cytometry. The concentrations of TNF (**G**), IL6 (**H**), IL1b (**I**) and KC (**J**) in BALF were determined 18 h after the administration. The data are quoted as the mean ± SEM. *, **: $p < 0.05$ and $p < 0.01$, respectively, in a t-test. The results are representative of three independent experiments ($n = 5$ mice/experiment).

3.6. Reducing Aggregation Limits Pulmonary Cytotoxicity Associated to Lung Administration of Nebulized Ab

Pharmaceutical development aims to design a high-quality product ensuring an efficacious and safe treatment along the life of the product. Hence, formulation and protein engineering are often adapted to limit Ab aggregation, especially considering chronic-based therapies. Different parameters, including addition of surfactant, have a protective effect, limiting Ab aggregation during nebulization [10]. Here, we added polysorbate 80 (PS80) in mIgG2b-1 formulation which significantly reduced its aggregation during nebulization (Supplementary Figure S7). The addition of surfactant did not significantly modify Ab particle size distribution (Supplementary Tables S4 and S5) or concentration (Supplementary Table S6) as compared to unformulated Ab. Single administration of nebulized mIgG2b-1 supplemented with 0.05% of PS80 abrogated the reduction of lung cell number (Figure 7C,D) and to a lesser extent of airway cell (Figure 7A,B) as compared to non-formulated mIgG2b-1. This was likely attributable to a reduction in cell death in the same compartment (Supplementary Figure S8). These results suggest that optimizing IgG formulation improved its molecular stability and might limit adverse effects on cell homeostasis.

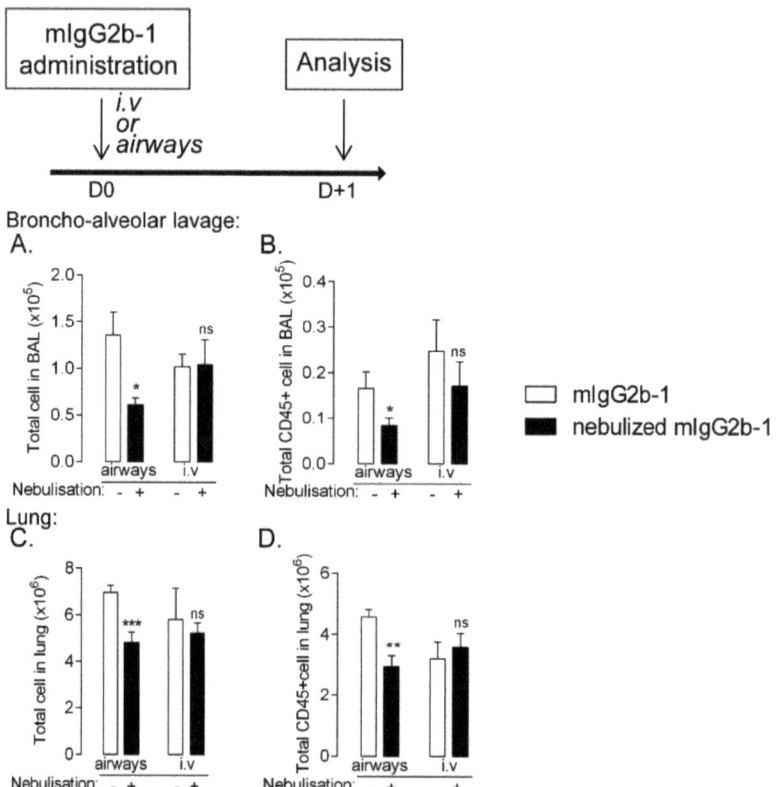

Figure 6. B6 mice received a 40 µL orotracheal instillation or 100 µL intravenous injection of mIgG2b-1 at 100 µg/mL either native (white bars) or nebulized (black bars). The total number of cells (**A,C**) and CD45+ cells (**B,D**) were quantified in BAL (**A,B**) and in the lungs (**C,D**) using flow cytometry, 18 h after the administration. The data are quoted as the mean ± SEM. *, **, ***: $p < 0.05$, $p < 0.01$ and $p < 0.001$, respectively, in a t-test. The results are representative of two independent experiments ($n = 5$ mice/experiment).

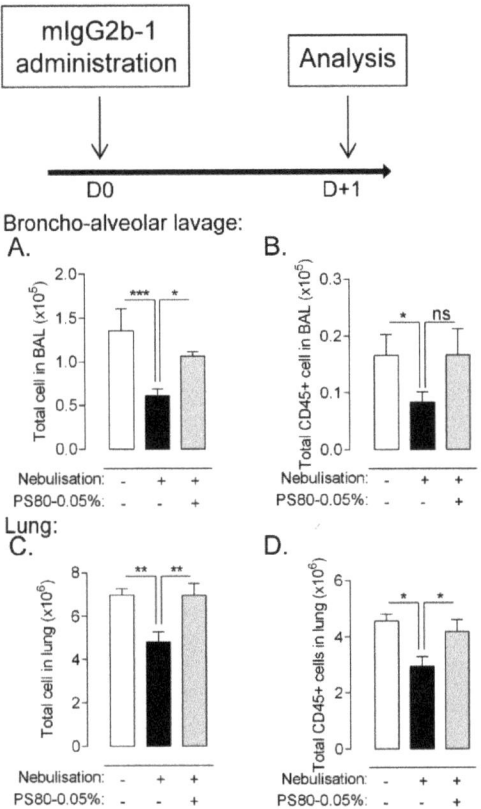

Figure 7. B6 mice received a 40 µL orotracheal instillation of mIgG2b-1 at 100 µg/mL either native (white bars), nebulized (black bars) or nebulized + 0.05%-PS80(gray bars). The total number of cells (**A,C**) and CD45+ cells (**B,D**) were quantified in BAL (**A,B**) and in the lungs (**C,D**) using flow cytometry, 18 h after the administration. The data are quoted as the mean ± SEM. *, **, ***: $p < 0.05$, $p < 0.01$ and $p < 0.001$, respectively, in a t-test. The results are representative of two independent experiments ($n = 5$ mice/experiment).

4. Discussion

Ab are highly sensitive to stresses encountered during their product development, manufacturing, storage or clinical use, and they often require high therapeutic doses, necessitating high concentration drug products with a higher risk of aggregation. Tracking aggregates prior and after Ab bioprocessing is essential to avoid risks for patients, treatment failure and ultimately termination of drug development/commercialization.

Protein aggregation has been widely demonstrated as an influential factor in the induction of adverse immunogenicity of biotherapeutics [35,36]. However, some of the stress conditions used in the literature are not representative of those experienced during product development, manufacturing, storage or clinical use, making the generated aggregates far different from those found in marketed products. This may hamper conclusions about the exact potency of protein aggregation in the occurrence of drug immunogenicity. Several intrinsic or extrinsic attributes of aggregates might work synergistically to induce immunogenicity. Among them, parameters related to the delivery route can affect the immune response associated with the administration of drugs. For example, subcutaneous delivery has been associated with higher immunogenicity than the intravenous route, for several biotherapeutics [37,38]. To our knowledge, there has not been any study conducted so far to assess the immunogenicity associated with lung administration of an aerosolized and aggregated Ab. We set out a dual experimental approach to investigate the quality and the extent of the immune responses induced by a nebulized and aggregated Ab using both in vitro and in vivo models. Here, we showed for the first time that the aggregates resulting from IgG nebulization induced immune cell over-activation and that their delivery to the lung markedly and durably impaired cell homeostasis.

Protein aggregation is a process of non-specific association of monomers through multiple physical and chemical pathways, which are well documented [39]. The characteristics of protein aggregates are variable in terms of particle size, number, morphology, chemical modifications, reversibility, conformation or hydrophobicity [40]. This phenotypic heterogeneity results from the various stresses applied to proteins and require specific analytical methods [41]. Aerosol generation involves the dispersion of liquid droplets into a gas. This process may be associated with physical stresses, including temperature variations and the generation of a massive air–liquid interface, which ultimately induce changes in protein conformation and lead to its aggregation [10]. We measured the aggregation of several human IgG submitted to aerosolization using a vibrating-mesh nebulizer, which is expected to be less deleterious than other nebulizers [42,43]. Flow cell microscopy and dynamic light scattering revealed that the number and size of aggregates were Ab dependent, confirming the results in the literature on the necessity of a case-by-case approach. Moreover, drastic differences were observed between commercial Abs (hIgG1-1 to 3) and murine Abs (mIgG2b-1 and -2), where the latter displayed higher aggregation upon nebulization. This may be explained by the fact that commercial Abs underwent advanced development programs and were thus selected for their limited aggregation potency. We next determined whether the aggregates found in the therapeutic product after nebulization may induce immunogenicity using an MoDC-based assay, which has been widely used to describe the potential immunogenicity of biotherapeutics or unwanted products [44]. Our analysis revealed that nebulized and aggregated hIgG1, in particular, hIgG1-1, were able to induce MoDC activation and maturation, as evidenced by the enhanced secretion in cytokines and increased expression of co-stimulatory proteins on MoDC. This response correlated with the fraction of micron-sized aggregates in the Ab aerosol. There are still discrepancies regarding the size and type of aggregates involved in the generation of immunogenic responses [45]. This depends on the type and strength of the stress applied and the multiple experimental protocols, which have been described [21,46]. Here, hIgG1-1 aerosol is mainly composed of small-sized particles (2–10 μm), which have been shown to enhance the immune response and be the most immunogenic [45,47].

One potential bias regarding Ab aggregation could be attributed to the aerosol collection step, which uses a polypropylene tube to re-pool aerosol droplets into a bulk liquid. Indeed, it has been evidenced that the aerosol collection device could influence protein stability, generating different aggregation profiles [11,48]. In this context, we used the VITROCELL technology, which was developed to improve the reliability of toxicological studies for aerosolized compounds on air–liquid interface cell cultures [49,50]. This system, which allows the direct deposition of aerosols on cells, avoids the collection step [51]. Our results showed that direct hIgG1-1 deposition on MoDCs resulted in cell activation, as evidenced by the similar increase in both cytokine production and expression of costimulatory proteins than those obtained with the nebulized-collected Ab. Thus, the collection system used here was considered relevant for these assays and was kept for the in vivo experiments.

Considering the complexity of the lung mucosal-associated immune system, it was necessary to use an animal model to predict the immunogenicity of nebulized Ab in vivo [52,53]. We chose murine antibodies to avoid a high immunogenic background response due to the non-specific activation of the mouse immune system by foreign proteins. In our study, we observed that single or repeated administration of a nebulized antibody in the lungs induced a significant contraction of the total and immune cell number in the airways starting quickly after the administration as compared to native Ab or saline controls. This was dependent on the number of aggregates as low aggregated Ab, filtered or PS80 preparation of nebulized Ab did not have any impact on cell number. Interestingly, at later time points, this contraction reached the lung parenchyma and the spleen, significantly reducing the number of both myeloid and lymphoid cells. We wondered whether this cell number reduction induced by the administration of nebulized Ab was associated with cell death. We observed that apoptosis was significantly increased in lung total cells and in leukocytes after the airway administration of nebulized Ab. Interestingly, these cellular injuries were dependent on the presence of aggregates, as Ab formulated with surfactant, known to limit aggregation [10], and even filtered nebulized Ab preparation did not promote cell death. These adverse effects were also dependent on the route of administration as nebulized Ab administered through the intravenous route was not associated with the same reduction in cell number. The complete understanding of the molecular and cellular mechanism associated with the massive cytotoxicity of nebulized and aggregated antibodies requires further investigations.

Protein aggregation underlies many chronic diseases where aggregates are thought to elicit injury, including cell apoptosis [54,55]. To the best of our knowledge, this is the first study reporting that extracellular therapeutic protein aggregates may sensitize the host to cytotoxicity. This cellular injury occurred in the absence of a pro-inflammatory response, which is contradictory with the current paradigm regarding the induction of innate immune responses by protein aggregates [13]. This discrepancy may come from the attributes of Ab aggregates associated with nebulization, as compared to those associated with other aggregation stresses, including the formation of neoepitopes, the immunomodulatory properties of the aggregates, the exposure of post-translational modifications or the generation of danger signals [56]. A complete understanding of the physical mechanisms accounting for the immunogenic properties of nebulized Ab aggregates is beyond the scope of this study. Immunogenicity may also be associated with the breakdown of self-tolerance rather than an active immune response [56]. It is particularly concordant with repeated exposure, which may occur during dosing regimens for chronic disease [36].

In conclusion, we demonstrated that aerosolization using a clinically-relevant nebulizer induced Ab aggregation and resulted in immune cell activation and immunocytotoxicity in vivo. Although there are still many questions to address to better understand the relationship between Ab aggregates and immunogenicity, our findings point to a significant role for the route of administration in the immunogenic/biological response associated to Ab aggregates. Further investigations will be required to determine the types and the number of aggregates and the role for the Fc domain in the immunocytotoxic response of Ab aggregates produced during nebulization. Our findings also highlight the importance to further explore the different methods (protein engineering, aerosolization process and formulations) to stabilize Ab during aerosolization to minimize risks for the patients.

Supplementary Materials: The following supporting information can be downloaded at: https://www.mdpi.com/article/10.3390/pharmaceutics14030671/s1, Figure S1: in vitro aerosol-MoDC exposure using Vitrocell; Figure S2: MoDC activation by nebulized mIgG2b-1; Figure S3: Lung cell immunophenotyping after administration of nebulized mIgG2b-1; Figure S4: Protein content in BALF after administration of nebulized mIgG2b-1; Figure S5: Apoptosis of lung and airway cells after administration of nebulized mIgG2b-2; Figure S6: Lung and airway cell count after i.v administration of nebulized mIgG2b-1; Figure S7: Effect of PS80 on the generation of aggregate after mIgG2b-1 nebulization; Figure S8: Lung cell count after administration of nebulized mIgG2b-1 supplemented with 0.05%-PS80; Table S1: Dynamic light scattering analysis of nebulized antibodies; Table S2: List of antibodies used for flow cytometry; Table S3: Phenotype of analyzed cells; Table S4: Particle size distribution (%) of nebulized antibodies; Table S5: Dynamic light scattering analysis of nebulized antibodies; Table S6: Nanodrop analysis of antibody concentration.

Author Contributions: T.S. and N.H.-V. conceived the study. T.S., E.B.-M., C.P., L.B., M.C., M.F., G.I., R.M., O.S., R.R. and N.H.-V. substantially contributed to the acquisition, analysis or interpretation of data. G.I. performed machine-learning analysis of histological sections. O.S. loaned the VITROCELL Cloud 12 system and provided expertise regarding the ALICE–cloud system. T.S. and N.H.-V. contributed to the manuscript draft, revision and critical review. All authors have read and agreed to the published version of the manuscript.

Funding: This work was supported by a public grant overseen by the French National Research Agency (ANR) as part of the "Investissements d'Avenir" program (LabEx MAbImprove, ANR-10-LABX-53-01) and by Region Centre as part of the "Intérêt Régional" program (grant Novantinh). T.S. was funded by a fellowship from ANR-10-LABX-53-01.

Institutional Review Board Statement: All animal experiments complied with the current European legislative, regulatory and ethical requirements and were approved by the local and national animal care and use committee (reference: APAFIS No.10200-2017061311352787).

Informed Consent Statement: Not applicable.

Data Availability Statement: The data supporting this article will be shared on reasonable request to the corresponding author.

Acknowledgments: We sincerely thank David Fraser (Biotech Communication SARL, France) for copy-editing services and Roxane Lemoine (Université of Tours, EA4245) for providing MoDC.

Conflicts of Interest: N.H-V. is co-founder and scientific expert for Cynbiose Respiratory. In the past two years, she received consultancy fees from Eli Lilly, Argenx, Novartis and research support from Sanofi and Aerogen Ltd. R.M-L. is Head of R&D, Science and Emerging Technologies in Aerogen. All other authors have no competing interests to declare.

References

1. Anselmo, A.C.; Gokarn, Y.; Mitragotri, S. Non-invasive delivery strategies for biologics. *Nat. Rev. Drug Discov.* **2019**, *18*, 19–40. [CrossRef] [PubMed]
2. Dall'Acqua, W.F.; Kiener, P.A.; Wu, H. Properties of human IgG1s engineered for enhanced binding to the neonatal Fc receptor (FcRn). *J. Biol. Chem.* **2006**, *281*, 23514–23524. [CrossRef] [PubMed]
3. Hart, T.K.; Cook, R.M.; Zia-Amirhosseini, P.; Minthorn, E.; Sellers, T.S.; Maleeff, B.E.; Eustis, S.; Schwartz, L.W.; Tsui, P.; Appelbaum, E.R.; et al. Preclinical efficacy and safety of mepolizumab (SB-240563), a humanized monoclonal antibody to IL-5, in cynomolgus monkeys. *J. Allergy Clin. Immunol.* **2001**, *108*, 250–257. [CrossRef] [PubMed]
4. Koleba, T.; Ensom, M.H. Pharmacokinetics of intravenous immunoglobulin: A systematic review. *Pharmacotherapy* **2006**, *26*, 813–827. [CrossRef]
5. Bodier-Montagutelli, E.; Mayor, A.; Vecellio, L.; Respaud, R.; Heuzé-Vourc'h, N. Designing inhaled protein therapeutics for topical lung delivery: What are the next steps? *Expert Opin. Drug Deliv.* **2018**, *15*, 729–736. [CrossRef]
6. Secher, T.; Dalonneau, E.; Ferreira, M.; Parent, C.; Azzopardi, N.; Paintaud, G.; Si-Tahar, M.; Heuzé-Vourc'h, N. In a murine model of acute lung infection, airway administration of a therapeutic antibody confers greater protection than parenteral administration. *J. Control. Release* **2019**, *303*, 24–33. [CrossRef]
7. Secher, T.; Mayor, A.; Heuzé-Vourc'h, N. Inhalation of Immuno-Therapeutics/-Prophylactics to Fight Respiratory Tract Infections: An Appropriate Drug at the Right Place! *Front. Immunol.* **2019**, *10*, 2760. [CrossRef]
8. Depreter, F.; Pilcer, G.; Amighi, K. Inhaled proteins: Challenges and perspectives. *Int. J. Pharm.* **2013**, *447*, 251–280. [CrossRef]
9. Hertel, S.P.; Winter, G.; Friess, W. Protein stability in pulmonary drug delivery via nebulization. *Adv. Drug Deliv. Rev.* **2015**, *93*, 79–94. [CrossRef]
10. Respaud, R.; Marchand, D.; Parent, C.; Pelat, T.; Thullier, P.; Tournamille, J.F.; Viaud-Massuard, M.C.; Diot, P.; Si-Tahar, M.; Vecellio, L.; et al. Effect of formulation on the stability and aerosol performance of a nebulized antibody. *mAbs* **2014**, *6*, 1347–1355. [CrossRef]
11. Bodier-Montagutelli, E.; Respaud, R.; Perret, G.; Baptista, L.; Duquenne, P.; Heuzé-Vourc'h, N.; Vecellio, L. Protein stability during nebulization: Mind the collection step! *Eur. J. Pharm. Biopharm.* **2020**, *152*, 23–34. [CrossRef] [PubMed]
12. Braun, A.; Kwee, L.; Labow, M.A.; Alsenz, J. Protein aggregates seem to play a key role among the parameters influencing the antigenicity of interferon alpha (IFN-alpha) in normal and transgenic mice. *Pharm. Res.* **1997**, *14*, 1472–1478. [CrossRef] [PubMed]
13. Joubert, M.K.; Hokom, M.; Eakin, C.; Zhou, L.; Deshpande, M.; Baker, M.P.; Goletz, T.J.; Kerwin, B.A.; Chirmule, N.; Narhi, L.O.; et al. Highly aggregated antibody therapeutics can enhance the in vitro innate and late-stage T-cell immune responses. *J. Biol. Chem.* **2012**, *287*, 25266–25279. [CrossRef]
14. Uchino, T.; Miyazaki, Y.; Yamazaki, T.; Kagawa, Y. Immunogenicity of protein aggregates of a monoclonal antibody generated by forced shaking stress with siliconized and nonsiliconized syringes in BALB/c mice. *J. Pharm. Pharmacol.* **2017**, *69*, 1341–1351. [CrossRef]

15. Mahlangu, J.N.; Weldingh, K.N.; Lentz, S.R.; Kaicker, S.; Karim, F.A.; Matsushita, T.; Recht, M.; Tomczak, W.; Windyga, J.; Ehrenforth, S.; et al. Changes in the amino acid sequence of the recombinant human factor VIIa analog, vatreptacog alfa, are associated with clinical immunogenicity. *J. Thromb. Haemost.* **2015**, *13*, 1989–1998. [CrossRef]

16. Holland, M.C.; Wurthner, J.U.; Morley, P.J.; Birchler, M.A.; Lambert, J.; Albayaty, M.; Serone, A.P.; Wilson, R.; Chen, Y.; Forrest, R.M.; et al. Autoantibodies to variable heavy (VH) chain Ig sequences in humans impact the safety and clinical pharmacology of a VH domain antibody antagonist of TNF-alpha receptor 1. *J. Clin. Immunol.* **2013**, *33*, 1192–1203. [CrossRef] [PubMed]

17. Ponce, R.; Abad, L.; Amaravadi, L.; Gelzleichter, T.; Gore, E.; Green, J.; Gupta, S.; Herzyk, D.; Hurst, C.; Ivens, I.A.; et al. Immunogenicity of biologically-derived therapeutics: Assessment and interpretation of nonclinical safety studies. *Regul. Toxicol. Pharmacol.* **2009**, *54*, 164–182. [CrossRef]

18. Schellekens, H. Bioequivalence and the immunogenicity of biopharmaceuticals. *Nat. Rev. Drug Discov.* **2002**, *1*, 457–462. [CrossRef] [PubMed]

19. Li, J.; Yang, C.; Xia, Y.; Bertino, A.; Glaspy, J.; Roberts, M.; Kuter, D.J. Thrombocytopenia caused by the development of antibodies to thrombopoietin. *Blood* **2001**, *98*, 3241–3248. [CrossRef]

20. Demeule, B.; Gurny, R.; Arvinte, T. Where disease pathogenesis meets protein formulation: Renal deposition of immunoglobulin aggregates. *Eur. J. Pharm. Biopharm.* **2006**, *62*, 121–130. [CrossRef]

21. Kiese, S.; Papppenberger, A.; Friess, W.; Mahler, H.C. Shaken, not stirred: Mechanical stress testing of an IgG1 antibody. *J. Pharm. Sci.* **2008**, *97*, 4347–4366. [CrossRef] [PubMed]

22. Fathallah, A.M.; Bankert, R.B.; Balu-Iyer, S.V. Immunogenicity of subcutaneously administered therapeutic proteins—A mechanistic perspective. *AAPS J.* **2013**, *15*, 897–900. [CrossRef] [PubMed]

23. Mahler, H.C.; Friess, W.; Grauschopf, U.; Kiese, S. Protein aggregation: Pathways, induction factors and analysis. *J. Pharm. Sci.* **2009**, *98*, 2909–2934. [CrossRef] [PubMed]

24. Lamichhane, A.; Azegamia, T.; Kiyonoa, H. The mucosal immune system for vaccine development. *Vaccine* **2014**, *32*, 6711–6723. [CrossRef]

25. Frank, D.W.; Vallis, A.; Wiener-Kronish, J.P.; Roy-Burman, A.; Spack, E.G.; Mullaney, B.P.; Megdoud, M.; Marks, J.D.; Fritz, R.; Sawa, T. Generation and characterization of a protective monoclonal antibody to *Pseudomonas aeruginosa* PcrV. *J. Infect. Dis.* **2002**, *186*, 64–73. [CrossRef]

26. Lenz, A.G.; Stoeger, T.; Cei, D.; Schmidmeir, M.; Semren, N.; Burgstaller, G.; Lentner, B.; Eickelberg, O.; Meiners, S.; Schmid, O. Efficient bioactive delivery of aerosolized drugs to human pulmonary epithelial cells cultured in air-liquid interface conditions. *Am. J. Respir. Cell Mol. Biol.* **2014**, *51*, 526–535. [CrossRef]

27. Spadaro, M.; Montone, M.; Cavallo, F. Generation and Maturation of Human Monocyte-derived DCs. *Bio-Protocol* **2014**, *4*, e1194. [CrossRef]

28. Arganda-Carreras, I.; Kaynig, V.; Rueden, C.; Eliceiri, K.W.; Schindelin, J.; Cardona, A.; Sebastian Seung, H. Trainable Weka Segmentation: A machine learning tool for microscopy pixel classification. *Bioinformatics* **2017**, *33*, 2424–2426. [CrossRef]

29. Zolls, S.; Tantipolphan, R.; Wiggenhorn, M.; Winter, G.; Jiskoot, W.; Friess, W.; Hawe, A. Particles in therapeutic protein formulations, Part 1: Overview of analytical methods. *J. Pharm. Sci.* **2012**, *101*, 914–935. [CrossRef]

30. EMEA Documentation. Guideline on Immunogenicity Assessment of Therapeutic Proteins. 2017. Available online: https://www.ema.europa.eu/en/documents/scientific-guideline/guideline-immunogenicity-assessment-therapeutic-proteins-revision-1_en.pdf (accessed on 18 January 2022).

31. FDA Documentation. Immunogenicity Assessment for Therapeutic Protein Products—Guidance for Industry. 2014. Available online: https://www.fda.gov/regulatory-information/search-fda-guidance-documents/immunogenicity-assessment-therapeutic-protein-products (accessed on 18 January 2022).

32. Galluzzi, L.; Bravo-San Pedro, J.M.; Kepp, O.; Kroemer, G. Regulated cell death and adaptive stress responses. *Cell. Mol. Life Sci.* **2016**, *73*, 2405–2410. [CrossRef]

33. Galluzzi, L.; Bravo-San Pedro, J.M.; Vitale, I.; Aaronson, S.A.; Abrams, J.M.; Adam, D.; Alnemri, E.S.; Altucci, L.; Andrews, D.; Annicchiarico-Petruzzelli, M.; et al. Essential versus accessory aspects of cell death: Recommendations of the NCCD 2015. *Cell Death Differ.* **2015**, *22*, 58–73. [CrossRef] [PubMed]

34. Vermes, I.; Haanen, C.; Steffens-Nakken, H.; Reutelingsperger, C. A novel assay for apoptosis. Flow cytometric detection of phosphatidylserine expression on early apoptotic cells using fluorescein labelled Annexin V. *J. Immunol. Methods* **1995**, *184*, 39–51. [CrossRef]

35. Moussa, E.M.; Panchal, J.P.; Moorthy, B.S.; Blum, J.S.; Joubert, M.K.; Narhi, L.O.; Topp, E.M. Immunogenicity of Therapeutic Protein Aggregates. *J. Pharm. Sci.* **2016**, *105*, 417–430. [CrossRef] [PubMed]

36. Ratanji, K.D.; Derrick, J.P.; Dearman, R.J.; Kimber, I. Immunogenicity of therapeutic proteins: Influence of aggregation. *J. Immunotoxicol.* **2014**, *11*, 99–109. [CrossRef]

37. Ross, C.; Clemmesen, K.M.; Svenson, M.; Sorensen, P.S.; Koch-Henriksen, N.; Skovgaard, G.L.; Bendtzen, K. Immunogenicity of interferon-beta in multiple sclerosis patients: Influence of preparation, dosage, dose frequency, and route of administration. *Ann. Neurol.* **2000**, *48*, 706–712. [CrossRef]

38. Hermeling, S.; Schellekens, H.; Crommelin, D.J.; Jiskoot, W. Micelle-associated protein in epoetin formulations: A risk factor for immunogenicity? *Pharm. Res.* **2003**, *20*, 1903–1907. [CrossRef]

39. Cromwell, M.E.; Hilario, E.; Jacobson, F. Protein aggregation and bioprocessing. *AAPS J.* **2006**, *8*, E572–E579. [CrossRef]

40. Joubert, M.K.; Luo, Q.; Nashed-Samuel, Y.; Wypych, J.; Narhi, L.O. Classification and characterization of therapeutic antibody aggregates. *J. Biol. Chem.* **2011**, *286*, 25118–25133. [CrossRef]
41. Wang, W. Protein aggregation and its inhibition in biopharmaceutics. *Int. J. Pharm.* **2005**, *289*, 1–30. [CrossRef]
42. Lightwood, D.; O'Dowd, V.; Carrington, B.; Veverka, V.; Carr, M.D.; Tservistas, M.; Henry, A.J.; Smith, B.; Tyson, K.; Lamour, S.; et al. The discovery, engineering and characterisation of a highly potent anti-human IL-13 fab fragment designed for administration by inhalation. *J. Mol. Biol.* **2013**, *425*, 577–593. [CrossRef]
43. Maillet, A.; Congy-Jolivet, N.; Le Guellec, S.; Vecellio, L.; Hamard, S.; Courty, Y.; Courtois, A.; Gauthier, F.; Diot, P.; Thibault, G.; et al. Aerodynamical, immunological and pharmacological properties of the anticancer antibody cetuximab following nebulization. *Pharm. Res.* **2008**, *25*, 1318–1326. [CrossRef]
44. Kraus, T.; Winter, G.; Engert, J. Test models for the evaluation of immunogenicity of protein aggregates. *Int. J. Pharm.* **2019**, *559*, 192–200. [CrossRef] [PubMed]
45. Carpenter, J.F.; Randolph, T.W.; Jiskoot, W.; Crommelin, D.J.; Middaugh, C.R.; Winter, G.; Fan, Y.X.; Kirshner, S.; Verthelyi, D.; Kozlowski, S.; et al. Overlooking subvisible particles in therapeutic protein products: Gaps that may compromise product quality. *J. Pharm. Sci.* **2009**, *98*, 1201–1205. [CrossRef] [PubMed]
46. Telikepalli, S.; Kumru, O.S.; Kim, J.H.; Joshi, S.B.; O'Berry, K.B.; Blake-Haskins, A.W.; Perkins, M.D.; Middaugh, C.R.; Volkin, D.B. Characterization of the physical stability of a lyophilized IgG1 mAb after accelerated shipping-like stress. *J. Pharm. Sci.* **2015**, *104*, 495–507. [CrossRef] [PubMed]
47. Xiang, S.D.; Scholzen, A.; Minigo, G.; David, C.; Apostolopoulos, V.; Mottram, P.L.; Plebanski, M. Pathogen recognition and development of particulate vaccines: Does size matter? *Methods* **2006**, *40*, 1–9. [CrossRef] [PubMed]
48. Hertel, S.; Friess, W.; Winter, G. Comparison of Aerosol Collection Methods for Liquid Protein Formulations. In Proceedings of the Respiratory Drug Delivery Europe 2011, Berlin, Germany, 3–6 May 2011.
49. Brandenberger, C.; Muhlfeld, C.; Ali, Z.; Lenz, A.G.; Schmid, O.; Parak, W.J.; Gehr, P.; Rothen-Rutishauser, B. Quantitative evaluation of cellular uptake and trafficking of plain and polyethylene glycol-coated gold nanoparticles. *Small* **2010**, *6*, 1669–1678. [CrossRef]
50. Brandenberger, C.; Rothen-Rutishauser, B.; Muhlfeld, C.; Schmid, O.; Ferron, G.A.; Maier, K.L.; Gehr, P.; Lenz, A.G. Effects and uptake of gold nanoparticles deposited at the air-liquid interface of a human epithelial airway model. *Toxicol. Appl. Pharmacol.* **2010**, *242*, 56–65. [CrossRef]
51. Rohm, M.; Carle, S.; Maigler, F.; Flamm, J.; Kramer, V.; Mavoungou, C.; Schmid, O.; Schindowski, K. A comprehensive screening platform for aerosolizable protein formulations for intranasal and pulmonary drug delivery. *Int. J. Pharm.* **2017**, *532*, 537–546. [CrossRef]
52. Shomali, M.; Freitag, A.; Engert, J.; Siedler, M.; Kaymakcalan, Z.; Winter, G.; Carpenter, J.F.; Randolph, T.W. Antibody responses in mice to particles formed from adsorption of a murine monoclonal antibody onto glass microparticles. *J. Pharm. Sci.* **2014**, *103*, 78–89. [CrossRef]
53. Freitag, A.J.; Shomali, M.; Michalakis, S.; Biel, M.; Siedler, M.; Kaymakcalan, Z.; Carpenter, J.F.; Randolph, T.W.; Winter, G.; Engert, J. Investigation of the immunogenicity of different types of aggregates of a murine monoclonal antibody in mice. *Pharm. Res.* **2015**, *32*, 430–444. [CrossRef]
54. Lim, J.; Yue, Z. Neuronal aggregates: Formation, clearance, and spreading. *Dev. Cell* **2015**, *32*, 491–501. [CrossRef] [PubMed]
55. Bucciantini, M.; Calloni, G.; Chiti, F.; Formigli, L.; Nosi, D.; Dobson, C.M.; Stefani, M. Prefibrillar amyloid protein aggregates share common features of cytotoxicity. *J. Biol. Chem.* **2004**, *279*, 31374–31382. [CrossRef] [PubMed]
56. Dingman, R.; Balu-Iyer, S.V. Immunogenicity of Protein Pharmaceuticals. *J. Pharm. Sci.* **2019**, *108*, 1637–1654. [CrossRef] [PubMed]

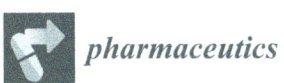

pharmaceutics

Article

Biopharmaceutical Assessment of Mesh Aerosolised Plasminogen, a Step towards ARDS Treatment

Lucia Vizzoni [1,2,†], Chiara Migone [1,†], Brunella Grassiri [1], Ylenia Zambito [1,3], Baldassare Ferro [4], Paolo Roncucci [4], Filippo Mori [5], Alfonso Salvatore [5], Ester Ascione [5], Roberto Crea [5], Semih Esin [6,7], Giovanna Batoni [6,7] and Anna Maria Piras [1,7,*]

1   Department of Pharmacy, University of Pisa, 56126 Pisa, Italy
2   Department of Life Sciences, University of Siena, 53100 Siena, Italy
3   Research Centre for Nutraceutical and Healthy Foods "NUTRAFOOD", University of Pisa, 56124 Pisa, Italy
4   Anestesia e Rianimazione, Azienda USL Toscana Nord Ovest, 57124 Livorno, Italy
5   Kedrion S.p.A., Via di Fondovalle, Loc. Bolognana, 55027 Gallicano, Italy
6   Department of Translational Research and New Technologies in Medicine and Surgery, University of Pisa, 56126 Pisa, Italy
7   Centre for Instrument Sharing of University of Pisa (CISUP), 56126 Pisa, Italy
*   Correspondence: anna.piras@unipi.it; Tel.: +39-050-2219704
†   These authors contributed equally to this work.

Citation: Vizzoni, L.; Migone, C.; Grassiri, B.; Zambito, Y.; Ferro, B.; Roncucci, P.; Mori, F.; Salvatore, A.; Ascione, E.; Crea, R.; et al. Biopharmaceutical Assessment of Mesh Aerosolised Plasminogen, a Step towards ARDS Treatment. *Pharmaceutics* **2023**, *15*, 1618. https://doi.org/10.3390/pharmaceutics15061618

Academic Editors: Michael Yee Tak Chow, Philip Chi Lip Kwok and Ivana D'Angelo

Received: 27 February 2023
Revised: 18 May 2023
Accepted: 26 May 2023
Published: 30 May 2023

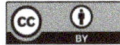
Abstract: Acute respiratory distress syndrome (ARDS) is a severe complication of lung injuries, commonly associated with bacterial, fungal and viral infections, including SARS-CoV-2 viral infections. ARDS is strongly correlated with patient mortality and its clinical management is very complex, with no effective treatment presently available. ARDS involves severe respiratory failure, fibrin deposition in both airways and lung parenchyma, with the development of an obstructing hyaline membrane drastically limiting gas exchange. Moreover, hypercoagulation is related to deep lung inflammation, and a pharmacological action toward both aspects is expected to be beneficial. Plasminogen (PLG) is a main component of the fibrinolytic system playing key roles in various inflammation regulatory processes. The inhalation of PLG has been proposed in the form of the off-label administration of an eyedrop solution, namely, a plasminogen-based orphan medicinal product (PLG-OMP), by means of jet nebulisation. Being a protein, PLG is susceptible to partial inactivation under jet nebulisation. The aim of the present work is to demonstrate the efficacy of the mesh nebulisation of PLG-OMP in an in vitro simulation of clinical off-label administration, considering both the enzymatic and immunomodulating activities of PLG. Biopharmaceutical aspects are also investigated to corroborate the feasibility of PLG-OMP administration by inhalation. The nebulisation of the solution was performed using an Aerogen® Solo™ vibrating-mesh nebuliser. Aerosolised PLG showed an optimal in vitro deposition profile, with 90% of the active ingredient impacting the lower portions of a glass impinger. The nebulised PLG remained in its monomeric form, with no alteration of glycoform composition and 94% of enzymatic activity maintenance. Activity loss was observed only when PLG-OMP nebulisation was performed under simulated clinical oxygen administration. In vitro investigations evidenced good penetration of aerosolised PLG through artificial airway mucus, as well as poor permeation across an Air–Liquid Interface model of pulmonary epithelium. The results suggest a good safety profile of inhalable PLG, excluding high systemic absorption but with good mucus diffusion. Most importantly, the aerosolised PLG was capable of reversing the effects of an LPS-activated macrophage RAW 264.7 cell line, demonstrating the immunomodulating activity of PLG in an already induced inflammatory state. All physical, biochemical and biopharmaceutical assessments of mesh aerosolised PLG-OMP provided evidence for its potential off-label administration as a treatment for ARDS patients.

Keywords: ARDS; COVID-19; SARS-CoV-2; C-ARDS; plasminogen; pulmonary delivery; lung in vitro model; immunomodulating activity

1. Introduction

Acute respiratory distress syndrome (ARDS) is described as noncardiogenic pulmonary oedema accompanied by severe lung inflammation, hypoxemia and decreased lung compliance. Respiratory failure is therefore the consequence of reduced alveolar–capillary oxygen transfer due to inflammation, vascular microthrombus and hyaline membrane/oedema in the alveoli [1,2].

For ARDS, there is no established gold standard for diagnosis, and it is still unknown whether the condition is caused by a single pathophysiologic mechanism or a number of processes with comparable clinical manifestations. As reported in the ATS/ERS criteria, from a histological point of view, ARDS is characterised by neutrophil infiltration, fluid in the alveoli and the presence of microthrombus, i.e., the triad of ARDS [3]. Increased pulmonary microvascular permeability can be brought about by several direct and indirect lung injuries, allowing protein-rich fluid to enter the alveolar spaces of the lung at normal hydrostatic pressures.

ARDS is a severe complication of lung injuries such as pneumonia, arising from either viral, fungus or bacterial infection. Furthermore, whatever the initial lung injury, patients with ARDS are greatly susceptible to secondary pulmonary infection [4,5]. Despite the improvement in our understanding of ARDS pathophysiology and treatment, the patient mortality rate remains extremely high (35–40%) [6]. ARDS can also result from SARS-CoV-2 infection, which mainly causes endothelial damages. Nearly 75% of COVID-19 patients admitted to intensive care units have thrombotic coagulopathy, and both the clinical picture and the pathologic results are consistent with occlusive microvasculature. When ARDS occurs as part of COVID-19, it is called COVID-19-related acute respiratory distress syndrome (C-ARDS). This new type of severe acute respiratory syndrome meets the Berlin 2012 ARDS definition, even if it seems to be a disease with different phenotypes [7]. The main distinction between C-ARDS and traditional ARDS is the preservation of the patients' respiratory mechanics in the face of severe hypoxemia. Indeed, the severity of ARDS is significantly associated with the mortality rate of critically ill patients [8], and recently [9], the significant correlation between hypercoagulation and inflammation (neutrophil infiltration and activation) was confirmed.

The main goal for treating ARDS is improved oxygenation and ventilation, often combining adjunctive (neuromuscular blocking agents, prone positioning) and pharmacological therapies [10]. As part of the therapy for the underlying disease (such as shock, trauma, sepsis, pneumonia, aspiration or burns), mechanical ventilation is critical for resolving life-threatening hypoxia and needs careful monitoring to avoid overinflation, barotrauma and cyclic closing/reopening of the alveoli [11]. Despite several clinical trials, few and often controversial positive results have been obtained. Salbutamol (conventionally applied for asthma and chronic obstructive pulmonary disease (COPD)) has shown poor tolerability and has been found to worsen ARDS patient outcomes [12]; simvastatin (an HMG-CoA reductase inhibitor) has shown no effects on ARDS outcomes [13]; and Interferon β-1a (inhibits tumour necrosis factor (TNF), exerts antiviral and antiproliferative properties) has led to no significant reduction in ARDS patient mortality [14]. For C-ARDS patients, only Favipiravir (anti-viral agent, inhibits the RNA-dependent RNA polymerase of RNA viruses) and Tocilizumab (humanised anti-human IL-6 receptor antibody) have shown a significant association with the course of severity of ARDS [15–17]. In contrast, the effectiveness of corticosteroids in viral ARDS remains controversial [18]. This scenario evidences an urgent need for a pharmacologically effective ARDS treatment. As such, the off-label administration of clinically relevant medicines appears to be worth pursuing [19].

Regardless of the initial aetiology, ARDS is characterised histologically by diffuse alveolar damage with interstitial and alveolar infiltration of neutrophils and macrophages [20]. The scientific community confirms that thrombolytic activity on fibrin depots in the lungs could enhance the ventilation–perfusion ratio of ARDS and C-ARDS patients [21]. However, these treatments are often administered parenterally, which involves a significant risk of systemic bleeding [22], whereas the inhalation pathway may reduce systemic exposure to fibrinolysis and promote a pulmonary loco-regional effect. The endogenous fibrinolytic system includes plasminogen (PLG) as a key component. PLG is a single-chain plasma protein (MW 92 kDa); it is the zymogen (inactive form) of the serine protease plasmin (fibrinolytic enzyme). PLG activators (t-PA and u-PA) convert PLG to plasmin, which lyses fibrin clots into eliminable products. Additionally, PLG contributes to the regulation of physiological processes like wound healing and operates as an immunomodulator in inflammation [23].

This work is part of a project aiming at consolidating the scientific evidence that supports the clinical pulmonary administration of PLG in ARDS patient. In particular, the work involves the off-label use of a PLG-based eye drop, namely, a human plasminogen orphan medicine (PLG-OMP, Orphan Medicinal Product number EU/3/07/461). PLG-OMP aerosolisation has been preliminary assessed, matching the Ph. Eur. requirements for a solution for aerosolisation [1]. However, part of the enzymatic activity was lost during either ultrasonic or jet nebulisation; it was found a limited correspondence between suitable lung-targeted aerodynamic distribution and activity performance. Since nebulisation techniques can affect the physical–chemical properties of labile drugs by generating heat and shear stresses [24] , the hypothesis of the present work is that mesh nebulisation could provide lower damaging stress but maintain lung-targeted aerodynamic features. Additionally, no previous pulmonary biopharmaceutical assessment of the zimogen protein PLG has been reported in the literature. To form the basis for PLG-OMP clinical off-label administration, a pulmonary biopharmaceutical evaluation is proposed here. Beyond the enzymatic activity, we also hypothesise that it is possible to take advantage of the immunomodulating effect of PLG. To verify the latter hypothesis, the nebulised PLG was tested for the first time on a cellular model of inflammation. The model was developed ad hoc to simulate the administration of the drug on a pre-established inflamed condition.

2. Materials and Methods

The workflow of the performed studies is reported in Scheme S1 (Supporting Info File).

2.1. Materials

Human plasminogen eye drops 1 mg/mL (PLG-OMP, Orphan Medicinal Product number EU/3/07/461 in EU and Orphan Designation number 10-3092 in US), Kedrion S.p.A. (Gallicano, (Lu) Italy). BIOPHEN™ Plasminogen LRT Ref 22151 (HYPHEN BioMed, Neuville-sur-Oise, France), Human PLG (Plasminogen) ELISA Kit, bicinchoninic acid assay (BCA), Toluene, Acetone, Citric Acid, Diethylenetriaminepentaacetic acid (DTPA), Egg Yolk Emulsion, gelatine from bovine skin type B, RPMI amino acid solution and type II mucin from porcine stomach were purchased from Sigma Aldrich (Milano, Italy). Clioxycarb O_2/CO_2 gas 95/5 by mol mixture was purchased from SOL S.p.A. (Monza, Italy). Human lung adenocarcinoma NCI-H441 epithelial cell line was purchased from the American Type Culture Collection LGC standards ((ATCC HTB-174), Milan, Italy) and propagated as indicated by the supplier. The murine macrophage cell line RAW 264.7 was purchased from the Cell Lines Service (Eppelheim, Germany) and propagated as indicated by the supplier. Dulbecco's phosphate-buffered saline (DPBS), fetal bovine serum (FBS), antibiotics (penicillin/streptomycin), RPMI-1640 medium and Dulbecco's Modified Eagles Medium (DMEM) were purchased from Sigma Aldrich (Milan, Italy). Cell proliferation reagent (WST-1) was provided by Roche diagnostic (Milan, Italy). Insulin-Transferrin-Selenium (ITS), Dexamethasone, Trypsin-EDTA and Triton X-100 were purchased from Sigma Aldrich (Italy). Haematoxylin and Eosin were purchased from Fluka (Buchs, Switzerland). Normal goat serum (NGS), primary antibody for *Zonula Occludens-1* (ZO-1), primary antibody for Occludin, primary antibody for E-cadherin, Alexa Fluor 594 anti-rabbit and Alexa Fluor 488 anti-mouse were purchased from Thermo Fisher Scientific (Waltham, MA, USA). Hank's buffer salts solution (HBSS10X) was obtained from Corning, Manassas (VI, USA) and 1 to ten diluted with deionised water when necessary. Multiplex LEGENDplex Mouse Macrophage/Microglia Panel Detection was obtained from Biolegend (Campoverde, Italy).

ProlongTM Diamond Antifade Mountant with DAPI were purchased from Thermo Fisher Scientific (Waltham, MA, USA).

2.2. Plasminogen (PLG-OMP) Aerosolisation

Aliquots of 5 mL of PLG-OMP were atomised using the Aerogen Solo® mesh nebuliser (Galway, Ireland). Nebulisation was performed in either air or oxygen-rich conditions by using 10 L/min flow of compressed air or 95% O_2 and 5% CO_2 molar mixture (clioxycarb), respectively. Nebulisation was conducted until no cloud was produced. Atomised samples were collected by condensation into a glass bioaerosol impinger (0–4 °C) [25]. Both the residual solutions in the nebuliser cup and the collected nebulised aliquots were submitted to biochemical characterisation (enzymatic activity and electrophoretic SDS-PAGE) and compared to the untreated PLG-OMP solutions (CTRL).

The presence of protein aggregates or fragments of PLG was evaluated by dynamic light scattering (DLS—Zetasizer Nano ZS, Malvern Panalytical Ltd., Malvern, UK). Protein analysis was performed by setting proteins as the material (RI 1.450; Absorption 0.001) and water as the dispersant (T 25 °C; RI 1.330), with a display range of 0.1–6000 and a threshold of 0.05–0.01. The molecular weight of the main protein peak and its mass percentage were obtained based on scattering intensity data. Protocol validation is reported in the Supplementary Information File (Figure S1).

2.3. Maintenance of Enzymatic Activity

A Plasminogen chromogenic kit (BIOPHEN™ Plasminogen LRT, HYPHEN BioMed) was applied to evaluate the PLG activity maintenance after nebulisation. The assay involves two reagents: streptokinase (R1) and a chromogenic substrate (R2). The PLG activity is measured following its specific activation by the addition of streptokinase; the complex plasminogen-streptokinase cleaves the plasmin-specific substrate SPm41, releasing para-nitroaniline (pNA) and absorbing at 405 nm. PLG activity was calculated on a calibration curve built by using untreated PLG-OMP 10–80 µg/mL samples (R^2 = 0.9902). A bicinchoninic acid assay (BCA) was used for the quantification of the protein content (PLG-OMP calibration curve 5–80 µg/mL; R^2 = 0.9997). The maintenance of the enzymatic activity of the nebulised samples was expressed as reported below, where the reference PLG-OMP product corresponded to 100% activity.

$$(\%) = 100 \times (\mu g/mL \text{ of active protein (Activity Assay)})/(\mu g/mL \text{ of total protein (BCA)}) \quad (1)$$

2.4. Protein Characterisation

SDS-PAGE was used to determine the native glutamic acid-plasminogen (Glu-PLG) and lysine-plasminogen (Lys-PLG). SDS-PAGE was performed under denaturing conditions with a 4–12% gel (Invitrogen, Carlsbad, CA, USA). PLG samples and home-made PLG standard were prepared with an LDS sample buffer 4× (Invitrogen) denaturing agent, followed by 5 min of heat denaturation at 95 °C. The gel was loaded with 4 µg of protein PLG samples, and the electrophoretic run lasted 55 min at 200 volts. The gel was captured using Chemidoc MP by the ImageLab software Lys-PLG. The results were expressed as a percentage of the band assigned to Glu-PLG or Lys-PLG in comparison to all bands in the line.

2.5. Droplet Distribution of Nebulised PLG-OMP

The aerodynamic evaluation of the aerosol clouds was performed by using a glass twin stage impinger (TSI), according to European Pharmacopoeia X ed., 2.9.18 Apparatus A procedure [26]. The B portion of the impinger was connected to the T-piece junction of the mesh nebuliser and a mechanical pump (Edwards RV5, Irvine, CA, USA) provided 60 L/min air flow. Fine droplets were captured between the TSI and the pump on a propylene filter (low resistance filter, PARI) and a cold trap. The upper and lower chambers of TSI were filled with 7 mL and 30 mL of 0.2 µm filtered Milli-Q water, respectively. PLG-

OMP (5 mL) was placed into the nebuliser cup. Before each nebulisation, 60 ± 5 L/min flow were guaranteed at the inlet to the throat, as measured with a flow meter (Brooks Instrument, Hatfield, PA, USA). The pump was started and, after 10 s, the nebuliser as well. At the end of nebulisation, the upper and lower stage solutions were collected individually and then washed with Milli-Q water. The collected protein was quantified by BCA. The procedure was repeated six times. The results for each of the two parts of the apparatus were expressed as a percentage of the total amount of active substance.

2.6. Penetration of Aerosolised PLG through Artificial Mucus

An in vitro mucus model was set, as reported by Costabile et al. 2016 [27]. The first to propose this composition was Ghani et al. [28], who developed a simulated mucus based on patients' sputum. Briefly, 1 mL of gelatine solution (10% w/v) was placed in each well of a 24-well plate, hardened at room temperature and stored at 4 °C until use. The artificial airway mucus was prepared by adding 250 µL of sterile egg yolk emulsion, 250 mg of mucin, 0.295 mg DTPA, 250 mg sodium chloride, 110 mg potassium chloride and 1 mL of RPMI to 50 mL of water [29]. Then, 1 mL of artificial mucus was placed on each of the hardened gelatine gels. PLG-OMP was directly nebulised for 30 s on each artificial mucus sample, and the plates were incubated maintaining 100% relative humidity so as to simulate a wet environment. At regular time intervals, the artificial mucus was withdrawn and separated from the gelatine gel. The PLG content in the gelatine and artificial mucus was quantified by specific Human PLG ELISA assay (Sigma-Aldrich).

2.7. Biological Investigation

In vitro biological evaluations were conducted on lung epithelial NCI-H441 cell line and on macrophage RAW 264.7 cell line. NCI-H441 cells were grown in RPMI-1640 medium (RPMI) with 1% pen/strep and 10% FBS at 37 °C in a 5% CO_2 atmosphere, while RAW 264.7 cells were grown in Dulbecco's Modified Eagles Medium (DMEM) with 1% pen/strep and 10% FBS at 37 °C in a 5% CO_2 atmosphere.

2.7.1. PLG Permeability across an In Vitro Model of Pulmonary Epithelium
Cytotoxicity Screening on NCI-H441 Cells by Tetrazolium Salts Assay (WST-1)

Cell viability studies were carried out on the NCI-H441 cell line in 96-well plates using the WST-1 test [30]. The cells were seeded in 96-well plates (4×10^4 cells/well). After 24 h, the culture medium was removed and replaced with test samples (PLG-OMP in the range of 4–900 µg/mL). After 4 h of incubation, media were removed, cells were washed twice with PBS and tetrazolium salt WST-1 (1/10 in medium) was added. The produced formazan was quantified after 4 h incubation at 450 nm with a microplate reader (BioTek 800/TS, Thermo Scientific, Walthman, MA, USA). Finally, the half-maximal inhibitory concentration (IC50) was determined.

In Vitro Air–Liquid Interface (ALI) Model

NCI-H441 cells were seeded onto a Transwell® insert (2.5×10^4 cells/well), and 600 µL of full medium was added into the basolateral chamber. After 48 h, the apical medium was removed (100 µL), leaving the apical surface of the cells exposed to air (air–liquid culture) while that of the basolateral chamber was replaced with cell medium containing 1% insulin transferrin selenium (ITS) and 200 nM dexamethasone. Cell monolayer formation was monitored by measuring the transepithelial electrical resistance (TEER) using a voltmeter with rod electrodes (Voltmeter Millicelles-ERS, Millipore, Molsheim, France). Monolayer formation and differentiation were verified by microscopy analysis of haematoxylin/eosin-stained samples and immunofluorescence analyses. For haematoxylin/eosin staining, the monolayers were washed with deionised water for 5 min, then haematoxylin (0.7% w/v, sodium iodate, aluminium ammonium sulphate 12 H_2O) was added and the mixture was incubated for 5 min. After washing with water, the samples were treated for 2 min with eosin (0.5% w/v in acidified 90% ethanol) for cytoplasm staining. Immunofluorescence staining of adhesion molecules, i.e., Zonula occludens-1 (ZO-1), E-cadherin and Occludin, was performed [31]. NCI-H441 monolayers were first fixed with 3.8% paraformaldehyde in PBS 1× for 1 h, treated with PBS 1×//Triton X-100 solution (0.2% v/v) for 15 min and blocked with normal goat serum (NGS, 1% w/v in PBS 1×) for 30 min. Anti-E-cadherin (1:100 in NGS), anti- ZO-1 (1:500) and anti-Occludin (1:50 in NGS) were applied separately on individual monolayer samples and incubated overnight at 4 °C. After washing with NGS solution (1% w/v in PBS 1×), samples were incubated for 2 h in the dark with the secondary antibody. Finally, samples were mounted on slides (ProlongTM Diamond Antifade Mountant with DAPI, Thermo Fisher Scientific). The samples were observed with a fluorescence laser scanning microscope (Nikon Eclipse Ts2R, Tokyo, Japan) using the following wavelengths: E-cadherin and Occludin λ_{ex} 499 nm/λ_{em} 519 nm, λ_{ex} 591 nm/λ_{em} 618 nm for ZO-1 and λ_{ex} 345 nm/λ_{em} 455 nm for nuclei (DAPI).

Assessment of Nebulised PLG Permeation through ALI Monolayer

Firstly, a cytotoxicity evaluation was performed. PLG-OMP was nebulised for 30 s directly on the apical portion of the NCI-H441 monolayers (n = 3) (Figure 1). The deposited PLG corresponded to 30.0 ± 0.06 µg of protein. Nebulised samples were then incubated for 2 h with 600 µL of HBSS 1×, placed in the basolateral chamber. At the end of the incubation time, the monolayers were rinsed with PBS 1×, and tetrazolium salt WST-1 (1/10 in medium) was added. The formazan produced was quantified at 450 nm.

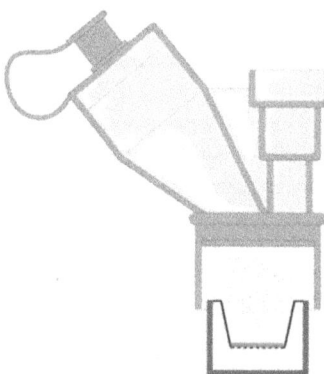

Figure 1. Setup for the direct nebulisation on an ALI monolayer with the Aerogen® Solo™ mesh nebuliser.

For permeation experiments, PLG-OMP was nebulised for 30 s on NCI-H441 ALI monolayers (n = 16) and then incubated with 600 µL of HBSS 1× in a basolateral chamber. At regular time intervals (30, 60, 90, 120 min), the HBSS was withdrawn and the permeated plasminogen was quantified by PLG ELISA assay (Sigma-Aldrich). Apparent permeability (Papp) was calculated from the linear correlation observed on a cumulative concentrations vs. time plot:

$$\text{Papp} = ((dC/dt)V)/(AC_0), \qquad (2)$$

where dC/dt is the line slope, V is chamber volume, A is the monolayer area and C_0 is the PLG concentration in PLG-OMP. The experiment was performed under sink conditions.

2.7.2. Immunomodulating Activity of Nebulised PLG

At first, cell viability studies were carried out on the RAW 264.7 cell line. Cells were seeded in 24-well plates at 10^6, 6.5×10^5 and 5×10^5 cells/well for cytotoxicity studies at 6, 18 and 24 h respectively. Then, 24 h after seeding, the culture medium was removed and replaced with test samples, either 5–20–50 µg/mL of PLG or 1 µg/mL LPS. After incubation, media were removed, and tetrazolium salt WST-1 (1/10 in medium) was added after washing with PBS 1×. The formazan produced was quantified at 450 nm with a microplate reader. Preliminary RAW 264.7 activation assays were performed using LPS in the range of 0.2–1 µg/mL. Cells (5×10^5) were seeded in 24-well plates and left to proliferate for 24 h prior to the incubation with LPS samples, which lasted a further 24 h. At the end of the incubation time, the supernatant was collected and analysed using the LEGENDplex Mouse Macrophage/Microglia Panel Detection multiplex system (Campoverde, Italy) for TNF-α, IL-1β and IL-6 quantification.

The evaluation of the maintenance of PLG immunomodulatory activity was performed as follows. RAW 264.7 cells were seeded in 24-well plates (10^6 cells/well) and left to proliferate for 24 h at 37 °C, 5% CO_2. The cells were incubated with LPS (0.2 µg/mL). After 6 h, PLG (5 µg/mL) and the nebulised PLG collected on a glass bioaerosol impinger (5 µg/mL) were added and incubated for additional 18 h. Cells treated with medium and with LPS only (0.2 µg/mL) were used as the negative and positive controls, respectively. At the end of the incubation time, the supernatant of each sample was collected and centrifuged at $300 \times g$ for 10 min at 4 °C. The obtained supernatants were evaluated for TNF-α, IL-1β and IL-6 quantification (LEGENDplex Mouse Macrophage/Microglia Panel, Campoverde, Italy). Data were normalised according to the total protein content. Cells were lysed with 100 µL of Ripa buffer, kept for 30 min at 4 °C under agitation and then centrifuged at $1000 \times g$ for 10 min. The supernatant was collected, and the total protein content was determined by BCA assay. Bovine serum albumin (BSA) was used as the standard for the calibration curve (2–100 µg/mL; $R^2 = 0.9994$).

2.8. Statistical Analysis

All the experiments were performed at least six times unless otherwise specified. Data are means ± SEM. The statistical significance between groups was determined by one-way ANOVA for paired samples, followed by Tukey–Kramer post hoc test. A $p < 0.05$, $0.001 < p < 0.01$ and $p < 0.001$ were considered significant, very significant and extremely significant, respectively.

3. Results

3.1. PLG Aerosolisation under Air or Oxidising Condition

The nebulisation of 5 mL of PLG-OMP was nearly complete, with only a small amount of lather on the device walls, corresponding to 0.146 ± 0.003 mg of undelivered protein. The aerosolisation took 26.8 ± 6.3 min at a flow rate of 0.19 ± 0.04 mL/min, in agreement with the user manual of Aerogen® Solo™. Furthermore, the collected nebulised samples, obtained under both air and oxygen conditions, showed no protein aggregates, with more than 98% of PLG remaining in its monomeric form (Figure S2, Supplementary Information File) and a calculated MW of 99.6 ± 3.7 KDa (nebulised in airflow) and 99.6 ± 5.2 KDa (nebulised in oxygen flow), in agreement with PLG-OMP data (MW 93.9 ± 4.2 kDa) tabulated MW (92 KDa) [32]. Concerning the enzymatic activity, it was unaffected by mesh nebulisation in air, with a percentage of activity maintenance of 93.8% ± 11.5 with respect to untreated PLG-OMP. In contrast, the presence of oxygen flow affected the activity of the protein, resulting in 59.4% ± 15.9 of activity maintenance with respect to untreated PLG-OMP.

In the aerosolised clouds, the distribution of the two isoforms, Glu-PLG and Lys-PLG, was assessed by SDS-PAGE. PLG-OMP is mainly composed of the natural glycoforms of plasminogen, Glu I and Glu II, having glutamic acid as the first amino acid in the chain (Glu-PLG). Lys-PLG is the most common shortened version of PLG, missing the first 77 amino acids and having lysine as the first amino acid of the chain. Lys-PLG is regarded as a product impurity or an undesirable pre-activation form. The Glu-PLG migrates as two distinct bands corresponding to the two glycoforms: Glu I and Glu II; if present, the Lys-PLG is seen as two separate distinct bands, Lys I and Lys II, derived from Glu I and Glu II, respectively. The replicates were run on gel and compared to standards (Figure S3 in the Supplementary Information File). The percentage of protein bands related to Lys-

Plasminogen was found to be 0% in all examined samples, whereas the bands of Glu-PLG forms were not altered for all samples (Table 1).

Table 1. SDS-PAGE investigation: percentage distribution of glycoforms Glu-I, Glu-II, Lys-I and Lys-II in nebulised PLG-OMP collected in a glass bioaerosol impinger under air (Neb PLG air) and oxygen (Neb PLG ox) currents. The samples ($n = 4$) were compared to untreated PLG-OMP (CTRL) and standards (STD Glu PLG, STD Lys PLG).

Samples	BAND% $\pm$ SD%			
	Glu-I	Glu-II	Lys-I	Lys-II
STD Glu PLG	66	35	-	-
STD Lys PLG	-	-	62	38
CTRL	65	35	-	-
Neb PLG air	64 $\pm$ 4.5	36 $\pm$ 7.9	-	-
Neb PLG ox	59 $\pm$ 8.8	39 $\pm$ 10.3	-	-

An aerodynamic assessment of the fine particles in the PLG-OMP aerosol cloud was performed using a glass impinger apparatus [26] and by dosing the PLG impacting in each TSI component by BCA assay. Most of the nebulised protein, corresponding to $90.5\% \pm 14.6$ of the total delivered dose, impacted the lower impinger stage. Beyond the ordinary aerodynamic particle cut-off size of 6.4 μm between the two stages [33], the TSI components can be divided into sub-regions correlating to specific tracts of the respiratory tree, such as oral cavity, pharynx and larynx of the upper respiratory tract, bronchi and the entire targeted lung area (lower respiratory tract) [34]. By adopting such a distribution, the delivered PLG could be portioned into percentages of protein impacting specific respiratory portions (Table 2). As expected, the highest amount of protein was found in the portion corresponding to lung.

Table 2. Nebulisation of 5 mL of PLG eye drops using Aerogen® Solo™ and air flow 10 L/min: percentage distribution of nebulised PLG in TSI portions according to the simulation of the respiratory tract.

Simulation of the Nebulised Protein Distribution	
TSI Portion	% $\pm$ SD
Junction (T-piece)	11.5 $\pm$ 9.7
Throat	0.2 $\pm$ 0.2
Lower respiratory tract	80.8 $\pm$ 5.7
Exhaled	10.2 $\pm$ 9.2

3.2. Aerosolised PLG Mobility in Simulated Mucus

To evaluate the tendency of PLG to diffuse through airway mucus, PLG-OMP was directly nebulised on an in vitro model consisting of a layer of artificial mucus deposited on solid gelatine [35]. As reported in Figure 2, PLG progressively diffused from the upper mucus layer to the lower gelatine gel, reaching a cumulative 20% value after 5 h ($p < 0.05$). The plasminogen was then distributed homogenously in the artificial mucus layer, passing for 1/5 in the gel layer below.

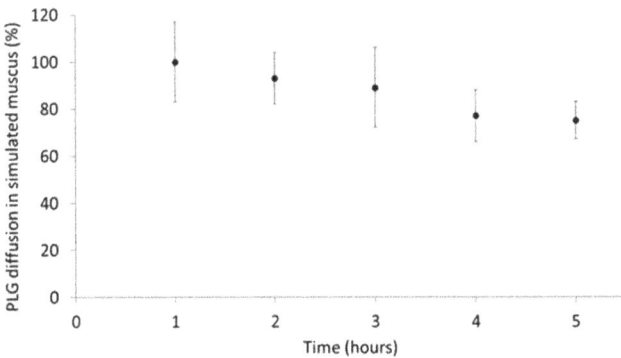

Figure 2. Diffusion kinetics of nebulised PLG in artificial mucus on a gelatine layer. PLG-OMP was deposited on the air side of the mucus layer, and every hour, both mucus and gelatine were treated to quantify the PLG content (ELISA). The diffusion percentage corresponds to the amount of PLG reaching the gel layer underneath.

3.3. PLG Permeability across a Monolayer

Firstly, cytotoxicity screening was performed on the NCI-H441 cell line. Exposing it to different PLG-OMP concentrations (4–900 µg/mL) showed an inhibiting concentration (IC_{50}) corresponding to 58.4 µg/mL (Figure 3). Untreated cells were used as the control.

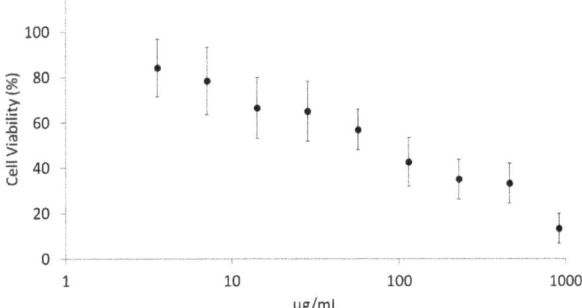

Figure 3. Cytotoxicity screening performed on NCI-H441 cells, exposed to PLG-OMP in the 4–900 µg/mL PLG concentration range. The values indicated in the figure are means ± SD ($n = 8$).

NCI-H441 cells are frequently used in drug disposition studies due to their ability to form confluent monolayers of polarised cells with high TEER [36]. The NCI-H441 monolayer was obtained in 8 days, as demonstrated by the TEER values. TEER was monitored from day 4 to day 12. An increase of the values was noticed, which then stabilised at around 600 Ω on the 8th day; the values then remained stable until the 11th day, and finally decreased on the 12th day (Figure S4a). Staining with haematoxylin/eosin was performed in order to evaluate the confluence of the cell monolayer. It was seen that at 7 days of culture, the cells were not yet able to form a complete monolayer (Figure S4b in the Supplementary Information File), while at 8 days of culture, the cells completely covered the surface of the Transwell® filter (Figure S4c). Furthermore, with prolonged culture times (10 and 12 days), the formation of a cell multilayer was observed (Figure S4d,e in the Supplementary Information File). In order to confirm cell differentiation by the presence of tight junction expressions, immunofluorescence was performed at 8 days of culture on NCI-H441 cultured in ALI conditions. A specific perimeter localisation of ZO-1, E-cadherin and Occludin expression, associated with cell differentiation, was observed (Figure S5).

PLG-OMP was directly nebulised on the ALI monolayer as a preliminary evaluation. The monolayer was placed in the second chamber of the TSI to collect the inhalable PLG droplets. However, the nebulisation time required to impact a measurable amount of PLG-OMP was too long, compromising the stability of the monolayer (data not displayed). As such, the direct PLG-OMP nebulisation on the Transwell® (Figure 1) was preferred. The biocompatibility of PLG-OMP directly nebulised on the ALI monolayer for 30 s was preliminarily verified (Figure S6 in the Supplementary Information File). The maintenance of TEER values over 600 Ω confirmed the integrity of the monolayer after PLG-OMP nebulisation and throughout the entire permeation experiment.

The permeation assay was carried out by nebulising PLG-OMP for 30 s (corresponding to 30.0 $\pm$ 0.06 μg of deposited protein) on each monolayer. PLG permeation was monitored using a specific Human PLG ELISA assay. A slow but progressive increase of PLG concentration was observed in the basolateral chamber, reaching a cumulative value of 26 ng after two hours, corresponding to 0.08% of the total deposited protein (Figure 4). The apparent permeability (Papp) of PLG across the monolayer was calculated as 3.82×10^{-9} cm/s.

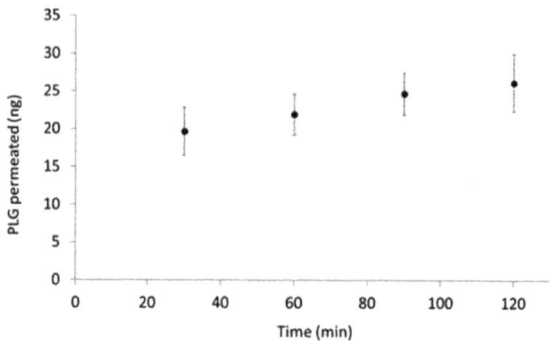

Figure 4. Permeation kinetics of nebulised PLG through the NCI-H441 ALI monolayer over time. PLG-OMP was directly nebulised on an in vitro model of the human alveolar epithelium [31]. At regular time intervals (30, 60, 90 and 120 min), the HBSS medium from the basolateral chamber was withdraw, and the PLG concentration was then determined by specific ELISA assay.

3.4. Maintenance of PLG Immunomodulatory Activity

A preliminary cell viability study performed on the RAW 264.7 cell line showed the absence of cytotoxicity for each PLG tested concentration, as well as for LPS 1 μg/mL (Figure S7 in the Supplementary Information File). Firstly, the LPS concentration screening (0.2–1 μg/mL) evidenced that the minimum concentration capable of stimulating the production of cytokines during 24 h incubation was LPS 0.2 μg/mL (Figure S8 in the Supplementary Information File). It was noticed that the TNF-α concentration values were not affected by increasing LPS concentration, resulting in a plateau. Differently, a dose–response relationship was evident for IL-6. An LPS concentration of 0.2 μg/mL, i.e., the lowest tested concentration capable of stimulating the macrophage cell line, was thus adopted for further studies.

RAW 264.7 cells were treated with LPS (24 h) and the nebulised PLG, collected on a glass bioaerosol impinger, was added 6 h post LPS addition. LPS alone and LPS with PLG-OMP eye drops (not nebulised) were used as a reference. From the results (Figure 5), it was observed that both PLG-OMP and the nebulised PLG-OMP reversed the effects of LPS activation by reducing the expression of pro-inflammatory cytokines IL-1β, IL-6 and TNFα. Notably, for IL-1β, both the nebulised product and PLG-OMP treatments significantly reduced its release (IL-1β 0.006 pg/μg and 0.003 pg/μg, respectively), compared to the positive control (IL-1β value of 0.016 pg/μg) (Figure 5a). Moreover, it was found that the nebulised product and PLG significantly decreased IL-6 secretion compared to the positive control (IL-6 values of 4.6 pg/μg and 3.07 pg/μg, respectively as compared to 7.6 pg/μg) (Figure 5b). The release of TNF-α from activated macrophages treated with either the nebulised product or PLG-OMP was also significantly affected, resulting in 41.9 pg/μg and 46.9 pg/μg, respectively. Those values were lower than what was recorded for the positive control (61.7 pg/μg) (Figure 5c).

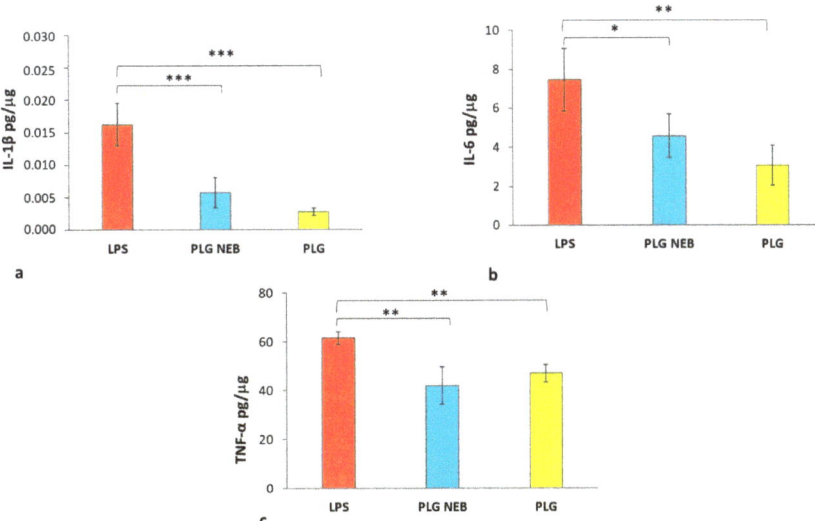

Figure 5. Maintenance of an immunomodulating effect on RAW 264.7 cells of nebulised PLG-OMP: assessment of pro-inflammatory cytokine secretion induced by 24 h stimulation with LPS (red), stimulated with LPS for 24 h and treated with either nebulised PLG-OMP (blue) or PLG-OMP (yellow). PLG NEB: aerosol cloud collected in a bio-impinger. PLG: untreated eye drops. (a) Expression of IL-1β, *** $p < 0.001$ vs. PLG NEB and PLG; (b) expression of IL-6, * $p < 0.05$ vs. PLG NEB, ** $0.001 < p < 0.01$ vs. PLG; (c) expression of TNF-α, ** $0.001 < p < 0.01$ vs. PLG NEB and PLG. Data were normalised in relation to the total protein concentration and expressed as pg of cytokine per μg of protein.

4. Discussion

Pulmonary delivery of PLG, through the off-label administration of PLG-OMP eye drops, has been considered as a possible therapy for C-ARDS patients [1]. During the COVID-19 pandemic, several drugs acting on the coagulopathy aspect of the disease were investigated. Mostly, heparin or tissue plasminogen activator/streptokinase were adopted under conventional routes of administration (sc. or i.v.), but a few researchers also considered the inhalation route. Due to pandemic resolution, study NCT04842292 [37], on nebulised heparin for COVID-19-associated Acute Respiratory Failure, terminated due to a lack of enrolment, whereas INHALE-HEP (NCT04723563) [38] was completed, although no results have been made available yet. Previous studies of patients with serious breathing problems due to pneumonia and other conditions found that nebulised heparin reduced the formation of small blood clots in the lungs, reduced the amount of injury to the lungs and hastened recovery, allowing patients to return home more quickly [39,40]. In 2019, a randomised controlled trial on nebulised streptokinase versus unfractionated heparin was conducted on patients with ARDS [41]. The study concluded that inhaled streptokinase could serve as rescue therapy in patients with severe ARDS. The therapy was found to improve oxygenation and lung mechanics more quickly than heparin or conventional management.

From a pharmaceutical technology perspective, nebulising a protein solution requires the monitoring of protein stability, the determination of droplet distribution and verification of activity maintenance. The generation of an aerosol exposes solutions and their components to physical stresses, often inducing protein unfolding and thermal degradation [42]. It is surprising that despite the presence of literature evidence of the effective clinical administration of nebulised proteins, reported descriptions of the used nebulisation devices have been poor. More efforts to indicate the most suitable administration setting in terms of the nebulisation device would improve the bench to bed translation of new medicines and off-label applications of already marketed ones. In a previous work, the jet and ultrasonic aerosolisation of PLG-OMP resulted in a significant loss of enzymatic activity. Only when the jet aerosolisation was set to the lowest air pressure, it was possible to preserve 89.8% of PLG proteolytic activity. However, the median diameter value ($dv_{(50)}$) resulted 9.2 ± 1.0 μm, which is not suited for pulmonary delivery [1]. Vibrating-mesh nebulisers, like the Aerogen® Solo™, employ perforated plates that vibrate to generate aerosols. Several studies have shown that no significant heat develops during atomisation, and the provided shear stress is lower than that of jet nebulisers. These devices are generally useful for delivering labile molecules, such as proteins [43]. In the present study, the mesh nebulisation of PLG-OMP was effective in preserving the chemical and physical features of PLG. Analyses of the protein in the collected clouds evidenced the maintenance of PLG in its monomeric form, with production of neither aggregates nor fragments, as demonstrated by DLS evaluations (Figure S2 in the Supplementary Information File). Moreover, the Glu-PLG glycoforms were maintained, with no cleavage to Lys-PLG (Table 1). The absence of Lys-PLG in aerosolised samples confirms the stability of PLG following mesh nebulisation. Regarding protein activity maintenance, it was totally preserved under normal aerosolisation conditions. Assuming that in cases of critical patient conditions, the off-label administration of PLG-OMP could occur in the presence of oxygen supply, the aerosolisation of PLG-OMP was also performed under an oxygen gas flow [44]. The nebulisation of PLG-OMP in the presence of oxygen led to significant decrease of PLG enzymatic activity (activity maintenance of 59.4% was recorded). Proteins are highly sensitive to oxidation, notably due to the modification of sulphur-containing amino acids Cys and Met, aromatic amino acids Trp, Tyr and Phe, as well as His, Pro, Lys and Arg [45]. The effect of oxidation depends on the oxidising stimuli and on the protein structure, varying from an effect on protein folding to the fragmentation of the sequence [46]. According to our DLS analysis, the protein was neither significantly aggregated nor fragmented, and the SDS-PAGE investigation evidenced no change in the PLG isoform distribution. Thus, the loss of activity may be attributed to the oxidative impact of oxygen on amino acid residues [47] essential for the enzymatic activity of PLG; however, the sequencing of the protein to define which amino acids are involved is beyond the scope of the present paper.

Aerosolised PLG showed an optimal in vitro deposition profile, with approximately 90% of the active ingredient impacting in the lower portions of the impinger. Under the Ph. Eur. setting, i.e., using a flow rate of 60 L/min through the impinger, the particle cut-off between upper and lower impingement chambers was 6.4 μm, indicating that particles smaller than 6.4 μm passed into the lower compartment [33]. The collected data are in agreement with previous reports on Aerogen® Solo™ mesh nebulisation, which describe mass median aerodynamic diameters of 4.4 μm and 2.7 μm for Aerogen® Solo™ and Aerogen® Solo™ with a T-piece device, respectively [48–50]. The results confirm that the clouds provided by these devices mainly impact the lower TSI compartment, suggesting the suitability of this approach for lung delivery in in vivo administration [34].

Two main aims of the future pulmonary administration of PLG are to take advantage of its loco-regional fibrinolytic action and to limit adverse effects due to systemic administration. To this end, airway mucus should not represent a barrier to PLG mobility, and PLG systemic absorption through alveolar permeation should be limited.

The mobility of nebulised drugs in artificial mucus is usually tested to verify that the layer of mucus that covers the respiratory epithelium does not represent a real physical barrier. The observed time-dependent transport of PLG through the simulated mucus suggested its homogeneous distribution toward the bronchoalveolar epithelium. The mobility observed for nebulised PLG was in agreement with literature reports, falling in between nanosized carriers, displaying about 5% penetration after 6 h [35], and small molecule drugs, reaching about 70% after 5 h [27].

The immortalised human lung adenocarcinoma cell line NCI-H441 (ATCC HTB-174), comprising epithelial lung distal cells, was selected in this study for biological evaluations [51]. The NCI-H441 cell line is frequently used in drug disposition studies due its ability to form confluent monolayers of polarised cells with high TEER [36], making it a valid in vitro model for permeation studies [31,51]. The permeability obtained for PLG (Papp 3.82×10^{-9} cm/s) is coherent with the Papp values determined for macromolecules with analogous molecular weights [36]. Low permeability of inhaled drugs is needed to extend their residence time in the lung, subsequently diminishing their diffusion through the lung epithelium toward the systemic circulation [52]. Thus, the low Papp value and the low amounts of PLG recovered in the basolateral chamber suggest a limited systemic absorption in vivo, supporting a hypothesised loco-regional enzymatic action.

Due to its main role as a zymogen of plasmin, PLG is closely associated with fibrinolysis, but PLG, its activators and its receptors play roles in various inflammation regulatory processes [53]. From this viewpoint, PLG administration could also help in the resolution of the severe lung inflammation that is typical of ARDS by direct interaction with macrophages. Macrophages have the ability to change into different phenotypes during inflammation, with a timely M1–M2 progression accompanying the inflammatory phases and resolution. M1 macrophages are involved in the beginning of inflammation and are responsible for inflammatory signalling, while M2 macrophages produce anti-inflammatory cytokines, thereby contributing to tissue healing [54]. Vago et al. [55] reported that the PLG receptors that are exposed on the macrophage cell surface bind plasminogen to enhance plasminogen activation. PLG and PLG receptors regulate key steps in the resolution of inflammation by affecting monocyte/macrophage migration, reprogramming macrophages toward an M2-like phenotype and reducing pro-inflammatory cytokine release.

LPS stimulation of RAW 264.7 macrophage cell line is generally applied as an in vitro model of inflammation [54,56], and LPS stimuli is also applied for in vivo ARDS animal models [57]. To simulate the in vivo effect of PLG treatment in an already induced inflammatory state, RAW 264.7 cells were treated with LPS for 24 h, but PLG was applied 6 h post LPS addition. Under the set conditions, PLG and LPS were simultaneously present for 18 h. It is known that LPS increases the production of urokinase-type plasminogen activator (uPA) in RAW 264.7 cells through the uPA core promoter domain [58]. uPA converts PLG into plasmin, and the plasmin produced can activate plasminogen/plasmin and plasmin/protease-activated receptor (PAR)-1 to modulate the inflammatory condition [59]. As reported in Figure 5, nebulised PLG treatment significantly reduced the production of relevant inflammatory mediators such as IL-1β, IL-6 and TNF-α in LPS-stimulated macrophages. Concerning the expression values of the investigated cytokines, striking differences were observed for TNF-α expression compared to those of IL-6 and IL1-β. According to the literature, the stimulus of LPS causes an immediate release of TNF-α, while IL-6 reached a peak after 6 h, mediated by TNF-α rather than LPS directly, indicating a cascading pattern after LPS stimulation in RAW 264.7 macrophages. This phenomenon may support the obtained results, where TNF-α showed elevated concentrations with respect to IL-6 [60]. Notably, the immunomodulating effect of PLG was evident for all tested cytokines and was preserved in the nebulised product. In addition, using human plasminogen minimises the risk of an immune response to non-human proteins, which could cause severe asthma/anaphylactic reactions when inhaled.

5. Conclusions

PLG-OMP mesh nebulisation effectively produced inhalable droplets for lung delivery of active PLG. In vitro investigations suggested a good safety profile of inhalable PLG, excluding high systemic absorption but indicating good mucus diffusion. The delivered protein maintained both its enzymatic activity and immunomodulating effect toward macrophages, which were activated by LPS inflammatory stimuli. All physical, biochemical and biopharmaceutical assessments of mesh aerosolised PLG-OMP are evidence for the potential of its off-label administration as treatment for ARDS patients. The locoregional deposition of PLG could provide fibrinolytic and anti-inflammatory actions, contributing to ARDS treatment. In vivo animal assessment represents the next step and will provide additional knowledge on PLG-OMP efficacy and dose correlations. Due to the simplicity of the PLG-OMP formulation (it is an eyedrop solution), the protein results susceptible to oxidation when the administration in oxygen current was simulated . Thus, in view of future clinical application, the concomitant administration of PLG-OMP aerosol and oxygen is discouraged, as it may result in a significant loss of enzymatic activity.

Supplementary Materials: The following supporting information can be downloaded at: https://www.mdpi.com/article/10.3390/pharmaceutics15061618/s1. Scheme S1. Workflow of the study. Protocol validation for protein aggregates and fragments [32,61,62], Figure S1. Correlation graph of Debye analysis, Figure S2. Protein Size distribution, Figure S3. SDS-PAGE assay, Figure S4. Micrograph of NCI-H441 cell monolayers, Figure S5. Representative fluorescence microscopy images of NCI-H441 cell ALI monolayers. Figure S6. Monolayer viability, Figure S7. Cell viability of RAW 264.7 cells at 6, 18 and 24 h, exposed to 5–20–50 µg/mL of PLG-OMP and LPS 1 µg/mL, Figure S8. Cytokines production by RAW 264.7 cells stimulated with different concentrations of LPS (0.2, 0.5, 0.8 and 1 µg/mL).

Author Contributions: Conceptualisation, F.M. and A.M.P.; Data curation, B.G., S.E. and G.B.; Formal analysis, L.V., C.M., B.G., A.S. and S.E.; Funding acquisition, B.F. and A.M.P.; Methodology, C.M., E.A. and S.E.; Resources, A.S.; Supervision, P.R., R.C. and A.M.P.; Validation, Y.Z., B.F. and G.B.; Visualisation, E.A.; Writing—original draft, L.V. and C.M.; Writing—review & editing, Y.Z., B.F., P.R., F.M., A.S., R.C., S.E., G.B. and A.M.P. All authors have read and agreed to the published version of the manuscript.

Funding: This research was funded by Regione Toscana, Ministero della Università e della Ricerca della Repubblica Italiana, PAR FSC 2007–2013, AEROPLAS-19 CUP I55F20000600007, Italy.

Institutional Review Board Statement: Not applicable.

Informed Consent Statement: Not applicable.

Data Availability Statement: The data presented in this study are available on request from the corresponding author.

Conflicts of Interest: The authors declare no conflict of interest. The company had no role in the design of the study.

References

1. Piras, A.M.; Zambito, Y.; Lugli, M.; Ferro, B.; Roncucci, P.; Mori, F.; Salvatore, A.; Ascione, E.; Bellini, M.; Crea, R. Repurposing of Plasminogen: An Orphan Medicinal Product Suitable for SARS-CoV-2 Inhalable Therapeutics. *Pharmaceuticals* **2020**, *13*, 425. [CrossRef]
2. Günther, A.; Ruppert, C.; Schmidt, R.; Markart, P.; Grimminger, F.; Walmrath, D.; Seeger, W. Surfactant alteration and replacement in acute respiratory distress syndrome. *Respir. Res.* **2001**, *2*, 353. [CrossRef]
3. Fujishima, S. Guideline-Based Management of Acute Respiratory Failure and Acute Respiratory Distress Syndrome. *J. Intensive Care* **2023**, *11*, 10. [CrossRef]
4. Luyt, C.-E.; Bouadma, L.; Morris, A.C.; Dhanani, J.A.; Kollef, M.; Lipman, J.; Martin-Loeches, I.; Nseir, S.; Ranzani, O.T.; Roquilly, A.; et al. Pulmonary Infections Complicating ARDS. *Intensive Care Med.* **2020**, *46*, 2168–2183. [CrossRef]
5. Bernard, G.R.; Artigas, A.; Brigham, K.L.; Carlet, J.; Falke, K.; Hudson, L.; Lamy, M.; Legall, J.R.; Morris, A.; Spragg, R. The American-European Consensus Conference on ARDS. Definitions, Mechanisms, Relevant Outcomes, and Clinical Trial Coordination. *Am. J. Respir. Crit. Care Med.* **1994**, *149*, 818–824. [CrossRef]

6. Eisner, M.D.; Thompson, T.; Hudson, L.D.; Luce, J.M.; Hayden, D.; Schoenfeld, D.; Matthay, M.A.; The Acute Respiratory Distress Syndrome Network. Efficacy of Low Tidal Volume Ventilation in Patients with Different Clinical Risk Factors for Acute Lung Injury and the Acute Respiratory Distress Syndrome. *Am. J. Respir. Crit. Care Med.* **2001**, *164*, 231–236. [CrossRef]

7. The ARDS Definition Task Force. Acute Respiratory Distress Syndrome: The Berlin Definition. *JAMA* **2012**, *307*, 2526–2533. [CrossRef]

8. Al Mutair, A.; Alhumaid, S.; Layqah, L.; Shamou, J.; Ahmed, G.Y.; Chagla, H.; Alsalman, K.; Alnasser, F.M.; Thoyaja, K.; Alhuqbani, W.N.; et al. Clinical Outcomes and Severity of Acute Respiratory Distress Syndrome in 1154 COVID-19 Patients: An Experience Multicenter Retrospective Cohort Study. *COVID* **2022**, *2*, 1102–1115. [CrossRef]

9. Stanford, S.; Roy, A.; Rea, C.; Harris, B.; Ashton, A.; Mangles, S.; Everington, T.; Taher, R.; Burns, D.; Arbuthnot, E.; et al. Pilot Study to Evaluate Hypercoagulation and Inflammation Using Rotational Thromboelastometry and Calprotectin in COVID-19 Patients. *PLoS ONE* **2023**, *18*, e0269738. [CrossRef]

10. Villar, J.; Ferrando, C.; Tusman, G.; Berra, L.; Rodríguez-Suárez, P.; Suárez-Sipmann, F. Unsuccessful and Successful Clinical Trials in Acute Respiratory Distress Syndrome: Addressing Physiology-Based Gaps. *Front. Physiol.* **2021**, *12*, 774025. [CrossRef]

11. Albaiceta, G.M.; Taboada, F.; Parra, D.; Blanco, A.; Escudero, D.; Otero, J. Differences in the Deflation Limb of the Pressure-Volume Curves in Acute Respiratory Distress Syndrome from Pulmonary and Extrapulmonary Origin. *Intensive Care Med.* **2003**, *29*, 1943–1949. [CrossRef] [PubMed]

12. Smith, F.G.; Perkins, G.D.; Gates, S.; Young, D.; McAuley, D.F.; Tunnicliffe, W.; Khan, Z.; Lamb, S.E. Effect of Intravenous β-2 Agonist Treatment on Clinical Outcomes in Acute Respiratory Distress Syndrome (BALTI-2): A Multicentre, Randomised Controlled Trial. *Lancet* **2012**, *379*, 229–235. [CrossRef]

13. McAuley, D.F.; Laffey, J.G.; O'Kane, C.M.; Perkins, G.D.; Mullan, B.; Trinder, T.J.; Johnston, P.; Hopkins, P.A.; Johnston, A.J.; McDowell, C.; et al. The HARP-2 Investigators, for the Irish Critical Care Trials Group. Simvastatin in the Acute Respiratory Distress Syndrome. *N. Engl. J. Med.* **2014**, *371*, 1695–1703. [CrossRef] [PubMed]

14. Ranieri, V.M.; Pettilä, V.; Karvonen, M.K.; Jalkanen, J.; Nightingale, P.; Brealey, D.; Mancebo, J.; Ferrer, R.; Mercat, A.; Patroniti, N.; et al. Effect of Intravenous Interferon β-1a on Death and Days Free From Mechanical Ventilation among Patients with Moderate to Severe Acute Respiratory Distress Syndrome: A Randomized Clinical Trial. *JAMA* **2020**, *323*, 725. [CrossRef] [PubMed]

15. Rahman, S.M.A.; Kabir, A.; Abdullah, A.B.M.; Alam, M.B.; Azad, K.A.K.; Miah, M.T.; Mowla, S.G.M.; Deb, S.R.; Amin, M.R.; Asaduzzaman, M. Safety and Efficacy of Favipiravir for the Management of COVID-19 Patients: A Preliminary Randomized Control Trial. *Clin. Infect. Pract.* **2022**, *15*, 100145. [CrossRef]

16. Menzella, F.; Fontana, M.; Salvarani, C.; Massari, M.; Ruggiero, P.; Scelfo, C.; Barbieri, C.; Castagnetti, C.; Catellani, C.; Gibellini, G.; et al. Efficacy of Tocilizumab in Patients with COVID-19 ARDS Undergoing Noninvasive Ventilation. *Crit. Care* **2020**, *24*, 589. [CrossRef]

17. Villar, J.; Ferrando, C.; Martínez, D.; Ambrós, A.; Muñoz, T.; Soler, J.A.; Aguilar, G.; Alba, F.; González-Higueras, E.; Conesa, L.A.; et al. Dexamethasone Treatment for the Acute Respiratory Distress Syndrome: A Multicentre, Randomised Controlled Trial. *Lancet Respir. Med.* **2020**, *8*, 267–276. [CrossRef]

18. Russell, C.D.; Millar, J.E.; Baillie, J.K. Clinical Evidence Does Not Support Corticosteroid Treatment for 2019-NCoV Lung Injury. *Lancet* **2020**, *395*, 473–475. [CrossRef]

19. Ferro, B.; Cinelli, R.; Vegnuti, L.; Piras, A.M.; Roncucci, P. The Potential Role of Aerosolized Phosphodiesterase 3 Inhibitor Enoximone in the Management of Coronavirus Disease 2019 Hypoxemia: A Case Report. *J. Aerosol Med. Pulm. Drug Deliv.* **2021**, *34*, 262–264. [CrossRef]

20. Yıldırım, F.; Yıldız Gülhan, P.; Şimşek, M. COVID-19 Related Acute Respiratory Distress Syndrome: Pathological, Radiological and Clinical Concordance. *Tuberk Toraks* **2021**, *69*, 360–368. [CrossRef]

21. Belen-Apak, F.B.; Sarıalioğlu, F. Pulmonary Intravascular Coagulation in COVID-19: Possible Pathogenesis and Recommendations on Anticoagulant/Thrombolytic Therapy. *J. Thromb. Thrombolysis* **2020**, *50*, 278–280. [CrossRef]

22. Camprubí-Rimblas, M.; Tantinyà, N.; Bringué, J.; Guillamat-Prats, R.; Artigas, A. Anticoagulant Therapy in Acute Respiratory Distress Syndrome. *Ann. Transl. Med.* **2018**, *6*, 36. [CrossRef]

23. Aisina, R.B.; Mukhametova, L.I. Structure and Function of Plasminogen/Plasmin System. *Russ. J. Bioorganic Chem.* **2014**, *40*, 590–605. [CrossRef]

24. Hertel, S.P.; Winter, G.; Friess, W. Protein Stability in Pulmonary Drug Delivery via Nebulization. *Adv. Drug Deliv. Rev.* **2015**, *93*, 79–94. [CrossRef]

25. Bodier-Montagutelli, E.; Respaud, R.; Perret, G.; Baptista, L.; Duquenne, P.; Heuzé-Vourc'h, N.; Vecellio, L. Protein Stability during Nebulization: Mind the Collection Step! *Eur. J. Pharm. Biopharm.* **2020**, *152*, 23–34. [CrossRef]

26. European Pharmacopoeia. *Preparations for Inhalation: Aerodynamic Assessment of Fine Particles*; Council of Europe: Strasbourg, France, 2014; pp. 276–286.

27. Costabile, G.; d'Angelo, I.; d'Emmanuele di Villa Bianca, R.; Mitidieri, E.; Pompili, B.; Del Porto, P.; Leoni, L.; Visca, P.; Miro, A.; Quaglia, F.; et al. Development of Inhalable Hyaluronan/Mannitol Composite Dry Powders for Flucytosine Repositioning in Local Therapy of Lung Infections. *J. Control. Release* **2016**, *238*, 80–91. [CrossRef]

28. Ghani, M.; Soothill, J.S. Ceftazidime, Gentamicin, and Rifampicin, in Combination, Kill Biofilms of Mucoid *Pseudomonas aeruginosa*. *Can. J. Microbiol.* **1997**, *43*, 999–1004. [CrossRef]

29. Marques, M.R.C.; Loebenberg, R.; Almukainzi, M. Simulated Biological Fluids with Possible Application in Dissolution Testing. *Dissolution Technol.* **2011**, *18*, 15–28. [CrossRef]
30. Chiellini, F. Perspectives on: In Vitro Evaluation of Biomedical Polymers. *J. Bioact. Compat. Polym.* **2006**, *21*, 257–271. [CrossRef]
31. Ren, H.; Birch, N.P.; Suresh, V. An Optimised Human Cell Culture Model for Alveolar Epithelial Transport. *PLoS ONE* **2016**, *11*, e0165225. [CrossRef]
32. Hayashi, M.; Matsuzaki, Y.; Shimonaka, M. Impact of Plasminogen on an in Vitro Wound Healing Model Based on a Perfusion Cell Culture System. *Mol. Cell. Biochem.* **2009**, *322*, 1–13. [CrossRef] [PubMed]
33. Hallworth, G.W.; Westmoreland, D.G. The Twin Impinger: A Simple Device for Assessing the Delivery of Drugs from Metered Dose Pressurized Aerosol Inhalers. *J. Pharm. Pharmacol.* **2011**, *39*, 966–972. [CrossRef] [PubMed]
34. Qi, A.; Friend, J.R.; Yeo, L.Y.; Morton, D.A.V.; McIntosh, M.P.; Spiccia, L. Miniature Inhalation Therapy Platform Using Surface Acoustic Wave Microfluidic Atomization. *Lab. Chip* **2009**, *9*, 2184–2193. [CrossRef] [PubMed]
35. Pellosi, D.S.; d'Angelo, I.; Maiolino, S.; Mitidieri, E.; d'Emmanuele di Villa Bianca, R.; Sorrentino, R.; Quaglia, F.; Ungaro, F. In Vitro/In Vivo Investigation on the Potential of Pluronic®Mixed Micelles for Pulmonary Drug Delivery. *Eur. J. Pharm. Biopharm.* **2018**, *130*, 30–38. [CrossRef]
36. Suresh, V. Permeability Properties of an In Vitro Model of the Alveolar Epithelium. *Cell. Mol. Bioeng.* **2021**, *14*, 653–659. [CrossRef]
37. Nebulized Heparin for COVID-19-Associated Acute Respiratory Failure. Available online: https://ClinicalTrials.gov/show/NCT04842292 (accessed on 12 April 2023).
38. Nebulized Heparin for the Treatment of COVID-19. Available online: https://ClinicalTrials.gov/show/NCT04723563 (accessed on 12 April 2023).
39. Serisier, D.J.; Shute, J.K.; Hockey, P.M.; Higgins, B.; Conway, J.; Carroll, M.P. Carroll. Inhaled Heparin in Cystic Fibrosis. *Eur. Respir. J.* **2006**, *27*, 354. [CrossRef]
40. van Haren, F.M.P.; Page, C.; Laffey, J.G.; Artigas, A.; Camprubi-Rimblas, M.; Nunes, Q.; Smith, R.; Shute, J.; Carroll, M.; Tree, J.; et al. Nebulised Heparin as a Treatment for COVID-19: Scientific Rationale and a Call for Randomised Evidence. *Crit. Care* **2020**, *24*, 454. [CrossRef]
41. Abdelaal Ahmed Mahmoud, A.; Mahmoud, H.E.; Mahran, M.A.; Khaled, M. Streptokinase Versus Unfractionated Heparin Nebulization in Patients with Severe Acute Respiratory Distress Syndrome (ARDS): A Randomized Controlled Trial with Observational Controls. *J. Cardiothorac. Vasc. Anesth.* **2020**, *34*, 436–443. [CrossRef]
42. Matthews, A.A.; Ee, P.L.R.; Ge, R. Developing Inhaled Protein Therapeutics for Lung Diseases. *Mol. Biomed.* **2020**, *1*, 11. [CrossRef]
43. Najlah, M.; Parveen, I.; Alhnan, M.A.; Ahmed, W.; Faheem, A.; Phoenix, D.A.; Taylor, K.M.G.; Elhissi, A. The Effects of Suspension Particle Size on the Performance of Air-Jet, Ultrasonic and Vibrating-Mesh Nebulisers. *Int. J. Pharm.* **2014**, *461*, 234–241. [CrossRef]
44. Dallas, R.H.; Rains, J.K.; Wilder, K.; Humphrey, W.; Cross, S.J.; Ghafoor, S.; Brazelton de Cardenas, J.N.; Hayden, R.T.; Hijano, D.R. The Aerogen®Solo Is an Alternative to the Small Particle Aerosol Generator (SPAG-2) for Administration of Inhaled Ribavirin. *Pharmaceutics* **2020**, *12*, 1163. [CrossRef]
45. Heinonen, M.; Gürbüz, G.; Ertbjerg, P. Oxidation of Proteins. In *Chemical Changes During Processing and Storage of Foods*; Elsevier: Amsterdam, The Netherlands, 2021; pp. 85–123. [CrossRef]
46. Kehm, R.; Baldensperger, T.; Raupbach, J.; Höhn, A. Protein Oxidation-Formation Mechanisms, Detection and Relevance as Biomarkers in Human Diseases. *Redox Biol.* **2021**, *42*, 101901. [CrossRef]
47. Gupta, A.; Yadav, V.; Yadav, J.S.; Rawat, S. Method Development and Photolytic Degradation Study of Doxofylline by RP-HPLC and LC-MS/MS. *Asian J. Pharm. Anal.* **2011**, *1*, 14–18.
48. Sayed, N.E.E.; Abdelrahman, M.A.; Abdelrahim, M.E.A. Effect of Functional Principle, Delivery Technique, and Connection Used on Aerosol Delivery from Different Nebulizers: An In-Vitro Study. *Pulm. Pharmacol. Ther.* **2021**, *70*, 102054. [CrossRef]
49. Sweeney, L.; McCloskey, A.P.; Higgins, G.; Ramsey, J.M.; Cryan, S.-A.; MacLoughlin, R. Effective Nebulization of Interferon-γ Using a Novel Vibrating Mesh. *Respir. Res.* **2019**, *20*, 66. [CrossRef]
50. McDermott, K.; Oakley, J.G. Droplet Size and Distribution of Nebulized 3% Sodium Chloride, Albuterol, and Epoprostenol by Phase Doppler Particle Analyzer. *Curr. Ther. Res.* **2021**, *94*, 100623. [CrossRef]
51. Salomon, J.J.; Muchitsch, V.E.; Gausterer, J.C.; Schwagerus, E.; Huwer, H.; Daum, N.; Lehr, C.-M.; Ehrhardt, C. The Cell Line NCl-H441 Is a Useful *in Vitro* Model for Transport Studies of Human Distal Lung Epithelial Barrier. *Mol. Pharm.* **2014**, *11*, 995–1006. [CrossRef]
52. Guo, Y.; Bera, H.; Shi, C.; Zhang, L.; Cun, D.; Yang, M. Pharmaceutical Strategies to Extend Pulmonary Exposure of Inhaled Medicines. *Acta Pharm. Sin. B* **2021**, *11*, 2565–2584. [CrossRef]
53. Baker, S.K.; Strickland, S. A Critical Role for Plasminogen in Inflammation. *J. Exp. Med.* **2020**, *217*, e20191865. [CrossRef]
54. Sugimoto, M.A.; Ribeiro, A.L.C.; Costa, B.R.C.; Vago, J.P.; Lima, K.M.; Carneiro, F.S.; Ortiz, M.M.O.; Lima, G.L.N.; Carmo, A.A.F.; Rocha, R.M.; et al. Plasmin and Plasminogen Induce Macrophage Reprogramming and Regulate Key Steps of Inflammation Resolution via Annexin A1. *Blood* **2017**, *129*, 2896–2907. [CrossRef]
55. Vago, J.P.; Sugimoto, M.A.; Lima, K.M.; Negreiros-Lima, G.L.; Baik, N.; Teixeira, M.M.; Perretti, M.; Parmer, R.J.; Miles, L.A.; Sousa, L.P. Plasminogen and the Plasminogen Receptor, Plg-RKT, Regulate Macrophage Phenotypic, and Functional Changes. *Front. Immunol.* **2019**, *10*, 1458. [CrossRef]

56. Grassi, L.; Pompilio, A.; Kaya, E.; Rinaldi, A.C.; Sanjust, E.; Maisetta, G.; Crabbé, A.; Di Bonaventura, G.; Batoni, G.; Esin, S. The Anti-Microbial Peptide (Lin-SB056-1)2-K Reduces Pro-Inflammatory Cytokine Release through Interaction with Pseudomonas Aeruginosa Lipopolysaccharide. *Antibiotics* **2020**, *9*, 585. [CrossRef] [PubMed]
57. Kaspi, H.; Semo, J.; Abramov, N.; Dekel, C.; Lindborg, S.; Kern, R.; Lebovits, C.; Aricha, R. MSC-NTF (NurOwn®) Exosomes: A Novel Therapeutic Modality in the Mouse LPS-Induced ARDS Model. *Stem Cell Res. Ther.* **2021**, *12*, 72. [CrossRef] [PubMed]
58. Das, R.; Burke, T.; Plow, E.F. Histone H2B as a Functionally Important Plasminogen Receptor on Macrophages. *Blood* **2007**, *110*, 3763–3772. [CrossRef] [PubMed]
59. Kanno, Y. The Role of Fibrinolytic Regulators in Vascular Dysfunction of Systemic Sclerosis. *Int. J. Mol. Sci.* **2019**, *20*, 619. [CrossRef] [PubMed]
60. Xiang, L.; Hu, Y.-F.; Wu, J.-S.; Wang, L.; Huang, W.-G.; Xu, C.-S.; Meng, X.-L.; Wang, P. Semi-Mechanism-Based Pharmacodynamic Model for the Anti-Inflammatory Effect of Baicalein in LPS-Stimulated RAW264.7 Macrophages. *Front. Pharmacol.* **2018**, *9*, 793. [CrossRef]
61. Tumolo, T.; Angnes, L.; Baptista, M.S. Determination of the Refractive Index Increment (Dn/Dc) of Molecule and Macromolecule Solutions by Surface Plasmon Resonance. *Anal. Biochem.* **2004**, *333*, 273–279. [CrossRef]
62. Barlow, G.H.; Summaria, L.; Robbins, K.C. Molecular Weight Studies on Human Plasminogen and Plasmin at the Microgram Level. *J. Biol. Chem.* **1969**, *244*, 1138–1141. [CrossRef]

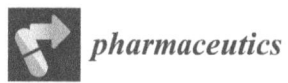

pharmaceutics

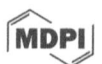

Article

A Supine Position and Dual-Dose Applications Enhance Spray Dosing to the Posterior Nose: Paving the Way for Mucosal Immunization

Amr Seifelnasr [1], Mohamed Talaat [1], Pranav Ramaswamy [1], Xiuhua April Si [2] and Jinxiang Xi [1,*]

[1] Department of Biomedical Engineering, University of Massachusetts, Lowell, MA 01854, USA
[2] Department of Mechanical Engineering, California Baptist University, Riverside, CA 92504, USA
* Correspondence: jinxiang_xi@uml.edu; Tel.: +1-978-934-3259

Abstract: Delivering vaccines to the posterior nose has been proposed to induce mucosal immunization. However, conventional nasal devices often fail to deliver sufficient doses to the posterior nose. This study aimed to develop a new delivery protocol that can effectively deliver sprays to the caudal turbinate and nasopharynx. High-speed imaging was used to characterize the nasal spray plumes. Three-dimensional-printed transparent nasal casts were used to visualize the spray deposition within the nasal airway, as well as the subsequent liquid film formation and translocation. Influencing variables considered included the device type, delivery mode, release angle, flow rate, head position, and dose number. Apparent liquid film translocation was observed in the nasal cavity. To deliver sprays to the posterior nose, the optimal release angle was found to be 40° for unidirectional delivery and 30° for bidirectional delivery. The flow shear was the key factor that mobilized the liquid film. Both the flow shear and the head position were important in determining the translocation distance. A supine position and dual-dose application significantly improved delivery to the nasopharynx, i.e., 31% vs. 0% with an upright position and one-dose application. It is feasible to effectively deliver medications to the posterior nose by leveraging liquid film translocation for mucosal immunization.

Keywords: nasal spray; liquid film translocation; supine position; wall liquid-holding capacity; nasopharynx; mucosal immunization

Citation: Seifelnasr, A.; Talaat, M.; Ramaswamy, P.; Si, X.A.; Xi, J. A Supine Position and Dual-Dose Applications Enhance Spray Dosing to the Posterior Nose: Paving the Way for Mucosal Immunization. *Pharmaceutics* **2023**, *15*, 359. https://doi.org/10.3390/pharmaceutics15020359

Academic Editors: Michael Yee Tak Chow and Philip Chi Lip Kwok

Received: 28 November 2022
Revised: 22 December 2022
Accepted: 17 January 2023
Published: 20 January 2023

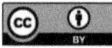
1. Introduction

Respiratory infectious diseases often enter the human body through the nose. SARS-CoV-2 preferentially binds to the ACE2-rich tissue cells in the posterior nose. Coronavirus can quickly replicate in the nasal mucosa, which has made it a frequent sampling site (i.e., for nasal swabs) in COVID-19 screening. Evidence has shown that viral binding and replication start in ciliated epithelial cells after being infected with virus-laden aerosols, and this process can last for 3~14 days without obvious symptoms [1]. The binding affinity between the coronavirus' S-protein and angiotensin-converting enzyme 2 (ACE2) is the crucial factor for viral transmission, while ACE2 is highly populated in nasal epithelial cells [2]. Lee et al. [3] mapped the distribution of subcellular ACE2 in human nasal epithelium. They observed the highest expression of ACE2 in ciliated epithelial cells and in descending order in goblet, club, and suprabasal cells. Moreover, the goblet cell in the nose is one of the three verified entry locations for SARS-CoV-2, which needs two coexisting proteins: ACE2 and type II transmembrane serine protease (TMPRSS2) [4,5]. The anterior one-third of the nose is lined with the stratified squamous epithelium, while the posterior two-thirds of the nose and nasopharynx are lined with mucus-producing goblet cells, columnar ciliated cells, and the suprabasal membrane [6].

Nasal sprays have been frequently used to administer influenza vaccines [7]. The elevated concentration of ACE2 in the posterior nose indicates that intranasal vaccines need to be dispensed to the posterior two-thirds of the nose and nasopharynx to be efficacious in eliciting mucosal immunization [8,9]. However, conventional nasal sprays fail to deliver drugs to the caudal turbinate and nasopharynx. Due to the geometrical complexity, most of the applied doses are deposited in the nasal vestibule and nasal valve, with only a small fraction passing the nasal valve filtration and reaching the turbinate region [10–13]. Many factors can contribute to the low doses in the posterior nose, for instance, spray properties, breathing conditions, the delivery method, and the nasal physiology [14]. Nasal spray properties that influence intranasal dosimetry include, but are not limited to, the spray discharge velocity, aerosol mean diameter and distribution, spray plume angle, release angle to the nostril, applied dose, and number of applications. The mean diameter of nasal spray droplets is much larger than those of nebulizers and metered dose inhalers, which range between 20 and 300 μm and whose deposition is predominantly governed by inertial impaction [15]. Cheng et al. evaluated the dose distributions from various nasal pumps in nasal casts reconstructed from magnetic resonance imaging (MRI) [16]. They found that wide plumes and/or large droplets give rise to higher deposition in the anterior nose, whereas narrow plume angles and/or small droplets enhance delivery to the turbinate region. Kundoor and Dalby studied the effects of the spray release angle in the range of 0°–90° with an increment of 15° [17]. The optimal release angle was found to be 60° in delivering the sprays to the middle turbinate. Liquid film translocation can also affect the dosimetry distribution because a liquid film can form, grow, and move from the accumulation of deposited droplets. It has been shown that liquid film translocation can substantially enhance the dosing to the olfactory cleft by adopting a head-to-floor position [18]. To achieve optimal protection against COVID-19 infection, a nasal device that can effectively deliver high doses of nasal sprays to the posterior nose is needed [19–25].

The objective of this study was to develop a method that can effectively deliver nasal sprays to the caudal turbinate and nasopharynx for mucosal immunization against infectious respiratory diseases. Various delivery parameters were tested in an image-based nasal airway model to understand the mechanisms underlying the liquid film translocation and identify the optimal delivery protocol. Specific aims included the following:

(1) Visualize the spatiotemporal development of the nasal sprays from different devices using a high-speed camera.
(2) Visualize the liquid film translocation in the nose with unidirectional delivery for various administration angles, head positions, and inhalation flow rates.
(3) Visualize the liquid film translocation with bidirectional delivery for various administration angles, head positions, inhalation flow rates, and the number of applications.
(4) Quantify the nasal spray deposition in the front nose, turbinate, and nasopharynx.
(5) Compare the performances among test cases and identify the optimal combination of the nasal device, delivery method, administration angle, inhalation flow rate, head position, and number of spray applications.

2. Materials and Methods

2.1. Study Design

Nasal spray delivery can be influenced by a variety of parameters (i.e., device, drug, patient, device, administration, and formulation related), and no individual parameter is universally accepted as a predictive index for the dosimetry distribution within the nasal cavity, making in vitro testing a necessity in studying nasal spray dosimetry. To evaluate the feasibility of delivering clinically significant doses to the posterior nose, the nasal dosimetry sensitivity to key influencing factors was tested in this study, including nasal devices, the delivery method, the administration angle, the inhalation flow rate, the head position, and the number of applications.

Three nasal spray devices were initially considered to select a candidate most favorable for posterior nose delivery: a saline nasal spray (Basic Care, with purified water, 0.65% sodium chloride, disodium phosphate, phenylcarbinol, monosodium phosphate, and benzalkonium chloride), the Xlear nasal spray (Xlear, with purified water, 11% xylitol, 0.85% sodium chloride, and grapefruit seed extract), and a refillable soft-mist spray inhaler

(Hengni, with purified water and 0.9% sodium chloride). To this aim, smaller droplet sizes and lower existing speeds were preferred. Because spray actuation is a highly transient process, high-speed imaging techniques were used to visualize the spray release and subsequent plume development.

It was hypothesized that bidirectional delivery could deliver more medications to the caudal turbinate and nasopharynx [26]. As such, the dosimetry of the nasal sprays was compared between these two delivery methods for different respiration flow rates and spray release angles. A baseline respiration flow rate of 30 L/min was implemented in the conventional unidirectional delivery, while a baseline flow rate of 11 L/min was used in bidirectional delivery. This difference was because the unidirectionally inhaled flow included flows through both nasal passages, while the bidirectional flow was the same flow that entered one nostril and exited from the other. A vacuum (Robinair 3 CFM, Warren, MI, USA) was connected to the nasopharynx to generate inhalation flows for unidirectional delivery and to the left nostril for bidirectional delivery, as illustrated in Figure 1a and Figure 1b, respectively. The inhalation flow rate was controlled using an inline flow meter (Omega, FL-510, Stamford, CT, USA). Considering that the spray-releasing angle could significantly affect the dosimetry mapping, five releasing angles ranging from 10° to 45° from the nostril normal were studied (Figure 1c).

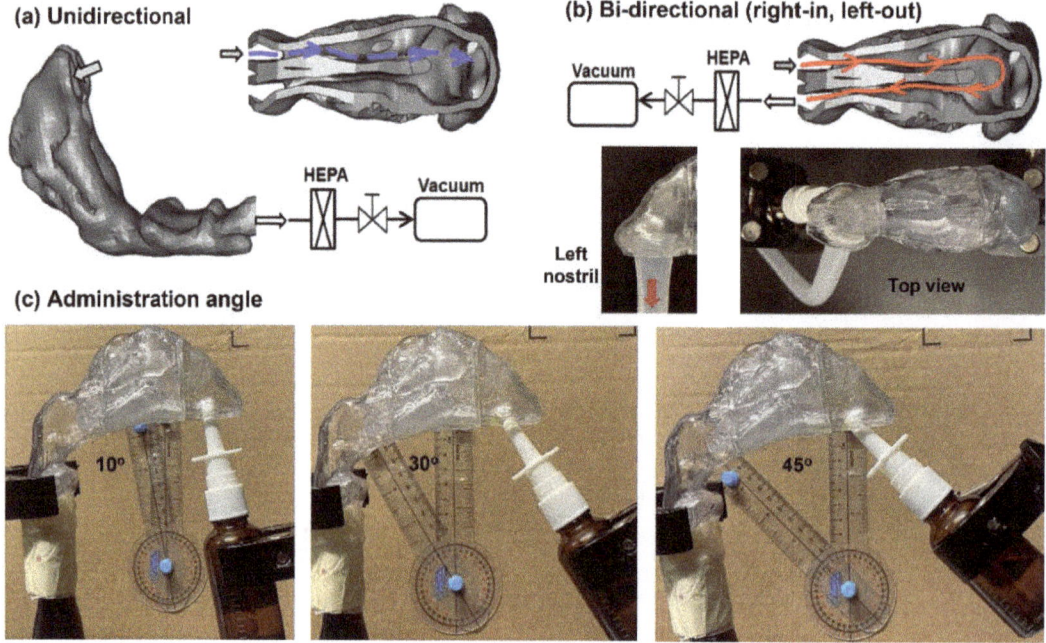

Figure 1. Nasal spray delivery diagram in (**a**) unidirectional mode, (**b**) bidirectional mode, and (**c**) administration angle to the right nostril: 10°, 30°, and 45°. To quantify the regional doses, the nasal cavity was divided into three parts: front nose, turbinate, and nasopharynx.

To study the head orientation effects, both the upright and supine positions were considered. To study the dosimetry after multiple applications, the nasal spray was applied either once or twice. The delivered doses were quantified by weighing the mass difference before and after spray administration. Regional deposition rates in the vestibule, turbinate, and nasopharynx were quantified and compared among test cases.

2.2. Nasal Airway Casts and Computational Model

A nasal airway model previously developed by Xi et al. [27] was used in this study. Briefly, the airway model was segmented from the MRI of a 53-year-old male (512 × 512-pixel resolution). A hollow-cast model was prepared using Magics (Materialise, Ann Abor, MI, USA) with a constant layer thickness of 4 mm and a feature detail size of 0.1 mm. Hollow-cast replicas were manufactured using transparent stereolithography (SLA) material (Somos WaterShed XC 11122) and a Stratasys Polyjet printer (Wenext, Shenzhen, China). A major advantage of using a transparent cast was that the instantaneous transport of the nasal sprays within the nasal cast could be visualized. To quantify the regional dosimetry, the hollow cast was divided into three components: front (nasal vestibule and valve), middle (turbinate), and back (nasopharynx). A step-shaped connector was created at the interface of each component, which had a width of 2.0 mm (half the wall thickness), a height of 2.5 mm, and a clearance of 0.2 mm so that the two parts could easily connect with each other. Transparent tape (Silicon Scar Tape) was applied to the interfaces to minimize the probability of leakage.

2.3. Visualization of Spray Plumes in Open Space

To understand the nasal spray patterns, a high-speed camera (Phantom VEO 1310, up to 11,000 fps acquisition rate) was used to visualize the dispersion of the spray plumes after being discharged into an open space. An LED light with up to 41,500 lumens (Mankerlight MK38) was adopted to illuminate the spray plumes. The acquisition speeds of the high-speed camera were varied in the range of 2000–6000 fps to select the best visualization effects in both the spatial and the temporal dispersion of the spray plumes [28].

2.4. UV-Illuminated Fluorescent Visualization of Spray Dynamics within the Nose

The behavior and fate of spray droplets in the nasal cast were visualized using 0.5% green ultraviolet (UV) reactive water-soluble fluorescent dye (GLO Effex, Murrieta, CA, USA) and a 385–395 nm LED light. Considering that liquid film translocation can be affected by surface smoothness (or roughness), a thin layer of silicone oil (MicroLubrol PMS-0125 Phenyl Methyl Silicone Oil, 125 CST Viscosity) was applied on the inner surface to simulate the mucus layer of human nasal airways. All tests were conducted in a dark room.

2.5. Regional Dose Quantification

The delivered doses in the front/middle/back of the nose were quantified using the weight difference ($\Delta W = W_1 - W_0$), and the deposition fraction was quantified as the ratio of ΔW to the applied dose [13]. The weight of the sectional cast was measured immediately before and after drug delivery, i.e., W_0 and W_1. A high-precision electronic scale (120 g/0.0001 g, Bonvoisin, A&D Medical, San Jose, CA, USA) was used to measure the weight. Photos of the deposition distribution with fluorescent dyes were taken in the transparent airway model. Each test case was repeated at least three times to evaluate the dosimetry variability.

2.6. Statistical Analysis

Minitab (State College, PA, USA) was used to conduct associated statistical analysis. One-way analysis of variance (ANOVA) was used to evaluate sample variability. The delivered doses were expressed as the mean ± standard deviation.

3. Results

3.1. High-Speed Imaging of Soft-Mist and Squeeze-Bottle Sprays

Figure 2a,b shows the spray generation and transport from two conventional nasal devices: a saline nasal spray and Xlear, respectively. The saline nasal spray generated much larger droplets; the droplet motions appeared to be predominately moving straightforward, with no apparent vortices (Figure 2a). The droplets from the Xlear nasal spray were apparently smaller in size than those from the saline nasal spray; the spray plume gradually developed into vortex flows (Figure 2b). However, large droplets were also observed immediately downstream of the Xlear spray nozzle (Figure 2b). High-speed images of the soft-mist nasal spray are shown in Figure 2c at varying instants after actuation, which generated smaller droplets with a more homogeneous size distribution. The droplet size distribution of the soft-mist spray was measured at 3 cm from the nozzle using the Malvern Spraytec, with D10 being 24.5 ± 0.3 μm (i.e., 10% of the sample is smaller than 24.5 ± 0.3 μm), D50 being 43.9 ± 0.7 μm, and D90 being 75.8 ± 2.9 μm. Considering that large droplets and straight droplet trajectories would lead to deposition mainly in the front nose from inertial impaction, the soft-mist spray bottle was chosen in the following investigations based on the rationale that smaller aerosols could reduce the front-nose deposition and increase the spray dispensing beyond the nasal valve.

(a) Saline nasal spray   **(b) Xlear nasal spray**

(c) Soft mist spray at three instants after administration

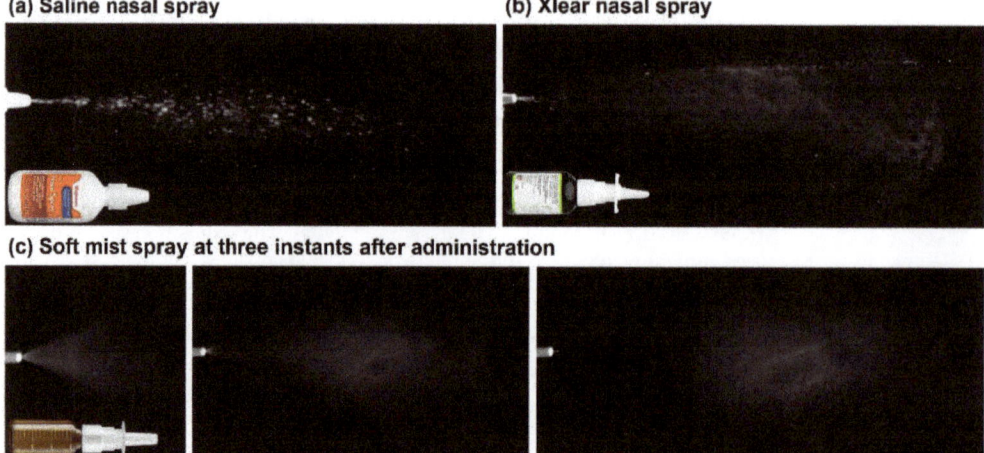

Figure 2. High-speed imaging of the three types of nasal sprays: (**a**) saline nasal spray, (**b**) Xlear, and (**c**) soft-mist spray (at three instants after administration).

3.2. Unidirectional Delivery

Figure 3 shows nasal spray deposition using the unidirectional delivery method with five device orientations from the vertical direction (i.e., spray release angles). For all device orientations considered, the majority of the nasal sprays deposited in the front nose, especially in the nasal valve region. Among them, the 40° orientation gave the optimal dose in the turbinate region. However, no perceivable dose was delivered to the nasopharynx.

Liquid film translocation was apparent in the nasal cavity during the nasal spray application. At 10° orientation, the nasal sprays were predominately deposited in the nasal vestibule, particularly the roof of the vestibular. There was clear liquid dripping downward due to gravity, as a significant dose of spray droplets was concentrated in this region. These droplets coalesced into patches of liquid films, and the self-weight of certain patches became large enough to overcome the surface tension and wall friction, causing the liquid film to drip along the gravitational direction. Liquid film translocation due to the flow shear stress at the air–liquid interface was also observed. In the case of 40° orientation, a thin liquid film moved from the middle turbinate toward the caudal turbinate, which eventually led to the formation of a large drop on the nose floor at the caudal turbinate (40°, Figure 3).

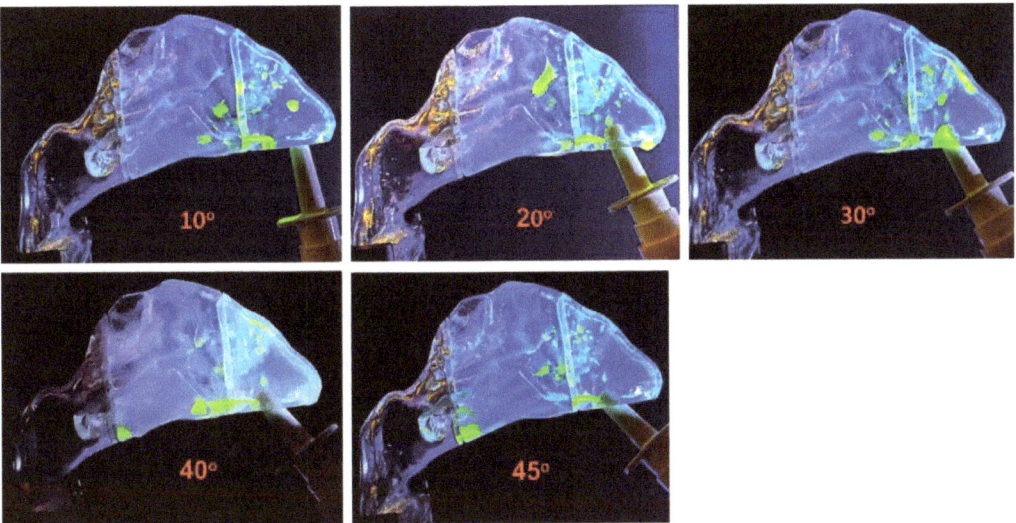

Figure 3. Nasal spray deposition distribution using the unidirectional delivery method for different administration angles: 10°, 20°, 30°, 40°, and 45°.

3.3. Bidirectional Delivery

3.3.1. Effects of Spray Administration Angles (Relative to the Nostril)

The nasal spray deposition using bidirectional delivery is shown in Figure 4 for different device orientation angles at a flow rate of 11 L/min. Considering that the sprays can deposit in both nasal passages using bidirectional delivery, photos were taken from both sides of the nose. The upper row in Figure 4 shows the right passage, into which the spray was applied; the lower row shows the left passage, where deposition occurred from the convection of small droplets and liquid translocation. Overall, the bidirectional delivery method delivered more doses beyond the nasal valve and to the middle and caudal turbinate. At a device orientation of 30°, a certain dose was also observed in the nasopharynx, which was not observed using unidirectional delivery. Moreover, different deposition patterns were observed between the bidirectional and unidirectional delivery methods (Figure 4 vs. Figure 3). This could be attributed to different flow dynamics, vortex fields, and associated wall shear (liquid-film-stabilizing force) and flow shear (destabilizing force), with more detailed explanations presented in Section 4.2.

Regarding the left passage, only a small quantity of nasal spray was observed in the posterior nose. This was because of liquid translocation either along the septum (middle wall) or channeled by the middle or inferior turbinate. Both turbinate projections resemble V-shaped open conduits, and the liquid within them is driven by the liquid self-weight or flow shear. Note that UV fluorescence was only visible when the UV concentration was high enough.

To evaluate the flow shear at the air–liquid interface, the dynamics of the liquid film during the first 0.33 s were compared in Figure 5 among three respiration flow rates (i.e., 0, 5.5, and 11 L/min). Clearly, a flow rate of 11 L/min and the resultant shear force exerted a more significant effect on the wall film stability and translocation compared to 5.5 L/min and 0 L/min. At 11 L/min, the nasal spray spread a longer distance at any instant considered herein than at 5.5 L/min and 0 L/min. However, more similarities were observed between 0 L/min and 5.5 L/min. Both showed a slow progression in spray deposition from a C-shaped strip to a horseshoe to a closed loop, which eventually merged into a dripping drop (Figure 5a,b). The drop stabilized in the middle turbinate, as illustrated by the negligible change in the deposition pattern from 5/30 s to 10/30 s. These similarities indicated that the flow shear at 5.5 L/min and gravity were not large enough to mobilize the liquid film to move much, despite a slightly longer distance of the film spreading than without a flow shear (last column, Figure 5b vs. Figure 5a). Conversely, the significantly enhanced liquid film spreading at 11 L/min indicated that the flow shear at 11 L/min succeeded in destabilizing the liquid film, which together with gravity surpassed the stabilizing forces from viscosity and surface tension. It was also observed that the mobilized wall film at 11 L/min stopped after traveling a certain distance and reached a new stabilized condition due to the decreasing liquid film thickness and gravity as it spread to other regions.

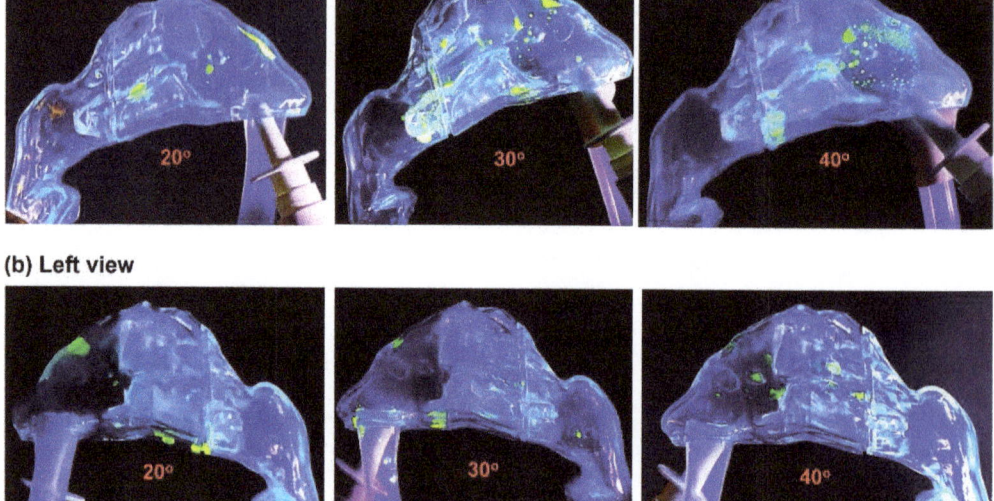

(a) Right view

(b) Left view

Figure 4. Nasal spray deposition distribution using the bidirectional delivery method for different administration angles: 20°, 30°, and 40°. (**a**) Right view and (**b**) left view. Enhanced deposition in the turbinate region was observed with an administration angle of 30°.

3.3.2. Effects of Dual-Spray Applications on Dosimetry

The airway wall has a limit to the amount of liquid it can hold, and this liquid-holding capacity varies with the slope and roughness of the wall. It is conjectured that a second application will deliver a higher percentage of the applied dose to the target. Because the first application has fulfilled the liquid-holding capacity of the airway wall leading to the target, all (or most of) the second dose should follow the same path and translocate to the target, with no (or negligible) loss to these walls. Figure 6a shows the liquid film translocation after the second dose when administered bidirectionally in a supine position and at a flow rate of 11 L/min. Apparently, more doses were found in the nasopharynx. As the first dose paved the way in the front nose and middle turbinate, the extra liquid mass streamed downward following the furrow between the inferior and the middle turbinate (referred to as turbinate furrow thenceforth; Figure 6a). This led to a large drop of sprays in the nasopharynx, which stabilized on the flat nasopharynx wall (0.33 s, Figure 6a).

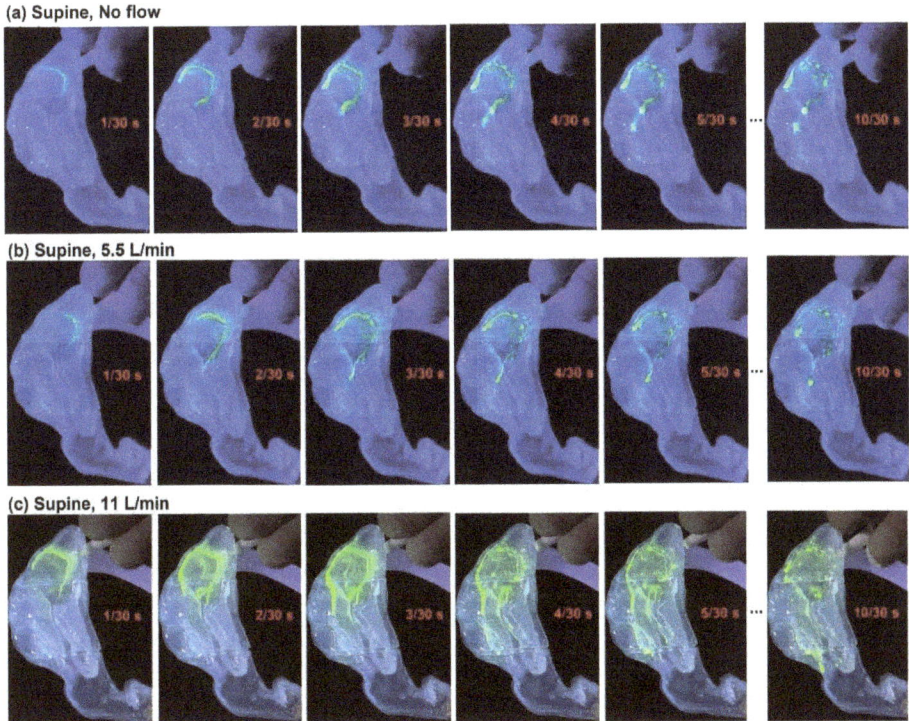

Figure 5. Liquid film translocation vs. time after administration using bidirectional delivery mode in a supine position under varying respiration flow rates: (**a**) no flow, (**b**) 5.5 L/min, and (**c**) 11 L/min.

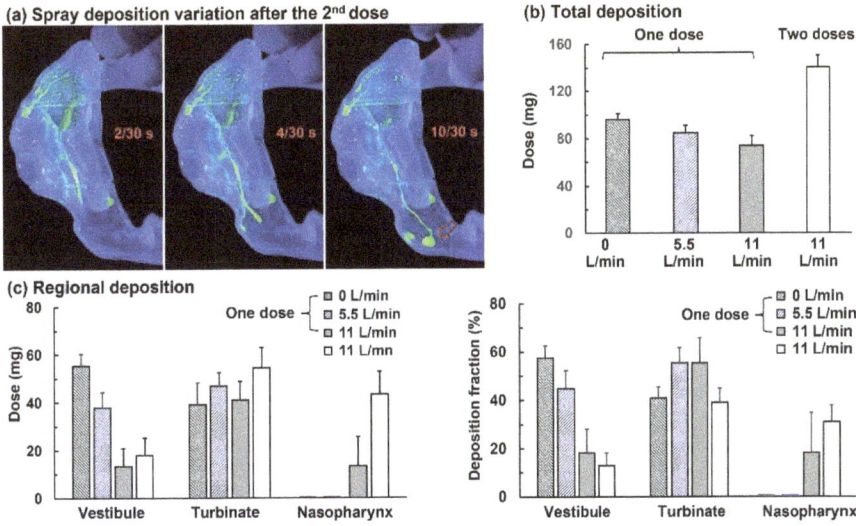

Figure 6. Nasal spray deposition with single- and dual-spray applications administered bidirectionally in a supine position: (**a**) liquid film translocation after applying two doses at a flow rate of 11 L/min, (**b**) total deposition, and (**c**) regional deposition at different flow rates.

A comparison of spray dosimetry among different flow rates, as well as between one and two doses, is shown in Figure 6b,c for total and regional deposition, respectively. The total deposition gradually decreased as the flow rate increased from 0 to 5.5 to 11 L/min (Figure 6b). This was as expected, considering that stronger convection would carry away more aerosol droplets out of the airway. Considering the regional deposition, the deposited mass in the anterior nose (vestibule) drastically decreased from 0 to 5.5 to 11 L/min, reflecting more intensified liquid film translocation with higher flow shear (Figure 6c). Insignificant variations in the turbinate deposition were observed among the three flow rates, as the extra mass beyond the vestibular liquid-holding capacity moved to the turbinate region, driven by gravity (and flow shear for 5.5 L/min and 11 L/min). No deposited mass was found in the nasopharynx when the flow shear was absent (0 L/min) or small (5.5 L/min), while a dose of 13.5 mg (or 18.2% of the total deposition) was found when the flow rate increased to 11 L/min (Figure 6c).

A second dose approximately doubled the total deposition at 11 L/min (Figure 6b) but more than tripled the deposition in the nasopharynx (left panel, Figure 6c). The fact that the first dose paved the way to the target and fulfilled the wall liquid-holding capacity made it easier for the second dose to reach the target with more spray mass than was otherwise needed to saturate the liquid film. This was evidenced by the deposited masses in the vestibule and turbinate (left panel, Figure 6c), which was only slightly higher in dual-dose vs. one-dose application for a given flow rate (11 L/min). As a result, a higher percentage of the total dose was delivered to the nasopharynx with dual-dose than with one-dose administration (30.9% vs. 18.2%; right panel Figure 6c; *p*-value = 0.044).

3.3.3. Head Positions (Supine)

Considering that the liquid-holding capacity of the turbinate furrows is sensitive to the head orientation, two head positions were evaluated that tilted up and down from the flat supine position by 20°, respectively. As shown in Figure 7a, when tilting the head up by 20° (equivalent to the head on a pillow), most of the spray droplets were deposited in the inferior turbinate and nasal floor. This was because the vestibule was aligned with the inferior turbinate along gravity in this case. Moreover, the liquid film spread a shorter distance than in the supine position because tilting the head up by 20° changed the turbinate furrow from vertical to a 70° slope. Applying the second dose delivered significantly more doses to the caudal turbinate, but a negligible dose was observed in the nasopharynx, as displayed in the middle panel of Figure 7a. The posterior nose dose (i.e., caudal turbinate and nasopharynx) with one-dose and dual-dose applications was 2.9 mg and 34.0 mg, respectively (right panel, Figure 7a).

Figure 7b shows the deposition distribution when the head was tilted back by 20°. Note that this would also change the turbinate furrow from vertical to a 70° slope, but the liquid film would touch the other side of the turbinate furrow and have a different liquid film stability. With one applied dose, the liquid film traveled down the turbinate furrow, with several drops reaching the nasopharynx (hollow red arrow, left panel, Figure 7b).

Applying another dose delivered more sprays to the caudal turbinate, particularly to the ridge of the caudal turbinate (solid red arrow, middle panel, Figure 7b). The turbinate deposition increased from 31.5 mg with one-dose application to 58.3 mg with dual-dose application; the nasopharynx deposition increased from 9.4 mg with one-dose application to 26.7 mg with dual-dose application (right panel, Figure 7b). Based on these observations, it was inferred that three factors are necessary for enhanced delivery to the posterior nose: (1) flow shear mobilizing the liquid film, (2) gravity aligning with the target, and (3) highly slanted turbinate furrows assisting the liquid film motion and minimizing the wall liquid-holding capacity. As a result, adopting a supine position or tilting the head backward by 20° is supposed to effectively deliver sprays to the posterior nose (Figures 6 and 7b).

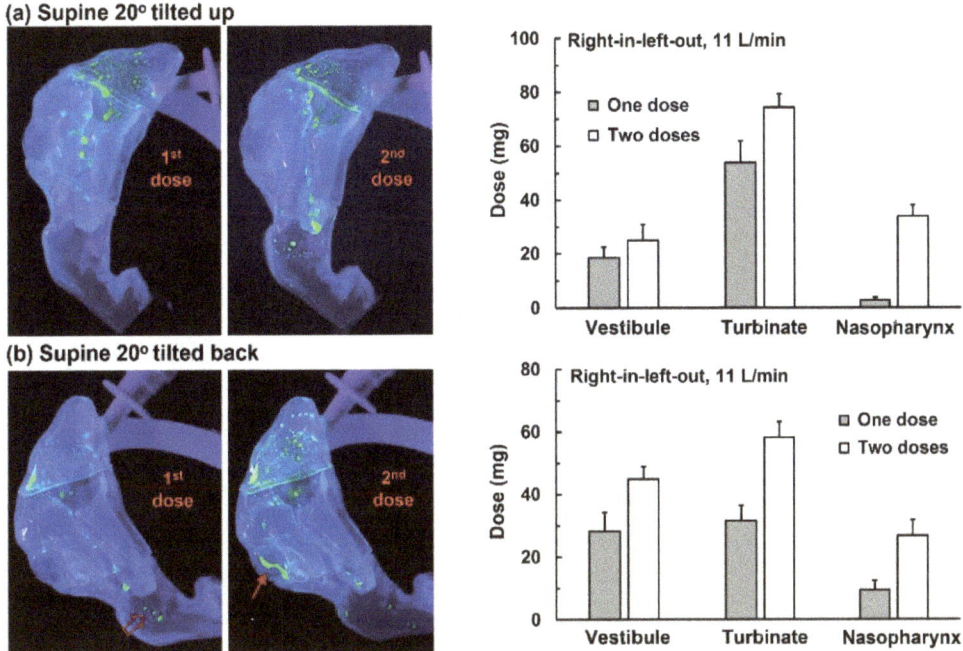

Figure 7. Head orientation effects on nasal spray deposition distribution: (**a**) supine 20° tilted up (head on a pillow) and (**b**) supine 20° tilted back.

3.4. Revisiting Unidirectional Delivery

Effects of Spray Administration Angles (Relative to the Nostril)

It was noted that these aforementioned three factors needed for enhanced delivery to the posterior nose could be valid for both bidirectional and unidirectional delivery methods as long as the flow shear is sufficient in mobilizing the liquid film. Thus, unidirectional delivery in a supine position with a high flow rate and multiple-dose applications could also give similarly enhanced doses to the target as bidirectional delivery.

Figure 8a,b displays the deposition pattern of unidirectional delivery at 30 L/min with one dose and two doses, respectively. The supine position appeared to significantly offset the liquid-film-stabilizing forces, which made it easier for the flow shear to mobilize the wall film. The increased gravitational component and reduced wall liquid-holding capacity in the supine position also facilitated the liquid film translocation toward the back of the nose, as illustrated by the increased nasopharynx dose (hollow red arrow, Figure 8a).

Applying a second dose further enhanced deposition in the nasopharynx (red arrow, Figure 8b). Moreover, liquid dripping was observed at the caudal tip of the turbinate (yellow arrow, Figure 8b), indicating that the liquid washed through the turbinate region. Quantitatively, applying a second dose more than doubled the deposition in the turbinate region (i.e., from 39.0 to 88.8 mg, p-value = 0.016) and nasopharynx (i.e., from 8.6 to 32.6 mg, p-value = 0.031), as shown in Figure 8c. It was also noted that the same factors (gravity and flow shear) that helped mobilize the liquid film could also reduce the maximal liquid film thickness, thus slightly decreasing the dose adhering to the same region.

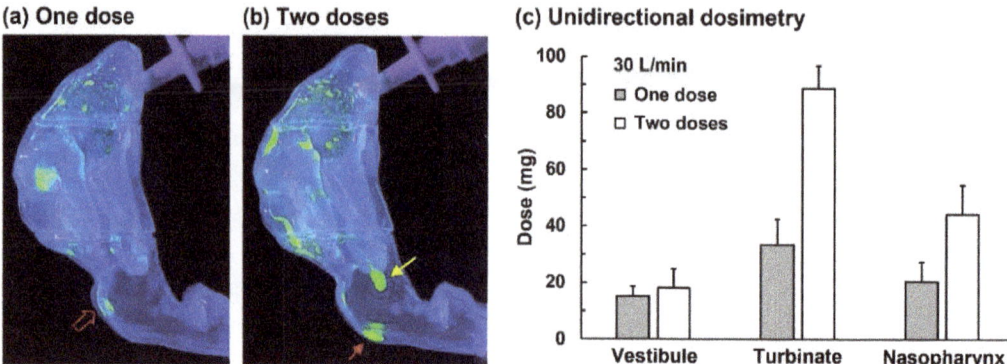

Figure 8. Nasal spray deposition distribution using unidirectional delivery in a supine position with a flow rate of 30 L/min with (**a**) one dose, (**b**) two doses, and (**c**) quantification of regional deposition fractions.

4. Discussion

4.1. Has the New Delivery System Delivered Sufficient Doses to the Posterior Nose?

In this study, we sought to develop an effective protocol for delivering nasal sprays to the posterior nose by testing different delivery modes, administration angles, inhalation flow rates, and the number of applications in a progressive manner. That is, after each parametric study, not only were the performances compared but also the underlying mechanisms were examined, hypotheses were checked, and new hypotheses were planned to be tested (more details in the following Section 4.2). With this progressive examination, it was found that a supine position and dual applications are able to significantly improve the doses delivered to the caudal turbinate and nasopharynx, which are the targets for mucosal immunization. Compared to the 0~5% of deposition fractions to these two regions using conventional nasal inhalers, the new protocol managed to deliver 31% of the dose to the nasopharynx alone (Figure 6c). This significant enhancement in posterior nose delivery can pave the way for mucosal immunization, for which low doses to the target using conventional methods have been a bottleneck to their wide clinical application, even though many nasally inhaled vaccines have been actively developed during the pandemic in the past 2 years [29–33].

Formulation viscosity can significantly affect spray generation and the subsequent dosimetry in the nose. Previous studies have demonstrated that a more viscous formulation would generate a spray with a narrower plume angle and large droplets, leading to a smaller spray area [34]. As a result, more doses would be deposited in the vestibule and anterior turbinate in comparison to formulations with lower viscosities [35,36]. Viscosity modifiers, such as mucoadhesive polymers, have often been added to nasal spray formulations to improve local delivery or cellular uptake [37,38]. In this study, saline solution was used that had a lower viscosity, which was expected to yield more distal deposition in the nose than using actual nasal formulations. In particular, slightly lower deposition in the nasopharynx was expected in clinical practice. Considering lipophilic drugs, suspension or emulsion formulations would form, which could affect the rate of both dissolution and film translocation [39]. Han et al. [40] measured the surface tension of various oral and nasal suspension formulations and reported a lower surface tension magnitude compared to saline water. Therefore, the liquid film on the nasal wall was expected to be less stable and more prone to translocate to the back of the nose.

4.2. Mechanisms Underlying Successful Posterior Nose Delivery

Controlled liquid film translocation was found to be the key to the success or failure of effective delivery to the caudal turbinate and nasopharynx. For a given delivery condition (device, administration angle, head position, etc.), liquid translocation from initial deposition sites to the target would be determined by three factors: First, whether a destabilizing force could mobilize or start the translocation of the liquid film; second, the translocation direction and distance followed gravity and were channeled by the nose topology; and lastly, the translocated mass depended on the applied mass over the liquid-holding capacity of the nasal wall.

Due to the large droplet sizes and high discharging velocities, nasal sprays often deposit in the anterior nose, particularly in the vestibule and nasal valve. Because of the highly localized deposition, liquid films form from these droplets as distinct or connected patches. However, whether these liquid film patches stay or move depends on the rivalry between the stabilizing and destabilizing forces. In this regard, surface tension (both liquid–air and liquid–wall) and viscosity (static wall fraction) were stabilizing forces, while gravity (i.e., tangential components of the liquid self-weight) and flow shear (at the air–liquid interface) were destabilizing forces. In this study, we observed negligible translocation when there was no inhalation flow (thus no flow shear), with most of the nasal spray being deposited in the anterior nose and staying there (Figure 5a). Increasing the flow rate increased the film translocation in both extent and traveling distance regardless of the delivery mode (Figure 5b,c). This indicated that flow-induced shear at the air–liquid interface could be the determining factor in mobilizing the liquid film, especially in regions where the stabilizing forces from surface tension and viscosity are only slightly larger than the destabilizing gravitational force [41–43].

How far the liquid film could move depended on the flow shear, gravity, and nose topology along the way. The liquid-holding capacity was influenced by both the wall slope and the local wall topological details. Previous studies have reported that the maximal liquid film thickness is reversely correlated with the wall slope angle [44,45]. A rough wall with geometrical irregularities could hold more liquid due to a large surface area for the intermolecular force, as well as a physical interlocking effect, leading to a higher static wall fraction [46]. Once the liquid film is mobilized, the kinematic wall shear would be much smaller due to the lubrication effects by transiting from static interlocking to laminar layer sliding (ref-lubrication) [47]. The motion of the liquid film will accelerate when moving down a slope and slow down when working against gravity. The liquid film may also stop as it fulfills the new walls' liquid-holding capacity while spreading until the liquid film is too thin to overcome the stabilizing forces. As a result, aligning gravity toward the target is a promising approach to maximize the delivered doses via film translocation, as demonstrated in Figures 5–7. Aligning the target with gravity has often been practiced in the treatment of rhinosinusitis [48]. Merkus et al. [49] recommended a head-to-floor position to enhance nasal spray delivery to the olfactory cleft after comparing four head positions: upright, supine-tilting-back, lying-on-one-side, and head-to-floor positions. Cannady et al. [50] reported that the head-to-floor position could deliver more drugs to the ethmoid cavity, maxillary sinus, and sphenoid sinus. Similarly, Mori et al. [51] observed that the lying-on-one-side (Kaiteki) position allows more nasal drops to reach the olfactory region. However, it is also cautioned that the practice of aligning gravity to the target is not guaranteed to deliver the maximal doses to the target, because the liquid motion is also subject to the wall geometrical details that can be either a blockage or a conduit to the liquid flow.

Once a path of liquid film translocation to the target was established (by adopting a specific device, delivery mode, administration angle, head position, etc.), the dose to the target could be controlled by applying multiple doses. As shown in Figures 6–8, a significantly higher dose from the second application was delivered to the posterior nose than from the first application, in the light of the fact that part of the first dose had been allocated to fill the wall liquid-holding capacity. However, too many applications would overflow the targeted regions and cause unwanted deposition in other regions [52,53].

4.3. Bidirectional vs. Unidirectional Modes

The experimental results in this study show that using the bidirectional route delivers higher doses to the caudal turbinate and nasopharynx than using the unidirectional route. With a single spray application, the optimal nasopharynx dose was 13.5 mg vs. 8.6 mg using the bidirectional and unidirectional methods, respectively (Figure 6c vs. Figure 8c). With a dual-dose application, the nasopharynx dose was 32.6 mg bidirectional ly vs. 43.3 mg unidirectionally (Figure 6c vs. Figure 8c).

Using a transparent nasal replica cast, it was clearly demonstrated that the liquid film translocation was far more intensified during bidirectional delivery than during unidirectional delivery, all other parameters being the same. Even though the exact reason underlying this difference was not clear at this moment, we speculated that this could be attributed to the distinct flow dynamics between these delivery methods, which further led to different wall shear (stabilizing force) and flow shear (destabilizing force). In the bidirectional route, the nasopharynx was closed and the airflow followed a U-shaped trajectory from the right nostril to the left nostril. Note that it is a natural reflex in humans that the soft palate is lifted up upon exhalation and blocks the oropharynx that connects the oral and nasal airways. As a result, the nasopharynx serves as a dead end, which generates an elevated pressure that diverts the airflow by $180°$ from one nasal passage to the other. It is likely that this forceful diversion in the flow direction creates a pressure-flow-shear field that is more prone to mobilizing the liquid film and driving the liquid film motion. Further studies are needed to prove/disprove this hypothesis and to unravel the exact reason responsible for the improved bidirectional dosimetry.

4.4. Limitations

This study can be further improved if more physiological factors can be considered, including a large cohort of nose models, more delivery scenarios, and compliant walls. Intranasal spray dosimetry is sensitive to nasal anatomical details; the inter-subject variability can be large and warrants future investigations [54–57]. It will be desirable to know the range or confidence level of the nasal dosage for a given device, formulation, and targeted patient population (e.g., child, adult, senior) [36,58–60]. Similarly, a limited number of delivery conditions were considered. By considering more test cases that cover the entire design space, a response surface can be developed, which can immediately provide an empirical estimation for any delivery scenarios [61]. Considering that nasal sprays generally have large droplet sizes and high exiting speeds, the inertial impaction will be the predominant deposition mechanism and the effects from compliant walls should be secondary [62,63]. Zeta potential analysis, which characterizes the droplet surface charge and is important in determining the stability of colloidal suspensions or emulsions, was not considered in this study based on the rationale that 0.9% saline water is a stable solution [64]. The droplet size distribution and physicochemical properties of the three nasal formulations were not fully characterized except the size distribution of the soft-mist nasal inhaler.

5. Conclusions

In this study, the feasibility of delivering high doses of nasal sprays to the caudal turbinate and nasopharynx was evaluated by experimentally testing different delivery methods, releasing angles, flow rates, head positions, and dosing numbers. The mechanisms underlying liquid film translocation were explored. Specific findings are as follows:

(1) For nasal spray delivery, liquid film translocation can be a more important factor than the initial deposition in determining the dosimetry distribution.
(2) Liquid film translocation is sensitive to the inhalation flow rate and head position.
(3) Liquid film translocation is more sensitive to the inhalation flow rate in bidirectional delivery than in unidirectional delivery and in a supine position than in the upright position.

(4) Factors favorable for posterior nose delivery include (1) flow shear mobilizing the liquid film, (2) gravity aligning with the target, and (3) slanted turbinate furrows assisting film motion and minimizing the wall liquid-holding capacity.

(5) A supine position and dual-dose application significantly enhance nasal spray deposition in the caudal turbinate and nasopharynx. A nasopharynx deposition fraction of 31% was achieved vs. no nasopharynx deposition in an upright position with a one-dose application.

Author Contributions: Conceptualization, X.A.S. and J.X.; methodology, A.S., M.T., X.A.S. and J.X.; software, A.S., X.A.S. and J.X.; validation, A.S., X.A.S. and J.X.; formal analysis, A.S. and J.X.; investigation, A.S., M.T. and P.R.; resources, X.A.S. and J.X.; data curation, A.S., M.T. and P.R.; writing—original draft preparation, J.X.; writing—review and editing, A.S. and X.A.S. All authors have read and agreed to the published version of the manuscript.

Funding: This research received no external funding.

Institutional Review Board Statement: Not applicable.

Informed Consent Statement: Not applicable.

Data Availability Statement: The data and images are available from the corresponding author (J.X.) upon request.

Acknowledgments: Jacob Stover is gratefully acknowledged for his assistance in experiments.

Conflicts of Interest: The authors declare no conflict of interest.

References

1. Hoffmann, M.; Kleine-Weber, H.; Schroeder, S.; Krüger, N.; Herrler, T.; Erichsen, S.; Schiergens, T.S.; Herrler, G.; Wu, N.-H.; Nitsche, A.; et al. SARS-CoV-2 cell entry depends on ACE2 and TMPRSS2 and is blocked by a clinically proven protease inhibitor. *Cell* **2020**, *181*, 271–280.e278. [CrossRef]
2. Sungnak, W.; Huang, N.; Bécavin, C.; Berg, M.; Queen, R.; Litvinukova, M.; Talavera-López, C.; Maatz, H.; Reichart, D.; Sampaziotis, F.; et al. SARS-CoV-2 entry factors are highly expressed in nasal epithelial cells together with innate immune genes. *Nat. Med.* **2020**, *26*, 681–687. [CrossRef]
3. Lee, I.T.; Nakayama, T.; Wu, C.-T.; Goltsev, Y.; Jiang, S.; Gall, P.A.; Liao, C.-K.; Shih, L.-C.; Schürch, C.M.; McIlwain, D.R.; et al. ACE2 localizes to the respiratory cilia and is not increased by ACE inhibitors or ARBs. *Nat. Commun.* **2020**, *11*, 5453. [CrossRef]
4. Ziegler, C.G.K.; Allon, S.J.; Nyquist, S.K.; Mbano, I.M.; Miao, V.N.; Tzouanas, C.N.; Cao, Y.; Yousif, A.S.; Bals, J.; Hauser, B.M.; et al. SARS-CoV-2 receptor ACE2 Is an interferon-stimulated gene in human airway epithelial cells and is detected in specific cell subsets across tissues. *Cell* **2020**, *181*, 1016–1035.e1019. [CrossRef]
5. Xu, K.; Shi, X.; Husted, C.; Hong, R.; Wang, Y.; Ning, B.; Sullivan, T.; Rieger-Christ, K.; Duan, F.; Marques, H.; et al. Smoking Modulates Different Secretory Subpopulations Expressing SARS-CoV-2 Entry Genes in the Nasal and Bronchial Airways. *Res. Sq.* **2021**, *12*, 18168. [CrossRef] [PubMed]
6. Berger, G.; Marom, Z.; Ophir, D. Goblet cell density of the inferior turbinates in patients with perennial allergic and nonallergic rhinitis. *Am. J. Rhinol.* **1997**, *11*, 233–236. [CrossRef]
7. Glezen, W.P. The new nasal spray influenza vaccine. *Pediatr. Infect. Dis. J.* **2001**, *20*, 731–732. [CrossRef]
8. Xi, J. Development and challenges of nasal spray vaccines for short-term COVID-19 protection. *Curr. Pharm. Biotechnol.* **2022**, *23*, 1671–1677. [CrossRef]
9. Nian, X.; Zhang, J.; Huang, S.; Duan, K.; Li, X.; Yang, X. Development of Nasal Vaccines and the Associated Challenges. *Pharmaceutics* **2022**, *14*, 1983. [CrossRef]
10. Waltz, E. How nasal-spray vaccines could change the pandemic. *Nature* **2022**, *609*, 240–242. [CrossRef]
11. Chavda, V.P.; Patel, A.B.; Vora, L.K.; Singla, R.K.; Shah, P.; Uversky, V.N.; Apostolopoulos, V. Nitric oxide and its derivatives containing nasal spray and inhalation therapy for the treatment of COVID-19. *Curr. Pharm. Des.* **2022**, *609*, 240–242. [CrossRef] [PubMed]
12. Paull, J.R.A.; Luscombe, C.A.; Castellarnau, A.; Heery, G.P.; Bobardt, M.D.; Gallay, P.A. Protective Effects of Astodrimer Sodium 1% Nasal Spray Formulation against SARS-CoV-2 Nasal Challenge in K18-hACE2 Mice. *Viruses* **2021**, *13*, 1656. [CrossRef]
13. Xi, J.; Yuan, J.E.; Zhang, Y.; Nevorski, D.; Wang, Z.; Zhou, Y. Visualization and quantification of nasal and olfactory deposition in a sectional adult nasal airway cast. *Pharm. Res.* **2016**, *33*, 1527–1541. [CrossRef]
14. Xi, J.; Si, X.A.; Kim, J.; Zhang, Y.; Jacob, R.E.; Kabilan, S.; Corley, R.A. Anatomical details of the rabbit nasal passages and their implications in breathing, air conditioning, and olfaction. *Anat. Rec.* **2016**, *299*, 853–868. [CrossRef]
15. Inthavong, K.; Fung, M.C.; Yang, W.; Tu, J. Measurements of droplet size distribution and analysis of nasal spray atomization from different actuation pressure. *J. Aerosol Med. Pulm. Drug Deliv.* **2015**, *28*, 59–67. [CrossRef] [PubMed]

16. Cheng, Y.S.; Holmes, T.D.; Gao, J.; Guilmette, R.A.; Li, S.; Surakitbanharn, Y.; Rowlings, C. Characterization of nasal spray pumps and deposition pattern in a replica of the human nasal airway. *J. Aerosol Med.* **2001**, *14*, 267–280. [CrossRef]
17. Kundoor, V.; Dalby, R.N. Effect of formulation- and administration-related variables on deposition pattern of nasal spray pumps evaluated using a nasal cast. *Pharm. Res.* **2011**, *28*, 1895–1904. [CrossRef]
18. Si, X.A.; Sami, M.; Xi, J. Liquid film translocation significantly enhances nasal spray delivery to olfactory region: A numerical simulation study. *Pharmaceutics* **2021**, *13*, 903. [CrossRef]
19. Abdelalim, A.A.; Mohamady, A.A.; Elsayed, R.A.; Elawady, M.A.; Ghallab, A.F. Corticosteroid nasal spray for recovery of smell sensation in COVID-19 patients: A randomized controlled trial. *Am. J. Otolaryngol.* **2021**, *42*, 102884. [CrossRef] [PubMed]
20. Guenezan, J.; Garcia, M.; Strasters, D.; Jousselin, C.; Lévêque, N.; Frasca, D.; Mimoz, O. Povidone Iodine mouthwash, gargle, and nasal spray to reduce nasopharyngeal viral load in patients with COVID-19: A randomized clinical trial. *JAMA Otolaryngol. Head Neck Surg.* **2021**, *147*, 400–401. [CrossRef]
21. Rubin, R. COVID-19 Vaccine Nasal Spray. *Jama* **2021**, *326*, 1138. [CrossRef] [PubMed]
22. Xi, J.; Si, X.A. A next-generation vaccine for broader and long-lasting COVID-19 protection. *MedComm (2020)* **2022**, *3*, e138. [CrossRef] [PubMed]
23. Hoseini-Tavassol, Z.; Ejtahed, H.S.; Soroush, A.R.; Sajjadpour, Z.; Hasani-Ranjbar, S.; Larijani, B. Natural derived nasal spray: A proposed approach for COVID-19 disease control. *Infect. Disord. Drug Targets* **2021**, *21*, e160921191568. [CrossRef] [PubMed]
24. Ku, Z.; Xie, X.; Hinton, P.R.; Liu, X.; Ye, X.; Muruato, A.E.; Ng, D.C.; Biswas, S.; Zou, J.; Liu, Y.; et al. Nasal delivery of an IgM offers broad protection from SARS-CoV-2 variants. *Nature* **2021**, *595*, 718–723. [CrossRef]
25. Chavda, V.P.; Vora, L.K.; Pandya, A.K.; Patravale, V.B. Intranasal vaccines for SARS-CoV-2: From challenges to potential in COVID-19 management. *Drug Discov. Today* **2021**, *26*, 2619–2636. [CrossRef]
26. Xi, J.; Wang, Z.; Nevorski, D.; White, T.; Zhou, Y. Nasal and olfactory deposition with normal and bidirectional intranasal delivery techniques: In vitro tests and numerical simulations. *J. Aerosol Med. Pulm. Drug Deliv.* **2017**, *30*, 118–131. [CrossRef]
27. Xi, J.; Kim, J.; Si, X.A.; Corley, R.A.; Zhou, Y. Modeling of inertial deposition in scaled models of rat and human nasal airways: Towards in vitro regional dosimetry in small animals. *J. Aerosol Sci.* **2016**, *99*, 78–93. [CrossRef]
28. Ochowiak, M.; Włodarczak, S.; Krupińska, A.; Matuszak, M. Particle Image Velocimetry based on Matlab and PIVlab for testing flow disturbing elements. In *Design, Simulation, Manufacturing: The Innovation Exchange*; Springer: Cham, Switzerland, 2021; pp. 268–276.
29. Xi, J.; Lei, L.R.; Zouzas, W.; April Si, X. Nasally inhaled therapeutics and vaccination for COVID-19: Developments and challenges. *MedComm* **2021**, *2*, 569–586. [CrossRef]
30. Moakes, R.J.A.; Davies, S.P.; Stamataki, Z.; Grover, L.M. Formulation of a Composite Nasal Spray Enabling Enhanced Surface Coverage and Prophylaxis of SARS-CoV-2. *Adv. Mater.* **2021**, *33*, e2008304. [CrossRef]
31. Lin, Y.; Yue, S.; Yang, Y.; Yang, S.; Pan, Z.; Yang, X.; Gao, L.; Zhou, J.; Li, Z.; Hu, L.; et al. Nasal spray of neutralizing monoclonal antibody 35B5 confers potential prophylaxis against severe acute respiratory syndrome coronavirus 2 (SARS-CoV-2) variants of concern (VOCs): A small-scale clinical trial. *Clin. Infect. Dis.* **2022**. [CrossRef]
32. Hemilä, H.; Chalker, E. Carrageenan nasal spray may double the rate of recovery from coronavirus and influenza virus infections: Re-analysis of randomized trial data. *Pharmacol. Res. Perspect.* **2021**, *9*, e00810. [CrossRef] [PubMed]
33. Castellarnau, A.; Heery, G.P.; Seta, A.; Luscombe, C.A.; Kinghorn, G.R.; Button, P.; McCloud, P.; Paull, J.R.A. Astodrimer sodium antiviral nasal spray for reducing respiratory infections is safe and well tolerated in a randomized controlled trial. *Sci. Rep.* **2022**, *12*, 10210. [CrossRef] [PubMed]
34. Pu, Y.; Goodey, A.P.; Fang, X.; Jacob, K. A Comparison of the Deposition Patterns of Different Nasal Spray Formulations Using a Nasal Cast. *Aerosol Sci. Technol.* **2014**, *48*, 930–938. [CrossRef]
35. Gao, M.; Shen, X.; Mao, S. Factors influencing drug deposition in thenasal cavity upon delivery via nasal sprays. *J. Pharm. Investig.* **2020**, *50*, 251–259. [CrossRef]
36. Sosnowski, T.R.; Rapiejko, P.; Sova, J.; Dobrowolska, K. Impact of physicochemical properties of nasal spray products on drug deposition and transport in the pediatric nasal cavity model. *Int. J. Pharm.* **2020**, *574*, 118911. [CrossRef] [PubMed]
37. Wong, Y.L.; Pandey, M.; Choudhury, H.; Lim, W.M.; Bhattamisra, S.K.; Gorain, B. Development of In-Situ Spray for Local Delivery of Antibacterial Drug for Hidradenitis Suppurativa: Investigation of Alternative Formulation. *Polymers* **2021**, *13*, 2770. [CrossRef]
38. Chaturvedi, M.; Kumar, M.; Pathak, K. A review on mucoadhesive polymer used in nasal drug delivery system. *J. Adv. Pharm. Technol. Res.* **2011**, *2*, 215–222. [CrossRef]
39. Rygg, A.; Hindle, M.; Longest, P.W. Absorption and Clearance of Pharmaceutical Aerosols in the Human Nose: Effects of Nasal Spray Suspension Particle Size and Properties. *Pharm. Res.* **2016**, *33*, 909–921. [CrossRef]
40. Han, K.; Woghiren, O.E.; Priefer, R. Surface tension examination of various liquid oral, nasal, and ophthalmic dosage forms. *Chem. Cent. J.* **2016**, *10*, 31. [CrossRef]
41. Katsiavria, A.; Bontozoglou, V. Stability of liquid film flow laden with the soluble surfactant sodium dodecyl sulphate: Predictions versus experimental data. *J. Fluid Mech.* **2020**, *894*, A18. [CrossRef]
42. Mirjalili, S.; Chan, W.H.R. Linear stability of a thin fluid film interacting with its surrounding bulk fluid. *Phys. Fluids* **2021**, *33*, 072104. [CrossRef]
43. Craster, R.V.; Matar, O.K. Dynamics and stability of thin liquid films. *Rev. Mod. Phys.* **2009**, *81*, 1131–1198. [CrossRef]

44. Yu, Y.Q.; Cheng, X. Experimental study of water film flow on large vertical and inclined flat plate. *Prog. Nucl. Energy* **2014**, *77*, 176–186. [CrossRef]
45. Kim, T.-S.; Kim, M.-U. The flow and hydrodynamic stability of a liquid film on a rotating disc. *Fluid Dyn. Res.* **2009**, *41*, 035504. [CrossRef]
46. Steinberg, C.; Liu, M.; Hung, D.L.S. A combined experimental–numerical study towards the elucidation of spray–wall interaction on step geometries. *Eng. Appl. Comput. Fluid Mech.* **2022**, *16*, 1866–1882. [CrossRef]
47. Du, R.; Zhang, A.; Du, Z.; Zhang, X. Molecular dynamics simulation on thin-film lubrication of a mixture of three alkanes. *Materials* **2020**, *13*, 3689. [CrossRef]
48. Meltzer, E.O.; Hamilos, D.L. Rhinosinusitis diagnosis and management for the clinician: A synopsis of recent consensus guidelines. *Mayo. Clin. Proc.* **2011**, *86*, 427–443. [CrossRef]
49. Merkus, P.; Ebbens, F.A.; Muller, B.; Fokkens, W.J. The 'best method' of topical nasal drug delivery: Comparison of seven techniques. *Rhinology* **2006**, *44*, 102–107.
50. Cannady, S.B.; Batra, P.S.; Citardi, M.J.; Lanza, D.C. Comparison of delivery of topical medications to the paranasal sinuses via "vertex-to-floor" position and atomizer spray after FESS. *Otolaryngol. Head Neck Surg.* **2005**, *133*, 735–740. [CrossRef]
51. Mori, E.; Merkonidis, C.; Cuevas, M.; Gudziol, V.; Matsuwaki, Y.; Hummel, T. The administration of nasal drops in the "Kaiteki" position allows for delivery of the drug to the olfactory cleft: A pilot study in healthy subjects. *Eur. Arch. Otorhinolaryngol.* **2016**, *273*, 939–943. [CrossRef]
52. Masiuk, T.; Kadakia, P.; Wang, Z. Development of a physiologically relevant dripping analytical method using simulated nasal mucus for nasal spray formulation analysis. *J. Pharm. Anal.* **2016**, *6*, 283–291. [CrossRef] [PubMed]
53. Bonart, H.; Rajes, S.; Jung, J.; Repke, J.-U. Stability of gravity-driven liquid films overflowing microstructures with sharp corners. *Phys. Rev. Fluids* **2020**, *5*, 094001. [CrossRef]
54. El Taoum, K.K.; Xi, J.; Kim, J.W.; Berlinski, A. In vitro evaluation of aerosols delivered via the nasal route. *Respir Care* **2015**, *60*, 1015–1025. [CrossRef]
55. Doughty, D.V.; Hsu, W.; Dalby, R.N. Automated actuation of nasal spray products: Effect of hand-related variability on the in vitro performance of Flonase nasal spray. *Drug Dev. Ind. Pharm.* **2014**, *40*, 711–718. [CrossRef]
56. Garcia, G.J.; Tewksbury, E.W.; Wong, B.A.; Kimbell, J.S. Interindividual variability in nasal filtration as a function of nasal cavity geometry. *J. Aerosol Med. Pulm. Drug Deliv.* **2009**, *22*, 139–155. [CrossRef] [PubMed]
57. Williams, G.; Suman, J.D. In vitro anatomical models for nasal drug delivery. *Pharmaceutics* **2022**, *14*, 1353. [CrossRef]
58. Zhou, Y.; Guo, M.; Xi, J.; Irshad, H.; Cheng, Y.-S. Nasal deposition in infants and children. *J. Aerosol Med.* **2014**, *26*, 110–116. [CrossRef]
59. Berlinski, A. Pediatric aerosol therapy. *Respir. Care* **2017**, *62*, 662–677. [CrossRef]
60. Kim, J.; Xi, J.; Si, X.; Berlinski, A.; Su, W.C. Hood nebulization: Effects of head direction and breathing mode on particle inhalability and deposition in a 7-month-old infant model. *J. Aerosol Med. Pulm. Drug Deliv.* **2014**, *27*, 209–218. [CrossRef]
61. Lu, J.; Xi, J.; Langenderfer, J.E. Sensitivity analysis and uncertainty quantification in pulmonary drug delivery of orally inhaled pharmaceuticals. *J. Pharm. Sci.* **2017**, *106*, 3303–3315. [CrossRef]
62. Djupesland, P.G. Nasal drug delivery devices: Characteristics and performance in a clinical perspective—A review. *Drug Deliv. Transl. Res.* **2013**, *3*, 42–62. [CrossRef] [PubMed]
63. Xi, J.; Wang, Z.; Si, X.A.; Zhou, Y. Nasal dilation effects on olfactory deposition in unilateral and bi-directional deliveries: In vitro tests and numerical modeling. *Eur. J. Pharm. Sci.* **2018**, *118*, 113–123. [CrossRef] [PubMed]
64. Far, J.; Abdel-Haq, M.; Gruber, M.; Abu Ammar, A. Developing Biodegradable Nanoparticles Loaded with Mometasone Furoate for Potential Nasal Drug Delivery. *ACS Omega* **2020**, *5*, 7432–7439. [CrossRef] [PubMed]

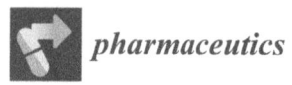 *pharmaceutics*

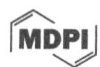

Article

Spray-Dried Powder Formulation of Capreomycin Designed for Inhaled Tuberculosis Therapy

Zitong Shao [1], Waiting Tai [2], Yingshan Qiu [1], Rico C. H. Man [1], Qiuying Liao [1], Michael Y. T. Chow [2], Philip C. L. Kwok [2] and Jenny K. W. Lam [1,3,*]

[1] Department of Pharmacology and Pharmacy, Li Ka Shing Faculty of Medicine, The University of Hong Kong, 21 Sassoon Road, Pokfulam, Hong Kong, China; u3006730@connect.hku.hk (Z.S.); u3004556@connect.hku.hk (Y.Q.); u3542606@connect.hku.hk (R.C.H.M.); liaoqy@connect.hku.hk (Q.L.)

[2] Advanced Drug Delivery Group, Sydney Pharmacy School, Faculty of Medicine and Health, The University of Sydney, Sydney, NSW 2006, Australia; wtai6746@uni.sydney.edu.au (W.T.); yee.chow@sydney.edu.au (M.Y.T.C.); philip.kwok@sydney.edu.au (P.C.L.K.)

[3] Advanced Biomedical Instrumentation Centre, Hong Kong Science Park, Shatin, New Territories, Hong Kong, China

* Correspondence: jkwlam@hku.hk

Citation: Shao, Z.; Tai, W.; Qiu, Y.; Man, R.C.H.; Liao, Q.; Chow, M.Y.T.; Kwok, P.C.L.; Lam, J.K.W. Spray-Dried Powder Formulation of Capreomycin Designed for Inhaled Tuberculosis Therapy. *Pharmaceutics* **2021**, *13*, 2044. https://doi.org/10.3390/pharmaceutics13122044

Academic Editors: Stefano Giovagnoli and Holger Grohganz

Received: 5 October 2021
Accepted: 26 November 2021
Published: 30 November 2021

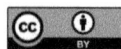
Abstract: Multi-drug-resistant tuberculosis (MDR-TB) is a huge public health problem. The treatment regimen of MDR-TB requires prolonged chemotherapy with multiple drugs including second-line anti-TB agents associated with severe adverse effects. Capreomycin, a polypeptide antibiotic, is the first choice of second-line anti-TB drugs in MDR-TB therapy. It requires repeated intramuscular or intravenous administration five times per week. Pulmonary drug delivery is non-invasive with the advantages of local targeting and reduced risk of systemic toxicity. In this study, inhaled dry powder formulation of capreomycin targeting the lung was developed using spray drying technique. Among the 16 formulations designed, the one containing 25% capreomycin (*w/w*) and spray-dried at an inlet temperature of 90 °C showed the best overall performance with the mass median aerodynamic diameter (MMAD) of 3.38 μm and a fine particle fraction (FPF) of around 65%. In the pharmacokinetic study in mice, drug concentration in the lungs was approximately 8-fold higher than the minimum inhibitory concentration (MIC) (1.25 to 2.5 μg/mL) for at least 24 h following intratracheal administration (20 mg/kg). Compared to intravenous injection, inhaled capreomycin showed significantly higher area under the curve, slower clearance and longer mean residence time in both the lungs and plasma.

Keywords: capreomycin; dry powder aerosol; inhalation; pulmonary delivery; spray drying; tuberculosis

1. Introduction

Tuberculosis (TB) is an airborne communicable disease caused by *Mycobacterium tuberculosis* (*Mtb*). It is one of the major causes of illness and death worldwide. As an unresolved public health threat, it is estimated that 10 million people fell ill with TB in 2019 [1]. Although the number of infections has slowly declined in recent years, the coronavirus disease 2019 (COVID-19) pandemic and the increasing number of human immunodeficiency virus (HIV) infections exert negative impact on global TB control [1]. The management of TB has become more challenging with the emergence of multi-drug-resistant TB (MDR-TB), which refers to the resistance to both isoniazid and rifampicin. Treatment of MDR-TB requires the use of second-line drugs that are mostly injectables with high toxicity and long treatment duration of at least nine months (typically up to 24 months) [1,2].

Capreomycin is a cyclic polypeptide antibiotic composed of four molecular analogues (IA, IB, IIA and IIB) isolated from *Streptomyces capreolus* [3]. It is a second-line anti-TB agent used for the treatment of MDR-TB. The mechanism of action of capreomycin is not completely clear but it is widely accepted that it inhibits bacterial protein synthesis by binding to the 70S ribosomal unit. It can interfere with several ribosomal functions, including the formation of the 30S subunit initiation complex and the translocation of tRNA [4,5]. Capreomycin needs to be repeatedly injected (up to five times per week) and is associated with severe adverse effects such as nephrotoxicity and ototoxicity. Therefore, long-term administration of capreomycin is a heavy load for patients, especially the elderly and those with renal impairment [6].

Pulmonary delivery is a non-invasive alternative route of drug administration for the treatment of pulmonary TB, including MDR-TB. By delivering the drug to the lung directly, high local drug concentration at the site of primary infection can be achieved. As a result, a lower dose is required, thereby minimising systemic exposure, improving drug efficacy and reducing the risk of drug resistance development [7]. Another advantage of inhaled TB therapy is that particles targeted to the lung can be phagocytosed by alveolar macrophages in which the *Mtb* colonized [8]. Compared to liquid formulations, dry powder formulations have better stability, which is convenient for storage and transportation. In addition, dry powder inhalers (DPIs) are easy to operate and allow the delivery of high doses, which are often required for antibiotics [9]. A few studies have reported the preparation of inhalable powder of capreomycin, some of which were formulated in liposomes or poly(lactic-*co*-glycolic acid) (PLGA) microparticles to control the particles size distribution for efficient lung deposition [10,11]. Hickey et al. produced spray-dried powder of capreomycin (as sulfate), in which 50% ethanol (v/v) was used as the solvent and L-leucine as dispersion enhancer [2,12–14]. Schoubben et al. blended spray-dried capreomycin (as sulfate) powders with lactose at a 1:50 ratio (w/w) to improve powder dispersibility [15]. Since TB therapy requires high dose of drug, it may not be practical to deliver capreomycin with such a large amount of excipient [16].

The aim of this study was to develop inhaled powder formulations of capreomycin that exhibit high drug loading, excellent aerosol performance and good pharmacokinetic profile compared to other previously reported formulations, in a method that is easy for scale-up without the use of organic solvent [2,8,10–15,17]. Mannitol was used in the present study as a bulking excipient to produce spray-dried powder of capreomycin for inhalation. It is frequently exploited as an excipient in spray-dried formulations with satisfactory aerosol performance and physical stability [9,18,19]. Formulations containing different drug contents were prepared by spray drying at different inlet temperatures in order to explore the effect on particle properties. The morphology, particle size distribution, aerosol performance, crystallinity and surface composition of the powder formulations were investigated. The optimal formulation was also identified to evaluate its pharmacokinetic profile in mice.

2. Materials and Methods

2.1. Materials

Capreomycin (Capastat® sulfate) was purchased from Yick-Vic Chemicals and Pharmaceuticals (Hong Kong, China). Mannitol (Pearlitol® 160) was purchased from Roquette (Lestrem, France). Analytical standard of capreomycin sulfate and trifluoroacetic acid (TFA) were obtained from Sigma-Aldrich (Poole, UK). Heptafluorobutyric acid (HFBA) of HPLC grade was obtained from Thermo Scientific Pierce (Rockford, IL, USA). All solvents and reagents were of analytical grade.

2.2. Preparation of Spray-Dried Powders

Capreomycin and mannitol were dissolved in 15 mL of ultra-pure water at four different drug: mannitol mass ratios of 1:4, 1:3, 1:2 and 1:1 to obtain a final solute concentration of 1% (w/v). Each formulation was spray-dried using a laboratory spray dryer (Büchi B-290, Labortechnik AG, Flawil, Switzerland) with the two-fluid nozzle (Büchi, with an internal diameter of 0.7 mm) at four different inlet temperatures of 60, 90, 120 and 150 °C. The nitrogen atomization flow rate was 742 L/h, the aspiration rate was 38 m^3/min (100%) and the liquid feed rate was 2.1 mL/min. A total of 16 formulations were prepared (Table 1). The spray-dried powders were stored in a desiccator with silica gel at room temperature until further analysis. The production yield was defined as the mass of powder collected after spray drying divided by the total feed solid mass.

Table 1. The composition of spray-dried powders prepared at different inlet temperature.

Sample Name	Capreomycin: Mannitol Ratio (w/w)	Capreomycin Percentage by Mass	Inlet Temperature (°C)
C$_{20}$_T60			60
C$_{20}$_T90			90
C$_{20}$_T120	1:4	20.0	120
C$_{20}$_T150			150
C$_{25}$_T60			60
C$_{25}$_T90			90
C$_{25}$_T120	1:3	25.0	120
C$_{25}$_T150			150
C$_{33}$_T60			60
C$_{33}$_T90			90
C$_{33}$_T120	1:2	33.3	120
C$_{33}$_T150			150
C$_{50}$_T60			60
C$_{50}$_T90			90
C$_{50}$_T120	1:1	50.0	120
C$_{50}$_T150			150

2.3. Drug Content

The drug content was determined as the measured amount of capreomycin with respect to the mass of the spray-dried powders. For each formulation, 1 mg of powder was weighed and dissolved in 5 mL of ultrapure water using a volumetric flask. The samples were filtered with 0.45 μm membrane filter (Nylon syringe filter, Membrane Solutions, Auburn, WA, USA) and quantified by high-performance liquid chromatography (HPLC) (Agilent 1260 Infinity; Agilent Technologies, Santa Clara, CA, USA). The HPLC method was adopted and modified according to a previous study [8]. In brief, a C18 column (5 μm, 4.6 × 250 mm, Agilent, Santa Clara, CA, USA) was used. The mobile phase was composed of 0.1% TFA aqueous solution (pH 2) and acetonitrile (95:5, v/v). The running flow rate was 1 mL/min. A volume of 50 μL sample was injected and capreomycin was detected by UV absorbance at 268 nm. Capreomycin IIA/IIB eluted at approximately 4.6 min while capreomycin IA/IB eluted at around 5.4 min. Total capreomycin was quantified by using a calibration curve with linearity (R^2 = 0.9999) between 3.0 μg/mL and 400.0 μg/mL.

2.4. Morphology Study

Scanning electron microscopy (SEM) (Hitachi S-4800, Hitachi High-technologies Crop., Tokyo, Japan) was used to study the morphology of the spray-dried powders. Samples were sputter-coated with gold-palladium alloy (approximately 11 nm) after being dispersed on the adhesive carbon discs. The coated sample was imaged at 5.0 kV.

2.5. Particle Size Distribution

The volumetric size distribution of the spray-dried powders was measured by laser diffraction (HELOS/KR incorporated with an inhaler module, Sympatec, Clausthal-Zellerfeld, Germany) as previously reported [20]. Approximately 5 mg of powder was loaded in gelatin capsules and dispersed from a Breezhaler® at a flow rate of 60 L/min and a pressure drop of 1.5 kPa. The 100 mm (R3) lens (measuring range 0.45–175 μm) was employed in the measurement. Each powder formulation was measured in triplicate. The tenth (D10), median (D50), and ninetieth (D90) percentile of the volumetric diameter were recorded. The span was calculated according to the formula (D90–D10)/D50.

2.6. In Vitro Aerosol Performance

The aerosol performance of the spray-dried powder was evaluated with a Next Generation Impactor (NGI) (Copley Scientific Limited, Nottingham, UK) without a pre-separator. For each formulation, a Size 3 gelatin capsule (Capsugel, Lonza, NSW, Australia) containing around 7 mg of spray-dried powders were placed in a Breezhaler®. The powders were dispersed at an airflow rate of 90 L/min for 2.7 s with a pressure drop of 3.5 kPa [20]. Before dispersion, the NGI plates were coated with the silicon lubricant (LPS Laboratories, Tucker, GA, USA). After dispersion, a volume of 4 mL ultrapure water was used to rinse and dissolve the powder in the capsule, inhaler, adaptor and each NGI plate separately. After filtering through a 0.45 μm membrane filter (Nylon syringe filter, Membrane Solutions, Auburn, WA, USA), the samples were assayed by HPLC as described above. The NGI experiments were performed in triplicate for each formulation. The recovered dose was defined as the total amount of powder in the capsule, inhaler, adaptor and all NGI stages assayed by HPLC in a single run. The emitted fraction (EF) referred to the fraction of the powder emitted from the inhaler with respect to the recovered dose. The fine particle dose (FPD) referred to the amount of powder with an aerodynamic diameter less than 5.0 μm, which was calculated by interpolation. Fine particle fraction (FPF) was the fraction of the fine particle dose with respect to the recovered dose. The mass median aerodynamic diameter (MMAD) was defined as the aerodynamic diameter at which 50% of the particles (collected from stage 1 to the micro-orifice collector) by mass are larger and 50% are smaller. The MMAD and geometric standard deviation (GSD) were calculated by a linear fit of the cumulative mass and aerodynamic cut-off diameter on a log scale.

2.7. Thermogravimetric Analysis (TGA)

Thermogravimetric analysis (TGA) was conducted to measure the residual moisture of the spray-dried powders. About 2 mg of each formulation was weighed into a 70 μL alumina crucible and heated from 25 to 150 °C at 10 °C/min with a 20 mL/min nitrogen flow in a TGA/DSC 1 STARe System (Mettler Toledo, Greifensee, Switzerland). The loss in mass indicated the residual moisture evaporated from the spray-dried powders.

2.8. Differential Scanning Calorimetry (DSC)

The thermal response profiles of each spray-dried powder formulation and raw materials were assessed by differential scanning calorimetry (DSC) (Model Q1000, TA Instruments, New Castle, DE, USA) as previously reported [21]. Between 1–3 mg of powder was loaded into an aluminum crucible, crimped with a non-perforated lid and heated from 20 °C to 200 °C at 10 °C /min under a 50 mL/min nitrogen purge.

2.9. Powder X-ray Diffraction (PXRD)

The crystalline structures of the spray-dried powders and raw materials were studied by X-ray powder diffraction (X'Pert Powder; Malvern Panalytical Ltd., Malvern, UK) as previously reported [20]. About 4 mg of powder was spread compactly on the sample plate and subjected to Cu-Kα radiation at a current of 45 mA and voltage of 40 kV under ambient temperature. The scattered X-rays were measured from 5 to 35° by a detector with a scan speed of 0.02° per second and a step size of 0.01°.

2.10. X-ray Photoelectron Spectroscopy (XPS)

The surface composition of the powders was examined by X-ray photoelectron spectroscopy (XPS) using a K-Alpha XPS system (Thermo Fisher Scientific, Waltham, MA, USA). Each sample was loaded onto carbon tape on the powder sample holder, followed by the measurement of the surface atomic concentration of carbon, oxygen, nitrogen, and sulfur. Hydrogen could not be detected by XPS so it was not measured. A monochromatic Al Kα

X-ray source was operated at 72 W with a spot size of 400 μm to obtain the spectra. The pass energy of the survey and region scans were 200 eV and 50 eV, respectively. Similar procedures and settings for XPS have been adopted in other studies [22–24]. During measurement, the pressure in the analysis chamber was about 2×10^{-7} mbar and the charging of the samples was compensated by an electron flood gun. Six spots on each sample were randomly selected for measurement. Since capreomycin was the only component in the spray-dried samples containing nitrogen, its surface coverage was determined by calculating the ratio of nitrogen atoms on the surface of the spray-dried particles to those on raw capreomycin. The rest of the surface of the spray-dried powders was covered by mannitol. The expected atomic percentage of nitrogen was calculated using the following equation by assuming a homogenous distribution of the components of the particle according to the theoretical ratio of the components in the formulation. (The molecular formula of capreomycin sulfate is $C_{24}H_{42}N_{14}O_8 \times H_2SO_4$ and the molecular weight is 752.8 g/mol).

$$Atomic\ \%_{nitrogen} = \left[\frac{\left(M\%_{capreomycin\ sulfate}/m_{capreomycin\ sulfate}\right)\left(N_{capreomycin\ sulfate}\right)+\left(M\%_{mannitol}/m_{mannitol}\right)\left(N_{mannitol}\right)}{\left(M\%_{capreomycin\ sulfate}/m_{capreomycin\ sulfate}\right)\left(Z_{capreomycin\ sulfate}\right)+\left(M\%_{mannitol}/m_{mannitol}\right)\left(Z_{mannitol}\right)}\right](100) \tag{1}$$

where $M\%$ is the mass percentage of a compound in the formulation, m the molecular weight of the compound, N the number of nitrogen atoms in the compound, and Z the total number of atoms in the compound excluding hydrogen.

2.11. Animal Study

BALB/c mice of either gender aged 7 to 9 weeks weighing between 18 to 30 g were employed in this study. The mice were obtained from the Centre for Comparative Medicine Research, The University of Hong Kong. They were housed in a 12-h light/12-h dark cycle with food and water supplied ad libitum. All the animal experiments were performed with the approval from the Committee on the Use of Live Animals in Teaching and Research, The University of Hong Kong (CULATR 4921-19, approved on 1 February 2019).

2.12. Pharmacokinetic Study

The mice were randomly divided into two treatment groups (n = 45 per group, five mice per time point, nine time points in total). The intravenous (IV) group received capreomycin (sulfate) solution prepared in normal saline (4 mg/mL) via tail vein injection at a dose of 20 mg/kg [2,13]. Intratracheal (IT) group received the C_{25}_T90 formulation as powder aerosol intratracheally as previously described [25]. In brief, the powder was loaded in a 200 μL gel loading pipette tip, which was connected with a three-way stopcock and 1 mL syringe. The pipette tip was inserted into the trachea of mice under anesthesia. The powder was dispersed into the lungs of mice by 0.6 mL of air in the syringe. After each powder insufflation, the pipette tip was removed and rinsed with 1 mL ultra-pure water. The rinsing solution was assayed by HPLC to calculate the residual mass of capreomycin in the tip. The delivered mass of capreomycin was calculated as drug content in the loaded mass of powder minus the residual mass of capreomycin in the tip. The insufflation efficiency (%) was the ratio of delivered mass of capreomycin to the loaded mass of capreomycin. According to a preliminary study, the insufflation efficiency of C_{25}_T90 formulation was around 80% (unpublished data). To achieve a dose comparable with the IV group, 25 mg/kg of capreomycin was initially loaded and administered in the IT group (around 2 mg powder for a 20 g mouse). The delivered dose within 17.5 to 22.5 mg/kg was considered successful administration, and mice that received dose outside this range were excluded. At 5 min, 15 min, 30 min, 1 h, 2 h, 4 h, 6 h, 8 h, and 24 h post-administration, the mice were euthanized with overdose pentobarbital (200 mg/kg). The whole blood was collected by cardiac puncture, followed by centrifugation at 13,000 rpm for 10 min to obtain the plasma. The lungs were collected and frozen in liquid nitrogen immediately. The plasma and lung tissues were stored at −80 °C until further analysis.

2.13. Extraction of Capreomycin

The extraction of capreomycin from plasma and tissue homogenates was performed according to a previous study [2] with minor modification. Tissue homogenates were obtained by homogenizing the tissue with sterile water. A volume of 1 μL perchloric acid was added to a microcentrifuge tube containing 100 μL of plasma or tissue homogenates to induce protein precipitation. The mixtures were vortexed for 10 min and centrifuged at $16,000 \times g$ for 10 min. The supernatant was collected and neutralized with 110 μL basic mix of 1:10 KOH/K_2HPO_4 solution. The obtained mixtures were then vortexed, followed by centrifugation at $16,000 \times g$ for 15 min. The supernatant was transferred to glass vials for HPLC analysis. A standard curve was obtained by spiking known concentrations of capreomycin (0.6 to 40.0 μg/mL) into blank plasma or blank lung tissue homogenate followed by treatment as mentioned above. HPLC was performed using a C18 column (5 μm, 4.6 × 250 mm, Agilent, Santa Clara, CA, USA) with a guard cartridge. In this HPLC method, HFBA replaced TFA to improve peak resolution of the samples. The mobile phase consisted of 0.1% HFBA in ultrapure water (solvent A) and 0.1% HFBA in HPLC grade acetonitrile (solvent B), pumped at 1 mL/min under the following gradient: 0 to 2 min, 80% A; 2 to 22 min, 80–20% A; 22 to 25 min, 20% A (*v/v*). A volume of 50 μL sample was injected and capreomycin was detected by UV absorption at 268 nm. Capreomycin eluted at approximately 9.7 min with this method. Linearity was demonstrated between 0.6 and 40.0 mg/mL ($R^2 = 0.998$).

2.14. Data Analysis

The FPF data evaluated by NGI was analyzed by one-way ANOVA followed by Tukey post hoc test by GraphPad Prism (version 8.0.1, GraphPad Software, San Diego, CA, USA). For the pharmacokinetics data, the maximum concentration of capreomycin (C_{max}) and time to obtain the maximum concentration (T_{max}) in plasma and lung tissues, the elimination rate constant (K_{el}), half-life ($t_{1/2}$), clearance (CL), area under the curve from 0 h to t (AUC_{0-t}), area under the curve from 0 h to infinity ($AUC_{0-\infty}$) and mean residence time (*MRT*) in plasma and lung tissue were calculated by noncompartmental methods (Phoenix WinNonlin, Certara, Princeton, NJ, USA). Pharmacokinetic parameters were analyzed by Student's *t*-test.

3. Results

3.1. Production Yield of Spray Drying

The production yield of spray drying was affected by both the capreomycin content in the formulation and the inlet temperature (Table 2). In general, as the capreomycin content increased, the production yield decreased. The inlet temperature of 60 °C (the lowest temperature employed in the study) resulted in the lowest production yield within the group of the same drug content. In the C_{20} and C_{25} groups, when the inlet temperature was 90 °C or above, formulations had relatively high yield of over 60%. Due to the low production yield of C_{50} group (all below 10%), the formulations in this group were not further investigated in the subsequent studies.

3.2. Drug Content and Residual Moisture

The measured drug content was close to the theoretical value in all tested formulations (Table 2). The residual moisture of spray-dried powders ranged from 0.48% to 3.13% (*w/w*). Low inlet temperature (60 °C) generally produced particles with higher moisture level than other formulations with the same capreomycin content. There was no clear trend between residual moisture and drug content.

3.3. Particle Morphology

As observed in the SEM images (Figure 1), spray-dried particles prepared at inlet temperature of 120 °C or below were generally spherical in shape with smooth surface and partially aggregated. When the drug content increased from 20% to 33% (*w/w*), the particles appeared to be progressively fused together to produce an interconnected structure, which was particularly prominent in C_{33}_T60 and C_{33}_T90 formulations. As the inlet temperature further increased to 150 °C, the particles were no longer spherical and instead showed a rough surface with large and irregularly shapes.

Table 2. The outlet temperature, production yield, drug content and residual moisture of spray-dried powders. Data for drug content was presented as mean ± standard deviation ($n = 3$). N.A. Not applicable. Due to the low production yield of C_{50} group, the spray-dried powders of this group were not further investigated.

Sample Name	Outlet Temperature (°C)	Production Yield (%, *w/w*)	Drug Content (%, *w/w*)	Residual Moisture (%, *w/w*)
C_{20}_T60	36–38	53.0	19.2 ± 0.4	2.2
C_{20}_T90	52–55	69.9	18.7 ± 1.4	1.2
C_{20}_T120	70–74	66.9	19.8 ± 0.3	1.6
C_{20}_T150	90–95	63.3	19.0 ± 0.6	1.4
C_{25}_T60	35–39	47.3	25.5 ± 0.3	2.3
C_{25}_T90	52–56	65.7	24.9 ± 0.6	0.7
C_{25}_T120	68–71	78.1	26.7 ± 0.4	1.5
C_{25}_T150	83–86	63.9	24.5 ± 0.8	0.5
C_{33}_T60	34–37	18.2	33.2 ± 0.6	3.1
C_{33}_T90	53–56	25.8	33.6 ± 0.4	2.8
C_{33}_T120	68–70	52.5	34.4 ± 0.8	2.0
C_{33}_T150	88–92	39.1	34.1 ± 0.2	2.8
C_{50}_T60	34–37	1.0	N.A.	N.A.
C_{50}_T90	52–57	6.9	N.A.	N.A.
C_{50}_T120	66–68	4.3	N.A.	N.A.
C_{50}_T150	84–87	7.2	N.A.	N.A.

3.4. Particle Size Distribution

The volumetric size distribution of spray-dried powder was measured by laser diffraction (Table 3). When the powder was prepared at a high inlet temperature of 150 °C, the particles were larger than those prepared at a lower inlet temperature, which was consistent with the SEM images. The T120 group exhibited the smallest volumetric diameter compared to those spray-dried with the same drug content at other inlet temperatures. Apart from T150 group, the higher inlet temperature, the smaller the particle size. In T60, T90 and T150 groups, when the content of capreomycin was increased to 33% (*w/w*), the particle size became larger. C_{20}_T120 showed the smallest D_{50} of 1.82 μm while C_{33}_T150 showed the largest D_{50} of 6.44 μm. Compared with other formulations, C_{25}_T150 and C_{33}_T150 showed a wider span (>2).

3.5. In Vitro Aerosol Performance

The aerosol performance of the spray-dried powders from NGI experiments are presented as EF, FPF (Figure 2) and MMAD (Table 3). All the spray-dried powders showed similar dispersion trends with EF approaching or over 80%. In the C_{20} and C_{33} groups, the powders prepared at an inlet temperature of 150 °C showed significantly lower FPFs than those prepared at 120 °C ($p < 0.05$, one-way ANOVA by Tukey post hoc test). In the C_{25} group, the FPF of C_{25}_T150 was significantly lower than all other formulations with the same drug content ($p < 0.05$ or 0.01, one-way ANOVA by Tukey post hoc test). All the formulations prepared at 120 °C or below had FPF values of over 50%. The MMAD of particles in the T150 group were larger than that of other formulations, which was consistent with the SEM images and volumetric diameter. Formulations that were prepared at 120 °C or below showed similar MMAD within the range of 3.4 to 5.3 μm regardless of the formulation composition, indicating that the inlet temperature should not be higher than 120 °C in order to produce inhalable powder. Among all the formulations investigated, C_{25}_T90 demonstrated the highest FPF of over 64% with the smallest aerodynamic diameter of 3.38 μm. Therefore, it was identified as the optimal formulation for the pharmacokinetic study.

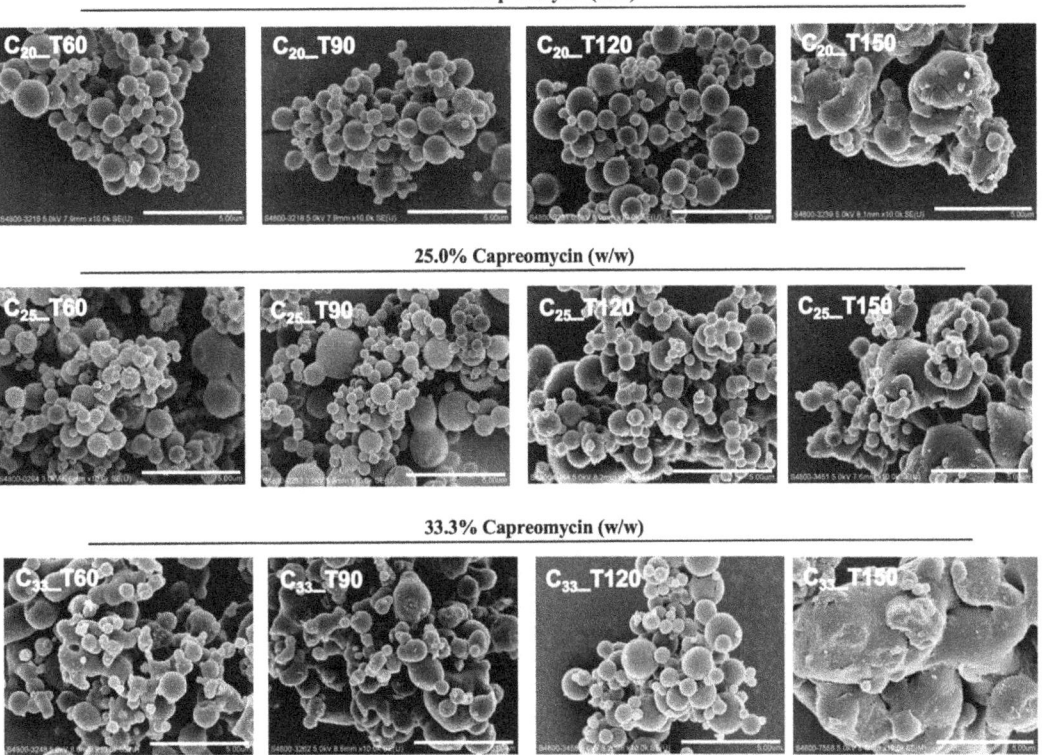

Figure 1. The scanning electron microscopy (SEM) images of spray-dried powder imaged at ×10,000 magnification, scale bar = 5 μm.

3.6. Thermoanalysis and Powder Crystallinity

All investigated formulations demonstrated a characteristic endothermic peak at 150 to 160 °C in the DSC study (Figure 3), whereas raw mannitol was reported to have a melting point at 166 to 168 °C [26]. This observation demonstrated a shift in melting point of mannitol in the presence of capreomycin. The higher the content of capreomycin, the lower the temperature of the endothermic peak. Formulations with the same content of capreomycin showed similar thermal behavior regardless of the inlet temperature of spray drying. The smaller particles size of mannitol after spray drying may also cause melting point depression [27]. According to the PXRD results (Figure 4), raw mannitol was highly crystalline and predominately in the β form, as indicated by the peaks at 10.5° and 14.7°(indicated by arrows) [28]. Formulations in the T120 group were also predominately in the β form (14.7°, indicated by the arrow in C_{20} group) while those in the T150 group exhibited α and β polymorphs, since they had the characteristic peaks not only at 14.7° but also at 13.6° (indicated by the arrow in C_{20} group) [28]. Interestingly, compared to the diffractogram of pure δ forms of $_D$-mannitol, the mannitol in T60 and T90 groups also contained the δ form (characteristic peak at 9.74° as the arrow indicated in C_{20} group) [28,29], which is thermodynamically less stable than the other two forms [29,30].

Table 3. Particle size distribution of spray-dried powders. The volumetric diameter was obtained from laser diffraction measurement (Flow rate: 60 L/min, inhaler: Breezhaler, capsule: gelatin). The median aerodynamic diameter (MMAD) and geometric standard deviation (GSD) was obtained from aerosol performance analysis (Next generation impactor, flow rate: 90 L/min, duration time: 2.7 s, inhaler: Breezhaler, capsule: gelatin). Data for volumetric diameter and aerodynamic size was presented as mean ± standard deviation ($n = 3$).

Sample	Volumetric Diameter				Aerodynamic Diameter	
	D_{10} (μm)	D_{50} (μm)	D_{90} (μm)	Span Value	MMAD (μm)	GSD
C_{20}_T60	1.21 ± 0.02	2.67 ± 0.02	5.20 ± 0.14	1.49 ± 0.03	4.29 ± 0.77	3.09 ± 0.14
C_{20}_T90	1.20 ± 0.02	2.52 ± 0.00	4.59 ± 0.10	1.35 ± 0.05	4.28 ± 0.85	3.30 ± 0.28
C_{20}_T120	0.76 ± 0.03	1.82 ± 0.06	3.47 ± 0.04	1.49 ± 0.07	4.58 ± 0.37	3.89 ± 0.33
C_{20}_T150	1.66 ± 0.04	5.36 ± 0.17	10.67 ± 0.44	1.68 ± 0.03	9.85 ± 1.15	4.02 ± 0.63
C_{25}_T60	1.32 ± 0.08	3.07 ± 0.09	6.51 ± 0.37	1.69 ± 0.07	4.46 ± 0.21	2.45 ± 0.25
C_{25}_T90	1.16 ± 0.01	2.62 ± 0.05	5.06 ± 0.16	1.49 ± 0.03	3.38 ± 0.22	2.83 ± 0.14
C_{25}_T120	0.97 ± 0.03	2.44 ± 0.04	4.80 ± 0.06	1.57 ± 0.03	4.28 ± 0.36	2.70 ± 0.25
C_{25}_T150	1.28 ± 0.04	5.16 ± 0.14	11.73 ± 0.22	2.03 ± 0.03	8.79 ± 0.38	2.72 ± 0.20
C_{33}_T60	1.57 ± 0.03	3.33 ± 0.02	6.83 ± 0.15	1.58 ± 0.05	5.29 ± 0.93	3.06 ± 0.06
C_{33}_T90	1.49 ± 0.05	3.16 ± 0.05	6.51 ± 0.24	1.59 ± 0.05	4.74 ± 1.14	3.08 ± 0.26
C_{33}_T120	1.08 ± 0.05	2.60 ± 0.11	5.17 ± 0.37	1.57 ± 0.07	4.32 ± 0.34	2.35 ± 0.31
C_{33}_T150	2.16 ± 0.21	6.44 ± 0.54	15.74 ± 2.83	2.10 ± 0.25	16.59 ± 2.66	3.87 ± 0.31

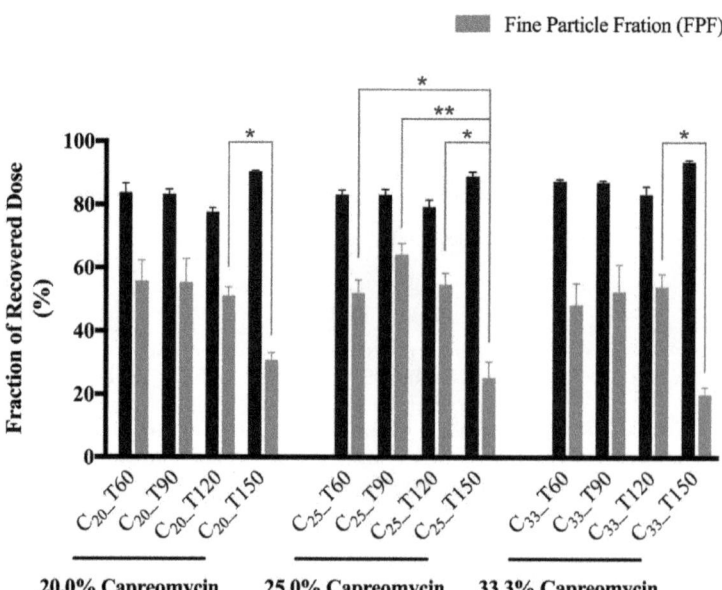

Figure 2. In vitro aerosol performance of spray-dried powders evaluated by the Next Generation Impactor (NGI). Data presented as mean ± standard deviation ($n = 3$). *p*-value indicated comparison of FPF between formulations with the same drug content (* and ** represents $p < 0.05$ and $p < 0.01$, respectively, one-way ANOVA followed by Tukey post hoc test).

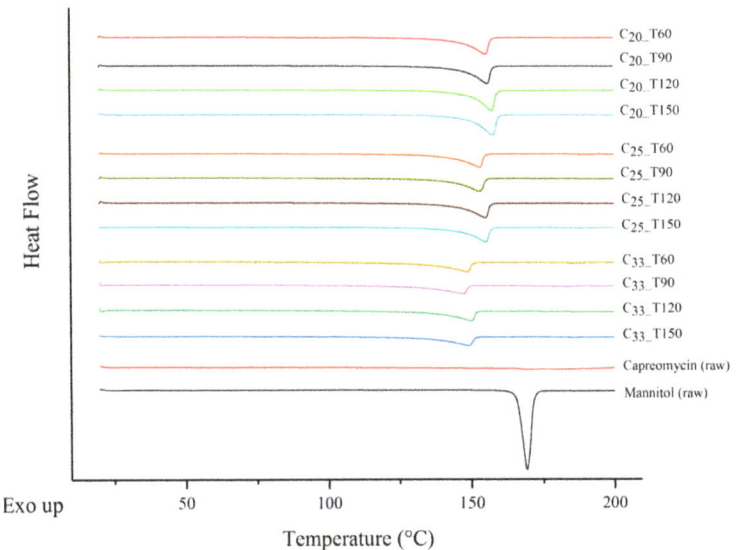

Figure 3. Differential scanning calorimetry (DSC) thermogram of spray-dried powders, raw capreomycin and raw mannitol. Negative peak represents endothermic events.

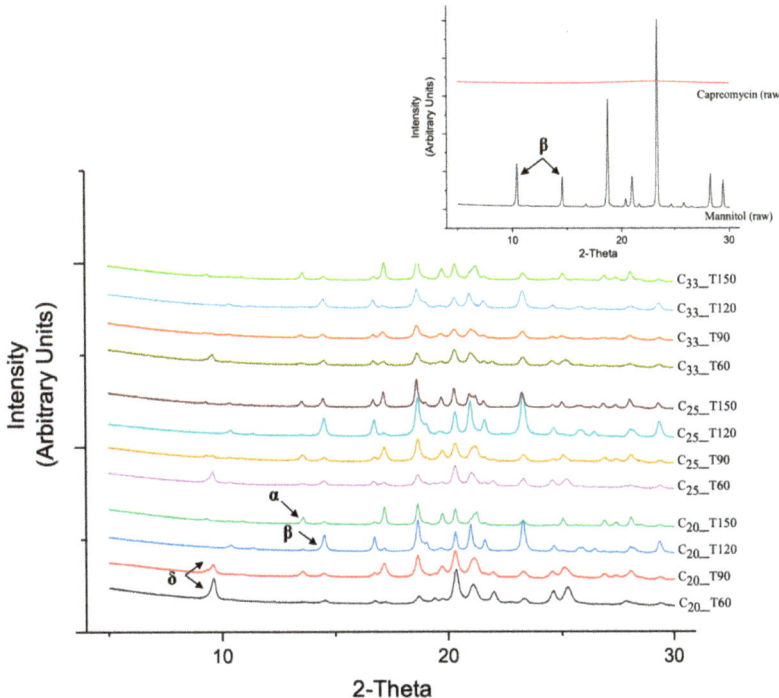

Figure 4. X-ray powder diffraction (PXRD) diffractogram of raw capreomycin, raw mannitol (right conner) and spray-dried powders (from 5° to 30°).

3.7. Surface Composition

The elemental composition of raw mannitol and capreomycin sulfate by the number of atoms in the molecules (Table 4), and the molar surface capreomycin sulfate composition of the spray-dried powders (Figure 5) were calculated. The experimentally measured fraction of carbon was higher than the theoretical one for both capreomycin sulfate and mannitol, while those of oxygen and nitrogen (in capreomycin sulfate only) were lower. The measured surface proportion of sulfur in capreomycin sulfate was close to the theoretical value. The theoretical molar proportion of capreomycin sulfate in C_{20}, C_{25} and C_{33} groups were 5.6%, 7.0%, and 9.3%, respectively. All spray-dried formulations displayed an enrichment of capreomycin on the surface of the particles. Among the formulations of the same drug content, those spray-dried at 90 °C had the lowest capreomycin sulfate surface coverage. Only formulations spray-dried at 120 °C showed a clear trend of increasing capreomycin sulfate surface coverage with the drug load, with C_{33}_T120 exhibiting the highest content of capreomycin sulfate on the surface (19.2% w/w). No clear trend was observed for other inlet temperatures.

Table 4. Theoretical and experimental percentages by the number of atoms of elements in pure capreomycin (as sulfate) and mannitol.

Element	Raw Capreomycin (as Sulfate)		Raw Mannitol	
	Theoretical	Experimental	Theoretical	Experimental
Carbon	47.1	57.2 ± 0.2	50.0	52.7 ± 0.2
Oxygen	23.5	19.0 ± 0.1	50.0	47.3 ± 0.2
Nitrogen	27.5	21.7 ± 0.1	-	-
Sulphur	2.0	2.1 ± 0.0	-	-

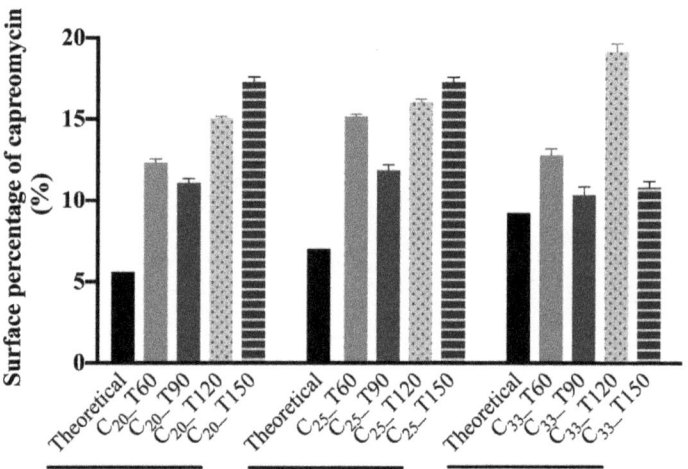

20.0% Capreomycin   25.0% Capreomycin   33.3% Capreomycin

Figure 5. Surface percentage of capreomycin in different spray-dried powders.

3.8. Pharmacokinetic Study

The pharmacokinetic profiles of capreomycin following IT and IV administration (as C_{25}_T90 powder and capreomycin solution, respectively) were compared (Figure 6) and the pharmacokinetics parameters in plasma and lung tissue were calculated by non-compartmental analysis (Table 5). In the plasma, the C_{max} was comparable between IT and IV group, approaching 80 µg/mL. Both groups achieved maximum capreomycin concentration within 10 min (T_{max}) after administration. However, the concentration of capreomycin declined at a slower rate in the IT group than the IV group until it was below the detection limit at 4 h. Although the K_{el} and $t_{1/2}$ of the two groups did not show any significant difference, the CL of the IT group was significantly lower than that of the IV group ($p < 0.001$ Student's t-test), and accordingly, the MRT in the IT group was significantly longer than in the IV group ($p < 0.01$ Student's t-test). The AUC_{0-t} and $AUC_{0-\infty}$ in IT group were around two-fold higher than that in the IV group ($p < 0.01$, Student's t-test). In the lung tissues, both IT and IV group achieved C_{max} within 20 min after administration. However, the C_{max} in the IT group was 40-fold higher than that in IV group ($p < 0.001$). The capreomycin concentration in the lung tissue of the IT group declined very slowly (significantly smaller K_{el} compared to the IT group, $p < 0.001$, Student's t-test) and the drug could still be detected after 24 h of administration. In contrast, capreomycin was no longer detectable in the lung 1 h after IV administration, with a significantly shorter MRT in the lung compared to the IT group ($p < 0.001$, Student's t-test). The CL in the lung tissue of IT group was significantly lower than that of the IV group ($p < 0.001$), while both AUC_{0-t} and $AUC_{0-\infty}$ of the IT group were 150-fold ($p < 0.01$, Student's t-test) and 220-fold ($p < 0.001$, Student's t-test) higher than that of the IV group, respectively.

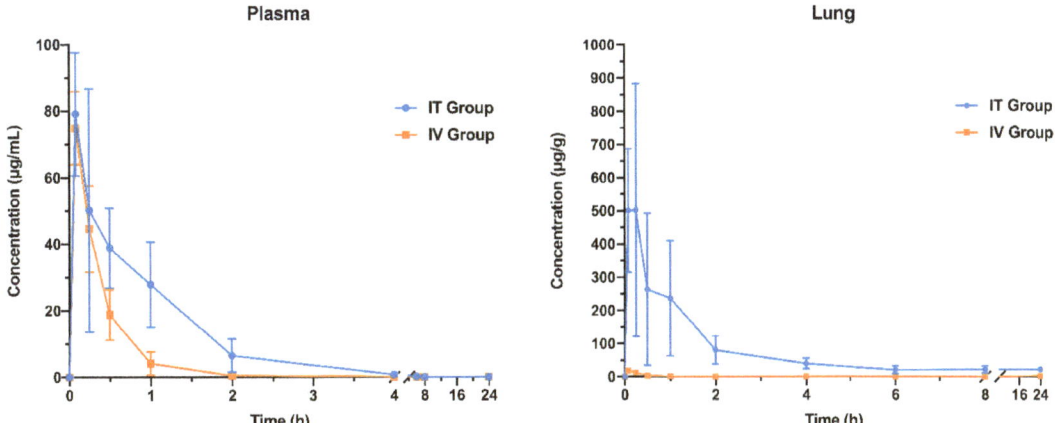

Figure 6. Pharmacokinetic study of spray-dried powder formulation of capreomycin on mice. The mice in intratracheal (IT) group were administered with capreomycin spray-dried powders (C_{25}_T90 formulation) intratracheally with a dosage range of 17.5–22.5 mg/kg (the average delivered dose was 20.54 ± 1.31 mg/kg). The mice in intravenous (IV) group were administered with capreomycin solution intravenously at a dose of 20 mg/kg. Data was presented as mean ± standard deviation. ($n = 5$ for each time point).

Table 5. Pharmacokinetic parameters obtained by noncompartmental analysis after administration of capreomycin by pulmonary or intravenous route. The mice in intratracheal (IT) group were administered with capreomycin spray-dried powders (C_{25}_T90 formulation) intratracheally with a dosage range of 17.5–22.5 mg/kg. The mice in intravenous (IV) group were administered with capreomycin solution intravenously at a dose of 20 mg/kg. Data was presented as mean ± standard deviation ($n = 5$).

Parameters [a]	Plasma		Lung	
	IT Group	IV Group	IT Group	IV Group
K_{el} (h^{-1})	1.15 ± 0.57	2.74 ± 1.67	0.07 ± 0.04 ***	2.37 ± 0.23 [b]
$t_{1/2}$ (h)	0.73 ± 0.33	0.34 ± 0.20	18.94 ± 20.67	0.29 ± 0.03 [b]
CL (mL/h·kg)	321.88 ± 81.65 ***	612.91 ± 93.46	12.99 ± 3.66 ***	2624.71 ± 157.19 [b]
AUC_{0-t} (µg·h/mL)	65.10 ± 16.37 **	32.55 ± 5.52	1061.88 ± 235.76 ***	6.71 ± 0.51
$AUC_{0-\infty}$ (µg·h/mL)	67.26 ± 16.92 **	33.78 ± 5.54	1726.37 ± 658.83 **	7.78 ± 0.46 [b]

Table 5. Cont.

Parameters [a]	Plasma		Lung	
	IT Group	IV Group	IT Group	IV Group
MRT (h)	0.79 ± 0.22 **	0.30 ± 0.11	6.62 ± 1.25 ***	0.23 ± 0.13
C_{max} (µg/mL) or (µg/g) [c]	80.08 ± 18.84	74.89 ± 10.94	739.13 ± 180.66 ***	18.23 ± 8.34
T_{max} (h)	0.15 ± 0.09	0.08 ± 0	0.27 ± 0.20	0.12 ± 0.07

[a] K_{el}, elimination rate constant; $t_{1/2}$, half-life; CL, clearance; AUC_{0-t}, area under the curve from 0 h to t; $AUC_{0-\infty}$, area under the curve from 0 h to infinity; MRT, mean residence time; C_{max}, maximum concentration; T_{max}, time at which C_{max} occurs. [b] In the lungs of mice in the IV group, the drug concentration fell below the detection limit quickly. Each mouse was allocated to one of the five groups in each time point according to their body weight. Two of the five mice showed drug concentration below the detection limit at 30 min post-administration, hence two sets of data did not have enough points to fit the linear model for the calculation of the predicted parameters by WinNonlin. Only three sets of data were presented. [c] The unit of C_{max} in the plasma was µg/mL and the unit of C_{max} in the lung tissue was µg/g. ** or *** Significant difference between IT group and IV group ($p < 0.01$ or $p < 0.001$, Student's t-test).

4. Discussion

Capreomycin is the first choice of the second-line anti-TB drugs for the treatment of MDR-TB. It is administered intramuscularly or intravenously up to 1.0 g per day, five times per week [16,31]. The high systemic exposure of capreomycin has led to nephrotoxicity and ototoxic effects in some patients [32,33]. To overcome the main challenge of toxicity and inconvenient administration, pulmonary drug delivery is an attractive administration route because it provides high drug concentration in the lungs and therefore decreases the dose required [31]. Inhaled therapy can reduce the risk of systemic adverse effects by targeting the drug directly to the lesion where *Mtb* typically reside. Despite the advantages of inhalation therapy against TB, there is no commercial inhalable product approved for TB. Spray drying is one of the most popular particle engineering technologies investigated for preparing inhalable dry powder of antibiotics, including antimicrobial peptides, for inhaled TB therapy [34–36]. It is a continuous process that is easy for scale-up and its closed system facilitates aseptic industrial production. Furthermore, spray drying has the advantage of having good control of particle size distribution, which is critical for inhaled formulations [37]. However, spray-dried powders tend to have low crystallinity, which often leads to particle aggregation and moisture absorption, rendering it unfavorable for long term storage [38].

Among the anti-TB drugs being investigated for inhalation, only one clinical study involved inhalable powders of capreomycin, in which safety, tolerability, and pharmacokinetic profile of a spray-dried formulation of capreomycin (containing drug to L-leucine at a mass ratio of 80:20) were evaluated in healthy subjects [14]. The inhaled formulation of capreomycin was well-tolerated, indicating that inhaled therapy of capreomycin is feasible. However, the production process involved the use of organic solvent (50% ethanol), and the hydrophobic L-leucine has dissolution issue. The use of organic solvent in the production process may increase the cost of manufacture with an increased risk of irritation to the pulmonary mucosa due to the residual solvent. Schoubbe et al. prepared capreomycin powder formulation with a nano-spray dryer [15]. According to the aerodynamic assessment evaluated by the twin-stage glass impinger with the Handihaler® at the flow rate of 60 L/min, the addition of lactose improved the respirable fraction of spray-dried capreomycin from 14% to 26%, but the large proportion of lactose in the formulation (capreomycin to lactose at 1:50 mass ratio) has limited the respirable dose of capreomycin. Compared with lactose, mannitol is a non-reducing sugar and less hygroscopic. Therefore it shows better compatibility and stability [39]. The safety of mannitol as inhalation excipient was well examined, and it has been used in commercial pharmaceutical protein formulations such as Exubera®, an inhaled insulin product approved by Food and Drug Administration (FDA) [39,40]. In addition, inhaled mannitol was also approved by the FDA as the active pharmaceutical ingredient (Bronchitol®) for the management of cystic fibrosis. This study aimed to develop a new inhaled powder formulation of capreomycin with mannitol by spray drying. Different drug contents and inlet temperatures during spray drying were investigated to identify the optimal formulation and spray drying conditions to produce capreomycin powders suitable for inhalation.

Both the drug content in the formulation and inlet temperature of spray drying can influence the production yield. When the temperature was low, drying was incomplete, leading to the adherence of droplets on the inner surfaces of the cyclone and hence low production yield [41–43]. In the C_{20}, C_{25} and C_{33} groups, the production yield was the highest at the inlet temperature of 120 °C, above which the yield started to decline. In the C_{50} group, there was a high content of capreomycin, which is amorphous in nature with high surface adhesive property [44]. As a result, the particles, in general, were more likely to adhere to the cyclone of the spray dryer instead of depositing in the collector vial. The inlet temperature also influenced the residual moisture in the spray-dried powder. As expected, spray drying at low temperature (inlet temperature of 60 °C) produced particles with higher residual moisture than other groups. No clear trend was observed in the residual moisture between T90, T120, and T150 groups. The result suggested that an inlet temperature of 60 °C was insufficient for proper drying, which led to the low production yield and high residual moisture.

The morphology of particles produced by spray drying was mainly affected by temperature rather than the capreomycin content. Unlike the T60, T90 and T120 formulations, particles of the T150 group were irregular in shape with rough surfaces. This can be explained by the different crystallization process of mannitol at different temperatures [45,46]. When the temperature reached a certain level (e.g., at 150 °C in this study), solvent evaporated very rapidly. The high solvent evaporation rate with a low crystallization nucleation rate rendered the feed liquid to become highly concentrated and viscous. As a result, larger mannitol crystals with rough surfaces were formed [45,46]. In contrast, the particles of T60, T90 and T120 groups were spherical, which have a small area-to-volume ratio that facilitates powder dispersion by reducing aggregation [47]. The particle size distribution was a decisive factor of the deposition site following inhalation. It is widely accepted that particles with median aerodynamic diameters in the range of 1 to 5 μm can efficiently deposit in the lower airways [48]. Formulation C_{25}_T90 had the smallest MMAD of 3.38 μm, indicating that this formulation is likely to achieve efficient lung deposition. The similar particle size between T60, T90 and T120 groups can be explained by the particle formation process [45,49,50]. During the drying process at lower inlet temperature (at 120 °C and below), the water evaporation rate was low, and the mannitol began to crystallize once it reached a critical concentration at the surface [45,49,50]. Therefore, the particles size was mainly determined by the droplet size. As the droplet size after atomization was similar between formulations with the same composition and spray drying parameters except for inlet temperature (which was not high enough to make any difference), the similar drying manner may produce particles with similar size [45,49,50]. In contrast, when the inlet temperature was high enough (at 150 °C or above), the solvent evaporated very rapidly, and the crystallization growth may be different due to supersaturation. The mannitol tended to crystallize with a secondary nucleation process, for instance, using other already crystalline particles in the spray dryer as seed, leading to a wide variation of particle size [45]. The particles in T150 groups with rough surface may also have different particle interaction compared to the smooth particles [45], hence affecting the resultant particle size.

Crystallinity plays an important role in the stability of powder formulation. For pure mannitol, the crystalline form was mainly determined by solvent evaporation rate during spray drying [45]. According to hot stage microscopy experiments in another study, when mannitol was heated to around 90 °C, the β form was dominant (95%); when mannitol was heated to a higher temperature of around 140 °C, a mixture of polymorphs containing both β form (85%) and α form (15%) were observed [45]. This phenomenon was consistent to our T120 and T150 groups. In the presence of capreomycin, the δ form of mannitol, which is the least stable crystalline form [51], was found in the formulations of T60 group and T90 group. Nonetheless, the mannitol in all spray-dried powders was crystalline, suggesting that they have good stability for long-term storage [52], but further investigation is needed.

In all spray-dried formulations, an enrichment of capreomycin at the particle surface was observed, which can be explained by the dimensionless Péclet number (*Pe*; Equation (2)):

$$Pe = \frac{\kappa}{8D_j} \tag{2}$$

where D_j is the solute diffusivity and κ is the evaporation rate [53,54]. A large *Pe* indicates a higher droplet surface recession rate than solute diffusion inwards during droplet evaporation, leading to surface enrichment by the molecule with slower diffusion rate [55]. At a given evaporation rate, the *Pe* of capreomycin is higher than that of mannitol due to its lower D_j, owing to its higher molecular weight and lower aqueous solubility, suggesting that capreomycin precipitated first and predominantly occupied at the surface. The XPS data were consistent with this phenomenon as more capreomycin was detected on the particle surface than expected in all spray-dried formulations. According to Equation (2), *Pe* increases with the evaporation rate, which can be achieved by increasing the inlet temperature of spray drying and changing the mass ratio of the components [56]. Therefore, drug surface coverage is expected to increase with the inlet temperature and drug load. However, the capreomycin sulfate surface coverage did not exactly follow this trend. The capreomycin sulfate surface coverage increased with drug loading in the formulation only at 120 °C but varied at other temperatures. The effects of drug loading, temperature, and their interaction on surface coverage have not been studied systematically. Mangal et al. studied the spray-dried polyvinylpyrrolidone with different concentrations of L-leucine (0, 2.5, 5, 7.5, 10, 12.5, and 15% w/w) [57]. Their XPS results showed that the surface coverage by L-leucine increased with its concentration and reached a plateau at 12.5% w/w. However, this observation may be formulation dependent. More research is required to establish the relationship between spray drying conditions, drug loading, and surface coverage.

Among all the formulations prepared in this study, C$_{25}$_T90 demonstrated the best aerosol properties in terms of FPF and MMAD with a reasonably good production yield. This formulation was selected for subsequent pharmacokinetic study in animals. The inhaled formulation of capreomycin was designed for high local concentration in the lung with reduced systemic adverse effects. The minimum inhibitory concentration (MIC) of capreomycin in liquid or on solid media is 1.25 to 2.5 µg/mL [58]. In the pharmacokinetic study, when administrated through pulmonary delivery, the capreomycin concentration in the lungs of mice were higher than the MIC and remained stable at around 20 µg/g from 6 to 24 h post-administration (8-fold higher than the MIC). As the lung is the primary site of *Mtb* infection, maintaining capreomycin concentration within the therapeutic window for an extended period in the lung can combat the bacteria more effectively [14]. Drug resistance can develop when the intracellular drug concentration does not reach the microbiologically active level during TB treatment [59]. Inhaled drug particles deposited in the deep lung would be ingested and phagocytosed by the alveolar macrophages and dendritic cells where the *Mtb* typically reside [8,60], resulting in high drug concentration in the infected cells. In addition, these drug-containing alveolar macrophages may migrate to the periphery of lung granulomas and facilitates the delivery of drug to the mycobacteria inside granulomas, where it was hard for the drug to achieve therapeutic concentration via circulation through injection [59]. According to the pharmacokinetics and pharmacodynamics studies of inhaled capreomycin particles in guinea pig model [2,12], animals receiving capreomycin by inhalation showed significantly higher drug concentration in the lungs and bronchoalveolar lavage fluid than intramuscular injection. Moreover, insufflation with high dose of capreomycin (14.5 mg/kg capreomycin) could lighten the bacterial burdens (CFU/mL) in the lungs more efficiently compared to intramuscular injection. High local drug concentration not only can reduce bacteria load in the lung, but more importantly, minimize the possibility of airborne transmission of bacteria to other individuals [59].

The inhaled formulation of capreomycin can achieve comparable drug concentration to capreomycin solution administrated by IV injection in the plasma through alveolar-capillary absorption, indicating that it can also treat extrapulmonary TB infection [14]. Capreomycin is associated with nephrotoxicity and ototoxicity, similar to the aminoglycosides [33,61]. The higher AUC in both the plasma and the lung obtained from the mice in IT group compared to IV group suggested that inhaled formulation of capreomycin showed higher bioavailability. To achieve comparable drug efficacy, a lower dose can be used, leading to less systemic exposure, and reduced adverse effects. The slower clearance and longer mean residence time in the mice of IT group indicated that capreomycin received by inhalation eliminated slower than by intravenous injection, which may help to reduce the dosing frequency. With the favorable aerosol properties and pharmacokinetic profile of C_{25}_T90 formulation, further study on its antibacterial effect in vivo is warranted.

5. Conclusions

Powder formulations containing different mass ratios of capreomycin to mannitol were prepared by spray drying at different inlet temperatures. Both factors influenced the production yield and residual moisture of the spray-dried powder. To achieve a good production yield, the formulation should have capreomycin content below 50% (w/w) and spray-dried at an inlet temperature of 90 °C or above. Except for the T150 groups, all spray-dried formulations in this study displayed spherical morphology with smooth surface and similar particle size distribution. Among all the formulations, C_{25}_T90 exhibited the best aerosol performance with the MMAD of 3.38 µm and FPF approaching 65%. This formulation not only showed better aerosol properties than the other two reported dry powder formulations of capreomycin but also with simpler and organic solvent-free preparation process. The pharmacokinetics study on healthy mice indicated that higher maximum concentration was achieved in the lung of mice receiving inhaled powder formulation than those receiving capreomycin solution by intravenous injection. Up to 24 h post-administration of the inhaled powder formulation, the drug concentration in the lungs was 8-fold higher than the MIC. Inhaled capreomycin formulations also showed slower clearance in the plasma than IV injection. While long-term stability and pharmacodynamic study remains to be investigated, this spray-dried formulation of capreomycin is promising for use in inhaled TB therapy.

Author Contributions: Conceptualization: Z.S. and J.K.W.L.; Methodology: Z.S. and J.K.W.L.; Formal analysis: Z.S., W.T. and M.Y.T.C.; Investigation: Z.S., W.T., Y.Q., R.C.H.M. and Q.L.; Resources: J.K.W.L. and P.C.L.K.; Writing-Original draft: Z.S. and W.T.; Writing-Review & Editing: J.K.W.L., M.Y.T.C. and P.C.L.K.; Supervision: J.K.W.L.; Funding acquisition: J.K.W.L. All authors have read and agreed to the published version of the manuscript.

Funding: This study was supported by the Health and Medical Research Fund (HMRF 18170972), Food and Health Bureau, The Government of the Hong Kong SAR; and Seed Funding for Strategic Interdisciplinary Research Scheme, The University of Hong Kong.

Institutional Review Board Statement: All the animal experiments were performed with the approval from the Committee on the Use of Live Animals in Teaching and Research, The University of Hong Kong (CULATR 4921-19, approved on 1 February 2019).

Informed Consent Statement: Not applicable.

Data Availability Statement: Data are available upon request.

Acknowledgments: This study was supported by the Health and Medical Research Fund (HMRF 18170972), Food and Health Bureau, The Government of the Hong Kong SAR; and Seed Funding for Strategic Interdisciplinary Research Scheme, The University of Hong Kong. The authors would like to thank the Electron Microscope Unit, The University of Hong Kong for the assistance in the SEM study.

Conflicts of Interest: The authors declare no conflict of interest.

References

1. World Health Organization. *Global Tuberculosis Report 2020*; World Health Organization: Geneva, Switzerland, 2020; p. 232.
2. Garcia-Contreras, L.; Muttil, P.; Fallon, J.K.; Kabadi, M.; Gerety, R.; Hickey, A.J. Pharmacokinetics of Sequential Doses of Capreomycin Powder for Inhalation in Guinea Pigs. *Antimicrob. Agents Chemother.* **2012**, *56*, 2612–2618. [CrossRef] [PubMed]
3. Liu, G.; Luan, B.; Liang, G.; Xing, L.; Huang, L.; Wang, C.; Xu, Y. Isolation and identification of four major impurities in capreomycin sulfate. *J. Chromatogr. A* **2018**, *1571*, 155–164. [CrossRef]
4. Johansen, S.K.; Maus, C.E.; Plikaytis, B.B.; Douthwaite, S. Capreomycin binds across the ribosomal subunit interface using tlyA-encoded 2′-O-methylations in 16S and 23S rRNAs. *Mol. Cell* **2006**, *23*, 173–182. [CrossRef]
5. Fu, L.M.; Shinnick, T.M. Genome-wide exploration of the drug action of capreomycin on Mycobacterium tuberculosis using Affymetrix oligonucleotide GeneChips. *J. Infect.* **2007**, *54*, 277–284. [CrossRef]
6. Reisfeld, B.; Metzler, C.P.; Lyons, M.A.; Mayeno, A.N.; Brooks, E.J.; DeGroote, M.A. A Physiologically Based Pharmacokinetic Model for Capreomycin. *Antimicrob. Agents Chemother.* **2012**, *56*, 926–934. [CrossRef]
7. Manion, J.A.R.; Cape, S.P.; McAdams, D.H.; Rebits, L.G.; Evans, S.; Sievers, R.E. Inhalable Antibiotics Manufactured Through Use of Near-Critical or Supercritical Fluids. *Aerosol Sci. Technol.* **2012**, *46*, 403–410. [CrossRef]
8. Pitner, R.A.; Durham, P.G.; Stewart, I.E.; Reed, S.G.; Cassell, G.H.; Hickey, A.J.; Carter, D. A Spray-Dried Combination of Capreomycin and CPZEN-45 for Inhaled Tuberculosis Therapy. *J. Pharm. Sci.* **2019**, *108*, 3302–3311. [CrossRef]
9. Shetty, N.; Park, H.; Zemlyanov, D.; Mangal, S.; Bhujbal, S.; Zhou, Q. Influence of excipients on physical and aerosolization stability of spray dried high-dose powder formulations for inhalation. *Int. J. Pharm.* **2018**, *544*, 222–234. [CrossRef]
10. Giovagnoli, S.; Blasi, P.; Vescovi, C.; Fardella, G.; Chiappini, I.; Perioli, L.; Ricci, M.; Rossi, C. Unilamellar vesicles as potential capreomycin sulfate carriers: Preparation and physicochemical characterization. *AAPS PharmSciTech* **2004**, *4*, 549–560. [CrossRef] [PubMed]
11. Schoubben, A.; Blasi, P.; Giovagnoli, S.; Ricci, M.; Rossi, C. Simple and scalable method for peptide inhalable powder production. *Eur. J. Pharm. Sci.* **2010**, *39*, 53–58. [CrossRef]
12. Garcia-Contreras, L.; Fiegel, J.; Telko, M.J.; Elbert, K.; Hawi, A.; ThomaS, A.; VerBerkmoes, J.; Germishuizen, W.A.; Fourie, P.B.; Hickey, A.J.; et al. Inhaled large porous particles of capreomycin for treatment of tuberculosis in a guinea pig model. *Antimicrob. Agents Chemother.* **2007**, *51*, 2830–2836. [CrossRef]
13. Fiegel, J.; Garcia-Contreras, L.; Thomas, M.; VerBerkmoes, J.; Elbert, K.; Hickey, A.; Edwards, D. Preparation and in vivo evaluation of a dry powder for inhalation of capreomycin. *Pharm. Res.* **2008**, *25*, 805–811. [CrossRef] [PubMed]
14. Dharmadhikari, A.S.; Kabadi, M.; Gerety, B.; Hickey, A.J.; Fourie, P.B.; Nardell, E. Phase I, Single-Dose, Dose-Escalating Study of Inhaled Dry Powder Capreomycin: A New Approach to Therapy of Drug-Resistant Tuberculosis. *Antimicrob. Agents Chemother.* **2013**, *57*, 2613–2619. [CrossRef] [PubMed]
15. Schoubben, A.; Giovagnoli, S.; Tiralti, M.C.; Blasi, P.; Ricci, M. Capreomycin inhalable powders prepared with an innovative spray-drying technique. *Int. J. Pharm.* **2014**, *469*, 132–139. [CrossRef]
16. Parumasivam, T.; Chang, R.Y.; Abdelghany, S.; Ye, T.T.; Britton, W.J.; Chan, H.K. Dry powder inhalable formulations for anti-tubercular therapy. *Adv. Drug Deliv. Rev.* **2016**, *102*, 83–101. [CrossRef]
17. Schoubben, A.; Blasi, P.; Giontella, A.; Giovagnoli, S.; Ricci, M. Powder, capsule and device: An imperative ménage à trois for respirable dry powders. *Int. J. Pharm.* **2015**, *494*, 40–48. [CrossRef]
18. Chow, M.Y.T.; Qiu, Y.; Lo, F.F.K.; Lin, H.H.S.; Chan, H.-K.; Kwok, P.C.L.; Lam, J.K.W. Inhaled powder formulation of naked siRNA using spray drying technology with l-leucine as dispersion enhancer. *Int. J. Pharm.* **2017**, *530*, 40–52. [CrossRef]
19. Qiu, Y.; Man, R.C.H.; Liao, Q.; Kung, K.L.K.; Chow, M.Y.T.; Lam, J.K.W. Effective mRNA pulmonary delivery by dry powder formulation of PEGylated synthetic KL4 peptide. *J. Control. Release* **2019**, *314*, 102–115. [CrossRef]
20. Liao, Q.; Lam, I.C.H.; Lin, H.H.S.; Wan, L.T.L.; Lo, J.C.K.; Tai, W.; Kwok, P.C.L.; Lam, J.K.W. Effect of formulation and inhaler parameters on the dispersion of spray freeze dried voriconazole particles. *Int. J. Pharm.* **2020**, *584*, 119444. [CrossRef]
21. Liang, W.; Chow, M.Y.T.; Chow, S.F.; Chan, H.-K.; Kwok, P.C.L.; Lam, J.K.W. Using two-fluid nozzle for spray freeze drying to produce porous powder formulation of naked siRNA for inhalation. *Int. J. Pharm.* **2018**, *552*, 67–75. [CrossRef]
22. Sharafi, A.; Yu, S.; Naguib, M.; Lee, M.; Ma, C.; Meyer, H.M.; Nanda, J.; Chi, M.; Siegel, D.J.; Sakamoto, J. Impact of air exposure and surface chemistry on Li–Li7La3Zr2O12 interfacial resistance. *J. Mater. Chem. A* **2017**, *5*, 13475–13487. [CrossRef]
23. Erdoğan, A.; Esen, M.; Simpson, R. Chemical Imaging of Human Fingermark by X-ray Photoelectron Spectroscopy (XPS). *J. Forensic Sci.* **2020**, *65*, 1730–1735. [CrossRef] [PubMed]
24. Corby, S.; Tecedor, M.-G.; Tengeler, S.; Steinert, C.; Moss, B.; Mesa, C.A.; Heiba, H.F.; Wilson, A.A.; Kaiser, B.; Jaegermann, W.; et al. Separating bulk and surface processes in NiOx electrocatalysts for water oxidation. *Sustain. Energy Fuels* **2020**, *4*, 5024–5030. [CrossRef]
25. Qiu, Y.S.; Liao, Q.Y.; Chow, M.Y.T.; Lam, J.K.W. Intratracheal Administration of Dry Powder Formulation in Mice. *Jove J. Vis. Exp.* **2020**, *161*, e61469. [CrossRef]
26. Whitesell, J.K. The Merck Index, 12th Edition, CD-ROM (Macintosh): An encyclopedia of chemicals, drugs & biologicals. *J. Am. Chem. Soc.* **1998**, *120*, 2209. [CrossRef]
27. Rim, P.B.; Runt, J.P. Melting point depression in crystalline/compatible polymer blends. *Macromolecules* **1984**, *17*, 1520–1526. [CrossRef]

28. Hulse, W.L.; Forbes, R.T.; Bonner, M.C.; Getrost, M. The characterization and comparison of spray-dried mannitol samples. *Drug Dev. Ind. Pharm.* **2009**, *35*, 712–718. [CrossRef] [PubMed]

29. Burger, A.; Henck, J.O.; Hetz, S.; Rollinger, J.M.; Weissnicht, A.A.; Stottner, H. Energy/temperature diagram and compression behavior of the polymorphs of D-mannitol. *J. Pharm. Sci.* **2000**, *89*, 457–468. [CrossRef]

30. Smith, R.R.; Shah, U.V.; Parambil, J.V.; Burnett, D.J.; Thielmann, F.; Heng, J.Y. The Effect of Polymorphism on Surface Energetics of D-Mannitol Polymorphs. *AAPS J.* **2017**, *19*, 103–109. [CrossRef]

31. Hickey, A.J.; Durham, P.G.; Dharmadhikari, A.; Nardell, E.A. Inhaled drug treatment for tuberculosis: Past progress and future prospects. *J. Control. Release* **2016**, *240*, 127–134. [CrossRef]

32. Muraoka, Y.; Hayashi, Y.; Minesita, T. Studies of capreomycin nephrotoxicity. *Toxicol. Appl. Pharmacol.* **1968**, *12*, 350–359. [CrossRef]

33. Shibeshi, W.; Sheth, A.N.; Admasu, A.; Berha, A.B.; Negash, Z.; Yimer, G. Nephrotoxicity and ototoxic symptoms of injectable second-line anti-tubercular drugs among patients treated for MDR-TB in Ethiopia: A retrospective cohort study. *BMC Pharmacol. Toxicol.* **2019**, *20*, 1–10. [CrossRef]

34. Arpagaus, C.; Meuri, M. Laboratory scale Spray drying of inhalable particles: A review. In Proceedings of the Respiratory Drug Delivery, Orlando, FL, USA, 25–29 April 2010; pp. 469–476.

35. Momin, M.A.M.; Tucker, I.G.; Das, S.C. High dose dry powder inhalers to overcome the challenges of tuberculosis treatment. *Int. J. Pharm.* **2018**, *550*, 398–417. [CrossRef]

36. Kwok, P.C.L.; Grabarek, A.; Chow, M.Y.T.; Lan, Y.; Li, J.C.W.; Casettari, L.; Mason, A.J.; Lam, J.K.W. Inhalable spray-dried formulation of D-LAK antimicrobial peptides targeting tuberculosis. *Int. J. Pharm.* **2015**, *491*, 367–374. [CrossRef]

37. Vishali, D.A.; Monisha, J.; Sivakamasundari, S.K.; Moses, J.A.; Anandharamakrishnan, C. Spray freeze drying: Emerging applications in drug delivery. *J. Control. Release* **2019**, *300*, 93–101. [CrossRef]

38. Weers, J.G.; Miller, D.P.; Tarara, T.E. Spray-Dried PulmoSphere Formulations for Inhalation Comprising Crystalline Drug Particles. *AAPS PharmSciTech* **2019**, *20*, 1–15. [CrossRef]

39. Saint-Lorant, G.; Leterme, P.; Gayot, A.; Flament, M.P. Influence of carrier on the performance of dry powder inhalers. *Int. J. Pharm.* **2007**, *334*, 85–91. [CrossRef]

40. Pilcer, G.; Amighi, K. Formulation strategy and use of excipients in pulmonary drug delivery. *Int. J. Pharm.* **2010**, *392*, 1–19. [CrossRef]

41. Kramek-Romanowska, K.; Odziomek, M.; Sosnowski, T.R.; Gradoń, L. Effects of Process Variables on the Properties of Spray-Dried Mannitol and Mannitol/Disodium Cromoglycate Powders Suitable for Drug Delivery by Inhalation. *Ind. Eng. Chem. Res.* **2011**, *50*, 13922–13931. [CrossRef]

42. Maury, M.; Murphy, K.; Kumar, S.; Shi, L.; Lee, G. Effects of process variables on the powder yield of spray-dried trehalose on a laboratory spray-dryer. *Eur. J. Pharm. Biopharm.* **2005**, *59*, 565–573. [CrossRef]

43. Littringer, E.M.; Mescher, A.; Eckhard, S.; Schröttner, H.; Langes, C.; Fries, M.; Griesser, U.; Walzel, P.; Urbanetz, N.A. Spray Drying of Mannitol as a Drug Carrier—The Impact of Process Parameters on Product Properties. *Dry. Technol.* **2012**, *30*, 114–124. [CrossRef]

44. Young, P.M.; Price, R. The influence of humidity on the aerosolisation of micronised and SEDS produced salbutamol sulphate. *Eur. J. Pharm. Sci.* **2004**, *22*, 235–240. [CrossRef] [PubMed]

45. Maas, S.G.; Schaldach, G.; Littringer, E.M.; Mescher, A.; Griesser, U.J.; Braun, D.E.; Walzel, P.E.; Urbanetz, N.A. The impact of spray drying outlet temperature on the particle morphology of mannitol. *Powder Technol.* **2011**, *213*, 27–35. [CrossRef]

46. Littringer, E.M.; Paus, R.; Mescher, A.; Schroettner, H.; Walzel, P.; Urbanetz, N.A. The morphology of spray dried mannitol particles—The vital importance of droplet size. *Powder Technol.* **2013**, *239*, 162–174. [CrossRef]

47. Maa, Y.-F.; Nguyen, P.-A.; Sweeney, T.; Shire, S.J.; Hsu, C.C. Protein Inhalation Powders: Spray Drying vs Spray Freeze Drying. *Pharm. Res.* **1999**, *16*, 249–254. [CrossRef] [PubMed]

48. Heyder, J.; Gebhart, J.; Rudolf, G.; Schiller, C.F.; Stahlhofen, W. Deposition of particles in the human respiratory tract in the size range 0.005–15 μm. *J. Aerosol Sci.* **1986**, *17*, 811–825. [CrossRef]

49. Elversson, J.; Millqvist-Fureby, A. Particle size and density in spray drying—effects of carbohydrate properties. *J. Pharm. Sci.* **2005**, *94*, 2049–2060. [CrossRef]

50. Elversson, J.; Millqvist-Fureby, A.; Alderborn, G.; Elofsson, U. Droplet and particle size relationship and shell thickness of inhalable lactose particles during spray drying. *J. Pharm. Sci.* **2003**, *92*, 900–910. [CrossRef]

51. Grohganz, H.; Lee, Y.Y.; Rantanen, J.; Yang, M. The influence of lysozyme on mannitol polymorphism in freeze-dried and spray-dried formulations depends on the selection of the drying process. *Int. J. Pharm.* **2013**, *447*, 224–230. [CrossRef]

52. Naini, V.; Byron, P.R.; Phillips, E.M. Physicochemical Stability of Crystalline Sugars and Their Spray-Dried Forms: Dependence upon Relative Humidity and Suitability for Use in Powder Inhalers. *Drug Dev. Ind. Pharm.* **1998**, *24*, 895–909. [CrossRef]

53. Vehring, R. Pharmaceutical particle engineering via spray drying. *Pharm. Res.* **2008**, *25*, 999–1022. [CrossRef] [PubMed]

54. Vehring, R.; Foss, W.R.; Lechuga-Ballesteros, D. Particle formation in spray drying. *J. Aerosol Sci.* **2007**, *38*, 728–746. [CrossRef]

55. Alhajj, N.; O'Reilly, N.J.; Cathcart, H. Designing enhanced spray dried particles for inhalation: A review of the impact of excipients and processing parameters on particle properties. *Powder Technol.* **2021**, *384*, 313–331. [CrossRef]

56. Lechanteur, A.; Evrard, B. Influence of Composition and Spray-Drying Process Parameters on Carrier-Free DPI Properties and Behaviors in the Lung: A review. *Pharmaceutics* **2020**, *12*, 55. [CrossRef] [PubMed]

57. Mangal, S.; Meiser, F.; Tan, G.; Gengenbach, T.; Denman, J.; Rowles, M.R.; Larson, I.; Morton, D.A.V. Relationship between surface concentration of l-leucine and bulk powder properties in spray dried formulations. *Eur. J. Pharm. Biopharm.* **2015**, *94*, 160–169. [CrossRef] [PubMed]
58. Donald, P.R.; McIlleron, H. Antituberculosis Drugs. In *Tuberculosis*; Schaaf, H.S., Zumla, A.I., Grange, J.M., Raviglione, M.C., Yew, W.W., Starke, J.R., Pai, M., Donald, P.R., Eds.; W.B. Saunders: Edinburgh, UK, 2009; pp. 608–617.
59. Muttil, P.; Wang, C.; Hickey, A.J. Inhaled drug delivery for tuberculosis therapy. *Pharm. Res.* **2009**, *26*, 2401–2416. [CrossRef]
60. Wolf, A.J.; Linas, B.; Trevejo-Nunez, G.J.; Kincaid, E.; Tamura, T.; Takatsu, K.; Ernst, J.D. Mycobacterium tuberculosis Infects Dendritic Cells with High Frequency and Impairs Their Function In Vivo. *J. Immunol.* **2007**, *179*, 2509–2519. [CrossRef] [PubMed]
61. World Health Organization. *Companion Handbook to the WHO Guidelines for the Programmatic Management of Drug-Resistant Tuberculosis*; World Health Organization: Geneva, Switzerland, 2014.

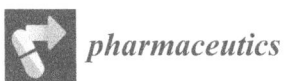 *pharmaceutics*

Article

Dry Powder Comprised of Isoniazid-Loaded Nanoparticles of Hyaluronic Acid in Conjugation with Mannose-Anchored Chitosan for Macrophage-Targeted Pulmonary Administration in Tuberculosis

Mahwash Mukhtar [1], Noemi Csaba [2,3], Sandra Robla [2,3], Rubén Varela-Calviño [4], Attila Nagy [5], Katalin Burian [6], Dávid Kókai [6] and Rita Ambrus [1,*]

[1]   Institute of Pharmaceutical Technology and Regulatory Affairs, Faculty of Pharmacy, University of Szeged, 6720 Szeged, Hungary; mahwash.mukhtar@szte.hu

[2]   Department of Pharmacology, Pharmacy and Pharmaceutical Technology, University of Santiago de Compostela, 15782 Santiago de Compostela, Spain; noemi.csaba@usc.es (N.C.); sandra.robla@outlook.es (S.R.)

[3]   Center for Research in Molecular Medicine and Chronic Diseases, University of Santiago de Compostela, 15782 Santiago de Compostela, Spain

[4]   Department of Biochemistry & Molecular Biology, School of Pharmacy, University of Santiago de Compostela, 15782 Santiago de Compostela, Spain; ruben.varela@usc.es

[5]   Wigner Research Centre for Physics, 1121 Budapest, Hungary; nagy.attila@wigner.hu

[6]   Department of Medical Microbiology, Albert Szent-Györgyi Medical School, University of Szeged, 6720 Szeged, Hungary; burian.katalin@med.u-szeged.hu (K.B.); kokai.david@med.u-szeged.hu (D.K.)

*   Correspondence: ambrus.rita@szte.hu

Citation: Mukhtar, M.; Csaba, N.; Robla, S.; Varela-Calviño, R.; Nagy, A.; Burian, K.; Kókai, D.; Ambrus, R. Dry Powder Comprised of Isoniazid-Loaded Nanoparticles of Hyaluronic Acid in Conjugation with Mannose-Anchored Chitosan for Macrophage-Targeted Pulmonary Administration in Tuberculosis. *Pharmaceutics* 2022, 14, 1543. https://doi.org/10.3390/pharmaceutics14081543

Academic Editors: Michael Yee Tak Chow and Philip Chi Lip Kwok

Received: 15 June 2022
Accepted: 20 July 2022
Published: 25 July 2022

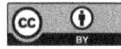

Abstract: Marketed dosage forms fail to deliver anti-tubercular drugs directly to the lungs in pulmonary Tuberculosis (TB). Therefore, nanomediated isoniazid (INH)-loaded dry powder for inhalation (Nano-DPI) was developed for macrophage-targeted delivery in TB. Mannosylated chitosan (MC) and hyaluronic acid (HA) with an affinity for the surface mannose and CD44 receptors of macrophages were used in conjugation to prepare hybrid nanosuspension by ionic gelation method using cross-linker, sodium tri-polyphosphate (TPP) followed by freeze-drying to obtain a dry powder composed of nanoparticles (INH-MC/HA NPs). Nanoformulations were evaluated for aerodynamic characteristics, cytotoxicity, hemocompatibility, macrophage phenotype analysis, and immune regulation. Cellular uptake imaging was also conducted to evaluate the uptake of NPs. The nanopowders did not pose any significant toxicity to the cells, along with good compatibility with red blood cells (RBCs). The pro-inflammatory costimulatory markers were upregulated, demonstrating the activation of T-cell response. Moreover, the NPs did not show any tolerogenic effect on the macrophages. Furthermore, confocal imaging exhibited the translocation of NPs in the cells. Altogether, the findings present that nano-DPI was found to be a promising vehicle for targeting macrophages.

Keywords: dry powder inhaler; immune regulation; inhalation; isoniazid; mannose conjugation; macrophage phenotype; next-generation impactor; tuberculosis

1. Introduction

Tuberculosis (TB) remains one of the main causes of death globally, which are estimated to be 1.2 to 1.4 million per year according to WHO, despite the advancement in therapeutics and diagnostics [1]. TB poses a serious socio-economic burden on developing and underdeveloped countries. Out of all the reported TB pathologies, pulmonary TB contributes to 80% of pathogenesis [2]. The onset of pulmonary TB occurs after the inhalation of *Mycobacterium tuberculosis* (M.Tb). Though M.Tb, microorganisms can be captured by mucous-secreting goblet cells in most instances, they bypass the mucociliary clearance system and are deposited by phagocytosis as a result of interaction between M.Tb surface lipoarabinomannan and surface mannose receptors of alveolar macrophages (AM). Hence,

M.Tb finds AM to be its niche for survival and reservoir for replication due to inhibition of phagosome-lysosome fusion [3]. Moreover, the TB microenvironment also facilitates the growth and survival of M.Tb. TB is spreading at an alarming rate due to a lack of patient-adherent therapeutic options and long-term duration of treatment (6 months) with standard therapy. Moreover, the mycobacteria in low proliferative phases and multi-drug resistant strains need more prolonged treatment of over 24 months. The only available option is the vaccine (Bacille Calmette-Guerin, BCG), but it also fails in people sensitized to M.Tb [4]. Among other challenges are the inadequate delivery of effective anti-tubercular agents to the site of infection along with an off-site accumulation of drugs leading to organ toxicity.

Conventional drug delivery systems fail to deliver anti-tubercular drugs to the alveolar region because of indirect delivery via blood. Consequently, innovative approaches need to be fabricated for effective pulmonary drug delivery without off-target accumulation. As the causative agent resides in the host AM, a suitable inhalation system with an excellent aerodynamic profile must be designed to achieve a targeted delivery, which might reduce the dosage frequency. Inhalable nanosystems have been widely and successfully investigated in the past as well with different compositions. Among them, the polymeric nanosystems are advantageous because of their attribute of encapsulating both the hydrophilic and hydrophobic drugs, controlled release profile, desirable pharmacokinetic outcomes, and ability to translocate across the biological barriers [5]. Polymeric nanocarriers comprised of polymers such as alginate, chitosan, [poly (DL-lactide-co-glycolide)] (PLGA), tri-block poly (ethylene glycol) (PEG)-poly (ε-caprolactone) (PCL), etc., have shown promising outcomes in the delivery of nanoparticles (NPs) to the lungs with localized drug release over a long time with minimal cytotoxicity and good therapeutic outcomes [6–11]. For this purpose, nanotechnology-based dry powder for inhalation (nano-DPIs) can be a promising opportunity that needs extensive research for bench-to-bedside availability.

Surprisingly, the registered patents (US20200289667A1, US20170319699A1) have already been exploiting the potential of NPs to target macrophages in different diseases. Moreover, the phagocytic feature of AM can be exploited by developing therapies targeted at intra-macrophage infections such as TB. This property can be probed by altering the physical, chemical, and surface characteristic of the NPs [12]. Thus, here we have developed a nano-DPI system using polymers for the optimistic therapy of TB. Antigen-presenting cells (APCs) such as macrophages have overexpression of surface receptors such as CD44 and mannose receptors that can be targeted by developing the nanosystems constituted of polymers serving as a ligand to these receptors. Mannose receptors have a pivotal function in the regulation of adaptive immune response. It is proposed that mannose receptor-mediated endocytosis of mannose conjugated nanoparticles can stimulate an enhanced immune response [13,14].

Based on the idea of targeting the surface receptors of macrophages, suitable polymers were chosen. Hyaluronic acid (HA) is an immune-compatible polymer that also protects against pulmonary injury [15] with an affinity for the CD44 receptors on the macrophages. HA also performs a vital role in the growth of epithelial cells and macrophages [16]. Similarly, chitosan (CS) is derived from marine source and demonstrates no toxicity to human cells along with biodegradability. Hence, it was the polymer of choice for mannose conjugation to synthesize mannosylated chitosan (MC). Oligosaccharides with terminal mannose on microorganisms can bind to the macrophage mannose receptor and allow their endocytic transport in the cells. This can be correlated with the use of mannose-conjugated polymeric nanoparticles for the intra-macrophage delivery of anti-tubercular drugs by exploiting surface mannose receptors for a T-cell immune response [17]. The use of MC not only facilitates mannose-targeted drug delivery but also promotes controlled drug release. Hence, in this work, we describe the pulmonary drug delivery nanopowder (the powders obtained after drying of the nanosuspensions) to potentially reach the infected AM by using biodegradable polymers. DPIs are propellant-free and cost-effective drug delivery devices for the pulmonary administration of drugs for local or systemic infections. The developed nanopowder was characterized in terms of the aerodynamic parameters and powder morphology. The nanopowder composed of MC and HA was compared with the CS and HA nanopowder in this study. The sole purpose of this comparative study was to evaluate if the synthetic polymer (MC) has any peculiar off-results in terms of cytotoxicity and T-cell pathway stimulation as compared to the natural CS.

2. Materials and Methods

2.1. Materials

Isoniazid (INH) [IUPAC: Isonicotinylhydrazide] from Pannon Pharma Kft (Hungary). Sodium hyaluronate equivalent to $1.5–1.8 \times 10^6$ Da (Hyaluronic acid) from Contipro Biotech (Czech Republic). Chitosan (CS) [75–85% deacetylated, low molecular weight, 50–190 kDa, Poly(D-glucosamine)] and 4',6-diamidino-2-phenylindole (DAPI) dye from Sigma-Aldrich (St. Louis, MO, USA). Macrophage Raw 264.7 and A549 cell lines were obtained from ATCC (Manassas, VA, USA). Granulocyte-macrophage colony-stimulating factor (GM-CSF), Allophycocyanin (APC)-conjugated anti-human CD83 (CD83-APC), and Phycoerythrin (PE)-conjugated anti-human CD80 (CD80-PE) were purchased from Miltenyi Biotec (Bergisch Gladbach, Germany). Ficoll-Paque ^{TM} PLUS (density 1.077 g/mL) was purchased from GE Healthcare Bioscience AB (Chicago, IL, USA). Dulbecco's modified Eagle's medium (DMEM) and Roswell Park Memorial Institute medium (RPMI-1640) were purchased from GIBCO® (Thermo Fischer Scientific, Bedford, MA, USA). Sodium tripolyphosphate (TPP) from Alfa Aesar (Thermofischer, Munich, Germany). Trifluoroacetic acid (Merk Schuchard OHG), 3-(4,5-dimethylthiazol-2-yl)-5-(3-carboxymethoxyphenyl)-2-(4-sulfophenyl)-2H-tetrazolium (MTS) cell proliferation assay kit was provided by BioVision (Milpitas, CA, USA). Sodium dodecyl sulfate (SDS), 3-(4,5-dimethylthiazol-2-yl)-2,5-diphenyltetrazolium bromide (MTT), and 4-Dimethylamino benzaldehyde were obtained from Sigma-Aldrich (Chemie GmbH, Steinheim, Germany). Fetal Bovine Serum (FBS) and PSG (100 u/mL penicillin, 0.1 mg/mL streptomycin, and 2 mM L-glutamine) were purchased from Invitrogen(Carlsbad, CA, USA). Glacial acetic acid (GAA) was purchased from Molar Chemicals Kft (Hungary). For in vitro experiments, sterile and autoclaved materials were used. All the chemicals were of high purity or reagent grade.

2.2. Synthetic Procedure

MC polymer was synthesized by our previously reported method [18]. The synthetic procedure is, however, briefly mentioned in the supplementary file. The number of mannose groups on MC was quantified after synthesis. In short, the polymer was hydrated and put into the 96-well plate. Totals of 20 µL of resorcinol, 100 µL of sulfuric acid, and 50 µL of pristane (2,6,10,14-tetramethyl-pentadecane) were added to each well. The well plate was kept at 90 °C for 20 min, and the optical density (OD) was read by a microplate reader (PerkinElmer, Waltham, MA, USA) at 450 nm.

2.3. Characterization of Polymer

The synthesized polymer MC was characterized by Fourier Transform infra-red spectroscope (FTIR) (Thermo Nicolet AVATAR 330, Waltham, MA, USA). IR spectra were acquired by the KBr disc method at 4 cm^{-1} resolution at the wavenumber range of 400–4000 cm^{-1} at room temperature (RT). Moreover, the ^{1}H NMR spectroscopy (Bruker BRX-500) was performed in deuterated DMSO to analyze the polymer.

2.4. Preparation of Nanoparticles

For the preparation of nanoparticles, the polymer MC was solubilized in 0.5 M glacial acetic acid solution, and HA was dissolved in water. The pH of the polymeric suspension was maintained at 4.9. Following the ionic gelation technique, TPP (0.5–2 mg/mL) was used as a cross-linker to facilitate the ionic interaction between the positively charged amino groups of MC and the anionic charge on HA [19]. TPP was added dropwise to the polymeric suspension consisting of HA and MC. After thorough stirring, INH (10 mg, 10%

of oral dose) was added dropwise to the polymeric nanosuspension. The nanosuspension was probe sonicated followed by stirring overnight to obtain a uniform consistency. A similar procedure was used to develop the CS-based nanosuspensions. Rhodamine-B (Rh-B)-labeled NPs were obtained by replacing INH with the fluorescent dye and later dialyzed against deionized water for three days to remove the unattached dye.

2.5. Freeze-Drying to Obtain Nanopowders

The prepared nanosuspensions were freeze-dried in Scanvac, Coolsafe 100-9 prototype apparatus (LaboGeneApS, Lynge, Denmark) to obtain the dry powders for inhalation. Four percent trehalose (v/v) was added to the liquid samples before lyophilization. The pressure of the chamber was maintained at 0.01 mbar throughout the process. Table 1 shows the process parameters recorded over time using a computer program attached to the instrument.

Table 1. Process parameters are taken into consideration during the process of freeze-drying.

Process	Time (h:min)	Chamber Pressure (mbar)	Product Temperature (°C)	Shelf Temperature (°C)
Freezing	01:30	-	−20	−40
	02:30		−20 to −26	
	03:45		−26 to −39	
Primary drying	04:00	0.01	−39 to −37	−25
	06:10		−37 to −31	−20
	09:40		−31 to −27	0
Secondary drying	16:00	0.01	−27 to −14	+9
	21:10		−14 to −6	+22
	40:15		−6 to −2	+30

2.6. Particle Size, Polydispersity Index (PDI), and Surface Charge

Parameters such as particle size, polydispersity index (PDI), and zeta potential were analyzed by the Malvern zeta sizer Nano ZS (Malvern instrument, Worcestershire, UK). The nanopowders were redispersed in purified water before analysis. All experiments were performed in triplicate and are expressed as mean ± SD.

2.7. Encapsulation Efficiency (EE)

The encapsulation efficiency (EE) of the nanosuspensions was evaluated by an indirect method using a supernatant. The supernatants were collected after centrifuging the nanosuspensions at 15,000 g for 30 min. The obtained supernatants were spectrophotometrically analyzed at 264 nm, and Equation (1) was used to calculate the % EE. The percentage of drug loading (DL) was also determined, which is the percentage of the actual mass of the drug loaded in the nanopowder to the total acquired mass of the nanopowder, as given by Equation (2)

$$\% \text{ Encapsulation Efficiency} = (\text{Total drug-Free drug})/(\text{Total drug}) \times 100 \qquad (1)$$

$$\% \text{ Drug Loading} = (\text{Mass of drug loaded in NPs})/(\text{Total mass of NPs}) \times 100 \qquad (2)$$

2.8. Morphological Examination

Nanopowders were studied for their surface morphology by using Scanning Electron Microscopy (SEM) (Hitachi S4700, Hitachi Scientific Ltd., Tokyo, Japan) at 2.0–5.0 kV. Throughout imaging, the pressure of the air was maintained at 1.3–13.0 mPa.

2.9. Colloidal Stability at Storage Conditions

The nanosuspensions before freeze-drying were kept at working and storage temperature (25 °C) for 1 month. The average particle size and PDI were determined after certain time points.

2.10. In Vitro Aerodynamic Profile by Next-Generation Impactor (NGI)

Next-Generation Impactor (NGI) (Copley Scientific Limited, Nottingham, UK) setup was employed for the assessment of the aerodynamic profile of the freeze-dried sample, INH-MC/HA NPs. Only the mannosylated sample was tested and compared with the results from previous studies by our group. This is the standard method for the determination of the size distribution of particles dispensed from DPIs on collection trays based on aerodynamic size. An optical microscopic method was conjoined with an impactor for the evaluation of particles deposited on each collection tray [20]. Figure 1 shows the measurement setup, which was used for the testing with the NGI. In the measurements, an in-house developed breath simulator generated the breathing waveform (red arrows), an induction port acted as the upper respiratory tract, and a vacuum pump (HCP5 High-capacity pump; Copley Scientific Ltd., Nottingham, UK) with a critical flow controller (TPK 2000; Copley Scientific Ltd., UK) maintained the constant flow along the blue arrows, which delivered the particles from the DPI to the impactor. The compressor compensated for the losses in the system. The mixing inlet (Copley Scientific Ltd., Nottingham, UK) provided the interface between the flow, which activated the DPI, and the main flow that delivered the particles to the NGI device. The NGI determines the aerodynamic size distribution of the particles by the impaction method. The sample flow rate of the NGI was maintained at 90 L/min, which was regularly checked during the measurements with a TSI 4000 thermal mass flow meter [20]. The direction of airflow indicated by arrows is similar to that of the working of the Aerodynamic Particle Sizer (Figure S1). The nanopowder equivalent to 10 mg INH (10% of the recommended oral dose) was loaded into the hydroxypropyl methylcellulose (HPMC) capsules (transparent, size 3, ACG) and was dosed through the Breezhaler® (Novartis) dry powder inhalator device. After the experiment was run, the fine particle fraction (FPF < 3) was calculated, which represents the percentage of particles smaller than 3 μm and denotes the settling of particles in the deeper parts of the lungs. The mass median aerodynamic diameter (MMAD) was also determined, which is defined as the median particle diameter of the particles settled in the NGI. This was evaluated by the logarithmic aerodynamic diameter of the particles between stages 2 and 3 versus the interpolation of the percentage undersize [21]. In general, MMAD is the cut-off diameter at which 50% of the deposited particles are smaller or larger by mass.

Moreover, the aerodynamic size was analyzed by time-of-flight measurements in an accelerated flow through an Aerodynamic Particle Sizer (APS-TSI 3321, Shoreview, MN, USA). As a breath simulator, we used an in-house developed pulmonary waveform generator. It uses a piston pump driven by a programmable logic controller (PLC)-controlled servo motor to generate the inhalation and exhalation air flows (Figure S1). The inhalation volume spans from 0.1 to 6800 cm^3. The time resolution of the inhalation profile can be set to 20, 50, and 100 ms. The inhalation waveform programmed into the breathing simulator was generated according to the literature (Figure S2) for the measurements [22,23].

2.11. Isolation of Monocytes and Differentiation into Macrophages

After informed consent was obtained, the heparinized blood was collected from the healthy donors. The identity of the donors was kept anonymous. The buffy coats were donated by the Organ and Blood Donation Agency (ADOS; Santiago de Compostela, Spain). The Ficoll density gradient separation method was employed to isolate peripheral blood mononuclear cells [24]. In brief, blood was poured into a 50 mL tube in the laminar flow cabinet. The blood was diluted with PBS (1:1) at maintained RT. This diluted blood was carefully added to Ficoll-Paque™ PLUS at a blood/Ficoll ratio of 2:1. Human peripheral blood mononuclear cells (PBMC) were isolated after centrifugation (Allegra X-12R, Beckman Coulter) at 400 g for 30 min at RT on deceleration mode. The upper layer was discarded, leaving behind the PBMC layer, which was carefully transferred to 50 mL centrifugation falcon tubes. The PBMC layer was washed with PBS using centrifugation at 300 g for 10 min to improve the purity by removing the remaining Ficoll media. The obtained cells were then resuspended in an R_2 medium (RPMI-1640 supplemented with 2% heat-inactivated

FBS and 1% of PSG). A total of 10 mL of the cells was seeded into a 75 cm^2 cell culture flask for 2 h (37 °C, 5% CO$_2$) by maintaining the density of cells at 1.2×10^6 cells/mL. After this time, the non-adherent cells, peripheral blood lymphocytes, were washed with PBS and the attached monocytes were cultured for 3 days in R$_{10}$ media (RPMI-1640 supplemented with 10% heat-inactivated FBS and 1% of PSG). After 3 days, the media was replaced with R$_{10}$ media (RPMI-1640 supplemented with 10% heat-inactivated FBS, 1% of PSG, and cytokines (GM-CSF at 100 ng/mL)) for the differentiation of monocytes to macrophages.

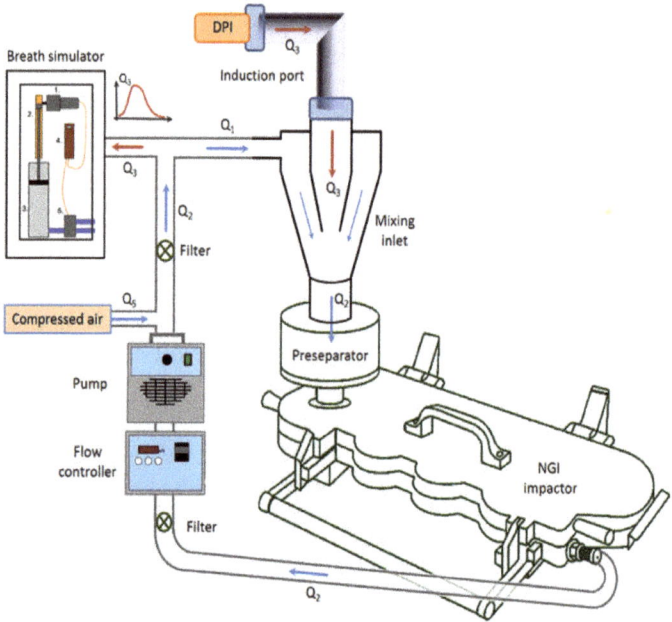

Figure 1. The schematic design and components of the measurement setup: DPI, induction port, NGI, vacuum pump with a critical flow controller, and mixing inlet.

2.12. Cytotoxicity Studies

Before experiments, the cell lines were cultured in Dulbecco's Modified Eagle Medium (DMEM) supplemented with 10% (v/v) fetal bovine serum (FBS) and 1% (v/v) penicillin-streptomycin-glutamine (PSG). The culture media was replaced after every 2–3 days to maintain the cell confluency. The cultured cells were incubated at 37 °C and 5% CO$_2$ in a humidifier chamber.

2.12.1. Cytotoxicity on A549 Cells

MTT assay was performed for the evaluation of the cytotoxic effect of NPs on the cells. A549 cells (adenocarcinoma human alveolar basal epithelial cells) were used as a model for alveolar type II cells, as these cells predominantly constitute the pulmonary alveolar epithelia [25]. For this purpose, A549 cells were seeded and cultured at a density of 4×10^4 cells/well in 96-well culture microplates. Later, the formulations, namely INH, blank CS/HA NPs, blank MC/HA NPs, INH-CS/HA NPs, and INH-MC/HA NPs, were added in different concentrations to the cultures and incubated for 24 h at 37 °C. After incubation for 24 h, 20 μL of MTT was added to each well, and the culture plates were again incubated for 4 h. Next, 100 μL of sodium dodecyl sulfate solution (10% in 0.01 M HCl) was added to the well plates to dissolve the formed formazan crystals. OD was measured using an EZ READ 400 ELISA reader (Biochrom, Cambridge, UK) at 550 nm (ref. 630 nm).

Untreated cells with 100% viability were used as a control. All the evaluations were performed in triplicate. The relative cell viability was calculated using the following Equation (3),

$$\text{Cell viability (\% control)} = (\text{Absorbance of sample})/(\text{Absorbance of control}) \times 100 \quad (3)$$

2.12.2. Cytotoxicity on Raw 264.7 Cells

Again, an MTT assay was performed to evaluate the cytotoxic effect of the formulations on the Raw 264.7 cells, which were cultured in the sterile flat-bottom 96-well tissue culture plates at a density of 1×10^4 cells/well for 24 h. The culture media was replaced with the different concentrations of nanopowder samples (100 μL final volume, dissolved in supplemented media) on the following day. Following incubation for 24 h, 10 μL of MTT (dissolved in phosphate buffer saline (PBS)) at 5 mg/mL concentration) was added to the wells. Well culture plates were incubated for 4 h at 37 °C without light. Afterward, the MTT solution was discarded, and the formazan crystals were dissolved by the addition of 100 μL of acid isopropanol (0.04 N HCl in isopropanol). The OD of the plates was read after 10 min at the wavelength of 570 nm (Reference wavelength 630 nm) using a microplate reader (Synergy H1 Hybrid Multi-Mode, BioTek, Winooski, VT, USA) to determine the cell viability using Equation (2). Untreated cells served as a negative control, and sodium dodecyl sulfate (SDS) was used as a positive control [26].

2.12.3. Cytotoxicity on Human Macrophages

An MTS assay was performed to determine the cytotoxic effect of INH, blank CS/HA NPs, blank MC/HA NPs, INH-CS/HA NPs, and INH-MC/HA NPs on the primary macrophage culture. Monocyte-differentiated macrophages were seeded onto the 96-well microplate at a density of 1.10×10^5 cells/mL and incubated for 24 h. Later, the media was replaced by the different concentrations of the samples and incubated for 24 h under standard sterile conditions (37 °C, 5% CO_2). A total of 10 μL of MTS reagent was then added to the well plates and incubated for 4 h. The absorbance was then measured at 490 nm using a microplate reader (Synergy H1 Hybrid Multi-Mode, BioTek, Winooski, VT, USA). Macrophages in culture media (0% toxicity) served as a negative control, and SDS was used as a positive control (100% toxicity). Equation (2) was used to calculate the viability of cells.

2.13. Confocal Imaging for Visualization of Uptake of NPs in A549 and Raw 264.7 Cells

The uptake of NPs was analyzed through confocal laser scanning microscopy. Briefly, A549 cells and Raw 264.7 cells (8×10^4 cells/mL) were seeded onto the individual Lab-Tek® chambered #1.0 Borosilicate cover glass system (0.8 cm^2/well). After 24 h, the cell culture media was replaced with 300 μL of Rh-B labeled NPs in a concentration of 10 μg/mL and incubated with cells for 2 h. The cells were washed thrice with PBS, and 4% paraformaldehyde was added to fix the cells and allowed to incubate for another 15 min. The cells were again washed with PBS three times followed by the addition of DAPI (300 μM, 1:500 in PBS) nucleus dye and incubated for 50 min. A549 and Raw 264.7 cells without the addition of formulations were used as controls. Following washing with PBS, the mounting media was added to the chamber, and imaging was performed by confocal microscope (Leica SP5, Mannheim, Germany). Rhodamine Ex: 546 nm/Em: 568 nm; DAPI Ex: 359 nm/Em: 457 nm.

2.14. Human Macrophage Phenotype Analysis

NPs were incubated with blood-derived macrophages in a 48-well plate at a final concentration of 10 μg/mL for 24 h. Cells were washed with PBS twice (400 g, 6 min at RT) to remove NPs. Later, the cells were resuspended in PBS and stained with an optimal concentration of different antibodies (CD83-APC and CD80-PE) for 25 min at −4 °C in the dark [27]. The cells were washed with PBS again (400 g, 6 min RT) and resuspended in PBS, and kept on ice until measurement. The level of maturation markers was then quantified by flow cytometry in a BD FACSCalibur cytometer. Flowing software (Cell Imaging Core, Turku Centre for Biotechnology) was used to analyze the data. The data have been shown as the ratio between the mean fluorescence intensity (MFI) of the corresponding markers in macrophages incubated with NPs and the MFI of macrophages incubated in culture media.

2.15. Tolerogenic Effect of NPs in Macrophages

2,3-Indoleamine dioxygenase (IDO) expression was assessed in the macrophages after their exposure to NPs. The enzyme, IDO, is involved in the catabolism of tryptophan, which is pivotal for the growth of microorganisms and, therefore, directly influences the T-cell tolerance [28]. Moreover, IDO is an immune-suppressive enzyme in macrophages with the function of catabolizing tryptophan into its metabolite, kynurenine, which is responsible for the apoptosis of Th1 cells in vitro. Hence, the IDO assay quantifies the kynurenine in culture media. The study was conducted to evaluate the tolerogenic response of the NPs on macrophages by using the described methods [29]. Briefly, cells were seeded onto a 48-well plate, followed by their incubation with different formulations in a final volume of 0.5 mL. Four hours before the end of the culture period, 1.25 µL of L-tryptophan (100 µM) was added to the medium. A total of 30% trifluoroacetic acid (2:1 v/v) was mixed with culture media (obtained after the centrifugation of cells at 10,000 g, 5 min at RT) to precipitate the cell debris in another round of centrifugation with the aforementioned parameters. Ehrlich Reagent was added to acquire supernatant, and absorbance was read using a microplate reader at 490 nm.

2.16. Hemolysis Assay

Fresh blood from four human donors was collected in the acid citrate dextrose (ACD)-containing tubes. The blood was washed thrice with PBS by centrifugation at 250 g for 5 min, and the red blood cells (RBCs) pellet was collected while the supernatant plasma was discarded. The obtained RBCs pellet was diluted with PBS, and the RBCs suspension was seeded onto a 96-well plate and incubated with NPs for 4 h and 24 h at 37 °C. Triton-X 100 (1% v/v) and PBS were kept as positive and negative controls, respectively. The absorbance of the samples was measured at 570 nm using a microplate reader (Synergy H1 Hybrid Multi-Mode, BioTek, Winooski, VT, USA), and % hemolysis was calculated using Equation (4),

$$\% \text{ hemolysis} = (\text{Absorbance of sample-Absorbance of negative control})/ (\text{Absorbance of positive control-Absorbance of negative control}) \times 100 \quad (4)$$

2.17. Statistical Analysis

All the experiments were performed in triplicate unless otherwise stated. All the results are expressed as mean ± standard deviation. GraphPad Prism v.6.01 software (GraphPad Software Inc., San Diego, CA, USA) was used for data analysis. A two-way ANOVA test in combination with Dunnett's multiple comparisons tests was used to present the difference between donor groups.

3. Results

3.1. Characterization of Polymer

The mannose groups on the MC polymer were quantified to be 232 ± 13 µM per gram. The NMR analysis (Figure 2) demonstrated the mannose conjugation to CS with a peak at 4.03 ppm (the methylene protons of the mannose sugar) [30]. The signals at 2.404 ppm corresponded to the protons of the CH_2-group, indicating the linking bridge (acetamido group) between mannose and chitosan by Schiff's base reductive amination [31]. The peak for the methyl group of the non-deacetylated part of CS was observed at 1.631 ppm, and the amine group of CS corresponded to 0.859 ppm [32].

Chitosan

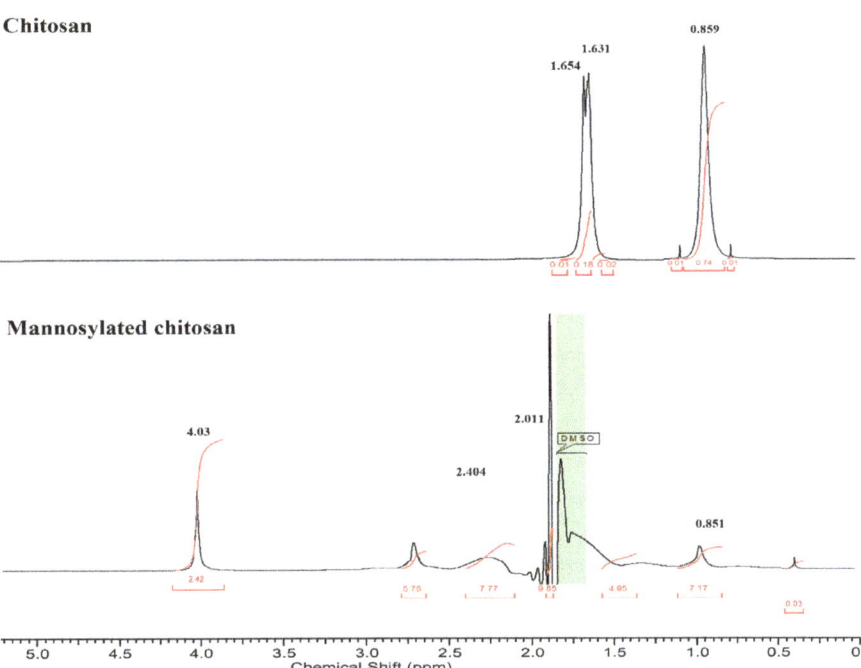

Mannosylated chitosan

Figure 2. NMR spectra of chitosan and mannosylated chitosan. The respective chemical shift peak signals are mentioned in bold. The red text presents the integral (or area) of the peak signals.

Moreover, FTIR spectra (Figure S3) presented the IR peak at 3351.69 cm^{-1}, corresponding to amide bond stretch in MC as a result of conjugation of mannose to the unmodified polymer. The peak at 1780 cm^{-1} presented COO symmetric stretching, and COO asymmetric stretching was seen at 1200 cm^{-1}. Further, the NH_2 band was observed at 1032.73 cm^{-1}, followed by the amide bond formation fingerprint peak in MC at 1100 cm^{-1} [33]. Moreover, the peak of mannose stretch can also be seen at 850 cm^{-1}. The peak at 1600 cm^{-1} was characteristic of $CO-NH_2$ in CS, whereas the peak at 3500 cm^{-1} demonstrated OH bond widening [34].

3.2. Freeze-Dried Nanopowders

The average particle size of the drug-loaded MC/HA NPs was found to be 303 ± 16.2 nm. In the past, nanoparticles within the size ranges of 200–350 nm have shown promising uptake into the macrophages [35–37]. Moreover, it has been reported that particles below 250 nm size present reduced uptake by the alveolar macrophages and pulmonary endothelial cells [38].

Besides the particle size, the PDI value, 0.179 ± 0.04, was also found to be promising for the INH-MC/HA NPs in comparison to the CS-based samples. The PDI value of less than 0.2 is considered to be ideal in the case of polymeric drug delivery nanovehicles [39]. Hence, the nanopowder was monodispersed with a narrow size distribution. The positive zeta potential was also considered favorable for the high stability of the nanopowders. Further, the cationic-charged moieties have high intracellular uptake efficiency in the macrophages, followed by pulmonary inhalation [40]. Table 2 enlists some parameters of the nanopowders.

3.3. Morphological Examination

SEM micrographs (Figure 3) displayed the smooth morphology of the freeze-dried nanopowders with a narrow size distribution from a working distance of 12.8 and 14.2 mm.

Likewise, the NPs were scattered uniformly. Blank-CS/HA NPs presented small patches of aggregation that might have been due to remnants of free TPP [41].

Table 2. Physicochemical attributes of nanopowders.

Samples	Average Particle Size (nm)	PDI	Zeta Potential (mV)	Encapsulation Efficiency (%)	Drug Loading (%)
CS/HA NPs	310 ± 21	0.231 ± 0.12	30.3 ± 9.05	-	-
INH-CS/HA NPs	342 ± 08	0.301 ± 0.17	29.5 ± 2.01	90.18 ± 1.01	23.5 ± 1.29
MC/HA NPs	298 ± 11	0.116 ± 0.01	30.6 ± 3.79	-	-
INH-MC/HA NPs	303 ± 16	0.179 ± 0.04	34.3 ± 6.03	92.31 ± 2.06	25.9 ± 2.11

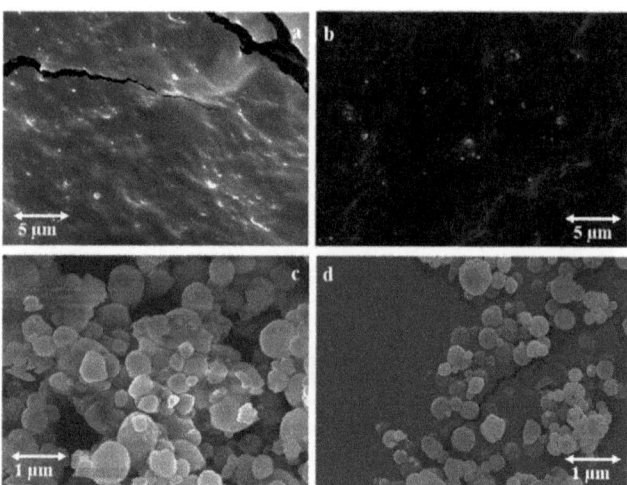

Figure 3. SEM micrographs of INH-CS/HA nanopowder (**a,c**) and INH-MC/HA NPs (**b,d**) were obtained separately with the 1 and 5 μm scale bars.

3.4. Colloidal Stability

The colloidal stability was evaluated for 1 month to demonstrate the minimum stability for operational purposes (Figure 4). Nanosuspensions demonstrated aggregation in the case of a long storage time. However, the average particle sizes were not significantly altered, which might be the reason for inconsistency in the individual readings. Moreover, the nanosuspensions were not sonicated before evaluations to get the real-time behavior. The PDI of the nanosuspensions was, therefore, increased proportionally to each time interval. However, most of the samples had PDI index values ≤ 0.5, which are considered appropriate for mono-disperse nanosystems [42]. Furthermore, freeze-drying was employed to guarantee long-term stability.

3.5. In Vitro Aerodynamic Profile

NGI was used to assess the aerodynamic size distribution of the particles from DPI via Breezhaler®. The amount of powder in each stage was determined by the optical method. The mannosylated dry powder sample demonstrated favorable results in terms of mass size distribution. First, the data were obtained from the APS by maintaining setting channel bounds according to the cut-off sizes of NGI plates. Later, the powder was evaluated for mass size distribution by NGI, and results were acquired based on the surface coverage of the collection plates. As shown in Figure S4, the highest fraction of particles in the dry powder system was within the range of 1.37–2.3 μm, as determined by APS with settings according to NGI. Later, the results obtained from NGI (Figure 5) confirm the data from APS, i.e., the size distribution was correlated to the previous measurement, and the average mass size distribution of the particles was within the same range of 1.37–2.3 μm, exhibiting deposition in the peripheral airways (terminal bronchioles and alveoli). The average of all the results (performed four times) is shown in Table S1. Thirty-five percent of FPF was found to be less than <3, highlighting that this ratio of the nanopowder was deposited in the deeper lung. MMAD was calculated to be 2.7 μm, which explains that a higher proportion of the particles demonstrated good aerodynamic behavior in terms of the surface properties of the particle.

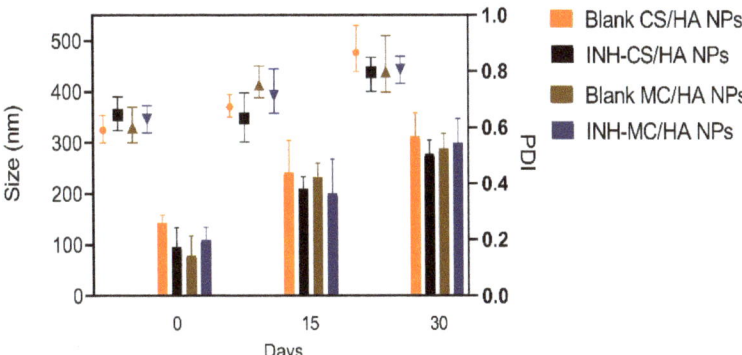

Figure 4. Stability of the nanosuspensions with the relative change in particle size (nm) and poly-dispersity index (PDI) at 15-day-intervals over one month. Results are expressed as mean ± S.D, performed in triplicate.

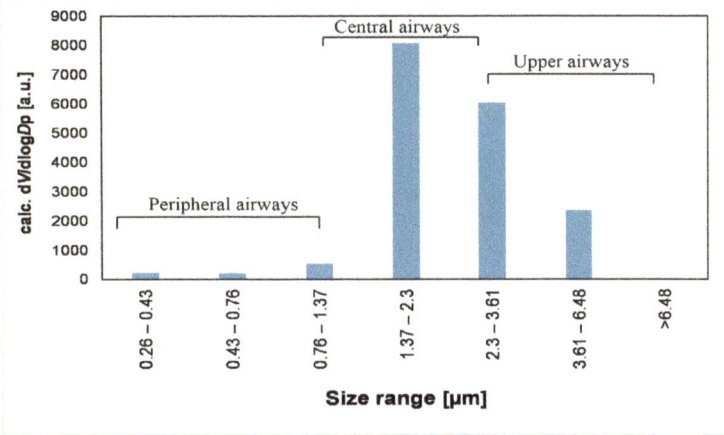

Figure 5. Mass size distribution of INH-MC/HA nanopowder as measured by the NGI using the data evaluation method based on the surface coverage of the collection plates.

3.6. Cytotoxicity Studies

An MTT assay was performed to investigate the cytotoxicity of the nanopowders and nascent INH on A549 and Raw 264.7 macrophages. After an exposure of 24 h with different concentrations of INH and nanopowders (0.01, 0.5, 1 mg/mL), it was evident that the A549 cell viability was pronounced for all samples (Figure 6a). The drug-loaded nanopowders demonstrated more than 80% viability for A549 cells. Blank MC/HA nanopowder showed remarkable results and was 100% in A549 cells. The cell viability for Raw 264.7 macrophages was concentration-dependent (Figure 6b). INH presented more than 50% viability at low concentrations of 0.5 and 0.01 mg/mL, which led to the evident conclusion that at higher doses, the drug is toxic to macrophages. Moreover, the cationic NPs display a high affinity toward macrophages, and hence the toxicity can increase depending on the concentration of NPs [43]. The MTT assay displayed a reduction in Raw 264.7 macrophage viability with increasing concentrations of polymers. However, all the concentrations were found to have more than 50% cell viability.

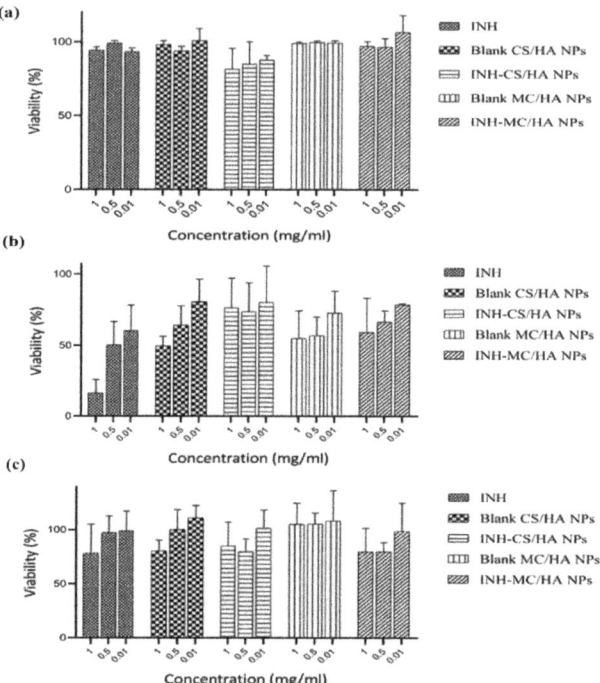

Figure 6. Effect of nanoformulations on the viability of A549 cells (**a**), Raw 264.7 macrophages (**b**), and primary culture of macrophages derived from human blood (**c**). The results were obtained after incubation of different concentrations of the nanoparticles (0.01, 0.5, 1 mg/mL) over 24 h. All the results were performed in triplicate and are expressed as mean ± S.D.

Likewise, the MTS assay, which was performed to access the impact of nanopowders on the metabolic activity of primary macrophages, revealed similar results. The % cell viability was evidently but not primarily dependent on the increase in the concentrations of the samples (Figure 6c). All the samples presented cell viability of ≥70%. These cytotoxicity data were obtained after 24 h incubation. The main purpose behind the viability studies on the primary cells was to evaluate the accurate concentration of the samples optimal for the human macrophage phenotype analysis.

3.7. Visualization of NPs in the A549 and Raw 264.7 Cells

Confocal laser scanning microscopy (CLSM) was employed for the qualitative assessment of the fluorescent-labeled Rh-B NPs. Figure 7 shows the shift in the intensity of fluorescence on the internalization of NPs as compared to the control (untreated cells). Human alveolar epithelial cells, A549, were also used to study the uptake behavior of NPs. It can be seen clearly that the internalization of NPs in the A549 cells was lower compared to the Raw 264.7 macrophages. This might be due to the well-established reason that A549 cells are not responsive to the NPs in a similar way to immune cells (macrophages) [44]. Immune cells, such as macrophages, identify antigens and NPs by phagocytosis, surface receptor-based endocytosis, and micropinocytosis. Supposedly, macrophages most likely responded through the surface receptors and hence translocated the moieties with mannose composition efficiently. The internalization intensity of the NPs was found to be higher in the case of MC/HA NPs as compared to CS/HA NPs (Figure S5), demonstrating the advantage of mannose conjugation to the polymer. Quantification of Rh-B-labeled NPs was also performed by flow cytometry (Figure S6).

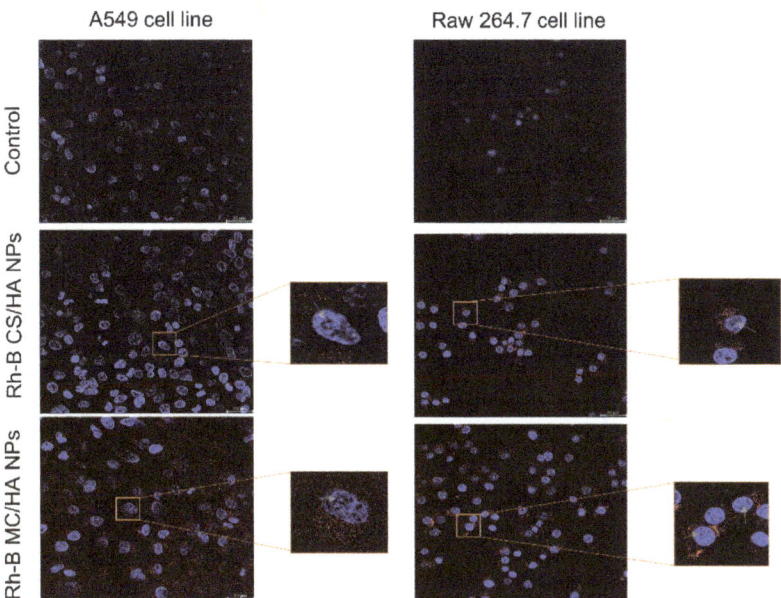

Figure 7. Cellular internalization study via confocal imaging. Confocal images of A549 cells and Raw 264.7 macrophages showing the internalization of Rhodamine-B labeled NPs (red) after an incubation of 2 h. The blue color indicates the nuclei staining with DAPI-dye. Rhodamine-B (Excitation λ_{max} = 546 nm, Emission λ_{max} = 568 nm), DAPI-dye (Excitation λ_{max} = 359 nm, Emission λ_{max} = 457 nm).

3.8. Human Macrophage Phenotype Analysis

The expression of T-lymphocyte costimulatory molecules (CD83 and CD80), the indicators of pro-inflammatory-activated phenotypes in macrophages, was evaluated by the incubation of NPs with macrophages for 2 h. The expression was analyzed by flow cytometry (Figure S7). CD83 is elevated and observed in the activated macrophages. CD80 is the prime costimulatory marker affecting cytokine secretion [45]. The delivery of antigen to macrophages upregulates the expression of CD83 and CD80, which are considered to induce T cell receptor signaling and activation. The expression was many folds higher for the MC/HA NPs when compared to other nanoformulations (average MFI = 1 for control). The results in Figure 8a show the relative comparison between the expression of CD83 and CD80 in macrophages derived from three different blood donors. On the whole, the findings demonstrate that blank and drug-loaded MC/HA NPs significantly upregulated the costimulatory markers in comparison to other NPs.

3.9. Tolerogenic Activity

IDO expression by macrophages influences peripheral tolerance and immune regulation. IDO assay was performed to determine if the NPs were inducing a tolerogenic phenotype on macrophages characteristic to the suppression of T-cells and the promotion of tolerance (contrary to pro-inflammatory response) (Figure 8b). It was analyzed by quantifying the IDO activity following incubation of NPs with macrophages. The NP samples demonstrated a similar response to that of control macrophages, establishing no tolerogenic effect of the NPs.

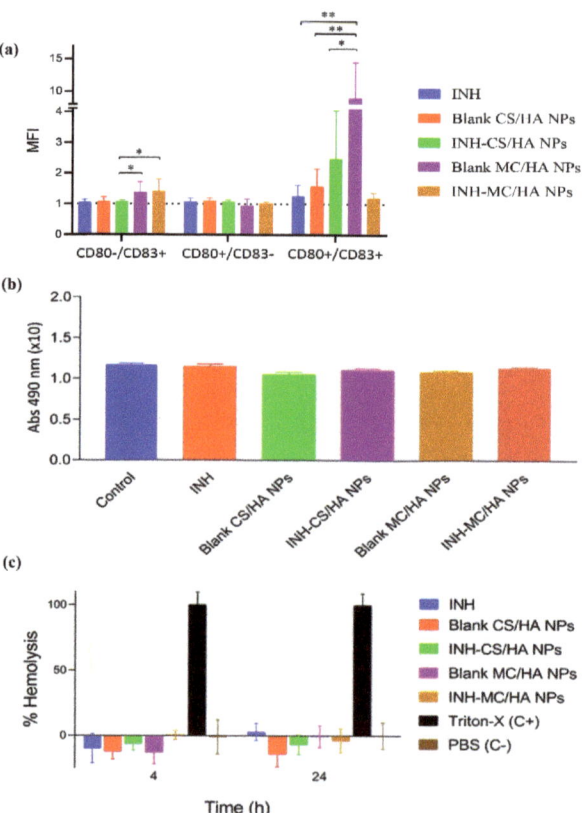

Figure 8. % Quantification of the expression of macrophage maturation markers, CD80 and CD83. All the results have been presented as mean fluorescence intensity (MFI) in macrophages incubated with NPs. The dotted line (MFI = 1) represents the signal from the macrophages incubated in culture (control). Data from blank MC/HA NPs were statistically significant (* $p < 0.05$, ** $p < 0.001$) (**a**), 2,3-Indoleamine dioxygenase (IDO) activity in macrophages cell culture (**b**), and in-vitro hemolysis assay after 4 and 24 h performed on fresh human blood obtained from donors after consent (**c**). All the results are expressed as mean ± SEM, $n = 3$ different blood donors ($p < 0.001$).

3.10. Hemolytic Activity

Hemolysis assay demonstrates the biocompatibility of NPs with RBCs to get insight into the behavior of formulations for in vivo applications. The % viability of RBCs was evaluated against the Triton-X (positive control) with 100% cell lysis. All the samples posed no toxicity on the RBCs, indicating biocompatibility with RBCs (Figure 8c). In this case, all the NPs samples were hemocompatible.

4. Discussion

The major obstacle in the treatment of TB is the inadequate availability of the drug in the affected organ. Therefore, a dosage form capable of delivering the effective drug concentration to the alveolar region of the lungs is the primary priority for the treatment of TB. In recent times, the use of nanotechnology has gained interest for organ-targeted drug delivery. The use of a nanotechnology-based aerosolization approach can limit off-site drug accumulation. Moreover, the nanocarriers show high residence time in the lungs because of the presence of mucous. Therefore, based on this rationale, dry powder for inhalation was developed in this study using nanotechnology. A hybrid nano-approach was utilized for the fabrication of nano-DPI by using two polymers, MC and HA. These polymers are non-toxic, non-thrombogenic, biodegradable, biocompatible, and non-immunogenic [46]. The limitations, such as mucociliary clearance of a large proportion of inhaled powders and exhalation of small-sized particles, can be overcome by using a ligand anchored polymeric drug delivery system. The ligand anchorage to the NPs can reduce the reticuloendothelial system (RES) uptake and improve the availability of the drug at the target site. Further, as mentioned previously, the mannose receptor is a C-type lectin that can identify the mannose-containing polymers with high affinity. Therefore, the mannosylated polymer was used in this study to improve the drug delivery in TB. Likewise, HA also presents a high affinity for the CD44 receptors on the surface of macrophages [47]. Therefore, these polymers were chosen for developing the macrophage-targeted nanoparticulate system. The cost-effective ionic gelation method was employed to prepare the polymeric nanosuspension, and anti-tubercular INH was loaded into the NPs, followed by freeze-drying with 4% trehalose as a cryoprotectant to yield dry powder. Freeze-drying removes the solvent from samples by sublimation of frozen content in the primary drying step and unfrozen solvents in the secondary drying step. The freeze-drying time is, however, dependent on the product height and hence varies with the sample volume [48].

The average particle size for the INH-MC/HA-loaded nano-DPI was found to be 303 ± 16.2 nm, with a monodisperse nature indicated by a PDI of 0.179. The surface zeta potential was 34.3 ± 6.03, showing good stability of the formulation. The % EE of the INH-CS/HA NPs and INH-MC/HA NPs was high, which might have been achieved because of the synthetic approach used for the NPs. The drug was loaded after the synthesis of NPs and hence was strongly adhered to the voids of the NPs. It has been observed that the use of the ionic gelation method yields NPs with a plexus, and the drug can be embedded within the matrices.

The prediction of the pharmacokinetic and pharmacodynamic (PK/PD) profile for the inhaled drugs can be a complicated protocol because of the complex pulmonary geometry. Hence, testing of the aerodynamic particle size distribution and deposition of the particles by NGI can narrow the gap between the in vitro and in vivo performance testing to accelerate research and development (R&D). The particles in the NGI are driven by the constant airflow towards different stages with defined cut-off diameters. The average mass size distribution was evaluated by NGI, operated according to European Pharmacopeial 2014 requirements. The results demonstrated that a high fraction of the particles had a size range of 1.37–2.3 µm, correlating to the deposition in stages 6 and 7 with the geometrical standard deviation (GSD) of 1.50. GSD determines the variation in diameters of particles within the aerosol cloud. Usually, the GSD values > 1.2 present the heterodispersive nature of the aerosols with broad particle size distribution [49]. The aerodynamic profile can further be improved by using the alternate drying procedure for the nanosuspensions to acquire the powder for inhalation, which has also been demonstrated by us in the past [50].

The cytotoxicity studies revealed that all the samples had high % cell viability and posed no toxicity to A549 cells, Raw 264.7 macrophage, and primary cultures. Likewise, the demonstration of hemolytic activity is essential because of the safety concerns of NPs. The in vitro hemolytic activity on RBCs is evaluated by spectrophotometric analysis of plasma-free hemoglobin derivatives after the incubation of NPs with blood. Centrifugation was performed to remove the undamaged RBCs. As established, the safe hemolytic ratio for biomaterials should be less than 5% according to ISO/TR 7406 [51]. In this study, all the formulations posed no toxicity to RBCs.

Principally, adaptive immune response mediated by T-cells is essential for the control of M.Tb. NPs did not interfere with the adaptive immune response and facilitated the T-cell signaling and activation. By the upregulation of the costimulatory molecule CD80, there is an elevation of interleukin-6 that exhibits pro-inflammatory activity and plays a role in the resistance against TB [52]. Correspondingly, CD83 plays a role in resolving immune responses in TB and is also essential during the differentiation of T-lymphocytes along with maintaining tolerance. The inhibition of CD83 alleviates the inflammation [53]. However, the developed NPs improved the expression of costimulatory markers.

The uptake of nanopowders by the A549 cells and Raw 264.7 macrophages was established by confocal microscopy. The nuclei of the cells were stained with DAPI dye to facilitate visual imaging. A549 cells (primarily comprised of alveolar basal epithelial cells) were used for studying the uptake of the NPs because the inhaled particles interact with the alveolar epithelia before engulfment by macrophages. MC/HA nanopowders presented high localization into the cells as compared to the CS/HA nanopowders. Altogether, the NPs were able to be translocated into the macrophages, which corroborated with the aim of the study. Further, the tolerogenic response was assessed for the nanopowders. The tolerogenic response is responsible for the immunosuppression that contradicts the T-cell response required in TB. Increased IDO activity by the macrophages suppresses effector T-cells and elevates regulatory T-cells, which then promotes immune tolerance [54], which is not favorable for the treatment of TB. The nanopowders did not exhibit any tolerogenic effect, as demonstrated by the IDO assay. All the results were compared with the CS/HA-based nanopowder for a thorough understanding of the various parameters that might otherwise be compromised by using MC polymer. Everything considered, the mannose-anchored nanoparticulate system is suitable for delivering anti-tubercular to the macrophages in the TB.

5. Conclusions

In this study, macrophage-targeted nanoparticles were developed to achieve higher retention at the site of a bacterial niche for promising therapy of TB. For this purpose, polymers were chosen because of their affinity for the surface receptor of macrophages for the uptake of encapsulated anti-tubercular inside the immune cells. The nanosystem INH-MC/HA was fabricated to be administered by inhalation via dry powder inhalers for efficient delivery to the lungs. The results reported that the nano dry powders had higher deposition in the deeper region of the lungs followed by pulmonary administration. The ability of NPs to interact with macrophages was conserved and amplified by using mannose-anchored chitosan along with HA. Altogether, nano-DPIs presented promising fundamental outcomes that might impact investigative studies in animals in the future.

Supplementary Materials: The following supporting information can be downloaded at: https://www.mdpi.com/article/10.3390/pharmaceutics14081543/s1.

Author Contributions: Conceptualization, M.M., R.A., and R.V.-C.; methodology, M.M. and S.R.; software, M.M., S.R., and A.N.; validation, M.M. and D.K.; formal analysis, M.M. and R.A.; investigation, D.K., K.B., S.R., and M.M.; resources, R.A., N.C., R.V.-C., S.R., and A.N.; writing—original draft preparation, M.M.; writing—review and editing, M.M., R.A., and K.B.; visualization, S.R., N.C., and M.M.; supervision, R.A.; project administration, R.A. and N.C.; funding acquisition, R.A. All authors have read and agreed to the published version of the manuscript.

Funding: This research was the funded by the Ministry of Innovation and Technology of Hungary from the National Research, Development, and Innovation Fund (Project No. TKP2021-EGA-32, financed under the TKP2021-EGA funding scheme).

Institutional Review Board Statement: All the institutional and national guidelines for obtaining and using blood were followed. Blood was drawn from all the subjects after informed consent. Permission was acquired from the Institutional Ethics Committee (Comité Ético de Investigación Clínica de Galicia, CEIC), approval number 2014/543, approval date 20 February 2015.

Informed Consent Statement: Informed consent was obtained from all subjects involved in the study. All the procedures were under the ethical standard of the institute and national committee on human experiments and the Declaration of Helsinki.

Data Availability Statement: Not applicable.

Acknowledgments: We acknowledge the Gedeon Richter Ltd.—GINOP project (2.2.1-15-2016-00007), TKP2021-EGA funding scheme and, Ministerio de Ciencia e Innovacion RETOS - PID2019-107500RB-I00 and Competitive Reference Groups, Consellería de Educación e Ordenación Universitaria, Xunta de Galicia, Ref: ED431C 2021/17.

Conflicts of Interest: The authors declare no conflict of interest.

References

1. Vieira, A.C.; Chaves, L.L.; Pinheiro, M.; Lima, S.C.; Neto, P.J.R.; Ferreira, D.; Sarmento, B.; Reis, S. Lipid Nanoparticles Coated with Chitosan Using a One-Step Association Method to Target Rifampicin to Alveolar Macrophages. *Carbohydr. Polym.* **2021**, *252*, 116978. [CrossRef] [PubMed]
2. Rawal, T.; Parmar, R.; Tyagi, R.K.; Butani, S. Rifampicin Loaded Chitosan Nanoparticle Dry Powder Presents an Improved Therapeutic Approach for Alveolar Tuberculosis. *Colloids Surf. B Biointerfaces* **2017**, *154*, 321–330. [CrossRef] [PubMed]
3. Mukhtar, M.; Pallagi, E.; Csóka, I.; Benke, E.; Farkas, Á.; Zeeshan, M.; Burián, K.; Kókai, D.; Ambrus, R. Aerodynamic Properties and in Silico Deposition of Isoniazid Loaded Chitosan/Thiolated Chitosan and Hyaluronic Acid Hybrid Nanoplex Dpis as a Potential Tb Treatment. *Int. J. Biol. Macromol.* **2020**, *165*, 3007–3019. [CrossRef] [PubMed]
4. Silva, J.P.; Gonçalves, C.; Costa, C.; Sousa, J.; Silva-Gomes, R.; Castro, A.G.; Pedrosa, J.; Appelberg, R.; Gama, F.M. Delivery of Llkkk18 Loaded into Self-Assembling Hyaluronic Acid Nanogel for Tuberculosis Treatment. *J. Control. Release* **2016**, *235*, 112–124. [CrossRef]
5. D'Angelo, I.; Conte, C.; Miro, A.; Quaglia, F.; Ungaro, F. Pulmonary Drug Delivery: A Role for Polymeric Nanoparticles? *Curr. Top. Med. Chem.* **2015**, *15*, 386–400. [CrossRef]
6. Ahmad, Z.; Pandey, R.; Sharma, S.; Khuller, G. Alginate Nanoparticles as Antituberculosis Drug Carriers: Formulation Development, Pharmacokinetics and Therapeutic Potential. *Indian J. Chest Dis. Allied Sci.* **2006**, *48*, 171.
7. Abdelghany, S.; Parumasivam, T.; Pang, A.; Roediger, B.; Tang, P.; Jahn, K.; Britton, W.J.; Chan, H.-K. Alginate Modified-Plga Nanoparticles Entrapping Amikacin and Moxifloxacin as a Novel Host-Directed Therapy for Multidrug-Resistant Tuberculosis. *J. Drug Deliv. Sci. Technol.* **2019**, *52*, 642–651. [CrossRef]
8. Scolari, I.R.; Páez, P.L.; Sánchez-Borzone, M.E.; Granero, G.E. Promising Chitosan-Coated Alginate-Tween 80 Nanoparticles as Rifampicin Coadministered Ascorbic Acid Delivery Carrier against Mycobacterium Tuberculosis. *Aaps Pharmscitech* **2019**, *20*, 67. [CrossRef]
9. Shah, S.; Cristopher, D.; Sharma, S.; Soniwala, M.; Chavda, J. Inhalable Linezolid Loaded Plga Nanoparticles for Treatment of Tuberculosis: Design, Development and in Vitro Evaluation. *J. Drug Deliv. Sci. Technol.* **2020**, *60*, 102013. [CrossRef]
10. Hakkimane, S.S.; Shenoy, V.P.; Gaonkar, S.L.; Bairy, I.; Guru, B.R. Antimycobacterial Susceptibility Evaluation of Rifampicin and Isoniazid Benz-Hydrazone in Biodegradable Polymeric Nanoparticles against Mycobacterium Tuberculosis H37rv Strain. *Int. J. Nanomed.* **2018**, *13*, 4303. [CrossRef]
11. Moretton, M.A.; Cagel, M.; Bernabeu, E.; Gonzalez, L.; Chiappetta, D.A. Nanopolymersomes as Potential Carriers for Rifampicin Pulmonary Delivery. *Colloids Surf. B Biointerfaces* **2015**, *136*, 1017–1025. [CrossRef] [PubMed]
12. Gustafson, H.H.; Holt-Casper, D.; Grainger, D.W.; Ghandehari, H. Nanoparticle Uptake: The Phagocyte Problem. *Nano Today* **2015**, *10*, 487–510. [CrossRef] [PubMed]
13. Yao, W.; Peng, Y.; Du, M.; Luo, J.; Zong, L. Preventative Vaccine-Loaded Mannosylated Chitosan Nanoparticles Intended for Nasal Mucosal Delivery Enhance Immune Responses and Potent Tumor Immunity. *Mol. Pharm.* **2013**, *10*, 2904–2914. [CrossRef] [PubMed]
14. Xu, B.; Zhang, W.; Chen, Y.; Xu, Y.; Wang, B.; Zong, L. Eudragit®L100-Coated Mannosylated Chitosan Nanoparticles for Oral Protein Vaccine Delivery. *Int. J. Biol. Macromol.* **2018**, *113*, 534–542. [CrossRef]
15. Hwang, S.; Kim, D.; Chung, S.; Shim, C. Delivery of Ofloxacin to the Lung and Alveolar Macrophages Via Hyaluronan Microspheres for the Treatment of Tuberculosis. *J. Control. Release* **2008**, *129*, 100–106. [CrossRef]
16. Sionkowska, A.; Gadomska, M.; Musiał, K.; Piątek, J. Hyaluronic Acid as a Component of Natural Polymer Blends for Biomedical Applications: A Review. *Molecules* **2020**, *25*, 4035. [CrossRef]
17. Jiang, H.-L.; Kang, M.L.; Quan, J.-S.; Kang, S.G.; Akaike, T.; Yoo, H.S.; Cho, C.-S. The Potential of Mannosylated Chitosan Microspheres to Target Macrophage Mannose Receptors in an Adjuvant-Delivery System for Intranasal Immunization. *Biomaterials* **2008**, *29*, 1931–1939. [CrossRef]
18. Mukhtar, M.; Szakonyi, Z.; Farkas, Á.; Burian, K.; Kókai, D.; Ambrus, R. Freeze-Dried Vs Spray-Dried Nanoplex Dpis Based on Chitosan and Its Derivatives Conjugated with Hyaluronic Acid for Tuberculosis: In Vitro Aerodynamic and in Silico Deposition Profiles. *Eur. Polym. J.* **2021**, *160*, 110775. [CrossRef]
19. Pornpitchanarong, C.; Rojanarata, T.; Opanasopit, P.; Ngawhirunpat, T.; Patrojanasophon, P. Catechol-Modified Chitosan/Hyaluronic Acid Nanoparticles as a New Avenue for Local Delivery of Doxorubicin to Oral Cancer Cells. *Colloids Surf. B Biointerfaces* **2020**, *196*, 111279. [CrossRef]
20. Attila, K. Optikai Mérési Módszerek Fejlesztése És Alkalmazása Az Aeroszolok Légúti Kiülepedésének Vizsgálatára. 2021. Available online: https://pea.lib.pte.hu/handle/pea/24067 (accessed on 14 June 2022).

21. Pomázi, A.; Buttini, F.; Ambrus, R.; Colombo, P.; Szabó-Révész, P. Effect of Polymers for Aerolization Properties of Mannitol-Based Microcomposites Containing Meloxicam. *Eur. Polym. J.* **2013**, *49*, 2518–2527. [CrossRef]
22. Abadelah, M.; Chrystyn, H.; Larhrib, H. Use of Inspiratory Profiles from Patients with Chronic Obstructive Pulmonary Disease (Copd) to Investigate Drug Delivery Uniformity and Aerodynamic Dose Emission of Indacaterol from a Capsule Based Dry Powder Inhaler. *Eur. J. Pharm. Sci.* **2019**, *134*, 138–144. [CrossRef] [PubMed]
23. Farkas, Á.; Szipőcs, A.; Horváth, A.; Horváth, I.; Gálffy, G.; Varga, J.; Galambos, K.; Kugler, S.; Nagy, A.; Szalai, Z. Establishment of Relationships between Native and Inhalation Device Specific Spirometric Parameters as a Step Towards Patient Tailored Inhalation Device Selection. *Respir. Med.* **2019**, *154*, 133–140. [CrossRef] [PubMed]
24. Posch, W.; Lass-Flörl, C.; Wilflingseder, D. Generation of Human Monocyte-Derived Dendritic Cells from Whole Blood. *JoVE J. Vis. Exp.* **2016**, *118*, e54968. [CrossRef] [PubMed]
25. Scordo, J.M.; Knoell, D.L.; Torrelles, J.B. Alveolar Epithelial Cells in Mycobacterium Tuberculosis Infection: Active Players or Innocent Bystanders? *J. Innate Immun.* **2016**, *8*, 3–14. [CrossRef]
26. Balzus, B.; Sahle, F.F.; Hönzke, S.; Gerecke, C.; Schumacher, F.; Hedtrich, S.; Kleuser, B.; Bodmeier, R. Formulation and Ex Vivo Evaluation of Polymeric Nanoparticles for Controlled Delivery of Corticosteroids to the Skin and the Corneal Epithelium. *Eur. J. Pharm. Biopharm.* **2017**, *115*, 122–130. [CrossRef]
27. Robla, S.; Prasanna, M.; Varela-Calviño, R.; Grandjean, C.; Csaba, N. A Chitosan-Based Nanosystem as Pneumococcal Vaccine Delivery Platform. *Drug Deliv. Transl. Res.* **2021**, *11*, 581–597. [CrossRef]
28. Braun, D.; Longman, R.S.; Albert, M.L. A Two-Step Induction of Indoleamine 2, 3 Dioxygenase (Ido) Activity During Dendritic-Cell Maturation. *Blood* **2005**, *106*, 2375–2381. [CrossRef]
29. Crecente-Campo, J.; Virgilio, T.; Morone, D.; Calviño-Sampedro, C.; Fernández-Mariño, I.; Olivera, A.; Varela-Calvino, R.; González, S.F.; Alonso, M.J. Design of Polymeric Nanocapsules to Improve Their Lympho-Targeting Capacity. *Nanomedicine* **2019**, *14*, 3013–3033. [CrossRef]
30. Rager, M.N.; Binet, M.R.; Ionescu, G.; Bouvet, O.M. 31p-Nmr and 13c-Nmr Studies of Mannose Metabolism in Plesiomonas Shigelloides: Toxic Effect of Mannose on Growth. *Eur. J. Biochem.* **2000**, *267*, 5136–5141. [CrossRef]
31. Yao, W.; Jiao, Y.; Luo, J.; Du, M.; Zong, L. Practical Synthesis and Characterization of Mannose-Modified Chitosan. *Int. J. Biol. Macromol.* **2012**, *50*, 821–825. [CrossRef] [PubMed]
32. Kumirska, J.; Czerwicka, M.; Kaczyński, Z.; Bychowska, A.; Brzozowski, K.; Thöming, J.; Stepnowski, P. Application of Spectroscopic Methods for Structural Analysis of Chitin and Chitosan. *Mar. Drugs* **2010**, *8*, 1567–1636. [CrossRef] [PubMed]
33. Mukhtar, M.; Zesshan, M.; Khan, S.; Shahnaz, G.; Khan, S.A.; Sarwar, H.S.; Pasha, R.A.; Ali, H. Fabrication and Optimization of Ph-Sensitive Mannose-Anchored Nano-Vehicle as a Promising Approach for Macrophage Uptake. *Appl. Nanosci.* **2020**, *10*, 4013–4027. [CrossRef]
34. Islam, S.; Arnold, L.; Padhye, R. Comparison and Characterisation of Regenerated Chitosan from 1-Butyl-3-Methylimidazolium Chloride and Chitosan from Crab Shells. *BioMed Res. Int.* **2015**, *2015*, 874316. [CrossRef] [PubMed]
35. Berton, M.; Allémann, E.; Stein, C.A.; Gurny, R. Highly Loaded Nanoparticulate Carrier Using an Hydrophobic Antisense Oligonucleotide Complex. *Eur. J. Pharm. Sci.* **1999**, *9*, 163–170. [CrossRef]
36. Gratton, S.E.; Ropp, P.A.; Pohlhaus, P.D.; Luft, J.C.; Madden, V.J.; Napier, M.E.; DeSimone, J.M. The Effect of Particle Design on Cellular Internalization Pathways. *Proc. Natl. Acad. Sci. USA* **2008**, *105*, 11613–11618. [CrossRef]
37. Hatami, E.; Mu, Y.; Shields, D.N.; Chauhan, S.C.; Kumar, S.; Cory, T.J.; Yallapu, M.M. Mannose-Decorated Hybrid Nanoparticles for Enhanced Macrophage Targeting. *Biochem. Biophys. Rep.* **2019**, *17*, 197–207. [CrossRef]
38. Azarmi, S.; Roa, W.H.; Löbenberg, R. Targeted Delivery of Nanoparticles for the Treatment of Lung Diseases. *Adv. Drug Deliv. Rev.* **2008**, *60*, 863–875. [CrossRef]
39. Danaei, M.; Dehghankhold, M.; Ataei, S.; Hasanzadeh Davarani, F.; Javanmard, R.; Dokhani, A.; Khorasani, S.; Mozafari, M. Impact of Particle Size and Polydispersity Index on the Clinical Applications of Lipidic Nanocarrier Systems. *Pharmaceutics* **2018**, *10*, 57. [CrossRef]
40. Jeon, S.; Clavadetscher, J.; Lee, D.-K.; Chankeshwara, S.V.; Bradley, M.; Cho, W.-S. Surface Charge-Dependent Cellular Uptake of Polystyrene Nanoparticles. *Nanomaterials* **2018**, *8*, 1028. [CrossRef]
41. Yang, W.; Fu, J.; Wang, T.; He, N. Chitosan/Sodium Tripolyphosphate Nanoparticles: Preparation, Characterization and Application as Drug Carrier. *J. Biomed. Nanotechnol.* **2009**, *5*, 591–595. [CrossRef] [PubMed]
42. Masarudin, M.J.; Cutts, S.M.; Evison, B.J.; Phillips, D.R.; Pigram, P.J. Factors Determining the Stability, Size Distribution, and Cellular Accumulation of Small, Monodisperse Chitosan Nanoparticles as Candidate Vectors for Anticancer Drug Delivery: Application to the Passive Encapsulation of [14c]-Doxorubicin. *Nanotechnol. Sci. Appl.* **2015**, *8*, 67. [CrossRef] [PubMed]
43. Tzankova, V.; Gorinova, C.; Kondeva-Burdina, M.; Simeonova, R.; Philipov, S.; Konstantinov, S.; Petrov, P.; Galabov, D.; Yoncheva, K. In Vitro and in Vivo Toxicity Evaluation of Cationic Pdmaema-Pcl-Pdmaema Micelles as a Carrier of Curcumin. *Food Chem. Toxicol.* **2016**, *97*, 1–10. [CrossRef]
44. Skuland, T.; Låg, M.; Gutleb, A.C.; Brinchmann, B.C.; Serchi, T.; Øvrevik, J.; Holme, J.A.; Refsnes, M. Pro-Inflammatory Effects of Crystalline-and Nano-Sized Non-Crystalline Silica Particles in a 3d Alveolar Model. *Part. Fibre Toxicol.* **2020**, *17*, 13. [CrossRef] [PubMed]

45. Maj, T.; Slawek, A.; Chelmonska-Soyta, A. Cd80 and Cd86 Costimulatory Molecules Differentially Regulate Ot-Ii Cd4+ T Lymphocyte Proliferation and Cytokine Response in Cocultures with Antigen-Presenting Cells Derived from Pregnant and Pseudopregnant Mice. *Mediat. Inflamm.* **2014**, *2014*, 769239. [CrossRef]
46. Chaudhary, K.R.; Puri, V.; Singh, A.; Singh, C. A Review on Recent Advances in Nanomedicines for the Treatment of Pulmonary Tuberculosis. *J. Drug Deliv. Sci. Technol.* **2022**, *69*, 103069. [CrossRef]
47. He, H.; Ghosh, S.; Yang, H. Nanomedicines for Dysfunctional Macrophage-Associated Diseases. *J. Control. Release* **2017**, *247*, 106–126. [CrossRef]
48. Adali, M.B.; Barresi, A.A.; Boccardo, G.; Pisano, R. Spray Freeze-Drying as a Solution to Continuous Manufacturing of Pharmaceutical Products in Bulk. *Processes* **2020**, *8*, 709. [CrossRef]
49. Bianco, F.; Salomone, F.; Milesi, I.; Murgia, X.; Bonelli, S.; Pasini, E.; Dellacà, R.; Ventura, M.L.; Pillow, J. Aerosol Drug Delivery to Spontaneously-Breathing Preterm Neonates: Lessons Learned. *Respir. Res.* **2021**, *22*, 71. [CrossRef]
50. Party, P.; Bartos, C.; Farkas, Á.; Szabó-Révész, P.; Ambrus, R. Formulation and in vitro and in Silico Characterization of "Nano-in-Micro" Dry Powder Inhalers Containing Meloxicam. *Pharmaceutics* **2021**, *13*, 211. [CrossRef]
51. Snima, K.; Jayakumar, R.; Unnikrishnan, A.; Nair, S.V.; Lakshmanan, V.-K. O-Carboxymethyl Chitosan Nanoparticles for Metformin Delivery to Pancreatic Cancer Cells. *Carbohydr. Polym.* **2012**, *89*, 1003–1007. [CrossRef] [PubMed]
52. Jiménez-Uribe, A.P.; Valencia-Martínez, H.; Carballo-Uicab, G.; Vallejo-Castillo, L.; Medina-Rivero, E.; Chacón-Salinas, R.; Pavón, L.; Velasco-Velázquez, M.A.; Mellado-Sánchez, G.; Estrada-Parra, S. Cd80 Expression Correlates with Il-6 Production in Thp-1-Like Macrophages Costimulated with Lps and Dializable Leukocyte Extract (Transferon®). *J. Immunol. Res.* **2019**, *2019*, 2198508. [CrossRef] [PubMed]
53. Islam, S.; Byun, H.-O.; Choi, B.; Sohn, S. Inhibition of Cd83 Alleviates Systemic Inflammation in Herpes Simplex Virus Type 1-Induced Behcet's Disease Model Mouse. *Mediat. Inflamm.* **2019**, *2019*, 5761392. [CrossRef]
54. Mellor, A.L.; Lemos, H.; Huang, L. Indoleamine 2, 3-Dioxygenase and Tolerance: Where Are We Now? *Front. Immunol.* **2017**, *8*, 1360. [CrossRef] [PubMed]

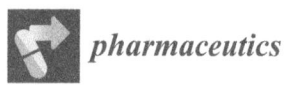

Article

Inhalable Mannosylated Rifampicin–Curcumin Co-Loaded Nanomicelles with Enhanced In Vitro Antimicrobial Efficacy for an Optimized Pulmonary Tuberculosis Therapy

Juan M. Galdopórpora [1], Camila Martinena [2], Ezequiel Bernabeu [1,3,4], Jennifer Riedel [1,4], Lucia Palmas [5], Ines Castangia [5], Maria Letizia Manca [5,*], Mariana Garcés [6], Juan Lázaro-Martinez [7], Maria Jimena Salgueiro [3], Pablo Evelson [6], Nancy Liliana Tateosian [2], Diego Andres Chiappetta [1,3,4] and Marcela Analia Moretton [1,3,4,*]

[1] Facultad de Farmacia y Bioquímica, Universidad de Buenos Aires, Buenos Aires 1113, Argentina; galdo.juan89@gmail.com (J.M.G.); eze_bernabeu@yahoo.com.ar (E.B.); jenn.driedel@gmail.com (J.R.); diegochiappetta@yahoo.com.ar (D.A.C.)
[2] Facultad de Ciencias Exactas y Naturales, Instituto de Química Biológica de la Facultad de Ciencias Exactas y Naturales (IQUIBICEN), CONICET, Universidad de Buenos Aires, Ciudad Universitaria, Buenos Aires 1113, Argentina; cami.b.m254@gmail.com (C.M.); nantateosian@gmail.com (N.L.T.)
[3] Consejo Nacional de Investigaciones Científicas y Técnicas (CONICET), Buenos Aires 1425, Argentina; mjsalguei@gmail.com
[4] Instituto de Tecnología Farmacéutica y Biofarmacia (InTecFyB), Universidad de Buenos Aires, Buenos Aires 1113, Argentina
[5] Department of Scienze della Vita e dell'Ambiente, University of Cagliari, 09124 Cagliari, Italy; luciapalmas@yahoo.it (L.P.); ines.castangia@unica.it (I.C.)
[6] Departamento de Química Analítica y Fisicoquímica, Cátedra de Química General e Inorgánica, Facultad de Farmacia y Bioquímica, Instituto de Bioquímica y Medicina Molecular (IBIMOL), CONICET, Universidad de Buenos Aires, Buenos Aires 1113, Argentina; msgarces87@gmail.com (M.G.); pevelson@gmail.com (P.E.)
[7] Departamento de Química Orgánica, Facultad de Farmacia y Bioquímica, Instituto de Química y Metabolismo del Fármaco (IQUIMEFA), CONICET, Universidad de Buenos Aires, Buenos Aires 1113, Argentina; jmlazaromartinez@gmail.com
* Correspondence: mlmanca@unica.it (M.L.M.); marcelamoretton@gmail.com (M.A.M.)

Citation: Galdopórpora, J.M.; Martinena, C.; Bernabeu, E.; Riedel, J.; Palmas, L.; Castangia, I.; Manca, M.L.; Garcés, M.; Lázaro-Martinez, J.; Salgueiro, M.J.; et al. Inhalable Mannosylated Rifampicin–Curcumin Co-Loaded Nanomicelles with Enhanced In Vitro Antimicrobial Efficacy for an Optimized Pulmonary Tuberculosis Therapy. *Pharmaceutics* 2022, 14, 959. https://doi.org/10.3390/pharmaceutics14050959

Academic Editors: Michael Yee Tak Chow and Philip Chi Lip Kwok

Received: 15 March 2022
Accepted: 25 April 2022
Published: 28 April 2022

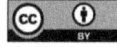

Abstract: Among respiratory infections, tuberculosis was the second deadliest infectious disease in 2020 behind COVID-19. Inhalable nanocarriers offer the possibility of actively targeting anti-tuberculosis drugs to the lungs, especially to alveolar macrophages (cellular reservoirs of the *Mycobacterium tuberculosis*). Our strategy was based on the development of a mannose-decorated micellar nanoformulation based in Soluplus® to co-encapsulate rifampicin and curcumin. The former is one of the most effective anti-tuberculosis first-line drugs, while curcumin has demonstrated potential anti-mycobacterial properties. Mannose-coated rifampicin (10 mg/mL)–curcumin (5 mg/mL)-loaded polymeric micelles (10% *w/v*) demonstrated excellent colloidal properties with micellar size ~108 ± 1 nm after freeze-drying, and they remain stable under dilution in simulated interstitial lung fluid. Drug-loaded polymeric micelles were suitable for drug delivery to the deep lung with lung accumulation, according to the in vitro nebulization studies and the in vivo biodistribution assays of radiolabeled (99mTc) polymeric micelles, respectively. Hence, the nanoformulation did not exhibit hemolytic potential. Interestingly, the addition of mannose significantly improved (5.2-fold) the microbicidal efficacy against *Mycobacterium tuberculosis* H37Rv of the drug-co-loaded systems in comparison with their counterpart mannose-free polymeric micelles. Thus, this novel inhaled nanoformulation has demonstrated its potential for active drug delivery in pulmonary tuberculosis therapy.

Keywords: polymeric micelles; Soluplus®; rifampicin; curcumin; tuberculosis; inhalable nanoformulation; active drug targeting; *Mycobacterium tuberculosis*

1. Introduction

Pulmonary drug delivery or "orally inhaled therapy" has been extensively tested in recent years due to the advantages of this administration route and the wide versatility on novel inhaled dosage forms [1]. The former includes (1) drug administration for both local (i.e., tuberculosis (TB), SARS coronavirus disease, chronic obstructive pulmonary disease and cystic fibrosis, pneumonia, asthma, lung cancer), and systemic diseases such as diabetes (Afrezza®) and migraine (Migranal®) [2,3], associated with a significant reduction of the systemic side-effects and hepatic first-pass metabolism; (2) the rapid onset of action; and (3) the possibility to specifically transport the drug in a precise site by the addition of sugar residues, polysaccharides, antibodies, peptides and small molecules capable of enhancing cellular uptake [4,5]

Different inhalable dosage forms such as solutions for nebulization [6] and dry powders for aerosolization [7] have been developed in the last decades aiming at optimizing the pulmonary therapy. One of the main drawbacks for inhalable dosage forms are the anatomical and physiological barriers (i.e., mucocilliary clearance, proteolytic enzymes and phagocytic cells) of the lungs [8]. In this context nanotechnology provides a feasible platform for the development of novel respirable drug delivery systems. For instance, fluticasone-loaded liposomes and cyclodextrins complexes [6]; chitosan/thiolated chitosan nanoparticles conjugated with hyaluronic acid loaded with isoniazid [4]; and antiviral-loaded polymeric nanoparticles for SARS-CoV-2 inhibition [9] highlight the nanotechnological platforms recently investigated for the treatment of lung diseases by means of inhaled therapy.

Among respiratory infections, TB is a chronic infectious disease that affects people globally. This disease is caused by *Mycobacterium tuberculosis* (Mtb). As reported by World Health Organization in 2021, TB was the second deadliest infectious disease in 2020 behind the COVID-19 global pandemic. Furthermore, 10 million cases were reported, and 1.5 million patients died because of TB infection [10].

Currently, TB is treated with a combined therapy that includes "first-line" anti-TB drugs as rifampicin (RIF), isoniazid, pyrazinamide and ethambutol for 6 months (short-term treatment). These "first-line" drugs are administered orally [11]. Nevertheless, side effects such as peripheral neurotoxicity, liver toxicity and renal toxicity affect both patient life-quality and adherence to the treatment. Consequently, these aspects lead to treatment failure and an increase of multi-drug resistant of TB strains [11].

In particular, RIF is the most effective first-line anti-TB drug, and it is currently classified as a borderline Class II drug by the Biopharmaceutics Classification System because of its low pH-dependent water solubility (2.56 mg/mL 25 °C, pH: 5.0) and low intestinal permeability [11]. Additionally, due to its low water solubility and poor chemical stability, there is a lack of liquid or aqueous RIF pharmaceutical dosage forms. Furthermore, simulation models of RIF pharmacokinetics/pharmacodynamics in lungs showed that the standard 600 mg RIF oral-dose could not prevent the development of drug resistance due to the low pulmonary RIF concentrations [12].

In this framework, novel inhalable RIF dosage forms are required in order to optimize TB therapy and enhance patient adherence. Moreover, previous studies have shown the potential of inhalable anti-TB drugs as a promising alternative to the current oral TB treatment [13]. Particularly, it is well known that Mtb is mainly hosted by alveolar macrophages (AMs), which exhibit in their surface mannose receptors (C-type lectin, CD206) involved in Mtb phagocytosis and responsible for the immune response in TB infections [14]. Patients with pulmonary TB showed an enhanced expression of the mannose receptor in both lung and pleural tissues [15]. Then, this receptor appears as an excellent target for an active drug delivery of anti-TB drugs to the Mtb cellular reservoirs.

Curcumin (CUR) is a polyphenol compound obtained from Curcuma longa root currently used as an oral nutraceutical [16] and as an anti-inflammatory agent in Ayurveda medicine. Nevertheless, CUR exhibits low aqueous solubility [17], which hampers the development of liquid CUR dosage forms.

Recently, the potential anti-mycobacterial properties of CUR have been investigated, since it is known that it can modulate the host immune response [18]. Furthermore, in a previous study, the association of curcumin and rifampicin by means of a nanotechnological system based on polyethylene sebacate nanoparticles has been formulated and tested for oral administration, confirming the ability of these systems to improve the in vitro mycobacterial clearance [19].

In a previous study, a respirable RIF-loaded nanocarrier based in Soluplus® polymeric micelles demonstrated to have a significantly improved in vitro microbicidal efficacy in comparison with the RIF solution [20]. Soluplus® is a graft copolymer of poly (vinyl caprolactam)-poly (vinyl acetate)-poly (ethylene glycol) (PEG) that showed good performance solubilizing poorly soluble drugs [15–17] and high micellar stability (due to its low CMC value). Hence, the present investigation was aimed at expanding the potential of this inhalable nanotechnological platform for an active drug targeting to the Mtb-infected macrophages. Given that, Soluplus® micelles decorated on the surface with mannose residues co-loading rifampicin and curcumin have been formulated and deeply characterized in terms of size, size distribution and morphology. Moreover, the in vitro nebulization aptitude of formulations and their aerodynamic diameter were evaluated along with their hemolytic potential. Finally, the microbicidal effectiveness of formulations and the micellar accumulation in the lungs has been investigated in vitro by using THP-1 infected (Mtb H37Rv) macrophages and in vivo by using Wistar rats, respectively.

2. Materials and Methods

2.1. Materials

Polyvinyl caprolactam–polyvinylacetate–PEG 6000 (Soluplus®, average MW~120,000 g/mol) was a kind gift of BASF (Buenos Aires, CABA, Argentina). Rifampicin (RIF) and dried bovine gelatin (Bloom 125, type B, average MW ~125,000 g/mol) were purchased from Parafarm® (CABA, Argentina). Curcumin (CUR), bovine serum albumin (BSA), concanavalin A (Con A, from Canavalia ensiformis, Jack Bean Type VI), mannose and mucin II (from porcine stomach) were acquired from Sigma-Aldrich (Buenos Aires, CABA, Argentina). All solvents were of grade and used following the manufacturer's instructions.

2.2. Gelatin/Mannose Formulation and Characterization

Gelatin–mannose (Gel(man)) was prepared using dried bovine gelatin and mannose as previously described with slight modifications [21]. Dried bovine gelatin (750 mg) was dispersed in 15 mL of distilled water at 45 °C under magnetic stirring (50 RPM) for 30 min. Meanwhile, mannose (80 mg) was solubilized in 10 mL of AcH/AcNa buffer (pH 4.20) under magnetic stirring (50 RPM) for 30 min. Afterwards, gelatin dispersion and mannose acid solution were mixed under magnetic stirring (100 RPM) at room temperature (25 °C) for 72 h. Finally, the resulting dispersion was dialyzed against distilled water using dialysis membranes (Spectra/Por®3 Dialysis Membrane, molecular weight cut off = 3500 Da, nominal flat width 18 mm, Merck SA, Buenos Aires, Argentina) over 1 h (replacing the external medium every 15 min) at room temperature. The dialyzed samples were then freeze-dried for 48 h at 0.03 mbar, using a freeze-dryer FIC-L05 (FIC, Scientific Instrumental Manufacturing, Buenos Aires, Argentina), to improve the stability of the sample in storage.

Gel(man) has been deeply characterized by means of different methods. Diamond ATR-FTIR (attenuated total reflectance Fourier-transform infrared spectroscopy) spectra were acquired using a Nicolet iS50 Advanced Spectrometer (Thermo Scientific, Waltham, MA, USA) with 64 scans and a resolution of 4 cm^{-1}. Proton Nuclear Magnetic Resonance (^{1}H-NMR) experiments were acquired with a Bruker Avance-III HD spectrometer equipped with a 14.1 T narrow bore magnet operating at Larmor frequencies of 600.09 MHz. Chemical shifts for ^{1}H (in ppm) are relative to $Si(CH_3)_4$. Gel(man) has been used to decorate Soluplus® micelles, and the presence of mannose residues on their surface/corona was evaluated using Concanavalin A (Con A) [22]. Briefly, Soluplus® was dispersed in phosphate buffer (pH 7.2) in order to obtain a final concentration of 10% w/v. Then, 100 mg of Gel(man) were added to the Soluplus® dispersion under magnetic stirring (50 RPM) until complete Gel(man) dispersion. Control Gel(man)-free Soluplus® micelles (10% w/v) were used for comparison. In a second step, bovine serum albumin (BSA, 90 mg) was added to the micellar dispersions with and without Gel(man) and Soluplus® (man)-micelles (2 mL). Samples were magnetically stirred for 30 min at 25 °C and diluted (1/2) with a Con A (10 µM) phosphate buffer solution (pH: 7.2). Finally, the micellar systems were magnetically stirred (100 RPM) for 2 h at room temperature, and the micellar size and size distribution was investigated by dynamic light scattering (DLS, scattering angle of θ = 173° to the incident beam, Zetasizer Nano-ZSP, ZEN5600, Malvern Instruments, Malvern, UK) at 25 °C (n = 5 ± S.D.).

2.3. Measurement of the Critical Micellar Concentration (CMC)

The CMC at 25 °C of Soluplus® and Soluplus®-Gel(man) (0.7% w/v) in water was assessed by dynamic light scattering (DLS), using a Zetasizer Nano-ZSP (ZEN5600, Malvern Instruments, Malvern, UK), at a scattering angle of Φ = 173° to the incident beam. Micellar aqueous dispersions were prepared to obtain a concentration range between 1×10^{-6} and 1% w/v. Samples were equilibrated for 24 h at 25 °C before their use. The CMC was graphically determined by plotting the derived count rate as a function of the polymer concentration (% w/v) [22].

2.4. Micellar Preparation and Drug Encapsulation

Soluplus® (1 g) was dispersed in distilled water (10 mL) under magnetic stirring (50 RPM, 1 h) at room temperature (25 °C) to obtain "drug-free-micelles" and stored overnight before the use. Soluplus® micelles decorated with Gel(man) so called "drug-free-(man)micelles", were prepared as well. The graft-copolymer (Soluplus®, 1 g) was dispersed in water (10 mL), and the appropriate amount of Gel(man) (25, 50, 70, 100 mg) was added under magnetic stirring (50 RPM) until complete and homogeneous dispersion.

In order to encapsulate both drugs, RIF and CUR, the solvent diffusion method was used, as previously described [17,20]. Briefly, RIF (100 mg) and CUR (50 mg) were dissolved in 20 mL of acetone; the solution was sonicated for 5 min (Digital Ultrasonic Cleaner, PS-10A 50/60 Hz, Shenzhen, China, 25 °C) and then added drop by drop using a programmable syringe infusion pump (PC11UB, APEMA, Buenos Aires, Argentina) to the aqueous dispersion of Soluplus® (10% w/v) at room temperature under constant magnetic stirring (50 RPM, 4 h) to let the complete evaporation of the organic solvent, as well. Afterwards, the volume of RIF–CUR co-loaded-micelles, so called "RIF–CUR-micelles", was repristinated at 10 mL using distilled water and samples were filtered using 0.45 µm, acetate cellulose filters (Microclar, Buenos Aires, Argentina), aiming at removing the undissolved/unentrapped drugs.

Drug-loaded, micelles-decorated mannose, so-called "RIF–CUR-(man)micelles", were prepared following the same procedure, with small modifications. In this case after the acetone evaporation, Gel(man) (25, 50, 70, 100 mg) was added under magnetic stirring at 25 °C until complete dispersion. Then, the procedure was performed as described above for the mannose-free, drug-loaded micelles.

Finally, drug-free and drug-loaded nanomicelles were freeze-dried for 24 h at 0.03 mbar using a freeze-dryer, FIC-L05 (FIC, Scientific Instrumental Manufacturing, Argentina), and stored in sealed amber glass vials until their use.

The concentrations of RIF and CUR in the samples were determined using a Shimadzu HPLC system (SIL-10A auto sampler, SCL-10A pump and SPD-10AV UV detector, Japan). All separations were achieved with an Atlantis-C18 reversed-phase column (4.6 mm × 150 mm, 3 µm particle size, Waters, Ireland) at a flow rate of 1 mL/min and at room temperature. The mobile phase consisted of acetonitrile:water (adjusted to pH 2.27 with orthophosphoric acid). For RIF measurement, the ratio of mobile phase was 54:44 (v/v), and the detection wavelength was 333 nm. The CUR detection wavelength was

425 nm, and the mobile phase was fixed at 44:56 (v/v). Twenty microliters of all the sample solutions were injected.

2.5. Measurement of Micellar Size and Morphological Characterization

Micellar size, size distribution and polydispersity index (PDI) of the nanoformulations was assessed at 25 °C by dynamic light scattering (DLS) using a Zetasizer Nano-ZSP (ZEN5600, Malvern Instruments, Malvern, UK) at a scattering angle of $\theta = 173°$ to the incident beam. Prior to the analysis, each sample was equilibrated at 25 °C. Finally, the results of hydrodynamic diameter (Dh) and PDI values were expressed as the average of five measurements ± S.D.

To assess the morphology of the RIF–CUR-loaded (10 mg/mL and 5 mg/mL) (man)micelles, a transmission electron microscopy (TEM) analysis was performed using a TEM apparatus (Philips CM-12 FEI Company, Eindhoven, The Netherlands). Freeze-dried samples were re-dispersed in distilled water (2 mL), and aliquots (5 μL) were negatively stained with 5 μL of uranyl acetate (2% w/v).

2.6. In Vitro Antioxidant Capacity Assays
2.6.1. DPPH Colorimetric Assay

The antioxidant activities of the different formulations were evaluated on the basis of the scavenging activity of the stable 2,2-diphenyl-1-picrylhydrazyl free radical (DPPH•). Aliquots of methanolic solutions (1 mg/mL) of the different formulations were incubated with 3 mL of a methanolic solution of DPPH• (25 mg/L). After 10 min, the absorbance of the mixture was measured at 517 nm. A calibration curve was prepared using Trolox (vitamin E analogue) as standard, and results were expressed as nmol Trolox Eq/mg sample and DPPH inhibition percentage [23].

2.6.2. ABTS Colorimetric Assay

Using 2,2-azino-bis-3-ethylbenzothiazoline-6-sulphonic acid, or ABTS, a radical cation can be generated. The ABTS is generated by reacting with a strong oxidizing (ABAP, 2 mM) agent with the ABTS salt (75 mM) for an hour at 45 °C. The reduction of the blue-green ABTS radical by hydrogen-donating antioxidants absorbs light at 734 nm in phosphate buffer. Aliquots of aqueous dispersions (1 mg/mL) of the different formulations were incubated with 3 mL of ABTS• solution. After 4 min, the absorbance of the mixture was measured at 734 nm. A calibration curve was prepared using Trolox (vitamin E analogue) as standard, and results were expressed as nmol Trolox Eq/mg sample and ABTS inhibition percentage [24].

2.7. In Vitro Nebulization Studies

The in vitro deposition of RIF and CUR (alone or in combination) was assessed using the next-generation impactor (NGI, Eur. Ph 7.2, Copley Scientific Ltd., Nottingham, UK) connected with the PariSX® air jet nebulizer and the ParyBoySX® compressor. Freeze-dried micelles (Soluplus® 10% w/v, Gel(man) 0.7%, RIF 10 mg/mL, CUR 5 mg/mL) were re-dispersed in 2 mL of water, manually shaken and placed in the nebulizer. The aerosolization process was performed for about 15 min directly into the throat of the New Generation Impactor (NGI). The corresponding dispersions in water at the same concentration of RIF, CUR or both were also nebulized and used as references. The amount of RIF and/or CUR deposited in each stage of the NGI along with the undelivered drug were collected by using methanol and analysed by using a spectrophotometer. Aerodynamic diameter (MMAD) and geometric standard deviation (GSD) values were calculated excluding the amount of drugs deposited in the induction port and were both extrapolated from the graph obtained by plotting the cumulative amount of particles with a diameter lower than the stated size of each stage as a percentage of each recovered drug versus the cut-off diameter, according to the European Pharmacopeia [25,26]. The total mass output (TMO%), the Fine Particle Dose (FPD), and the Fine Particle Fraction (FPF), which represent the percentage of drug recovered in the NGI versus the amount initially placed in the nebulizer, the amount of drug contained in droplets of size less than 5 μm, and the percentage of droplets with size less than 5 μm, respectively, were measured as previously reported [27].

2.8. Stability of the Micellar Systems in Simulated Interstitial Lung Fluid

The in vitro physicochemical stability of the inhalable RIF–CUR-micelles with and without mannose residues was investigated after dilution. Simulated Interstitial Lung Fluid (SILF) was obtained by dissolving 9.85 mg $MgCl_2$, 603.2 mg NaCl, 40.4 mg KCl, 43.6 mg Na_2HPO_4, 259.6 mg $NaHCO_3$, 8.3 mg Na_2SO_4, 35.9 mg $CaCl_2$, 60.7 mg $C_2H_3NaO_2$ and 11.5 mg of sodium citrate in 100 mL of distilled water (pH 7.40) [28]. Freeze-dried RIF–CUR (10 mg/mL and 5 mg/mL)-(man)micelles (10% w/v) and freeze-dried RIF–CUR-(10 mg/mL and 5 mg/mL)-micelles (10% w/v) were re-dispersed in distilled water (2 mL) and then diluted (1/50) in SILF. Micellar size distribution and PDI were assessed at 0, 1, 2, 3 and 24 h after dilution at 37 °C by dynamic light scattering using a Zetasizer Nano-ZSP, ZEN5600 (Malvern Instruments, Malvern, UK) at a scattering angle of θ = 173° to the incident beam (n = 5 ± S.D.).

2.9. In Vitro Drug Release Study

The CUR and RIF cumulative in vitro release from the nanomicelles with (0.7% w/v) and without Gel(man) was studied by using dialysis method in SILF (pH 7.4) with the addition of ethanol (30% v/v) [17] as external medium. Lyophilized micellar systems were redispersed in distilled water and further diluted with distilled water in order to achieve concentrations of 1 mg/mL for RIF and 0.5 mg/mL for CUR. Later, 0.5 mL aliquots (500 μg of RIF and 250 μg of CUR) were placed into dialysis membranes (3500 Da, Spectra/Por®3 Dialysis Membrane, molecular weight cut off = 3500, nominal flat width 18 mm, Waltham, MA, USA), which were then placed inside Falcon® conical tubes containing the external medium (12 mL). The system was incubated at 37 °C for 1, 2, 3, 4, 6, 8 and 24 h by inversion using a sample rotator (Mini Labroller LabNet rotator, St. Louis, MO, USA, 40 RPM). For every timepoint, the external medium was completely replaced with fresh and pre-heated medium. The amount of RIF and CUR was determined by RP-HPLC-UV-Vis, as previously described (Section 2.4). Assays were performed in triplicate, and results are expressed as average ± S.D.

2.10. In Vitro Hemolytic Assay

Hemolytic cytotoxic effects of the prepared micelles were determined in vitro. Fresh blood from control rats was collected in hemolysis tubes containing 3.2% of sodium citrate (1:9). Red blood cells (RBCs) were separated by centrifugation at 3500 RPM for 10 min and then acquired and washed with saline solution (NaCl 0.9% w/v). Afterwards, samples were centrifuged 3 times (3500 RPM, 10 min, MiniSpin® plus™, Eppendorf, Hamburg, Germany), and the supernatant was discarded while the pellets were diluted with saline solution to reach the final concentration of 10% w/v to be used to evaluate the hemolytic activity of the formulations. The hemolytic assay was performed as previously described [29], with slight modifications. Saline solution was used as the negative control (0% lysis), and distilled water as the positive control (100% lysis), employing a 1/2 dilution with the RBCs suspension.

Freeze-dried samples (RIF, RIF–CUR-(man)micelles and drug-free-(man)micelles) were re-dispersed in distilled water (2 mL) and then diluted (1/2) with the RBCs suspension. The final RIF concentrations were 1, 5, 10 and 20 μg/mL. They were incubated at 37 °C for 3 h by inversion using a sample rotator (Mini Labroller LabNet rotator, USA, 40 RPM); then, samples were centrifuged for 10 min at 3500 RPM (800 RCF) (MiniSpin® plus™, Eppendorf, Germany). The supernatant was processed, and hemoglobin released was measured at 541 nm by means of visible spectroscopy (8452A Diode Array Spectrophotometer, Hewlett

Packard, Palo Alto, CA, USA). Later, the hemolysis percentage was calculated using the following equation:

$$\text{Hemolysis (\%)} = (\text{Abs sample} - \text{Abs negative})/(\text{Abs positive} - \text{Abs negative}) \times 100$$

where Abs negative and Abs positive correspond to the absorbance of the erythrocytes treated with saline solution and distilled water, respectively. Animal experiments and animal care were approved by the Animal Care Committee of School of Pharmacy of the University of Buenos Aires (REDEC-2021-2792-E-UBA-DCT_FFYB). Assays were performed in triplicate and expressed as mean ± S.D.

2.11. In Vivo Micellar Lung Accumulation Assay

2.11.1. Radiolabeling Procedure of Soluplus® (Man)Micelles

Freeze-dried micelles were re-dispersed in distilled water (2 mL), and then they were radiolabeled using stannous chloride (SnCl2; analytical grade Merck, Germany) as the reducing agent, as previously reported, with slight modifications [20]. Briefly, 1 mL of the aqueous micellar dispersion (3 mg/mL) was prepared and then mixed with 25 μL of and acidic solution (pH = 3.0, acidified with HCl 0.1 N) of SnCl2 (1 mg/mL) and 300 μL of freshly prepared sodium pertechnetate (Na99mTcO4; 1.5 mCi) eluted from an a99Mo/99mTc generator (Laboratorios Bacon SAIC, Villa Martelli, Argentina). The pH of the final dispersion was adjusted up to 7.0 using NaOH (0.1% *w/v* aqueous solution), and it was maintained for 60 min at room temperature in a closed chamber aiming at reducing the exposition of the samples to air.

2.11.2. Radiolabeling Efficiency and Stability

The obtained 99mTc-(man)micelles were assayed for both labeling efficiency and radiochemical purity. Ascending chromatography was performed to detect free TcO4−, using Instant Thin Layer Chromatography-Silica Gel (ITLC-SG, Varian, Palo Alto, CA, USA) as the stationary phase and acetone as the mobile phase. The same stationary phase (ITLC-SG) but a different mobile phase (mixture of pyridine:acetic acid:water, 3:5:1.5) were used to detect 99mTc-radiocolloids and hydrolysate. The same procedure was used to test the effectiveness and stability of the after-incubation of 99mTc-(man)micelles in vitro using a saline solution at room temperature and in rat plasma at 37 °C for 24 h.

2.11.3. Biodistribution Studies: Ex Vivo and Scintigraphic Procedures

Experimental tests with animals were completed according to the experimental protocol approved by the ethical committee of the School of Pharmacy and Biochemistry, University of Buenos Aires (REDEC-2021-2792-E-UBA-DCT_FFYB). Female Sprague-Dawley rats (6 weeks of age; 200 ± 10 g) were provided by the animal house (School of Pharmacy and Biochemistry, University of Buenos Aires). Animals were allowed to acclimate for at least 48 h before the experiment, housed in stainless steel cages with free access to both food and water and 12 h of light/dark cycles. Before the experiment, animals were anesthetized using ketamine–xilazine (90 mg/kg–5 mg/kg), and the radiolabeled micelles were administered by means of a surgical puncture tracheotomy (~0.3 mg micelles per rat, ~50 μCi); then, the animals were maintained at a supine position (45°) and with heads up during the first hour of the biodistribution assay. After 1 and 24 h of the administration procedure, the rats in each group (n = 5) were anesthetized using isofluorane 2% (Cassara, Buenos Aires, Argentina) and subjected to a static scintigraphy to detect the distribution of the radiolabeled (man)micelles by a view gamma camera, which was equipped with a high-resolution parallel hole's collimator. Images were then processed with OHIO NUCLEAR, software IM512P (Alfanuclear, Buenos Aires, Argentina).

At the end of the experiment, rats were euthanized; blood samples were taken, and the organs of interest (liver, spleen, lungs, kidneys, heart, intestine and stomach) were removed, washed and weighted. The radioactivity in each organ was measured in a calibrated well type gamma counter (Alfanuclear, Argentina), and the results have been expressed as % of the injected dose of tissue, where decay correction was considered for the calculation.

2.12. Microbicidal Efficacy against Mycobacterium tuberculosis

2.12.1. Bacterial Growth Conditions

Mycobacterium tuberculosis H37Rv (Mtb H37Rv) was grown in Middlebrook 7H9 broth or on 7H10 agar with 0.5% Tween 20, 0.2% glycerol, and albumin–dextrose–catalase–oleic acid supplement. Cultures were harvested at an exponential growing phase at 37 °C. To disaggregate clumps, mycobacteria were sonicated at 2.5 W output for 4 min (Elma d-7700 Singentrans sonic), then centrifuged for 10 min at $300 \times g$, and the supernatant was diluted in PBS. Finally, the OD at 600 nm was determined. The bacterial growth of Mtb H37Rv and any experiment involving the pathogenic strain were performed in BSL3 security cabinets at the ANLIS-Malbran Institute, Buenos Aires, Argentina.

2.12.2. Cell Culture and Infection

Human monocyte cell line (THP-1, ATCC TIB-202) was purchased from the American Type Culture Collection (Manassas, VA, USA). RPMI-1640 (Gibco, 22400–071) supplemented with 10% FBS (Gibco, 10437028), L-glutamine (2 mM; Sigma, G5792), penicillin-streptomycin and 2-mercaptoethanol (0.05 mM; Gibco) was used as the medium. Cells were cultured at 37 °C in a humidified atmosphere with 5% CO_2. Macrophages were obtained by adding 10 ng/mL of phorbol-12-myristate-13-acetate (PMA; EMD Biosciences, La Jolla, CA, USA) for 48 h in 96-wells flat-bottom plates. After differentiation, THP-1 cells were infected with Mtb H37Rv (MOI 10) for 2 h. Then, cells were washed twice with warm RPMI and cultured in a complete medium without penicillin-streptomycin and in presence of (i) freeze-dried drug-free Soluplus® (10% w/v) micelles, (ii) freeze-dried RIF-(10 mg/mL)-micelles (10% w/v) and (iii) freeze-dried RIF–CUR (10 mg/mL and 5 mg/mL)-micelles (10% w/v) in the presence and absence of Gel(man) 0.7% w/v for 48 h. The final drug concentrations investigated were: (i) RIF (5 μg/mL) and (ii) CUR (2.5 μg/mL). Freeze-dried micelles were re-dispersed in distilled water (1 mL) before their use.

2.12.3. Colony-Forming Unit Assay

THP-1 differentiated into macrophages and infected with Mtb H37Rv were washed 2 times with (200 μL) of warm PBS and lysed with 0.05% Triton X-100 in PBS. The serial dilution of adherent cells lysates was made, and 10 μL aliquots were inoculated (in triplicate) on Middlebrook 7H10 agar plates supplemented with oleic acid–albumin–dextrose–catalase (OADC BD BBL Middelebrook cat 212351. 10% v/v). Plates were incubated for 3 weeks, and colonies were counted from dilutions yielding 10-100 visible colonies.

2.12.4. Statistical Analysis

Statistical analysis was performed by one-way ANOVA test and Tukey's multiple comparisons post-hoc test using GraphPadPrism version 6.01 for Windows (GraphPad Software, San Diego, CA, USA).

Statistical analysis concerning the colony-forming unit was performed by means of analysis of variance (ANOVA) and the post-hoc Tukey multiple comparisons test ($p < 0.05$).

3. Results and Discussion

3.1. Gelatin–Mannose Preparation and Characterization

One of the main goals of the present investigation was the development of a novel inhalable micellar formulation for an active drug targeting macrophages. In this way, the enhancement of the anti-TB therapy has been in the spot in recent years, mainly associated with the lack of patient adherence to the oral pharmacological treatment and the development of MDR-Mtb strains.

It has been found that the mannose receptor of the AMs is involved in the immune response after TB infection [14], and its over-expression has been reported in pulmonary

TB patients [15]. Thus, this receptor can be considered an excellent target for an active drug delivery therapy to the cellular Mtb reservoirs in the lungs.

In this framework, we prepared mannose-modified gelatin in order to decorate the surface of the co-loaded (RIF and CUR) micellar nanoformulations. Gelatin is a natural biopolymer encoded as a GRAS material by the FDA [30]. Gelatin has been extensively employed in pharmaceutical, cosmetic and food industries and in drug/gene delivery systems since it is a biodegradable, biocompatible and low immunogenic polymer, with a great potential of chemical modifications to fine tune its biofunctional properties [31]. Further combining gelatin with other biomaterials has been explored as an attractive strategy to develop novel nano-drug delivery systems, such as poli(epsilon caprolactone)/gelatin based nanofibers [32]. Even more, the nanotechnological approach of employing mannosylated gelatin nanoparticles has been investigated as an attempt to modify the surface of nanoformulations for an improved anti-TB therapy employing linezolid [33].

Herein, we successfully developed mannose-modified gelatin as it could be observed by ATR-FTIR and ^{1}H-NMR studies. Firstly, the ATR-FTIR spectrum for gelatin shows the characteristic peaks of the amide I (C=O stretching vibrations), amide II (N–H bending vibrations) and amide III (C–N stretching vibrations) at 1630, 1535 and 1241 cm^{-1}, respectively (Figure 1A) [34]. Then, the ATR-FTIR spectra for gelatin and mannose-modified gelatin show an important difference in the stretching bands between 1200 and 1100 cm^{-1} with a new band at 1136 cm^{-1} associated to the C–O–C asymmetric stretching vibration frequency of mannose (Figure 1A,B) [35]. This situation is completely different from a physical mixture between gelatin with 5% mannose where the sum of the bands in the IR spectrum of the components is evident (Figure 1C). Although the nature of the interaction between both molecules cannot be known from the experiment, it is seen that the stretching of the C-O bonds typically found for mannose is present in the modified gelatin sample with a width and intensity different from the reference monosaccharide (Figure 1B–D).

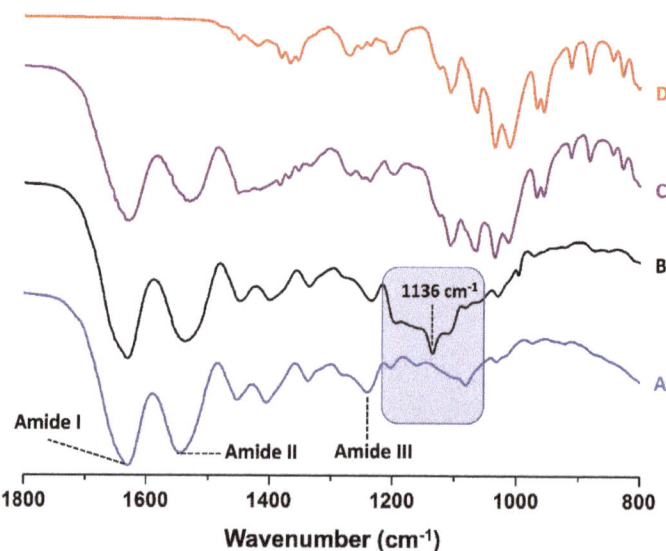

Figure 1. ATR-FTIR spectra for gelatin (A), mannose-modified gelatin (B), physical mixture of gelatin with 5% mannose (C) and mannose (D).

Then, and in order to identify the nature of the interaction between mannose and gelatin, ^{1}H-NMR experiments in deuterated water (D$_2$O) were performed for the pure components and for the modified gelatin (Figure 2).

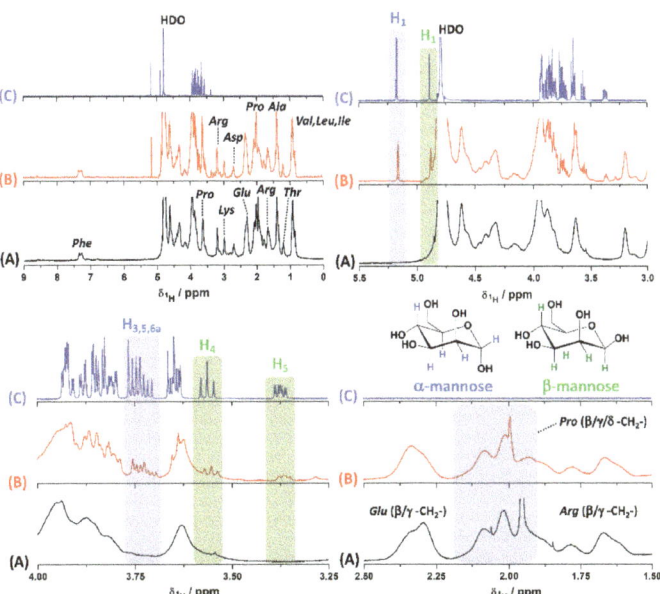

Figure 2. ^{1}H-NMR spectra for gelatin (A), mannose-modified gelatin (B) and mannose (C) dissolved in D$_2$O. Different regions are shown for each of the samples for better understanding. The hydrogens of the α- and β-anomers for D-mannose are drawn with different colors for the assignments of the NMR signals.

It can be observed in the different ^{1}H-NMR regions that mannose is present. Furthermore, the presence of the anomers (α and β) for the monosaccharide is observed at proton chemical shifts (δ^{1}H) of 5.1 and 4.8, respectively. In addition, some other hydrogens can be assigned for the rest of the molecule for each anomer, as indicated in Figure 2 [36]. Although the spectrum for gelatin is complex due to the diverse amino acid composition, the aromatic region does not show resonance signals, associated with the formation of an imine or Schiff's base (δ^{1}H 7–9 ppm) [37], among the components of interest. The only signal present at δ^{1}H~7.4 ppm is assigned to the hydrogens of the phenylalanine residues present in both gelatin and mannose-modified gelatin [38]. On the other hand, changes associated with proline residues close to δ^{1}H~2 ppm are evidenced, which could indicate a molecular interaction between gelatin and mannose that also affects glutamic acid residues at δ^{1}H~2.3 ppm. In a comparative way, it can be observed how the signals for the arginine residues (δ^{1}H = 1.5–1.8 ppm) do not undergo changes in the presence of mannose. Additionally, the observed changes in the NMR spectrum may be the result of the changes or rearrangement in the gelatin structure after the interaction with mannose.

To complement the analysis, it was possible to estimate the mannose ratio in the modified gelatin. For the quantitative NMR analysis, the signals for the anomeric mannose hydrogens were considered, and they were related to the hydrogens for the methylene protons of the lysine residues next to the ε-amino group at δ^{1}H = 2.9 ppm (-CH$_2$-NH$_2$). In this way, and considering that the average content of *Lys* in gelatin samples is 4% [39], 4.2% mannose was determined for the modified gelatin sample according with the area of the NMR signals.

Further, a study with a water-soluble lectin (Con A) was also explored in order to evaluate the presence of mannose residues on the micellar surface after the incorporation of Gel(man) to the Soluplus$^®$ micellar dispersion. Con A selectively binds to α-D-mannosyl and α-D-glucosyl residues due to its tetrameric form (with four independent sugar-binding sites) above pH = 7.0 [40]. In this way, the presence of mannose residues on the surface of the nanoformulation would lead to the formation of large aggregates in comparison with the micellar system without the addition of mannose. Indeed, this lectin has been explored to confirm the surface mannosylation of different nano-sized carriers [41].

As could be observed in Table 1, before the addition of Con A, Soluplus® micelles and Soluplus® (man)micelles (dispersed in phosphate buffer pH 7.2) demonstrated unimodal size distributions of 158.1 ± 3.5 nm and 270.1 ± 31.3 nm, respectively. Furthermore, the PDI values observed were 0.205 and 0.275 for the micellar systems with or without mannose, respectively.

Table 1. Micellar size and size distribution (PDI) of Soluplus® micelles and Soluplus® (man)micelles (10% w/v) in presence and absence of Con A after incubation (2 h) at 25 °C. Data are expressed as mean ± S.D. (n = 5).

Sample	Con A Presence	PDI (±SD)	Dh (nm) (±SD)					
			Peak 1	Intensity (%)	Peak 2	Intensity (%)	Peak 3	Intensity (%)
Soluplus® micelles	-	0.205 (0.006)	158.1 (3.5)	100.0	-	-	-	-
	+	0.201 (0.005)	161.8 (4.6)	100.0				
Soluplus® (man)micelles	-	0.275 (0.013)	270.1 (31.3)	100.0	-	-	-	-
	+	0.359 (0.008)	246.5 (5.1)	94.2	4370 (392)	5.3	11.2 (19.4)	0.6

However, after the incubation with the lectin, a change in the size distribution pattern for the Soluplus® (man)micelles could be observed. In this case, a bimodal size distribution with a main size peak of 265.5 ± 5.1 nm and a second size population of 4370 ± 392 nm was observed, along with an increment in the polydispersity of the sample (PDI 0.359), suggesting the formation of large aggregates due to the presence of mannose moieties on the micellar surface.

This change of the size distribution was not observed for those Soluplus® micelles without the addition of mannose. In this case, there was still only one size population (161.8 ± 4.6 nm) with a narrow size distribution (PDI 0.201) after Con A incubation. Similar results were observed after the incubation of Con A with mannosylated PEG-based polymeric micelles [41].

3.2. Micellar Preparation, Drug Encapsulation and Physicochemical Stability under Dilution

Polymeric micelles (PMs) are amphiphilic, self-assembled nanocarriers that represent an attractive platform for drug delivery [42]. Due to self-aggregation in water, which occurs above the critical micellar concentration (CMC), PMs are characterized by a hydrophobic core and a hydrophilic corona, which provide both stability to the nanocarrier (due to hydrophilic corona) and lipophilic drug encapsulation (within their hydrophobic core) [17,22,42]. One of the biomaterials highlighted for PMs preparation is known as Soluplus®. Previously, we successfully demonstrated that this biopolymer is able to encapsulate hydrophobic drugs as RIF [20], CUR and PTX [17,22] (conforming simple and mixed micelles) to optimize tuberculosis and cancer therapy. These micellar systems exhibited excellent colloidal properties combined with high physicochemical stability under dilution. The last beings of great clinical importance since micellar systems are dynamic colloidal nanocarriers, which could undergo dis-assembling upon dilution after administration [43]

In particular, a Soluplus®-based micellar (3% w/v) nanoformulation with RIF (10 mg/mL) was developed as a respirable nanocarrier with an optimized in vitro microbicidal efficacy versus a RIF solution [20]. In this framework, we aimed to expand the potential of this nanoformulation by the co-encapsulation with an antioxidant drug as CUR and the surface decoration of the nanocarrier with mannose residues for an active drug targeting macrophages. In this case, CUR was incorporated due to its potential anti-mycobacterial properties associated with the host immune response modulation [18].

In a first step, we successfully developed a Soluplus® micellar system (10% w/v) within RIF (10 g/mL) and CUR (5 mg/mL) employing a solvent-diffusion technique. Samples remain translucent to the naked eye with a bright red color due to the presence of RIF and CUR without the presence of any aggregates (Figure 3). It is worth stressing that an increment of the Soluplus® concentration from 3% w/v to 10% w/v was required for the co-encapsulation of both RIF and CUR. Then, the RIF concentration was 10 mg/mL since it is clinically relevant for a pulmonary dosage form taking into account that the RIF concentration in an inhalable formulation could be approximately 100-fold lower than in an oral dosage form [44].

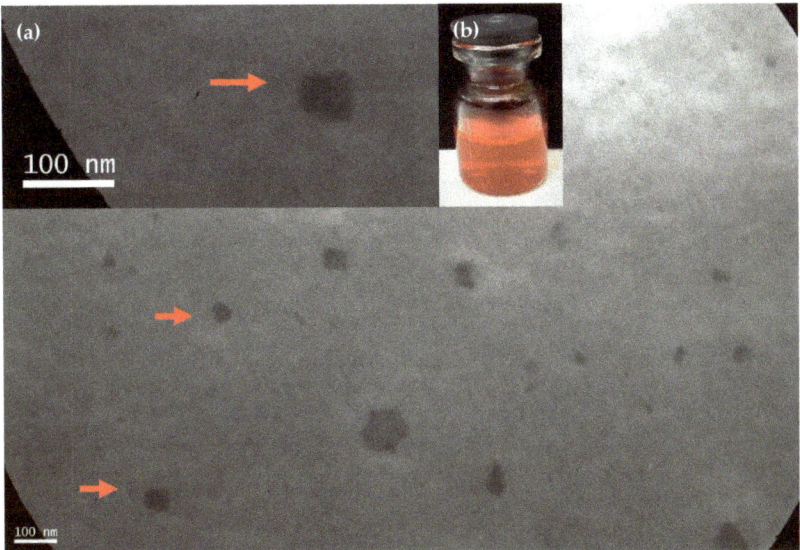

Figure 3. TEM micrograph of RIF–CUR (10 mg/mL and 5 mg/mL)-(man)(0.7% w/v)-micelles (10% w/v). Red arrows point out the polymeric micelles. Scale bar: 100 nm. Photo Inset: (**a**) Magnification of TEM micrograph and (**b**) macroscopic aspect of the drug-loaded micellar dispersion after re-dispersion in distilled water.

Furthermore, it was observed that 5 mg/mL of CUR was the highest drug concentration that could be employed in order to maintain the colloidal stability of the micellar system. Higher CUR concentrations led to micellar aggregation and drug precipitation over time (data not shown).

The DLS analysis at 25 °C showed that this nanoformulation exhibited an adequate colloidal stability with one size population and a narrow size distribution before (82.2 ±1.7 nm; PDI: 0.221) and after (81.2 ± 2.1 nm; PDI: 0.138) freeze-drying. A similar trend was observed for the drug-free micellar systems (Table 2). It is worth stressing that the drug incorporation within the micellar core did not lead to an increase of the micellar size. This behavior may be connected to the dynamic nature of the PMs where the final hydrodynamic diameter is mainly associated with the combination of biomaterial and the encapsulated drugs. Similar results were observed after CUR encapsulation in paclitaxel-loaded Soluplus®/TPGS mixed micelles [17]. At this first approach, micellar nanoformulations showed good post lyophilization aspects, with easy redispersion in distilled water without any macroscopic aggregates.

Table 2. Micellar size and size distribution (PDI) of free and drug-loaded Solupus micelles (10% w/v) with and without mannose at 25 °C, before and after lyophilization. Data are expressed as mean ± S.D. (n = 5).

Nanoformulation	Gel(man) Concentration (%)	Before Lyophilization		After Lyophilization	
		Size (nm) (±S.D.)	PDI (±S.D.)	Size (nm) (±S.D.)	PDI (±S.D.)
Drug-free-micelles	-	114.1 (1.2)	0.194 (0.002)	124.0 (1.3)	0.217 (0.006)
	0.25	137.2 (4.1)	0.213 (0.009)	127.4 (0.3)	0.257 (0.006)
Drug-free-	0.5	149.1 (1.8)	0.226 (0.003)	145.6 (4.4)	0.264 (0.007)
(man)micelles	0.7	287.6 (28.3)	0.414 (0.015)	164.5 (6.7)	0.257 (0.009)
	1.0	345.0 (68.7)	0.444 (0.003)	120.6 (4.7)	0.207 (0.009)
RIF–CUR-micelles	-	82.2 (1.7)	0.221 (0.007)	81.2 (2.1)	0.138 (0.020)
	0.25	122.2 (3.7)	0.224 (0.003)	113.7 (1.7)	0.215 (0.011)
RIF–CUR-	0.5	147.8 (4.6)	0.244 (0.010)	101.8 (3.8)	0.218 (0.009)
(man)micelles	0.7	197.6 (7.4)	0.312 (0.042)	108.1 (0.9)	0.208 (0.001)
	1.0	360.2 (11.2)	0.288 (0.004)	366.7 (5.5)	0.424 (0.011)

In a second step, based in previous investigations employing nanocarrier coating with a mannose-based surfactant for a respirable nanoformulation [45], we performed a pre-formulation assay in order to determine the amount of Gel(man) (0.25–1% w/v) that could be employed to surface-coating the micellar system without affecting its colloidal stability in terms of size and size distribution.

For those systems in the absence of RIF and CUR, it could be observed that the coating with mannose led to an increment of the micellar size and PDI values. For instance, micellar size increased from 114.1 ± 1.2 nm (without mannose) to 287.6 ± 28.3 nm (Gel(man) 0.7% w/v) and 345.0 ± 68.7 nm (Gel(man) 1% w/v) before lyophilisation. A similar trend was followed by the PDI values (Table 2). It is worth stressing that the Dh determination includes the micellar corona along with its associated solvent molecules from the external medium. Hence, the addition of hydrophilic additives as polymers could interact with the micellar corona, according with their water affinity, and this interaction would influence the final Dh values. An example of this kind of interaction is the addition of glycols and PEG 400 to poloxamers and poloxamines [46].

Interestingly, after the freeze-drying process, a decrement of the polydisperity and the micellar size of the nanoformulations with PDI values between 0.207 and 0.257 was observed for those systems with a higher (between 0.7% and 1% w/v) content of Gel(man). This effect could be related to a micellar contraction phenomenon after the lyophilization process due to the dynamic nature of the PMs. With lower Gel(man) concentrations, the lyophilisation process did not alter either the PDI values or the micellar size (Table 2).

These results demonstrated that the colloidal stability of Soluplus® (man)micelles could be enhanced after freeze-drying. In this way, higher amounts of Gel(man) could be incorporated to actively target the cellular reservoirs of the Mtb.

A similar trend was observed after Gel(man) addition to the co-loaded (RIF and CUR) micellar dispersions before lyophilisation. The increment of Gel(man) concentration led to an increment of both micellar size and size distribution with only one size population. For instance, the micellar size increased from 122.2 ± 3.7 nm to 360.2 ± 11.2 nm for 0.25% w/v and 1% w/v of Gel(man), respectively. Nevertheless, after freeze-drying, only those micellar dispersions with the higher Gel(man) content (1% w/v) showed a sharp increment of micellar size and polydispersity (size and PDI). This could be associated with micellar aggregation and drug precipitation over time.

On the contrary, Soluplus® (man)micelles with Gel(man) concentrations between 0.25% and 0.7% w/v demonstrated lower hydrodynamic diameters and narrow PDI values than their counterparts before freeze-drying (Table 2).

Overall, the drug-co-loaded micellar nanoformulation with the higher Gel(man) concentration (0.7% w/v) that demonstrated an adequate colloidal stability after freeze-drying was chosen for further analysis.

Pharmaceutics **2022**, *14*, 959

Taking into account the dynamic nature of the PMs, we aimed to further predict their aggregation behavior after pulmonary administration. To reach this objective, we diluted (1/50) the drug-loaded nanoformulations with Simulated Interstitial Lung Fluid (SILF) at 37 °C.

Initially, as could be observed in Table 3, there was a decrement of the Dh values after the PMs dilution in SILF in comparison with the un-diluted systems in distilled water (Table 2). This reduction of the micellar size could be expended due to the dynamic equilibrium between copolymer monomers in the bulk and those being part of the polymeric micelles. Upon dilution, the number of monomers of the micelles could decrease in order to maintain the free amphiphilic molecules of the bulk. Then, a reduction of the micellar size could be observed [47].

Table 3. Micellar size and size distribution of the RIF(10 mg/mL)-CUR (5 mg/mL)-loaded micelles (10% w/v) with and without mannose at 37°C in simulated interstitial lung medium (SILF, pH 7.4, sample dilution 1/50) over 24 h. Data are expressed as mean ± S.D. (n = 5).

Nanoformulation	Time (h)	Size (nm) (±S.D.)		PDI (±S.D.)
		Peak 1	Intensity (%)	
RIF–CUR-micelles	0	56.04 (0.48)	100.0	0.044 (0.007)
	1	58.15 (0.51)	100.0	0.040 (0.008)
	2	58.09 (0.08)	100.0	0.042 (0.009)
	3	57.49 (0.51)	100.0	0.037 (0.011)
	24	62.69 (0.45)	100.0	0.056 (0.008)
RIF–CUR-(man)micelles	0	61.26 (0.65)	100.0	0.103 (0.016)
	1	61.35 (0.27)	100.0	0.068 (0.008)
	2	61.44 (0.36)	100.0	0.075 (0.011)
	3	60.08 (0.37)	100.0	0.063 (0.004)
	24	68.13 (1.10)	100.0	0.080 (0.009)

On the other hand, both micellar systems (in the absence and presence of mannose) demonstrated colloidal stability after their dilution in SILF over time, as only one size population with a narrow size distribution was detected over 24 h. Moreover, there was only a slight size increase from 56.04 ± 0.48 nm (0 h) to 62.69 ± 0.45 nm (24 h) for RIF–CUR-micelles. A similar trend was followed by the RIF–CUR-(man)micelles where micellar size increased from 61.26 ± 0.65 nm (0 h) to 68.13 ± 1.10 nm (24 h). In this framework, these results showed that the micellar dispersions (regardless of the presence of mannose) exhibited colloidal stability under dilution, standing as a potential nanoformulation for pulmonary administration.

Finally, a morphological characterization of the RIF (10 mg/mL)-CUR (5 mg/mL)-(man) (0.7% w/v) micelles (10% w/v) was assessed by TEM visualization. As can be observed in Figure 3, micelles demonstrated a spherical shape as previously described for Soluplus®-based PMs [20]. This morphology provides to the nanoformulation a great potential for drug intracellular accumulation since spherical colloidal nanocarriers could be easily up-taken by macrophages [48].

3.3. CMC Determination

The CMC value is the concentration at which amphiphilic molecules occupy the total of the air/water interface and start forming micelles. In the present study, the CMC was detected from a graph in which the derived count rate as a function of Soluplus® or Soluplus®(man) (0.7% w/v) concentration (% w/v) was plotted, where the CMC value (% w/v) was observed as having a sharp increase in the derived count rate.

No difference in CMC value was observed for either treatment. The CMC value for drug-free micelles was 0.000541% w/v, and the CMC value for drug-free (man)-micelles was 0.000495% w/v. In this case, low CMC values were observed, which ensures micellization even under diluted conditions [47].

3.4. Nebulization Studies

Micelles containing RIF, CUR or both, RIF–CUR-(man)micelles, along with the corresponding drug dispersions, were nebulized using an air jet nebulizer (PariSX®) connected to the NGI, and both in vitro deposition and aerodynamic diameter of droplets were measured to evaluate their suitability and effectiveness as pulmonary delivery systems. As can be seen in Table 4, the aerodynamic diameter of all nanosystems was ≤3 μm, without significant differences between the micellar systems and the drug dispersions, suggesting that during the nebulization process, the device was capable of forming small droplets with the appropriate size for pulmonary administration. Indeed, as previously reported, the devices mainly used for pulmonary administration may generate particles with different aerodynamic diameters, but only the smaller ones (MMAD between 1 and 5 μm) are deposited by gravitational settling in the deeper part of the lungs, while those with MMAD > 5 μm are generally recovered in the upper airways (mouth, trachea and main bronchi) by inertial impaction [27].

Table 4. Total mass output (TMO%), fine particle dose (FPD, mg), fine particle fraction (FPF, %) and mass median aerodynamic diameter (MMAD) of nanosystems nebulized by using the next generation impactor (NGI). FPD and FPF values are shown as mean ± S.D. of three experiments; MMAD values are shown as mean ± geometric standard deviation.

Sample	Total Mass Output (%)	Fine Particle Dose (FPD) (mg)	Fine Particle Fraction (FPF) (%)	Aerodynamic Diameter (± Geometric Standard Deviation)
RIF	86 ± 6	8 ± 3	46 ± 4	1.27 ± 1.18
CUR	88 ± 7	2 ± 0.5	19 ± 3	2.18 ± 1.70
RIF + CUR	89 ± 12	8 ± 2	30 ± 4	2.52 ± 1.88
RIF-micelles	100 ± 3	15 ± 2	75 ± 15	1.26 ± 1.17
CUR-micelles	89 ± 2	5 ± 1	57 ± 6	2.14 ± 1.68
RIF–CUR-micelles	83 ± 6	15 ± 3	62 ± 9	1.65 ± 1.41
RIF–CUR-(man)micelles	81 ± 7	13 ± 2	52 ± 6	2.10 ± 1.66

As previously reported [49], the process of jet nebulization involves repeated cycles of aerosol formation and recapture in the nebulizer reservoir before the sample leaves the device, during which shearing forces are applied to the tested formulations, and for this reason, the carrier characteristics and stability play a key role for its use as a system for pulmonary administration. The nebulizer content, by using both nanosystem and dispersions, was not completely aerosolized being that the highest (~100%) total mass output (TMO) was obtained by nebulizing RIF-micelles, while the lowest (~81%) was by nebulizing RIF–CUR-(man)micelles (Table 4). This is probably due to the higher viscosity of the last system, which reduces the efficiency of the device along with the amount of drug nebulized. Any significant differences were detected between nanosystems and dispersions, suggesting the good aptitude of both to be nebulized. However, the suitability of RIF, CUR or both to be nebulized was improved by their incorporation into the nanosystems, as only the formulations containing Soluplus® alone or combined with Gel(man) were capable of reaching the latest stages of the impactor in a high amount and percentage, which mimic the deeper airways. Indeed, the FPD and the FPF obtained by nebulizing the dispersions was lower and always less than 50% (Table 4). Overall results suggest that the micellar formulations, especially RIF–CUR-(man)micelles, seem to be ideal systems capable of effectively delivering both drugs to the deep lung.

3.5. In Vitro Antioxidant Capacity

An experimental Mtb-infection model in guinea pigs demonstrated oxidative stress conditions associated to endothelial damage mediated by free radicals and an insufficient serum total antioxidant capacity, similarly to the human TB disease [50]. On this matter, CUR properties could contribute to adverse lung effects associated with TB infection together with RIF antibiotic activity. As expected, the antioxidant activity of Cur was very high since its capability of scavenging a variety of reactive oxygen species including superoxide anion radical, hydrogen peroxide, hydroxyl radical, singlet oxygen, nitric oxide and other organic free radicals is well known [17]. Indeed, the addition of an antioxidant therapy to the conventional TB treatment could improve the disease outcome [50]. Hence CUR co-encapsulation with RIF within the mannose-decorated micelles could represent a potential alternative to optimize pulmonary TB therapy.

Numerous methods are used to evaluate antioxidant activities of natural compounds in formulations, foods and biological systems. Two free radicals that are commonly used to assess antioxidant activity in vitro are 2,2-azinobis (3-ethylbenzothiazoline-6-sulfonic acid) (ABTS) and 2,2-diphenyl-1-picrylhydrazyl (DPPH). The ABTS assay measures the relative ability of antioxidants to scavenge the ABTS generated in the aqueous phase, while DPPH is a stable free radical used in organic phases [23].

In the present investigation, the total antioxidant capacity of the different formulations was assessed by monitoring their ability to scavenge ABTS˙ or DPPH. Every tested sample containing CUR was able to show antioxidant properties in both assays.

Interestingly, on ABTS˙ experiments, CUR dispersions (2239 ± 153 nmol Trolox Eq/mg, ABTS˙ inhibition $18.6 \pm 1.6\%$) showed less antioxidant activity compared to the co-loaded micellar systems ($23,075 \pm 205$ nmol Trolox Eq/mg, ABTS˙ inhibition ~100%) (Table 5). A similar behavior was observed for the RIF–CUR-(man)micelles ($20,404.0 \pm 663.0$ nmol Trolox Eq/mg, ABTS˙ inhibition ~100%). For both micellar systems, with and without mannose, the total antioxidant capacity was significantly higher ($p < 0.0001$) than CUR and RIF dispersions (Table 5). The high water affinity of polymeric micelles on aqueous phases due to their hydrophilic corona allows CUR to exert its antioxidant properties, compared to poor solubility observed on CUR dispersions. Similarly, RIF solution showed antioxidant capacity (938 ± 212 nmol Trolox Eq/mg, ABTS˙ inhibition $5.5 \pm 0.6\%$), which was significantly ($p < 0.05$) improved once incorporated into the PMs (3918 ± 104, ABTS˙ inhibition $16.0 \pm 0.4\%$). Similar results were observed for the RIF + CUR dispersion (4523.0 ± 214 nmol Trolox Eq/mg, ABTS˙ inhibition $35.5 \pm 1.7\%$) and the drug-co-loaded micelles in the absence and presence of mannose (Table 5).

Table 5. Antioxidant activity of nanoformulations (drug-free, RIF-micelles, RIF–CUR-micelles and RIF–CUR-(man)micelles) and drugs dispersion (CUR, RIF and RIF + CUR), calculated as the inhibition percentage of ABTS radical. Data are expressed as mean ± S.D. (n = 6).

Sample	Total Antioxidant Capacity (nmol Trolox Eq/mg Sample)	ABTS˙ Inhibition (%)
RIF	938.0 ± 212.0	5.5 ± 0.6
CUR	2239.0 ± 153.0	18.6 ± 1.6
RIF+ CUR	4523.0 ± 214.0	35.5 ± 1.7
Drug-free micelles	ND	ND
RIF-micelles	3918.0 ± 104.0 #	16.0 ± 0.4
RIF–CUR-micelles	$23,075.0 \pm 205.0$ *	99.0 ± 1.0
RIF–CUR-(man)micelles	$20,404.0 \pm 663.0$ *	99.0 ± 6.0

Note: Multiple comparisons were performed using one-way ANOVA and Tukey's multiple comparisons post-hoc test. ND: not detected. * $p < 0.0001$ vs. RIF, CUR, drug-free micelles and RIF-micelles. # $p < 0.05$ vs. RIF.

In contrast, due to its high solubility on methanol phases, CUR was observed to have an increased antioxidant activity using the DPPH˙ test compared to ABTS˙ (2678 ± 193 nmol Trolox Eq/mg, DPPH inhibition $49.7 \pm 7.4\%$). This antioxidant capacity was increased (3440.0 ± 5.7 nmol Trolox Eq/mg, DPPH inhibition $96.2 \pm 0.7\%$) for the solution of RIF + CUR. Micelles containing CUR and RIF showed an increased activity compared to CUR solutions before (3633 ± 68 nmol Trolox Eq/mg, DPPH inhibition $75.6 \pm 1.3\%$) and after (3302.0 ± 83.0 nmol Trolox Eq/mg, DPPH inhibition $61.6 \pm 1.8\%$) mannose addition (Table 6). Once again, there was a significant increment in the total antioxidant activity of RIF ($p < 0.0001$) and CUR ($p < 0.05$) after their encapsulation within the polymeric nanocarriers versus free drugs (Table 6).

Table 6. Antioxidant activity of nanoformulations (drug-free, RIF-micelles, RIF–CUR-micelles and RIF–CUR-(man)micelles) and drugs solutions (CUR, RIF and RIF + CUR), calculated as the inhibition percentage of DDPH radical. Data are expressed as mean ± S.D. (n = 6).

Sample	Total Antioxidant Capacity (nmol Trolox Eq/mg Sample)	DPPH· Inhibition (%)
RIF	595.0 ± 76.0	18.6 ± 2.9
CUR	2678.0 ± 193.0 #	49.7 ± 7.4
RIF + CUR	3440.0 ± 5.7	96.2 ± 0.7
Drug-free micelles	ND	1.0 ± 0.4
RIF-micelles	120.0 ± 37.0	25.2 ± 5.6
RIF–CUR-micelles	3633.0 ± 68.0 *	75.6 ± 1.3
RIF–CUR-(man)micelles	3302.0 ± 83.0 *	61.6 ± 1.8

Note: Multiple comparisons were performed using one-way ANOVA and Tukey's multiple comparisons post-hoc test. ND: not detected. * $p < 0.0001$ vs. RIF, drug-free micelles and RIF-micelles. # $p < 0.05$ vs. RIF–CUR-micelles and RIF–CUR-(man)micelles.

Furthermore, both assays demonstrated that the antioxidant properties of CUR were not affected by its co-encapsulation within PMs.

3.6. In Vitro Drug Release

To better understand the potential of the nanoformulations to deliver RIF and CUR to the lungs, the in vitro drug releases were evaluated in SILF at 37 °C over 24 h employing a dialysis method.

On the one hand, results demonstrated that RIF could be successfully released from the polymeric matrix. For instance, 50.4% of RIF was release over 4 h along with a sustained and complete drug release (~100%) at 24 h for the RIF–CUR-micelles. Interestingly, the mannose surface decoration slightly slowed the RIF release from those micellar systems. As can be observed in Figure 4, there was a drug cumulative release of 46.08% after 4 h and 84.2% over 24 h.

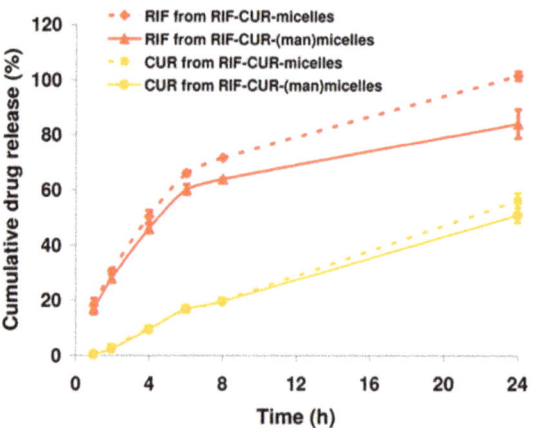

Figure 4. In vitro RIF and CUR release profiles from RIF–CUR-micelles and RIF–CUR-(man)micelles (10% *w/v*) at pH 7.4 (SILF, 37 °C) over 24 h. Results are expressed as mean ± standard deviation (S.D.) (n = 3). RIF and CUR concentrations were 10 mg/mL and 5 mg/mL, respectively.

On the other hand, the release of CUR was significantly different from that of RIF, regardless of the presence of mannose. Indeed, a slowed drug release was observed in comparison with RIF over 24 h. For instance, after 8 h, 19.9% and 19.7 % of CUR was released in the release medium from Soluplus® micelles and Soluplus® (man)micelles, respectively. Then, after 24 h, CUR release was 56.2% and 51.1% from the micellar systems with and without mannose, respectively (Figure 4), confirming a reduced effect of mannose on the CUR release. These results suggested a high affinity between the lipophilic CUR and the hydrophobic micellar core, as previously observed after CUR encapsulation into PMs employing Soluplus® [17].

3.7. Hemolysis Assay

For a respirable nanoformulation, it is important to investigate its hemolytic potential, since drugs will interact with the lung capillary network and the bloodstream after their pulmonary administration [51].

This is the main reason why the in vitro hemolytic performance of the RIF–CUR-(man)-micelles, its drug-free counterpart and a RIF solution were compared. The maximum drug concentration assayed (20 µg/mL) was higher than the therapeutic drug concentrations in blood [52].

As can be seen in Figure 5, there was no hemolytic effect with the micellar dispersions and the RIF solution at the different drug concentrations assayed. For instance, a hemolytic percentage of 0.61 ± 0.28 and 0.81 ± 0.28 was observed for RIF–CUR-(man)micelles and drug-free-(man)micelles, respectively, for the highest concentration of RIF (20 µg/mL) (Figure 5). Interestingly, the RIF solution exhibit a hemolytic percentage of 2.17 ± 0.09 at the same concentration (20 µg/mL) (Figure 5).

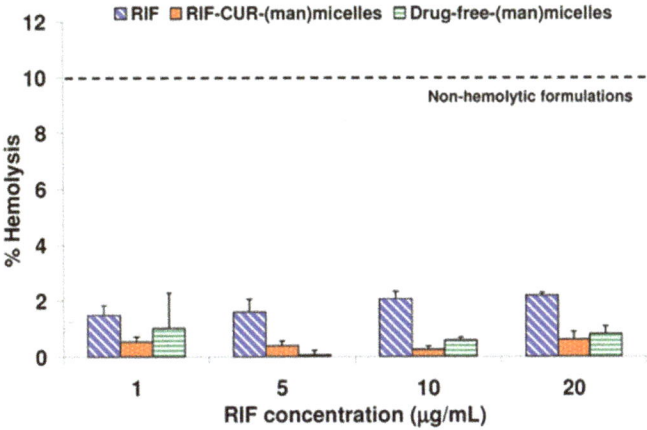

Figure 5. Percentages of hemolysis of RIF, drug-free-(man)micelles and RIF–CUR-(man)micelles at various concentrations after incubation for 3 h at 37 °C. Results are expressed as mean ± S.D. (n = 3).

In this framework, every formulation (mannose-decorated micellar systems and drug solution) demonstrated to be safe (non-hemolytic), taking into account guidance for the in vitro hemolysis [53]. This guidance states that pharmaceutical formulations with hemolysis percentages below 10% are considered as non-hemolytic.

3.8. Micellar Lung Accumulation

Previously, we reported the lung accumulation over 24 h of Soluplus® micelles (3% w/v) [20]. Hence, in order to investigate the fate of the (man)micelles (10% w/v) after their intratracheal administration in Wistar rats, micellar systems were radiolabeled with 99mTc. For this purpose, a non-invasive technique was employed by means of acquiring radioisotopic planar images. Before the in vivo biodistribution assays, it was confirmed that the micellar radiolabeling was efficient (98%) where the concentration of predictable impurities remains under accepted limits [54]. Furthermore, it was observed that radiochemical purity was >95% in serum samples, denoting no release of 99mTc over 24 h

Herein, biodistribution assays demonstrated that although the technical procedure was performed carefully to introduce the 99mTc-(man)micelles in the trachea, and animals remained in a 45° position during the biodistribution time, some of the administered dose was regurgitated, and the biodistribution profile showed the results of two administration pathways: oral and intratracheal. For the intratracheal-administered (leftover) fraction (55% of the administered dose), 10 % was still at the administered point with tracheal deposition, since no rinse was made following administration, and 45% reached the lungs after 1 h of the administration (Figure 6A). The other regurgitated fraction (45% of the administered dose) was distributed in the stomach (15%) and intestines (30%) by the same time (Figure 6A). Interestingly, after 24 h, the radiolabeled micellar system washed out from the trachea towards the lungs, where it remained by 53% of lung deposition and no tracheal accumulation (Figure 6B). On the other hand, stomach and intestines uptake drastically decreased over 24 h (up to 15%) due to fecal elimination. Altogether, the results showed that almost 100% of the 99mTc-(man)micelles that reached the lungs remained there 24 h after the administration.

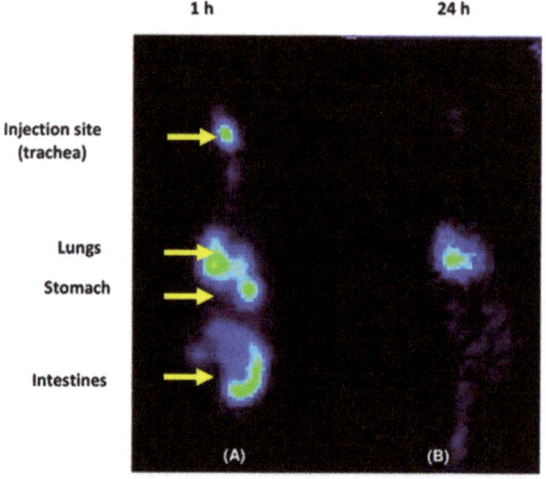

Figure 6. Biodistribution of 99mTc radiolabeled Soluplus® (man)micelles (1.85 MBq). Static images were acquired 1 (**A**) and 24 h (**B**) post intratracheal administration by means of a surgical puncture tracheotomy. Anesthesia: isofluorane. After 24 h post-administration, almost 100% of the 99mTc (man)micelles of the intratracheal route remained in the lungs (color intensity in the image is not corrected by physical decay of the signal).

In this framework, the potential as an inhalable nanoformulation for TB therapy is highlighted due to the ability of the micellar systems to accumulate in lungs over time.

3.9. Microbicidal Efficacy against Mycobacterium tuberculosis

After developing a colloidal RIF–CUR-based micellar nanoformulation, which could be nebulized to reach the deep lung and accumulated there over 24 h with non-hemolytic effects, we aimed to evaluate its in vitro microbicidal efficacy. For this purpose, we employed derived macrophages (THP-1) infected with Mtb (H37Rv strain) by means of multiplicity of infection (MOI, 10). Samples were diluted to obtain a RIF final concentration of 5 µg/mL, since this is a comparable RIF concentration to therapeutic drug blood concentrations [52].

As it could be observed in Figure 7, the drug-free-micelles did not decrease the colony forming units (CFU) of infected macrophages, suggesting that the biomaterial did not exhibit microbicidal efficacy against Mtb H37Rv. Nevertheless, there was a decrement of CFU after macrophage incubation with RIF-micelles. These results are being in good concordance with previous studies employing RIF-loaded Soluplus® micelles (3% w/v) [20].

Furthermore, the addition of CUR to the micellar system demonstrated a significant decrement (2.0-fold, $p < 0.05$) of the CFU versus RIF-micelles. These results suggest that the presence of CUR enhanced the antimicrobial efficacy of the nanoformulation, which is probably related to CUR's capacity to induce caspase-3-dependat apoptosis and autophagy in derived THP-1 macrophages [55]. Similar results were assessed after co-loading of RIF and CUR in polyethylene sebacate nanoparticles for oral administration [19].

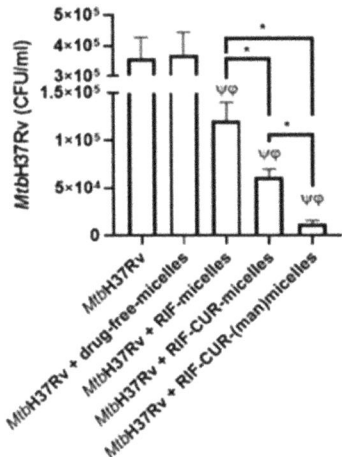

Figure 7. Intracellular survival of *Mycobacterium tuberculosis* H37Rv in RIF-(10 mg/mL) micelles (10% w/v), RIF–CUR (10 mg/mL and 5 mg/mL)-micelles, RIF–CUR (10 mg/mL and 5 mg/mL)-(man)micelles and drug-free-micelles treated THP-1 cells. Macrophages derived from THP-1 cells line (1 × 106 cells/mL) were infected with Mtb H37Rv (MOI: 10). After 2 h of infection, the culture medium was replaced, and cells were cultured with RIF-micelles (5 µg/mL), RIF–CUR-micelles (5 µg/mL and 2.5 µg/mL) or RIF–CUR-(man)micelles (5 µg/mL and 2.5 µg/mL) for 48 h. Then, cells were washed and lysed for mycobacterial colony-forming units (CFU) determination. Data are presented as means of bacterial viability (CFU expressed as percentage of the control) ± standard error of the mean (SEM), * $p < 0.05$; φ $p < 0.001$; ψ $p < 0.001$. p values were calculated using one-way ANOVA with post hoc Tukey's multiple comparisons test.

Furthermore, promising results were observed after the mannose coating of the RIF–CUR-micelles. In this case, a significant decrement ($p < 0.05$, 5.2-fold) of the CFU in comparison with their mannose-free counterpart was observed. Furthermore, an approximately 10-fold decrement of the CFU was observed for the mannosylated systems versus RIF-micelles (Figure 7). Similar results were observed for mannosylated nanoparticles covalently linked with isoniazid where the mannosylation strategy effectively promoted the complete bacterial eradication in comparison with the free drug and mannose-free nanoparticles [56]. Furthermore, mannosylated solid lipid nanoparticles loaded with isoniazid also demonstrated an enhanced intracellular antibiotic efficacy in vivo [57]. In this way, previous studies have demonstrated that mannosylation improves the macrophage uptake of solid lipid nanoparticles associated with the presence of the membrane mannose receptor in human THP1 macrophages [58].

The overall results highlight the potential of our mannosylated nanoformulation for an active drug targeting macrophages, leading to an improved inhalable anti-TB therapy.

4. Conclusions

A respirable co-loaded micellar system for an active RIF and CUR delivery to macrophages was successfully developed. To the best of our knowledge, this is the first time that RIF and CUR were co-loaded in a mannose surface-decorated micellar system for pulmonary administration.

Pharmaceutics **2022**, *14*, 959

The micellar dispersion coated with mannose demonstrated an excellent colloidal stability even after dilution in SILF. Furthermore, the antioxidant properties of CUR were not affected by its encapsulation within PMs. Our nanoformulation did not exhibit hemolytic potential, and it was suitable for nebulization and drug delivery to the deep lung, according to its aerodynamic diameter. In vivo biodistribution studies confirmed the lung accumulation of the radiolabeled PMs over 24 h. Furthermore, the in vitro microbicidal efficacy against Mtb H37Rv was clearly enhanced after mannose coating. In this context, the potential of our mannose-coated RIF–CUR-nanoformulation for an optimized pulmonary anti-TB therapy was confirmed. Further studies employing an in vivo TB-infection model will be performed to investigate the anti-TB performance of this nanoformulation to optimize TB pulmonary therapy.

Author Contributions: Conceptualization: M.A.M. and D.A.C.; Methodology: J.M.G., C.M., J.R., E.B., I.C., M.L.M., J.L.-M., M.G., M.J.S., P.E., N.L.T., M.A.M. and D.A.C.; Formal analysis: J.M.G., C.M., J.R., E.B., L.P., I.C., M.L.M., J.L.-M., M.G., M.J.S., P.E., N.L.T., M.A.M. and D.A.C.; Investigation: J.M.G., C.M., J.R., E.B., L.P., I.C., M.L.M., J.L.-M., M.G., M.J.S., P.E., N.L.T., M.A.M. and D.A.C.; Writing—Original Draft: J.M.G., I.C., M.L.M.; J.L.-M., M.G., M.J.S., P.E., N.L.T., M.A.M. and D.A.C.; Writing—Review and Editing: I.C., M.L.M.; M.A.M. and D.A.C. All authors have read and agreed to the published version of the manuscript.

Funding: This research received no external funding.

Institutional Review Board Statement: The animal study protocol was approved by the Animal Care Committee of School of Pharmacy of the University of Buenos Aires (REDEC-2021-2792-E-UBA-DCT_FFYB).

Informed Consent Statement: Not applicable.

Acknowledgments: The authors thank the Universidad de Buenos Aires (Grants UBACyT 2002017010 0362BA and PIDAE 2018 (SP28–FFYB–CHIA). Juan Galdoporpora is supported by a postdoctoral scholarship of CONICET. Camila Martinena is supported by a doctoral scholarship of CONICET. Jennifer Riedel is supported by a doctoral scholarship of UBA. Ezequiel Bernabeu, Juan Manuel Lázaro-Martinez, Nancy Tateosian, Pablo Evelson, Mariana Garces, Diego A. Chiappetta and Marcela A. Moretton are partially supported by CONICET, Argentina.

Conflicts of Interest: The authors declare no conflict of interest.

References

1. García-Fernández, A.; Sancenón, F.; Martínez-Máñez, R. Mesoporous silica nanoparticles for pulmonary drug delivery. *Adv. Drug Deliv. Rev.* **2021**, *177*, 113953. [CrossRef] [PubMed]
2. Goldberg, T.; Wong, E. Afrezza (Insulin Human) Inhalation Powder: A New Inhaled Insulin for the Management of Type-1 or Type-2 Diabetes Mellitus. *Pharm. Ther.* **2015**, *40*, 735–741.
3. United States Food and Drug Administration (FDA). Available online: https://www.accessdata.fda.gov/drugsatfda_docs/label/2019/020148Orig1s025lbl.pdf (accessed on 12 March 2022).
4. Mukhtar, M.; Pallagi, E.; Csóka, I.; Benke, E.; Farkas, Á.; Zeeshan, M.; Burián, K.; Kókai, D.; Ambrus, R. Aerodynamic properties and in silico deposition of isoniazid loaded chitosan/thiolated chitosan and hyaluronic acid hybrid nanoplex DPIs as a potential TB treatment. *Int. J. Biol. Macromol.* **2020**, *165*, 3007–3019. [CrossRef] [PubMed]
5. Al Hajj, N.; Chee, C.F.; Wong, T.W.; Rahman, N.A.; Abu Kasim, N.H.; Colombo, P. Lung cancer: Active therapeutic targeting and inhalational nanoproduct design. *Expert Opin. Drug Deliv.* **2018**, *15*, 1223–1247. [CrossRef]
6. Dogbe, M.G.; Mafilaza, A.Y.; Eleutério, C.V.; Cabral-Marques, H.; Simões, S.; Gaspar, M.M. Pharmaceutical Benefits of Fluticasone Propionate Association to Delivery Systems: In Vitro and In Vivo Evaluation. *Pharmaceutics* **2019**, *11*, 521. [CrossRef]
7. Eedara, B.B.; Alabsi, W.; Encinas-Basurto, D.; Polt, R.; Mansour, H.M. Spray-Dried Inhalable Powder Formulations of Therapeutic Proteins and Peptides. *AAPS PharmSciTech* **2021**, *22*, 1–12. [CrossRef]
8. Thakur, A.K.; Chellappan, D.K.; Dua, K.; Mehta, M.; Satija, S.; Singh, I. Patented therapeutic drug delivery strategies for targeting pulmonary diseases. *Expert Opin. Ther. Patents* **2020**, *30*, 375–387. [CrossRef]
9. Sanna, V.; Satta, S.; Hsiai, T.; Sechi, M. Development of targeted nanoparticles loaded with antiviral drugs for SARS-CoV-2 inhibition. *Eur. J. Med. Chem.* **2022**, *231*, 114121. [CrossRef]
10. World Health Organization (WHO). Global Tuberculosis Report 2021. Available online: https://www.who.int/teams/global-tuberculosis-programme/tb-reports/global-tuberculosis-report-2021 (accessed on 12 March 2022).

Pharmaceutics 2022, 14, 959

11. Grotz, E.; Tateosian, N.; Amiano, N.; Cagel, M.; Bernabeu, E.; Chiappetta, D.A.; Moretton, M.A. Nanotechnology in Tuberculosis: State of the Art and the Challenges Ahead. *Pharm. Res.* **2018**, *35*, 213. [CrossRef]
12. Goutelle, S.; Bourguignon, L.; Maire, P.H.; Van Guilder, M.; Conte, J.E.; Jelliffe, R.W. Population Modeling and Monte Carlo Simulation Study of the Pharmacokinetics and Antituberculosis Pharmacodynamics of Rifampin in Lungs. *Antimicrob. Agents Chemother.* **2009**, *53*, 2974–2981. [CrossRef]
13. Misra, A.; Hickey, A.J.; Rossi, C.; Borchard, G.; Terada, H.; Makino, K.; Fourie, P.B.; Colombo, P. Inhaled drug therapy for treatment of tuberculosis. *Tuberculosis* **2011**, *91*, 71–81. [CrossRef] [PubMed]
14. Gazi, U.; Martinez-Pomares, L. Influence of the mannose receptor in host immune responses. *Immunobiology* **2009**, *214*, 554–561. [CrossRef] [PubMed]
15. Suzuki, Y.; Shirai, M.; Asada, K.; Yasui, H.; Karayama, M.; Hozumi, H.; Furuhashi, K.; Enomoto, N.; Fujisawa, T.; Nakamura, Y.; et al. Macrophage mannose receptor, CD206, predict prognosis in patients with pulmonary tuberculosis. *Sci. Rep.* **2018**, *8*, 1–9. [CrossRef] [PubMed]
16. Imaizumi, A. Highly bioavailable curcumin (Theracurmin): Its development and clinical application. *PharmaNutrition* **2015**, *3*, 123–130. [CrossRef]
17. Riedel, J.; Calienni, M.N.; Bernabeu, E.; Calabro, V.; Lázaro-Martinez, J.M.; Prieto, M.J.; Gonzalez, L.; Martinez, C.S.; Alonso, S.D.V.; Montanari, J.; et al. Paclitaxel and curcumin co-loaded mixed micelles: Improving in vitro efficacy and reducing toxicity against Abraxane®. *J. Drug Deliv. Sci. Technol.* **2021**, *62*, 102343. [CrossRef]
18. Barua, N.; Buragohain, A.K. Therapeutic Potential of Curcumin as an Antimycobacterial Agent. *Biomolecules* **2021**, *11*, 1278. [CrossRef]
19. Jahagirdar, P.S.; Gupta, P.K.; Kulkarni, S.P.; Devarajan, P.V. Intramacrophage Delivery of Dual Drug Loaded Nanoparticles for Effective Clearance of Mycobacterium tuberculosis. *J. Pharm. Sci.* **2020**, *109*, 2262–2270. [CrossRef]
20. Grotz, E.; Tateosian, N.L.; Salgueiro, J.; Bernabeu, E.; Gonzalez, L.; Manca, M.L.; Amiano, N.; Valenti, D.; Manconi, M.; García, V.; et al. Pulmonary delivery of rifampicin-loaded soluplus micelles against Mycobacterium tuberculosis. *J. Drug Deliv. Sci. Technol.* **2019**, *53*, 101170. [CrossRef]
21. Costa, A.M.M.M.; Sarmento, B.; Seabra, V. Mannose-functionalized solid lipid nanoparticles are effective in targeting alveolar macrophages. *Eur. J. Pharm. Sci.* **2018**, *114*, 103–113. [CrossRef]
22. Moretton, M.A.; Bernabeu, E.; Grotz, E.; González, L.; Zubillaga, M.; Chiappetta, D.A. A glucose-targeted mixed micellar formulation outperforms Genexol in breast cancer cells. *Eur. J. Pharm. Biopharm.* **2017**, *114*, 305–316. [CrossRef]
23. Dobrecky, C.; Marchini, T.; Ricco, R.; Garcés, M.; Gadano, A.; Carballo, M.; Wagner, M.L.; Lucangioli, S.; Evelson, P. Antioxidant activity of flavonoid rich fraction of Ligaria cuneifolia. *Chem. Biodivers* **2020**, *17*, e2000302. [CrossRef] [PubMed]
24. Ilyasov, I.R.; Beloborodov, V.L.; Selivanova, I.A.; Terekhov, R.P. ABTS/PP decolorization assay of antioxidant capacity reaction pathways. *Int. J. Mol. Sci.* **2020**, *21*, 1131. [CrossRef] [PubMed]
25. Manca, M.L.; Valenti, D.; Sales, O.D.; Nacher, A.; Fadda, A.M.; Manconi, M. Fabrication of polyelectrolyte multilayered vesicles as inhalable dry powder for lung administration of rifampicin. *Int. J. Pharm.* **2014**, *472*, 102–109. [CrossRef]
26. Manconi, M.; Manca, M.L.; Valenti, D.; Escribano, E.; Hillaireau, H.; Fadda, A.M.; Fattal, E. Chitosan and hyaluronan coated liposomes for pulmonary administration of curcumin. *Int. J. Pharm.* **2017**, *525*, 203–210. [CrossRef]
27. Manca, M.; Ferraro, M.; Pace, E.; Di Vincenzo, S.; Valenti, D.; Fernàndez-Busquets, X.; Peptu, C.; Manconi, M. Loading of Beclomethasone in Liposomes and Hyalurosomes Improved with Mucin as Effective Approach to Counteract the Oxidative Stress Generated by Cigarette Smoke Extract. *Nanomaterials* **2021**, *11*, 850. [CrossRef] [PubMed]
28. Derbali, R.M.; Aoun, V.; Moussa, G.; Frei, G.; Tehrani, S.F.; Del'Orto, J.C.; Hildgen, P.; Roullin, V.G.; Chain, J.L. Tailored Nanocarriers for the Pulmonary Delivery of Levofloxacin against Pseudomonas aeruginosa: A Comparative Study. *Mol. Pharm.* **2019**, *16*, 1906–1916. [CrossRef]
29. Qiu, L.; Qiao, M.; Chen, Q.; Tian, C.; Long, M.; Wang, M.; Li, Z.; Hu, W.; Li, G.; Cheng, L.; et al. Enhanced effect of pH-sensitive mixed copolymer micelles for overcoming multidrug resistance of doxorubicin. *Biomaterials* **2014**, *35*, 9877–9887. [CrossRef]
30. United States Food and Drud Administration (FDA). Available online: http://wayback.archive-it.org/7993/20171031062708/https://www.fda.gov/Food/IngredientsPackagingLabeling/GRAS/SCOGS/ucm261307.htm (accessed on 12 March 2022).
31. Elzoghby, A.O. Gelatin-based nanoparticles as drug and gene delivery systems: Reviewing three decades of research. *J. Control. Release* **2013**, *172*, 1075–1091. [CrossRef]
32. Lv, F.; Wang, J.; Xu, P.; Han, Y.; Ma, H.; Xu, H.; Chen, S.; Chang, J.; Ke, Q.; Liu, M.; et al. A conducive bioceramic/polymer composite biomaterial for diabetic wound healing. *Acta Biomater.* **2017**, *60*, 128–143. [CrossRef]
33. Patil, K.; Bagade, S.; Bonde, S. In-vitro and ex-vivo characterization of novel mannosylated gelatin nanoparticles of linezolid by Quality-by-Design approach. *J. Drug Deliv. Sci. Technol.* **2020**, *60*, 101976. [CrossRef]
34. Chen, Y.; Lu, W.; Guo, Y.; Zhu, Y.; Lu, H.; Wu, Y. Superhydrophobic coatings on gelatin-based films: Fabrication, characterization and cytotoxicity studies. *RSC Adv.* **2018**, *8*, 23712–23719. [CrossRef]
35. Pană, A.-M.; Ştefan, L.-M.; Bandur, G.; Sfîrloagă, P.; Gherman, V.; Silion, M.; Popa, M.; Rusnac, L.-M. Novel Glycopolymers Based on d-Mannose and Methacrylates: Synthesis, Thermal Stability and Biodegradability Testing. *J. Polym. Environ.* **2013**, *21*, 981–994. [CrossRef]
36. Kosaka, A.; Aida, M.; Katsumoto, Y. Reconsidering the activation entropy for anomerization of glucose and mannose in water studied by NMR spectroscopy. *J. Mol. Struct.* **2015**, *1093*, 195–200. [CrossRef]

37. Li, J.; Li, B.; Liu, M. One-step synthesis of mannose-modified polyethyleneimine copolymer particles as fluorescent probes for the detection of Escherichia coli. *Sens. Actuators B Chem.* **2018**, *280*, 171–176. [CrossRef]
38. Ding, W.; Sun, J.; Lian, H.; Xu, C.; Liu, X.; Zheng, S.; Zhang, D.; Han, X.; Liu, Y.; Chen, X.; et al. The Influence of Shuttle-Shape Emodin Nanoparticles on the Streptococcus suis Biofilm. *Front. Pharmacol.* **2018**, *9*, 227. [CrossRef]
39. Kariduraganavar, M.Y.; Kittur, A.A.; Kamble, R.R. *Polymer Synthesis and Processing*, 1st ed.; Elsevier Inc.: Amsterdam, The Netherlands, 2014. [CrossRef]
40. Štimac, A.; Šegota, S.; Sikirić, M.D.; Ribić, R.; Frkanec, L.; Svetličić, V.; Tomić, S.; Vranešić, B.; Frkanec, R. Surface modified liposomes by mannosylated conjugates anchored via the adamantly moiety in the lipid bilayer. *Biochim. Biophys. Acta* **2012**, *1818*, 2252. [CrossRef]
41. Moretton, M.A.; Chiappetta, D.A.; Andrade, F.; das Neves, J.; Ferreira, D.; Sarmento, B.; Sosnik, A. Hydrolyzed Galactomannan-Modified Nanoparticles and Flower-Like Polymeric Micelles for the Active Targeting of Rifampicin to Macrophages. *J. Biomed. Nanotechnol.* **2013**, *9*, 1076–1087. [CrossRef]
42. Cagel, M.; Tesan, F.C.; Bernabeu, E.; Salgueiro, M.J.; Zubillaga, M.B.; Moretton, M.A.; Chiappetta, D.A. Polymeric mixed micelles as nanomedicines: Achievements and perspectives. *Eur. J. Pharm. Biopharm.* **2017**, *113*, 211–228. [CrossRef]
43. Owen, S.C.; Chan, D.P.; Shoichet, M.S. Polymeric micelle stability. *Nano Today* **2012**, *7*, 53–65. [CrossRef]
44. Prakash, S.; Katiyar, S.; Bihari, S. Low-dose inhaled versus standard dose oral form of anti-tubercular drugs: Concentrations in bronchial epithelial lining fluid, alveolar macrophage and serum. *J. Postgrad. Med.* **2008**, *54*, 245–246. [CrossRef]
45. Truzzi, E.; Leite Nascimento, T.; Iannuccelli, V.; Costantino, L.; Martins Lima, E.; Leo, E.; Siligardi, C.; Lassinantti Gualtieri, M.; Maretti, E. In Vivo Biodistribution of Respirable Solid Lipid Nanoparticles Surface-Decorated with a Mannose-Based Surfactant: A Promising Tool for Pulmonary Tuberculosis Treatment? *Nanomaterials* **2020**, *10*, 568. [CrossRef] [PubMed]
46. Moretton, M.A.; Cohen, L.; Lepera, L.; Bernabeu, E.; Taira, C.; Höcht, C.; Chiappetta, D.A. Enhanced oral bioavailability of nevirapine within micellar nanocarriers compared with Viramune ®. *Colloids Surf. B Biointerfaces* **2014**, *122*, 56–65. [CrossRef] [PubMed]
47. Bonde, G.V.; Ajmal, G.; Yadav, S.K.; Mittal, P.; Singh, J.; Bakde, B.V.; Mishra, B. Assessing the viability of Soluplus®self-assembled nanocolloids for sustained delivery of highly hydrophobic lapatinib (anticancer agent): Optimisation and in-vitro characterisation. *Colloids Surf. B Biointerfaces* **2019**, *185*, 110611. [CrossRef] [PubMed]
48. Zheng, M.; Yu, J. The effect of particle shape and size on cellular uptake. *Drug Deliv. Transl. Res.* **2015**, *6*, 67–72. [CrossRef]
49. Melis, V.; Manca, M.L.; Bullita, E.; Tamburini, E.; Castangia, I.; Cardia, M.C.; Valenti, D.; Fadda, A.M.; Peris, J.E.; Manconi, M. Inhalable polymer-glycerosomes as safe and effective carriers for rifampicin delivery to the lungs. *Colloids Surf. B Biointerfaces* **2016**, *143*, 301–308. [CrossRef]
50. Palanisamy, G.S.; Kirk, N.M.; Ackart, D.F.; Shanley, C.A.; Orme, I.M.; Basaraba, R.J. Evidence for Oxidative Stress and Defective Antioxidant Response in Guinea Pigs with Tuberculosis. *PLoS ONE* **2011**, *6*, e26254. [CrossRef]
51. Zhou, Y.; Niu, B.; Wu, B.; Luo, S.; Fu, J.; Zhao, Y.; Quan, G.; Pan, X.; Wu, C. A homogenous nanoporous pulmonary drug delivery system based on metal-organic frameworks with fine aerosolization performance and good compatibility. *Acta Pharm. Sin. B* **2020**, *10*, 2404–2416. [CrossRef]
52. Clemens, D.L.; Lee, B.-Y.; Xue, M.; Thomas, C.R.; Meng, H.; Ferris, D.; Nel, A.E.; Zink, J.I.; Horwitz, M.A. Targeted Intracellular Delivery of Antituberculosis Drugs to Mycobacterium tuberculosis-Infected Macrophages via Functionalized Mesoporous Silica Nanoparticles. *Antimicrob. Agents Chemother.* **2012**, *56*, 2535–2545. [CrossRef]
53. Amin, K.; Dannenfelser, R.-M. In vitro hemolysis: Guidance for the pharmaceutical scientist. *J. Pharm. Sci.* **2006**, *95*, 1173–1176. [CrossRef]
54. Bringhammar, T. Quality assurance of radiopharmaceuticals. In *Technetium-99 M Pharmaceuticals. Preparation and Quality Control in Nuclear Medicine*; Zolle, I., Ed.; Springer: Berlin/Heidelberg, Germany, 2007; pp. 67–71.
55. Bai, X.; Oberley-Deegan, R.E.; Bai, A.; Ovrutsky, A.R.; Kinney, W.H.; Weaver, M.; Zhang, G.; Honda, J.R.; Chan, E.D. Curcumin enhances human macrophage control of Mycobacterium tuberculosis infection. *Respirology* **2016**, *21*, 951–957. [CrossRef]
56. Lunn, A.M.; Unnikrishnan, M.; Perrier, S. Dual pH-Responsive Macrophage-Targeted Isoniazid Glycoparticles for Intracellular Tuberculosis Therapy. *Biomacromolecules* **2021**, *22*, 3756–3768. [CrossRef] [PubMed]
57. Ma, C.; Wu, M.; Ye, W.; Huang, Z.; Ma, Z.; Wang, W.; Wang, W.; Huang, Y.; Pan, X.; Wu, C. Inhalable solid lipid nanoparticles for intracellular tuberculosis infection therapy: Macrophage-targeting and pH-sensitive properties. *Drug Deliv. Transl. Res.* **2021**, *11*, 1218–1235. [CrossRef] [PubMed]
58. Vieira, A.C.C.; Chaves, L.L.; Pinheiro, M.; Lima, S.; Ferreira, D.; Sarmento, B.; Reis, S. Mannosylated solid lipid nanoparticles for the selective delivery of rifampicin to macrophages. *Artif. Cells Nanomed. Biotechnol.* **2018**, *46*, 653–663. [CrossRef] [PubMed]

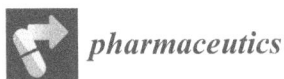

Article

Angiotensin-(1–7) Peptide Hormone Reduces Inflammation and Pathogen Burden during *Mycoplasma pneumoniae* Infection in Mice

Katie L. Collins [1,†], Usir S. Younis [2,†], Sasipa Tanyaratsrisakul [2], Robin Polt [3], Meredith Hay [4], Heidi M. Mansour [5,6,7] and Julie G. Ledford [2,5,8,*]

1   Department of Immunobiology, College of Medicine, The University of Arizona, Tucson, AZ 85724, USA; collins.katieleanne@gmail.com
2   Asthma and Airway Disease Research Center, Tucson, AZ 85724, USA; usirsyounis@gmail.com (U.S.Y.); sasipat@email.arizona.edu (S.T.)
3   Departments of Chemistry and Biochemistry, College of Science, The University of Arizona, Tucson, AZ 85721, USA; polt@u.arizona.edu
4   Department of Physiology, College of Medicine, The University of Arizona, Tucson, AZ 85724, USA; mhay@email.arizona.edu
5   BIO5 Institute, The University of Arizona, Tucson, AZ 85719, USA; mansour@pharmacy.arizona.edu
6   Department of Medicine, Division of Translational & Regenerative Medicine, College of Medicine, The University of Arizona, Tucson, AZ 85724, USA
7   Departments of Pharmacology/Toxicology and Pharmaceutical Sciences, College of Pharmacy, The University of Arizona, Tucson, AZ 85724, USA
8   Department of Cellular and Molecular Medicine, College of Medicine, The University of Arizona, Tucson, AZ 85721, USA
*   Correspondence: jledford@email.arizona.edu or jagledford@gmail.com; Tel.: +1-520-626-0276
†   These authors contributed equally to this work.

Citation: Collins, K.L.; Younis, U.S.; Tanyaratsrisakul, S.; Polt, R.; Hay, M.; Mansour, H.M.; Ledford, J.G. Angiotensin-(1–7) Peptide Hormone Reduces Inflammation and Pathogen Burden during *Mycoplasma pneumoniae* Infection in Mice. *Pharmaceutics* **2021**, *13*, 1614. https://doi.org/10.3390/pharmaceutics13101614

Academic Editors: Philip Chi Lip Kwok and Michael Yee Tak Chow

Received: 17 August 2021
Accepted: 1 October 2021
Published: 4 October 2021

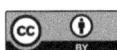
Abstract: The peptide hormone, angiotensin (Ang-(1–7)), produces anti-inflammatory and protective effects by inhibiting production and expression of many cytokines and adhesion molecules that are associated with a cytokine storm. While Ang-(1–7) has been shown to reduce inflammation and airway hyperreactivity in models of asthma, little is known about the effects of Ang-(1–7) during live respiratory infections. Our studies were developed to test if Ang-(1–7) is protective in the lung against overzealous immune responses during an infection with *Mycoplasma pneumonia* (Mp), a common respiratory pathogen known to provoke exacerbations in asthma and COPD patients. Wild type mice were treated with infectious Mp and a subset of was given either Ang-(1–7) or peptide-free vehicle via oropharyngeal delivery within 2 h of infection. Markers of inflammation in the lung were assessed within 24 h for each set of animals. During Mycoplasma infection, one high dose of Ang-(1–7) delivered to the lungs reduced neutrophilia and *Muc5ac*, as well as *Tnf-α* and chemokines (*Cxcl1*) associated with acute respiratory distress syndrome (ARDS). Despite decreased inflammation, Ang-(1-7)-treated mice also had significantly lower Mp burden in their lung tissue, indicating decreased airway colonization. Ang-(1–7) also had an impact on RAW 264.7 cells, a commonly used macrophage cell line, by dose-dependently inhibiting TNF-α production while promoting Mp killing. These new findings provide additional support to the protective role(s) of Ang1-7 in controlling inflammation, which we found to be highly protective against live Mp-induced lung inflammation.

Keywords: angiotensin-(1–7); *Mycoplasma pneumoniae*; asthma; inflammation; macrophages

1. Introduction

Angiotensin-(1–7) or Angiotensin$_{1-7}$, here forth referred to as Ang-(1–7), is an endogenous peptide that is produced from Angiotensin II by angiotensin-converting enzyme 2 (ACE2). Ang-(1–7) has been shown to inhibit inflammatory actions of Angiotensin II through interactions with the Mas receptor. This axis is known to counteract and balance the vasoconstrictive effects of the renin-angiotensin system [1]. Recent studies have described how Ang-(1–7) opposes this inflammatory pathway, and as such, long-term administration of Ang-(1–7) has been shown to reduce oxidative stress and pro-inflammatory cytokine production in animal models [1]. Additional clinical positive effects on Ang-(1–7) reported include prevention of cardiac output reduction, cardiomyocyte size normalization, interstitial fibrosis and lung fibrosis reduction, decreased collagen deposition, and prevention of oxidative damage in vessels [2–5]. Papinska et al. proposed that Ang-(1–7) treatment inhibits all of the contributing factors that lead to structural remodeling in the lungs [1]. Other efforts have also delved into mechanistic pathways by which the ACE2/Ang-(1-7)/Mas axis acts to inhibit certain inflammatory pathways, one of which is thought to be directly involved in suppressing ERK and NF-κB-dependent signaling pathways [6,7].

A key regulator of heart, vascular, kidney, and brain function is the ACE2 enzyme, which is an important component of the well-described renin–angiotensin system (RAS) [8]. The ACE-AngII-AT1R system is thought to be opposed physiologically, and balanced by the ACE2–Ang-(1-7)-Mas system [9–11]. These two separate enzymatic pathways of RAS are thought to be involved in functionally balancing reactive oxygen species (ROS), nitric oxide (NO) production and inflammation, in several areas of the body, including peripheral tissues and the brain [8,9,12]. The beneficial and tissue protective effects of Ang-(1–7) are generated by Ang-(1–7) binding to the G-protein-coupled Mas receptor. Studies in our labs have shown that Ang-(1–7) and its derivatives decrease IL-6, IL-7, TNF-α, and macrophage influx into the brain [13], and reversed cognitive impairment caused by systemic inflammatory disease caused by heart failure. Studies by others have shown activation of the ACE2–Ang-(1-7)-Mas system is associated with inhibition of the ERK1/2 pathway [14] and inhibition of leukocyte influx and inflammatory tissue damage.

Mas receptors are present in the lung epithelium, and with regard to resolving pulmonary inflammation, connections between Ang-(1–7) and the Mas receptor have been observed [15]. Research is ongoing to better understand the mechanisms of the ACE2/Ang-(1-7)/Mas axis and the role these cellular and molecular actions play within acute lung injury and lung fibrogenesis [16]. Along these lines, studies have also demonstrated the importance of the Mas receptor-dependent anti-inflammatory effects of Ang-(1–7) in the OVA model of allergic airways disease [6,17,18]. A considerable number of in vivo studies demonstrates the beneficial actions of the ACE2/ANG-(1–7) axis in acute lung injury in several animal models [19–21].

Outside of the respiratory system, Ang-(1–7) has also shown function as a vasodilator with anti-thrombotic and anti-proliferative effects in pre-clinical trials [3,22]. These biological characteristics have suggested potential indications of Ang-(1–7) as a therapeutic drug option for cardiovascular disease conditions, such as hypertension, as well as a prospective cancer therapy [23,24]. Formulations of Ang-(1–7) have been administered in several clinical trials for the treatment of a variety of conditions, including pre-eclampsia, as well as for ovarian cancer patients undergoing chemotherapy [25,26]. We have previously published results showing cognitive protection following treatment with the native and glycosylated-Ang-(1-7), in our model of inflammation-induced cognitive impairment [13,27].

Additional studies from our group have shown that Ang-(1–7) derivatives decrease TNF-α, IL-7, IL-6, MCP1, and G-CSF while increasing the protective cytokine, IL-10, and inhibiting macrophage influx into the brain [13]. Cytokine release syndrome (CRS) or "cytokine storm" is defined as a massive systemic inflammatory response that can be triggered by a variety of factors including viruses, influenza, bacterial infections, and certain antibody-based therapeutic drugs, most common among these being chimeric antigen receptor (CAR)-T cell infusion in hematological patients [28]. The trigger stimulus typically results in the lysis of immune cells and release of IFN−γ and TNF−α. This in turn results in a feed-forward cascade of the release of pro-inflammatory cytokines from macrophages and endothelial cells leading to a cytokine storm [28]. In the CAR-T cell associated CRS patients, IL-6 is thought to be the driver in clinical symptoms with tocilizumab, a monoclonal antibody directed against IL-6 receptors, as a first line of therapy [29,30]. Given that Ang-(1–7) and derivatives are pluripotent and known to inhibit many of the cytokines activated in the "cytokine storm", our study was set up to test the efficacy of Ang-(1–7) in controlling inflammation during live pulmonary infection with Mp.

Infection with the Mp, also known as "walking pneumonia", is a common cause of respiratory illnesses in children and often leads to exacerbations in asthma and COPD patients [31–34]. Colonization of Mp in the airway is a potent inducer of TNF-α production and is associated with increased neutrophilia in the lung [31]. The objective of the present study was to determine if treatment with Ang-(1–7) peptide would provide protective and anti-inflammatory effects in Mp-challenged mice. We discovered that when given within 2 h of Mp infection, one dose of Ang-(1–7) delivered to the lungs significantly reduced neutrophilia and *Muc5AC*, as well as TNF-α and KC. Despite decreased inflammation, Ang-(1–7) treatment also resulted in significantly lower Mp burden in the lung tissue, which in vitro studies suggest may be through Ang-(1-7)-dependent enhanced macrophage killing mechanisms. To the authors' knowledge, this study is the first to report these findings.

2. Methods

2.1. Animal Models

BALB/c male mice (~22–27 grams) were purchased from Jackson labs (Bar Harbor, ME, USA) for use in this model of Mp infection. Each experimental group was approximately 6–8 weeks of age and included of a vehicle group, a Mp infection only group, a Mp infection given a low dose Ang-(1–7) (Sigma, St. Louis, MO, USA) treatment group, and a Mp infection given high dose Ang-(1–7) treatment group. All animals were sacrificed after 24 h of infection for analysis of inflammation. The study was repeated twice with an n = 10 for each experimental condition. All studies were on protocols approved and in accordance with the University of Arizona Institutional Animal Care and Use Committee (IACUC) on protocol number 15-575, with approval dates 2/06/2018 and 2/06/2021.

2.2. Pathogen-Challenge and Drug Treatment

Mp was given via intranasal instillation at 1×10^8 Mp delivered in 50 µL per mouse, as previously described [35]. The experimental vehicle group, which did not receive the Mp, received a dose of sterile saline via intranasal instillation. Ang-(1–7) was given two hours post-infection via forced oropharyngeal instillation at a low dose of 0.3 mg/kg and a high dose of 1.0 mg/kg, while mice were under isoflurane anesthesia. Doses of Ang-(1–7) were based on previous publications in which Ang-(1–7) was active in repressing inflammation in murine models in the 0.3 and 1.0 mg/kg range [6,13]. Forced oropharyngeal delivery is used in place of traditional intratracheal incisions as we have previously shown [36]. All members performing this procedure have been trained with Evan's blue dye to insure their technique results in lung delivery, and not delivery to the gut. The animals that were not treated with Ang-(1–7) received sterile saline via oropharyngeal instillation. Bronchoalveolar lavage (BAL) fluid and lungs from the mice were harvested twenty-four hours post-infection for cellular analysis, qPCR, ELISA, and histological analysis of inflammatory biomarkers.

2.3. Bronchoalveolar Lavage (BAL) Fluid Cell Counts and Cell Differentiation

Twenty-four hours post-infection, mice were euthanized through intraperitoneal injection of a lethal dose of urethane. Lungs were gently flushed with 1.25 mL of PBS (0.1 mM EDTA) to obtain bronchoalveolar lavage fluid (BALF) via a cannulated trachea. The cell-free lavage fluid was used to assess cytokines and chemokines. BALF cells were enumerated by an automated cell counter (Countess, Thermo Fisher Scientific, Waltham, MA, USA) with Trypan blue exclusion for cell viability. Differential cell counts were assessed by use of the Easy III Stain Kit.

2.4. Lung Tissue Preparation for Histological Analysis

Both left and right lung lobes were collected from each mouse subject following BALF collection. Right lung lobes were collected and processed for RNA extraction. Left lung lobes were preserved by immersion in 10% formalin. Left lung lobes were transferred to immersion in 70% ethanol at least 3 days following collection of samples. Left lung samples were processed for hematoxylin and eosin (H&E) staining, and sections of each lung sample were scored in a blinded manner according to a standard scale: 0 = only alveolar macrophages were detected throughout entire tissue section; 1 = very few neutrophils observed throughout entire tissue section; 2 = neutrophils present in alveolar airspaces only; 3 = neutrophils observed in alveolar airspaces and in lymphatics; 4 = neutrophils observed in alveolar airspaces, in lymphatics and in the lumen of large airways.

2.5. RT-PCR Analysis

Right lung lobe tissue was collected from each subject and processed for RNA extraction, cDNA synthesis, and real-time polymerase chain reaction (RT-PCR) analysis. Bio-Rad^{TM} (Bio-Rad laboratories, Hercules, CA, USA) cDNA Synthesis kit was used to synthesize DNA from 1 μg of total RNA. Quanta bio PerfeCTa SYBR Green Supermix (Quanta BioSciences, Gaithersburg, MD, USA) was used to perform RT-PCR. The gene expression of Mp P1-adhesin, TNF-α, Muc5ac, and KC were measured in mice lung tissue by RT-PCR. The mammalian housekeeper gene cyclophilin was used for expression level normalization.

2.6. Growth and Stimulation of RAW 264.7 Cells

RAW 264.7 cells were purchased from ATCC (TIB-71^{TM}, Manassas, VA, USA) and grown according to standard conditions. For TNF-α stimulation, RAW cells were grown until confluent in 24-well culture plates (~500,000 cell per well). On the day of challenge, media was removed and replaced with media containing differing doses of Ang-(1–7) or vehicle control, 30 min prior to Mp stimulation. Mp was added at a MOI of 10:1 and allowed to stimulate cells for 4 h, after which the media was removed and TNF-α levels determined by ELISA. For Mp killing assays, RAW cells were seeded at a density of ~100,000 cells per well into a 96-well tissue culture plate and allowed to adhere (~4 h). Media was removed and prepared Mp was added at a MOI of 2:1 (200,000 Mp to 100,000 seeded cells) with increasing doses of Ang-(1–7) or vehicle control (saline). After 18 h, a 10-μL sample was taken from each well, diluted 1:100 in SP4 media and plated on PPLO agar plates. After 2 weeks of incubation at 35 °C with no CO_2, Mp counts were enumerated with the aid of a microscope at 4x magnification. At the dosing range used for these studies, Ang-(1–7) did not appear to directly impact Mp growth alone as no differences in colony counts were detected when Ang-(1–7) was added to Mp alone in the range of 0–0.5 μg/mL. Cell viability was assessed over a 24-h period, in which increasing doses of Ang-(1–7) were added by Trypan blue exclusion with the aid of an automated cell counter (Countess, Thermo Fisher Scientific, Waltham, MA, USA). Doses were examined in triplicate wells.

2.7. ELISA Analysis

Media from the RAW cell studies (diluted 1:10–1:100) were examined for TNF-α protein levels according to standard methods of the Mouse TNF-α ELISA MAX Deluxe Set protocol (R&D Biosystems, Minneapolis, MN, USA).

2.8. Statistical Analysis

Prism software (GraphPad, version 8.1.2) was used for all statistical analyses. Data comparisons and analysis for significance was performed using ordinary one-way ANOVA with Turkey's multiple comparisons test. Reported significance if * $p < 0.05$, ** $p < 0.01$, *** $p < 0.001$, and **** $p < 0.0001$.

3. Results

3.1. Effect of Ang-(1–7) on Inflammatory Cells in the BALF Post Mp-Infection

Infection with *Mycoplasma pneumoniae* resulted in a significant decrease in the percentage of macrophages, while increasing the percentage of neutrophils present in the BALF as compared to non-infected controls (Figure 1A,C). The total number of macrophages remained consistent (Figure 1B); however, the total number of neutrophils in the Mp-infected only group was significantly increased compared to non-infected vehicle control (Figure 1D). The group receiving the high dose (1.0 mg/kg) Ang-(1–7) treatment following Mp infection had significantly fewer neutrophils, as measured as a percentage of cells recovered and by total neutrophil counts as compared to the Mp infection only group (Figure 1C,D). The group receiving a low dose (0.3 mg/kg) Ang-(1–7) treatment had a significant decrease in the total number of neutrophils as compared to the group with Mp infection only (Figure 1D).

3.2. Effect of Ang-(1–7) on Mp Burden in Lung Tissue

Colonization and infection by Mp occurs through adhesion of the bacteria to cells in the host respiratory tract [37]. Adhesin-P1, an Mp specific adhesin protein, was used to quantify the Mp burden from lung samples of the infected mice [35]. The expression of adhesin-P1 was measured by PCR. As shown in Figure 2, there was a significant decrease in Mp burden among both the low and high dose Ang-(1–7) treatment groups when compared to Mp infected only mice.

3.3. Effect of Ang-(1–7) on Muc5ac, Cytokines, and Chemokines during Mp Infection

Typical markers associated with Mp infection were assessed to determine if Ang-(1–7) would have an impact on inflammation: the mucin gene *Muc5AC*, the cytokine TNF-α, and the neutrophil recruiting KC (*Cxcl1*). Both low dose and high dose Ang-(1–7) treatments led to significantly decreased *Tnf-α* and *Cxcl1* gene expression in lung tissue following Mp infection (Figure 3A,B). *Cxcl1* levels were elevated 12 h after Mp infection, which were significantly decreased by the high dose of Ang-(1-7). While *Cxcl1* levels were lower by 24 h of infection compared to 12 h of infection, Ang-(1–7) treated groups continued to have reduced expression at both the low and high doses. Mp infection led to a slight increase in *Muc5AC* by 24 h; however, both Mp-infected groups treated with either low or high doses of Ang-(1–7) had significantly lower *Muc5ac* gene expression in lung tissue as compared to Mp-infected (Figure 3C).

3.4. Effect of Ang-(1–7) Treatment on Lung Tissue Inflammation in Histological Sections

In order to determine if Ang-(1–7) impacted tissue inflammation during acute Mp infection, left lung sections were processed for H&E staining, and sections of each lung sample were scored according to standard scale. From the four treatment groups described above, sections of each lung sample were scored in a blinded manner according to a standard scale: 0 = only alveolar macrophages were detected throughout entire tissue section; 1 = very few neutrophils observed throughout entire tissue section; 2 = neutrophils present in alveolar airspaces only; 3 = neutrophils observed in alveolar airspaces and in lymphatics; 4 = neutrophils observed in alveolar airspaces, in lymphatics, and in the lumen of large airways. Mice treated with Ang-(1–7) during Mp infection, at both low and high doses, had significantly less lung tissue inflammation compared to Mp-infected mice given vehicle (Figure 4).

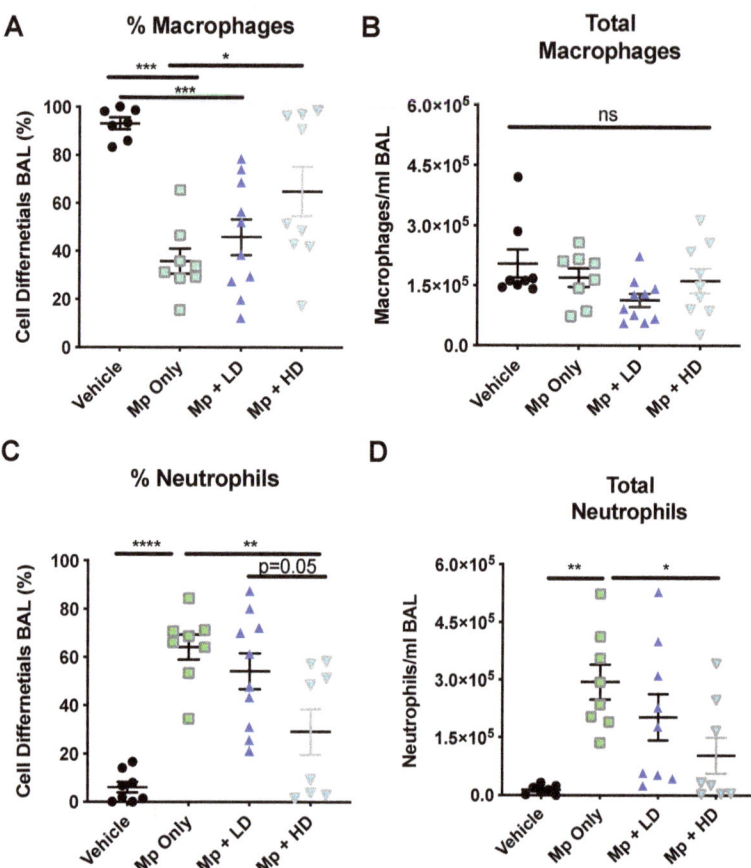

Figure 1. The effect of Ang-(1–7) on inflammatory cell recruitment in *Mycoplasma pneumoniae*–challenged BALB/c mice. A–D) Mice were infected with Mp (or vehicle control) and 2 h later were treated with Ang-(1–7) at high (1 mg/kg body weight) or low (0.3 mg/kg body weight) doses. Total cells present in the BALF were assessed by differential staining. (**A**) The percentage, (**B**) total macrophages, (**C**) the percentage, and (**D**) total neutrophils present in the BAL 24 h post infection are reported. Data are expressed in mean ± SEM. n = 8–10 mice/group, two independent experiments combined. * $p < 0.05$, ** $p < 0.01$, *** $p < 0.001$, **** $p < 0.0001$ by one-way ANOVA for multiple comparisons.

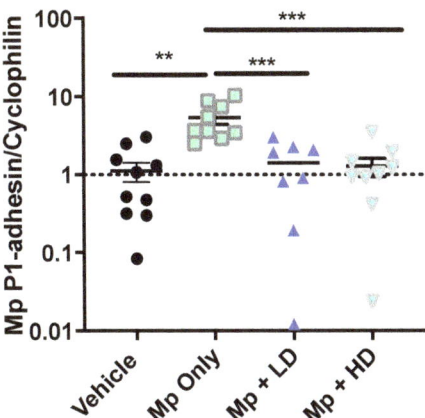

Figure 2. The effect of Ang-(1–7) on *Mycoplasma pneumoniae* burden in lung tissue. Mp burden was determined in lung tissue by RT-PCR for Mp-specific *P1-adhesin* gene expression relative to housekeeper, *Cyclophilin*. Data are expressed in mean ± SEM. n = 8–10 mice/group, two independent experiments combined. ** $p < 0.01$, *** $p < 0.001$ by one-way ANOVA for multiple comparisons.

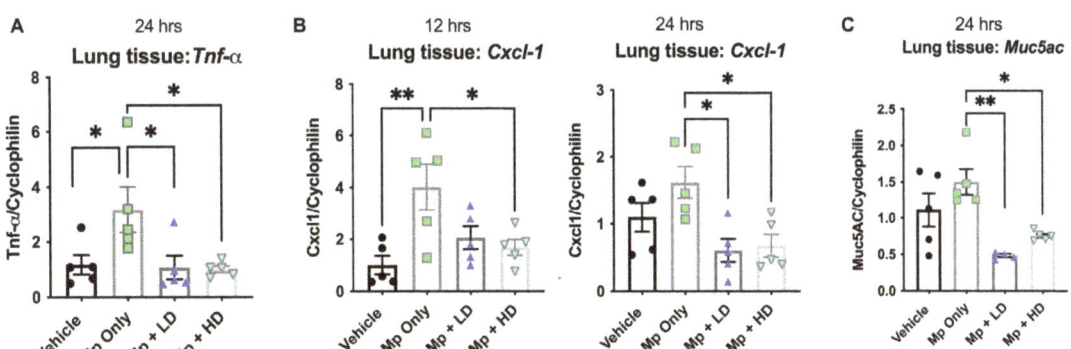

Figure 3. The effect of Ang-(1–7) on indices of inflammation during infection with *Mycoplasma pneumoniae*. (**A**) *Tnf-α*, (**B**) *Cxcl1* (KC), and (**C**) *Muc5AC* gene expression were examined in lung tissue by RT-PCR in a subset of mice at either 12 h or 24 h post infection, as indicated. Data are expressed in mean ± SEM, relative to housekeeper gene expression. n = 5 mice/group and representative of two independent experiments. * $p < 0.05$, ** $p < 0.01$ by one-way ANOVA.

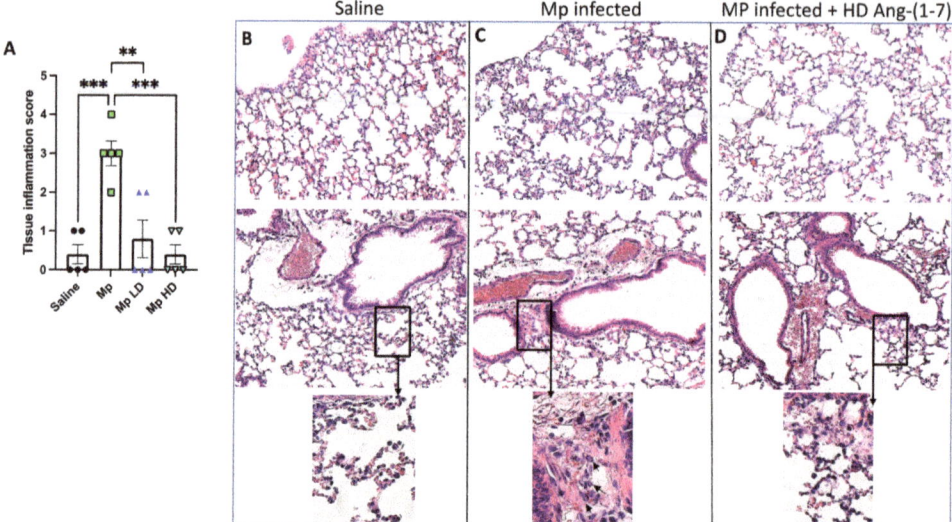

Figure 4. The effect of Ang-(1–7) on pulmonary inflammation in H&E stained slides of sectioned mouse lung. (**A**) Average grade scores for each experimental group. Data are expressed in mean ± SEM. n = 5 mice/group. Representative H&E stained lung sections at 20X magnification from (**B**) saline vehicle, (**C**) Mp infection only (arrows in boxed enlargement indicate neutrophils), (**D**) Mp infection with high dose Ang-(1–7) treatment. ** $p < 0.01$, *** $p < 0.001$ by one-way ANOVA for multiple comparisons.

3.5. Ang-(1–7) Dose-Dependently Inhibits TNF-α Secretion from RAW 264.7 Cells Following Mp Challenge

Since macrophages are the predominant producers of TNF-α during airway infection, we sought to determine if Ang-(1–7) would have an impact on Mp-induced TNF-α production in vitro. For these studies, we used a common macrophage cell line, RAW 264.7, which is known to produce high levels of TNF-α. As shown in Figure 5A, Ang-(1–7) had no impact on TNF-α secretion at low doses; however, starting at doses of 5 μg/mL or higher, we did see an inhibition of TNF-α by RAW 264.7 cells. We based our Ang-(1–7) dose response to be within the limits of cell tolerability, as this peptide has not shown toxicity at levels up to 1000 μg/mL in five other cell lines, as recently published [38]. In line with these results, Ang-(1–7) did not reduce RAW 264.7 cell viability at any of the doses tested over a 24 h period (Figure 5B).

3.6. Ang-(1–7) Dose-Dependently Promotes Killing of Mp by RAW Cells In Vitro

We next set out to investigate if Ang-(1–7) had an impact on Mp-killing activity in RAW 264.7 cells. In our study, we compared the killing efficiency of RAW cells with and without Ang-(1–7) over an 18 h incubation period. While RAW cells effectively reduced Mp CFUs in media by 25% in 18 h, RAW cells given Ang-(1–7) had a greater reduction in Mp CFUs in a dose-dependent manner, with the lowest dose reducing 48% (* $p < 0.05$ versus RAW cells + vehicle) and the highest dose reducing Mp by 75% (**** $p < 0.0001$ versus RAW cells + vehicle) (Figure 5C). At the dosing range used for these studies, Ang-(1–7) did not appear to directly impact Mp growth alone as no differences in colony counts were detected when Ang-(1–7) was added to Mp alone in the range of 0–0.5 μg/mL (not shown).

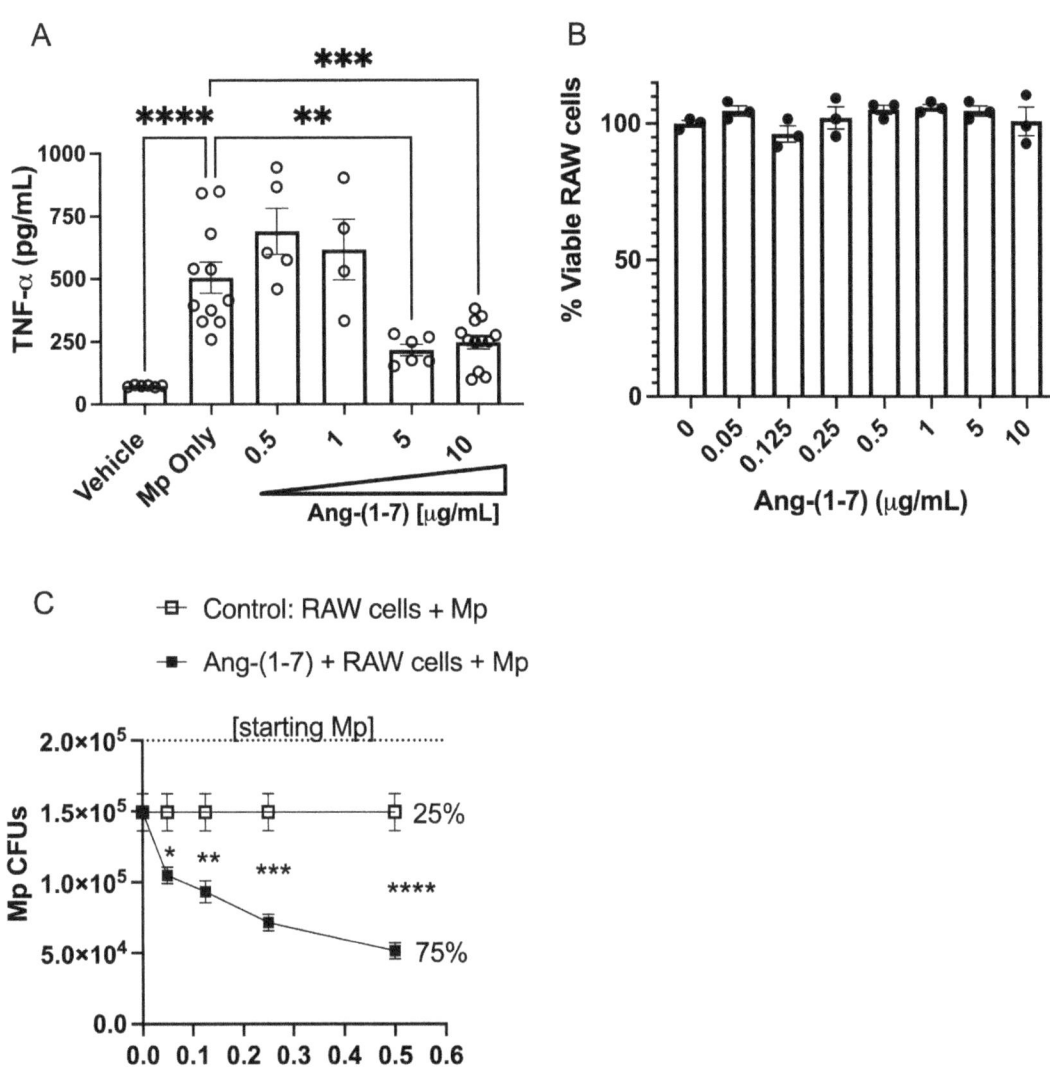

Figure 5. The impact of Ang-(1–7) on macrophage function. (**A**) RAW cells were stimulated with Mp (MOI 10:1) for 4 h in the presence or absence of increasing doses of Ang-(1-7). Cell-free supernatants were assessed for TNF-α by ELISA. n = minimum of two repeats with triplicates for each. (**B**) RAW cells were incubated with increasing doses of Ang-(1–7) in triplicate for 24 h and viability assessed by Trypan blue exclusion using a Countess cell counter. (**C**) RAW cells were stimulated with Mp (MOI of 2:1) with increasing doses of Ang-(1–7) or vehicle control (saline) for 18 h, after which a sample was taken from each well, diluted 1:100 in SP4 media and plated on PPLO agar plates. CFUs were counted after 2 weeks of growth. n = minimum of two repeats with triplicates for each. * $p < 0.05$, ** $p < 0.01$, *** $p < 0.001$, **** $p < 0.0001$ by the *t*-test for each respective dose.

4. Discussion

The role of Ang-(1–7) in reducing allergic inflammation in animal models has been previously reported; however, the role of this protective peptide hormone in treating infections common among many chronic asthma sufferers has not been described. *Mycoplasma pneumoniae* is known to colonize the airways of patients considered to have chronic asthma, and this underlying bacterial infection is thought to contribute to asthma exacerbations among these patients. Therefore, we thought it would be important to understand how secondary illnesses common among asthmatics affect the efficacy of a potentially new drug being considered for the treatment of asthma.

Our research aimed to address how Ang-(1–7) would perform during acute infection with Mp. The main findings of this study indicate that Ang-(1–7) has the ability to provide protection in an experimental mouse model of acute Mp infection by ameliorating inflammatory phenotypes within 24 h of infection. We chose to test Ang-(1–7) delivery to the lungs, as we believed this would have the greatest impact to controlling inflammation. However, additional therapeutic routes, including oral or aerosol delivery via nebulizer, which would be congruent with options for humans, should be explored. In support of this, our colleagues recently reported excellent aerosol dispersion performance of Ang-(1–7) with a human DPI device and in vitro human cell viability assays showed that Ang-(1–7) was biocompatible and safe for different human respiratory cells [38]. We chose to only assess Ang-(1–7) treatment when given shortly (within 2 h) after an infectious challenge. While our findings indicate that high doses of Ang-(1–7) led to decreased infiltrating neutrophils, as well as the cytokines and chemokines that can recruit them, *TNF-α* and *Cxcl1*, we recognize in humans it would be more translatable to give Ang-(1–7) treatment after symptoms of "walking pneumoniae" are more evident, which could occur several days after exposure. Future studies should address the timing for Ang-(1–7) dosing to see how long after Mp infection, delivery of Ang-(1–7) is still efficacious to increase the availability in clinical practices.

Mp infections among asthmatic patients have been associated with a dramatic spike in levels of TNF-α [39]. We provide evidence that Ang-(1–7) treatment can significantly reduce levels of TNF-α at the RNA and protein levels during Mp infection. In addition, Ang-(1–7) dose-dependently reduced TNF-α production or secretion from Mp-stimulated RAW 264.7 cells, which are a macrophage cell line. While RAW 264.7 cells are well utilized in the field for drug screening, future studies should test Ang-(1–7) on primary macrophage populations from humans to validate our findings. Since macrophages are the predominant producers of TNF-α during respiratory infection, it is relevant that Ang-(1–7) can work directly on these cells during Mp stimulation. Reducing any downstream impacts of TNF-α driven inflammation would likely have additional positive impacts for asthmatic patients beyond those we detected and should be examined in future studies.

Similarly, mucus production is an important factor when evaluating treatments for asthma, as mucus hyper-secretion into the airway lumen obstructs airways and worsens asthma symptoms [40]. Along these lines, we found that *Muc5AC* gene expression was significantly decreased during Mp infection following treatment with Ang-(1–7). Interestingly, the level of *Muc5AC* was repressed by Ang-(1–7) during infection below the levels normally present without infection. This suggests that Ang-(1–7) may have an inhibitory impact of on mucin production in the absence of infection, which should be further studied. While an increase in mucin production was not evident at this early timepoint, future directions should examine the impact of Ang-(1–7) treatment in longer models of Mp infection to see if the reduced *Muc5AC* gene expression results in deceased mucin production in lung sections. Examination of lung histological sections revealed enhanced neutrophilia in airways of Mp infected mice, while those treated with Ang-(1–7) were more similar to untreated controls. So not only did Ang-(1–7) results in fewer neutrophils migrating into the lung lumen, it also impacted neutrophils migrating into the lung tissue.

Along with providing a promising therapeutic option for the treatment of asthma, the results of this study also indicate that Ang-(1–7) treatment may be helpful for controlling inflammation during Mp infection, and in the clearance of Mp. While fewer neutrophils were detected in the Ang-(1–7) treatment groups, the Mp burden was also decreased. This was somewhat surprising given that neutrophils would contribute to Mp killing in the lungs. This finding of fewer neutrophils and reduced Mp burden, suggest that another compensatory mechanism for pathogen removal may have been activated. Those could include more activation of macrophages prone for pathogen killing or an induction of epithelial-driven antimicrobial host defense.

We next conducted studies to see if Ang-(1–7) had any direct antimicrobial impact on Mp and we found that Ang-(1–7) alone was not able to reduce Mp CFUs over a two-week growth period (data not shown). However, Mp-killing studies in RAW 264.7 cells in the presence or absence of increasing concentrations of Ang-(1–7) indicated that RAW cells had increased Mp-killing efficiency with increases doses of Ang-(1-7). This suggests that Ang-(1–7) may have a therapeutic potential in stimulating macrophages to better eliminate pathogens in the lungs. Since Ang-(1–7) and analogs are known to reduce ROS and promote NO production, it is likely this Ang-(1–7) activity contributes to the enhanced Mp-killing function by macrophages. Future studies should evaluate this possible mechanism and the ability of Ang-(1–7) to assist in clearance of other infectious agents common among asthmatics, such as human rhinovirus (HRV) and respiratory syncytial virus (RSV) [41].

While most commonly known as a vasodilator agent with important roles in the cardiovascular system, Ang-(1–7) has also emerged with anti-oxidant, anti-inflammatory, and anti-fibrotic effects in several model systems [6,42]. Importantly, Ang1-7 inhibits production and expression of many cytokines and adhesion molecules associated with a cytokine storm [43,44] and delivery of exogenous Ang1-7 has been shown to improve oxygenation and can be safely delivered to humans [25,45,46]. In line with these studies, we add that not only does Ang-(1–7) reduce inflammation during live respiratory infection with Mp, it also leads to a significant reduction in Mp pathogen burden and reduction of mucin production in the airways.

5. Conclusions

To our knowledge, this is the first study to demonstrate the effects of Ang (1-7) peptide in Mp lung infection and offer mechanistic insight into macrophage killing mechanisms. Taken with the many previous studies in various models in which Ang-(1–7) peptide has anti-inflammatory activity, our studies not only support these findings, but also bring to light a potentially novel indication, i.e., as a therapeutic for the treatment of respiratory infections.

Author Contributions: K.L.C., U.S.Y., S.T. carried out the experiments. M.H., R.P. and H.M.M. provided technical expertise, background knowledge, and reagents. K.L.C., U.S.Y. and J.G.L. performed the statistical analysis. K.L.C. and J.G.L. wrote the manuscript. All authors have read and agreed to the published version of the manuscript.

Funding: HL142769, AI135935, R01NS091238.

Institutional Review Board Statement: All studies were conducted on protocols approved by (and in accordance with) the University of Arizona Institutional Animal Care and Use Committee (IACUC), protocol number 15-575, with approval dates 2 June 2018 and 2 June 2021.

Informed Consent Statement: Not applicable.

Data Availability Statement: Not applicable.

Acknowledgments: Not applicable.

Conflicts of Interest: The authors have no conflict of interest to declare.

References

1. Kostenis, E.; Milligan, G.; Christopoulos, A.; Sanchez-Ferrer, C.F.; Heringer-Walther, S.; Sexton, P.; Gembardt, F.; Kellett, E.; Martini, L.; Vanderheyden, P.; et al. G-Protein–Coupled Receptor Mas Is a Physiological Antagonist of the Angiotensin II Type 1 Receptor. *Circulation* **2005**, *111*, 1806–1813. [CrossRef]
2. Papinska, A.M.; Soto, M.; Meeks, C.J.; Rodgers, K.E. Long-term administration of angiotensin (1-7) prevents heart and lung dysfunction in a mouse model of type 2 diabetes (db/db) by reducing oxidative stress, inflammation and pathological remodeling. *Pharmacol. Res.* **2016**, *107*, 372–380. [CrossRef] [PubMed]

3.   Freeman, E.J.; Chisolm, G.M.; Ferrario, C.M.; Tallant, E.A. Angiotensin-(1-7) Inhibits Vascular Smooth Muscle Cell Growth. *Hypertension* **1996**, *28*, 104–108. [CrossRef] [PubMed]
4.   Guo, L.; Yin, A.; Zhang, Q.; Zhong, T.; O'Rourke, S.T.; Sun, C. Angiotensin-(1–7) attenuates angiotensin II-induced cardiac hypertrophy via a Sirt3-dependent mechanism. *Am. J. Physiol. Circ. Physiol.* **2017**, *312*, H980–H991. [CrossRef] [PubMed]
5.   Kittana, N. Angiotensin-converting enzyme 2-Angiotensin 1-7/1-9 system: Novel promising targets for heart failure treatment. *Fundam Clin. Pharmacol.* **2018**, *32*, 14–25. [CrossRef] [PubMed]
6.   El-Hashim, A.Z.; Renno, W.M.; Raghupathy, R.; Abduo, H.T.; Akhtar, S.; Benter, I.F. Angiotensin-(1-7) inhibits allergic inflammation, via the MAS1 receptor, through suppression of ERK1/2- and NF-κB-dependent pathways. *Br. J. Pharmacol.* **2012**, *166*, 1964–1976. [CrossRef]
7.   Li, Y.; Cao, Y.; Zeng, Z.; Liang, M.; Xue, Y.; Xi, C.; Zhou, M.; Jiang, W. Angiotensin-converting enzyme 2/angiotensin-(1-7)/Mas axis prevents lipopolysaccharide-induced apoptosis of pulmonary microvascular endothelial cells by inhibiting JNK/NF-κB pathways. *Sci. Rep.* **2015**, *5*, 8209. [CrossRef]
8.   Santos, R.A.S.; Ferreira, A.J.; Verano-Braga, T.; Bader, M. Angiotensin-converting enzyme 2, angiotensin-(1–7) and Mas: New players of the renin–angiotensin system. *J. Endocrinol.* **2012**, *216*, R1–R17. [CrossRef]
9.   Ferrario, C.M. Angiotensin-converting enzyme 2 and angiotensin-(1-7): An evolving story in cardiovascular regulation. *Hypertension* **2006**, *47*, 515–521. [CrossRef]
10.   Raizada, M.K.; Ferreira, A.J. ACE2: A New Target for Cardiovascular Disease Therapeutics. *J. Cardiovasc. Pharmacol.* **2007**, *50*, 112–119. [CrossRef] [PubMed]
11.   Vickers, C.; Hales, P.; Kaushik, V.; Dick, L.; Gavin, J.; Tang, J.; Godbout, K.; Parsons, T.; Baronas, E.; Hsieh, F.; et al. Hydrolysis of Biological Peptides by Human Angiotensin-converting Enzyme-related Carboxypeptidase. *J. Biol. Chem.* **2002**, *277*, 14838–14843. [CrossRef]
12.   Lazartigues, Y.F.A.J.L.L.E.; Feng, Y.; Lavoie, J. The Two fACEs of the Tissue Renin-Angiotensin Systems: Implication in Cardiovascular Diseases. *Curr. Pharm. Des.* **2007**, *13*, 1231–1245. [CrossRef]
13.   Hay, M.; Polt, R.; Heien, M.L.; Vanderah, T.W.; Largent-Milnes, T.M.; Rodgers, K.; Falk, T.; Bartlett, M.J.; Doyle, K.P.; Konhilas, J. A Novel Angiotensin-(1-7) Glycosylated Mas Receptor Agonist for Treating Vascular Cognitive Impairment and Inflammation-Related Memory Dysfunction. *J. Pharmacol. Exp. Ther.* **2019**, *369*, 9–25. [CrossRef]
14.   Wang, Y.; Qian, C.; Roks, A.J.; Westermann, D.; Schumacher, S.-M.; Escher, F.; Schoemaker, R.G.; Reudelhuber, T.L.; Van Gilst, W.H.; Schultheiss, H.-P.; et al. Circulating Rather Than Cardiac Angiotensin-(1-7) Stimulates Cardioprotection After Myocardial Infarction. *Circ. Hear. Fail.* **2010**, *3*, 286–293. [CrossRef]
15.   Karnik, S.S.; Singh, K.D.; Tirupula, K.; Unal, H. Significance of angiotensin 1-7 coupling with MAS1 receptor and other GPCRs to the renin-angiotensin system: IUPHAR Review 22. *Br. J. Pharmacol.* **2017**, *174*, 737–753. [CrossRef]
16.   Gopallawa, I.; Uhal, B.D. Molecular and cellular mechanisms of the inhibitory effects of ACE-2/ANG1-7/Mas axis on lung injury. *Curr. Top. Pharmacol.* **2014**, *18*, 71–80. [CrossRef]
17.   Magalhaes, G.; Barroso, L.C.; Reis, A.; Rodrigues-Machado, M.G.; Gregório, J.; Motta-Santos, D.; Oliveira, A.C.; Perez, D.A.; Barcelos, L.S.; Teixeira, M.M.; et al. Angiotensin-(1–7) Promotes Resolution of Eosinophilic Inflammation in an Experimental Model of Asthma. *Front. Immunol.* **2018**, *9*, 58. [CrossRef] [PubMed]
18.   Magalhaes, G.; Rodrigues-Machado, M.D.G.; Motta-Santos, D.; Alenina, N.; Bader, M.; Santos, R.A.S.; Barcelos, L.S.; Campagnole-Santos, M.J. Chronic allergic pulmonary inflammation is aggravated in angiotensin-(1–7) Mas receptor knockout mice. *Am. J. Physiol. Cell. Mol. Physiol.* **2016**, *311*, L1141–L1148. [CrossRef] [PubMed]
19.   Chen, Q.; Liu, J.; Wang, W.; Liu, S.; Yang, X.; Chen, M.; Cheng, L.; Lu, J.; Guo, T.; Huang, F. Sini decoction ameliorates sepsis-induced acute lung injury via regulating ACE2-Ang (1-7)-Mas axis and inhibiting the MAPK signaling pathway. *Biomed. Pharmacother.* **2019**, *115*, 108971. [CrossRef] [PubMed]
20.   Chen, Q.F.; Kuang, X.D.; Yuan, Q.F.; Hao, H.; Zhang, T.; Huang, Y.H.; Zhou, X.Y. Lipoxin A attenuates LPS-induced acute lung injury via activation of the ACE2-Ang-(1-7)-Mas axis. *Innate Immun.* **2018**, *24*, 285–296. [CrossRef] [PubMed]
21.   Melo, E.M.; Del Sarto, J.; Vago, J.P.; Tavares, L.P.; Rago, F.; Gonçalves, A.P.F.; Machado, M.G.; Aranda-Pardos, I.; Valiate, B.V.; Cassali, G.D.; et al. Relevance of angiotensin-(1-7) and its receptor Mas in pneumonia caused by influenza virus and post-influenza pneumococcal infection. *Pharmacol. Res.* **2021**, *163*, 105292. [CrossRef] [PubMed]
22.   McKinney, C.A.; Fattah, C.; Loughrey, C.; Milligan, G.; Nicklin, S.A. Angiotensin-(1–7) and angiotensin-(1–9): Function in cardiac and vascular remodelling. *Clin. Sci.* **2014**, *126*, 815–827. [CrossRef] [PubMed]
23.   Fraga-Silva, R.A.; Costa-Fraga, F.P.; De Sousa, F.; Alenina, N.; Bader, M.; Sinisterra, R.; Santos, R.A.S. An orally active formulation of angiotensin-(1-7) produces an antithrombotic effect. *Clinics* **2011**, *66*, 837–841. [CrossRef] [PubMed]
24.   Gallagher, P.E.; Tallant, E.A. Inhibition of human lung cancer cell growth by angiotensin-(1-7). *Carcinogenesis* **2004**, *25*, 2045–2052. [CrossRef] [PubMed]
25.   Pham, H.; Schwartz, B.M.; Delmore, J.E.; Reed, E.; Cruickshank, S.; Drummond, L.; Rodgers, K.E.; Peterson, K.J.; Dizerega, G.S. Pharmacodynamic stimulation of thrombogenesis by angiotensin (1-7) in recurrent ovarian cancer patients receiving gemcitabine and platinum-based chemotherapy. *Cancer Chemother. Pharmacol.* **2013**, *71*, 965–972. [CrossRef]
26.   Stanhewicz, A.; Alexander, L.M. Local angiotensin-(1-7) administration improves microvascular endothelial function in women who have had preeclampsia. *Am. J. Physiol. Integr. Comp. Physiol.* **2020**, *318*, R148–R155. [CrossRef]

27. Hay, M.; Vanderah, T.W.; Samareh-Jahani, F.; Constantopoulos, E.; Uprety, A.R.; Barnes, C.A.; Konhilas, J. Cognitive impairment in heart failure: A protective role for angiotensin-(1-7). *Behav. Neurosci.* **2017**, *131*, 99–114. [CrossRef]

28. Shimabukuro-Vornhagen, A.; Gödel, P.; Subklewe, M.; Stemmler, H.J.; Schlößer, H.A.; Schlaak, M.; Kochanek, M.; Böll, B.; von Bergwelt-Baildon, M.S. Cytokine release syndrome. *J. Immunother Cancer* **2018**, *6*, 56. [CrossRef]

29. Kotch, C.; Barrett, D.; Teachey, D.T. Tocilizumab for the treatment of chimeric antigen receptor T cell-induced cytokine release syndrome. *Expert Rev. Clin. Immunol.* **2019**, *15*, 813–822. [CrossRef]

30. Murthy, H.; Iqbal, M.; Chavez, J.C.; A Kharfan-Dabaja, M. Cytokine Release Syndrome: Current Perspectives. *ImmunoTargets Ther.* **2019**, *8*, 43–52. [CrossRef]

31. Atkinson, T.P.; Balish, M.F.; Waites, K.B. Epidemiology, clinical manifestations, pathogenesis and laboratory detection of Mycoplasma pneumoniae infections. *FEMS Microbiol. Rev.* **2008**, *32*, 956–973. [CrossRef]

32. Carr, T.F.; Kraft, M. Chronic Infection and Severe Asthma. *Immunol Allergy Clin. North. Am.* **2016**, *36*, 483–502. [CrossRef]

33. Kraft, M.; Hamid, Q. Mycoplasma in severe asthma. *J. Allergy Clin. Immunol.* **2006**, *117*, 1197–1198. [CrossRef]

34. Kraft, M.; Cassell, G.H.; Pak, J.; Martin, R.J. Mycoplasma pneumoniae and Chlamydia pneumoniae in asthma: Effect of clarithromycin. *Chest* **2002**, *121*, 1782–1788. [CrossRef] [PubMed]

35. Johnson, M.D.L.; Younis, U.S.; Menghani, S.V.; Addison, K.J.; Whalen, M.; Pilon, A.L.; Cress, A.E.; Polverino, F.; Romanoki, C.E.; Kraft, M.; et al. CC16 Binding to α4β1 integrin protects against *Mycoplasma pneumoniae* infection. *Am. J. Respir Crit Care Med.* **2021**, *203*, 1410–1418. [CrossRef] [PubMed]

36. Ledford, J.G.; Voelker, D.R.; Addison, K.J.; Wang, Y.; Nikam, V.S.; Degan, S.; Kadasamy, P.; Tanyaratsrisakul, S.; Fischer, B.M.; Kraft, M.; et al. Genetic variation in SP-A2 leads to differential binding to Mycoplasma pneumoniae membranes and regulation of host responses. *J. Immunol.* **2015**, *194*, 6123–6132. [CrossRef] [PubMed]

37. Kashyap, S.; Sarkar, M. Mycoplasma pneumonia: Clinical features and management. *Lung India.* **2010**, *27*, 75–85. [CrossRef] [PubMed]

38. Alabsi, W.; Acosta, M.F.; Al-Obeidi, F.A.; Hay, M.; Polt, R.; Mansour, H.M. Synthesis, Physicochemical Characterization, In Vitro 2D/3D Human Cell Culture, and In Vitro Aerosol Dispersion Performance of Advanced Spray Dried and Co-Spray Dried Angiotensin (1-7) Peptide and PNA5 with Trehalose as Microparticles/Nanoparticles for Targeted Respiratory Delivery as Dry Powder Inhalers. *Pharmaceutics* **2021**, *13*, 1278. [PubMed]

39. Razin, S.; Yogev, D.; Naot, Y. Molecular biology and pathogenicity of mycoplasmas. *Microbiol Mol. Biol Rev.* **1998**, *62*, 1094–1156. [CrossRef]

40. Evans, C.M.; Kim, K.; Tuvim, M.J.; Dickey, B.F. Mucus hypersecretion in asthma: Causes and effects. *Curr. Opin. Pulm. Med.* **2009**, *15*, 4–11. [CrossRef]

41. Darveaux, J.I.; Lemanske, R.F. Infection-Related Asthma. *J. Allergy Clin. Immunol. Pr.* **2014**, *2*, 658–663. [CrossRef]

42. Benter, I.F.; Yousif, M.; Dhaunsi, G.S.; Kaur, J.; Chappell, M.C.; Diz, D.I. Angiotensin-(1–7) Prevents Activation of NADPH Oxidase and Renal Vascular Dysfunction in Diabetic Hypertensive Rats. *Am. J. Nephrol.* **2007**, *28*, 25–33. [CrossRef] [PubMed]

43. Rodrigues Prestes, T.R.; Rocha, N.P.; Miranda, A.S.; Teixeira, A.L.; Simoes e-Silva, A.C.; Oliveira, A.C.; Carvalho Bittencourt de Oliveira, F.; Gonçalves, R. The Anti-Inflammatory Potential of ACE2/Angiotensin-(1-7)/Mas Receptor Axis: Evidence from Basic and Clinical Research. *Curr. Drug Targets* **2017**, *18*, 1301–1313. [CrossRef] [PubMed]

44. de Carvalho Santuchi, M.; Dutra, M.F.; Vago, J.P.; Lima, K.M.; Galvao, I.; de Souza-Neto, F.P.; Morais e Silva, M.; Oliveira, A.C.; de Oliveira, F.C.; Gonçalves, R.; et al. Angiotensin-(1-7) and Alamandine Promote Anti-inflammatory Response in Macrophages In Vitro and In Vivo. *Mediators Inflamm.* **2019**, *2019*, 2401081. [CrossRef] [PubMed]

45. Rodgers, K.E.; Oliver, J.; diZerega, G.S. Phase I/II dose escalation study of angiotensin 1-7 [A(1-7)] administered before and after chemotherapy in patients with newly diagnosed breast cancer. *Cancer Chemother. Pharmacol.* **2006**, *57*, 559–568. [CrossRef]

46. Savage, P.D.; Lovato, J.; Brosnihan, K.B.; Miller, A.A.; Petty, W.J. Phase II Trial of Angiotensin-(1-7) for the Treatment of Patients with Metastatic Sarcoma. *Sarcoma* **2016**, *2016*, 1–7. [CrossRef]

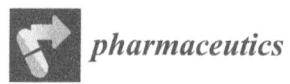

Article

The Influence of Formulation Components and Environmental Humidity on Spray-Dried Phage Powders for Treatment of Respiratory Infections Caused by *Acinetobacter baumannii*

Wei Yan [1], Ruide He [2], Xiaojiao Tang [2], Bin Tian [3], Yannan Liu [4], Yigang Tong [5], Kenneth K. W. To [1] and Sharon S. Y. Leung [1,*]

[1] School of Pharmacy, Faculty of Medicine, The Chinese University of Hong Kong, Hong Kong Shatin, NewTerritories, Hong Kong, China; 1155114125@link.cuhk.edu.hk (W.Y.); kennethto@cuhk.edu.hk (K.K.W.T.)
[2] Livzon Pharmaceutical Group Co., Ltd., Zhu Hai 519090, China; heruide2021@163.com (R.H.); tangxiaojiaoxfx@163.com (X.T.)
[3] Department of Pharmaceutical Sciences, School of Food and Biological Engineering, Shanxi University of Science and Technology, Weiyang University Park, Xi'an 710021, China; tianbin@sust.edu.cn
[4] Emergency Medicine Clinical Research Center, Beijing Chao-Yang Hospital, Capital Medical University, Beijing 100069, China; yannan_liu@foxmail.com
[5] Beijing Advanced Innovation Center for Soft Matter Science and Engineering (BAIC-SM), College of Life Science and Technology, Beijing University of Chemical Technology, Beijing 100029, China; tongyigang@mail.buct.edu.cn
* Correspondence: sharon.leung@cuhk.edu.hk; Tel.: +852-3943-9795

Citation: Yan, W.; He, R.; Tang, X.; Tian, B.; Liu, Y.; Tong, Y.; To, K.K.W.; Leung, S.S.Y. The Influence of Formulation Components and Environmental Humidity on Spray-Dried Phage Powders for Treatment of Respiratory Infections Caused by *Acinetobacter baumannii*. *Pharmaceutics* **2021**, *13*, 1162. https://doi.org/10.3390/pharmaceutics13081162

Academic Editors: Michael Yee Tak Chow, Philip Chi Lip Kwok and Jaehwi Lee

Received: 29 May 2021
Accepted: 15 July 2021
Published: 28 July 2021

Publisher's Note: MDPI stays neutral with regard to jurisdictional claims in published maps and institutional affiliations.

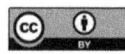

Abstract: The feasibility of using respirable bacteriophage (phage) powder to treat lung infections has been demonstrated in animal models and clinical studies. This work investigated the influence of formulation compositions and excipient concentrations on the aerosol performance and storage stability of phage powder. An anti-*Acinetobacter baumannii* phage vB_AbaM-IME-AB406 was incorporated into dry powders consisting of trehalose, mannitol and L-leucine for the first time. The phage stability upon the spray-drying process, room temperature storage and powder dispersion under different humidity conditions were assessed. In general, powders prepared with higher mannitol content (40% of the total solids) showed a lower degree of particle merging and no sense of stickiness during sample handling. These formulations also provided better storage stability of phage with no further titer loss after 1 month and <1 log titer loss in 6 months at high excipient concentration. Mannitol improved the dispersibility of phage powders, but the in vitro lung dose dropped sharply after exposure to high-humidity condition (65% RH) for formulations with 20% mannitol. While previously collected knowledge on phage powder preparation could be largely extended to formulate *A. baumannii* phage into inhalable dry powders, the environmental humidity may have great impacts on the stability and dispersion of phage; therefore, specific attention is required when optimizing phage powder formulations for global distribution.

Keywords: phage therapy; spray drying; bacterial lung infections; environmental humidity; aerosol performance; inhalation

1. Introduction

With the overuse and misuse of antibiotics, antimicrobial resistance (AMR) has become one of the greatest threats to human health worldwide [1]. To guide research efforts aiming to develop new treatment strategies, the World Health Organization (WHO) published the first global priority pathogen list in 2017 [2]. Among all identified bacteria, *Acinetobacter baumannii* has been ranked as the number one critical-priority pathogen, emphasizing the extent of the threats posed to human health and the urgency for new treatment strategies. In fact, *A. baumannii* is generally regarded as a low-virulence pathogen. However, it has such an exceptional ability to acquire resistance to antibiotics that the resistance rates of multidrug-resistant (MDR), extensively drug-resistant (XDR), and pandrug-resistant (PDR) *A. baumannii* were 50.2%, 28.5%, and 14.0%, respectively, presenting a significant clinical challenge in choosing appropriate treatment regimens [3]. Last-line antibiotics, such as polymyxins and carbapenems, have been increasingly used as the only therapeutic option for life-threatening infections [4], but outbreaks of PDR *A. baumannii* have been increasing reported worldwide with a mortality rate of 26.0–55.7% [5].

Bacteriophage (phage) therapy is now being re-introduced in Western countries [6] and has been listed as one of the top alternatives to address the AMR threat [3]. The safety and efficacy of phage in treating patients against drug-resistant *A. baumannii* have been demonstrated in multiple cases of life-saving therapeutic use [7–9]. With pneumonia being one of the most frequent clinical manifestations of *A. baumannii* infection, increasing attention has been given to the investigation of the effectiveness of *A. baumannii* phage in treating lung infections [10–14]. Although nebulization has been the method of choice for phage delivery to the lung in the clinical setting, dry powder formulations are preferred to liquid formulations in terms of storage, transportation and administration [15].

Recently, spray drying has been demonstrated as a promising single-step process in producing inhalable phage dry powder formulations using low-cost excipients, such as trehalose, lactose, mannitol and leucine, showing a sufficiently long storage stability ($\leq$1 log titer loss in 12 months) under refrigerated or room temperatures in low-humidity conditions (<20% RH) [16–21]. The efficacy of intratracheally administered spray-dried phage powder against lung infection caused by *Pseudomonas aeruginosa* has been demonstrated in a murine model [22]. To the best of our knowledge, there are no reports on formulating *Acinetobacter* phage into inhalable powders. As previous reports highlighted that the detrimental effects to phage upon the production process and storage conditions are phage dependent and excipient context specific [18,20,23], current knowledge obtained for *Pseudomonas* and other phages might not be directly applicable for *A. baumannii* phage. In the present study, our primary objective is to investigate the feasibility of extending the collected knowledge to produce inhalable *Acinetobacter* phage powders for inhaled therapy. A two-factor three-level factorial design [24] was used to evaluate the impacts of the two identified formulation factors, formulation compositions and total solid content, on the phage stability and in vitro aerosol performance of produced powders, using an *A. baumannii* phage vB_AbaM-IME-AB406 (AB406 in short) as a model phage.

As phages were usually stabilized with amorphous sugar in the powder form, their handling and storage in low-humidity conditions (RH < 20%) are required to minimize the occurrence of recrystallization. However, excessive environmental moisture could be relevant in patients' homes or healthcare settings, especially in areas with subtropical climates such as Hong Kong and southern USA, where the average RH $\geq$ 65% all year round [25–27]. To estimate the impacts of high humidity on the administration of phage powders, we measured the in vitro aerosolization performance of phage powders after incubating at RH 65% for a certain period, mimicking a scenario where patients fail to administer the medication immediately after unpacking.

2. Materials and Methods

2.1. Materials

A lytic *Myoviridae* phage, AB406, active against *A. baumannii* was isolated and characterized by the Beijing Institute of Microbiology and Epidemiology. High titer phage lysate was obtained and titered using well-established protocols [28]. The phage lysate was then purified by anion-exchange chromatography using a CIMmultus™ QA 1 mL Monolithic Column (BIA Separations, Slovenia) [29]. The phage elution was dialyzed with phosphate-buffered saline (PBS, Sigma–Aldrich, St. Louis, MO, USA) and the obtained phage titer was 1.1×10^{10} pfu/mL. The host *A. baumannii* strain, MDR-AB2, was isolated from the sputum sample of a patient with pneumonia at PLA Hospital 307. The powder matrix systems were composed of different amounts of D-(+)-Trehalose dihydrate, mannitol and L-leucine (Sigma–Aldrich, USA).

2.2. Design of Experiment–Factorial Design

A two-factor three-level (3^2) full factorial design (Design Expert software version 12.0.1.0) [30] was used to investigate the influence of two factors on the stabilization of AB406 phage in the dry powder form and its dispersibility. The studied factors were as follows: A—trehalose to mannitol ratio (80:0, 60:20 and 40:40); B—total solid content (20, 40 and 60 mg/mL), as shown in Table 1. The range of trehalose to mannitol ratio was selected based on our previous reports on *Pseudomonas* phage [17] that a higher mannitol content would cause significant titer loss. The range of total solid content was selected based on our preliminary data on producing powder with a size distribution fall within the inhalable range ($\leq$5 μm) [31] using the same excipient systems without phage. Formulations were prepared randomly according to the Design Expert software, but reordered in order here to improve readability. Three separate batches of powders were produced for each formulation. The responses studied were as follows: phage viability after a 6-month storage period at room temperature and RH < 20%; fine particle fraction of phage (FPF) for dispersion performed under normal conditions (<35%) and dispersing after incubating at 65% RH for 1 h.

Table 1. Formulation compositions and powder characteristics.

Formulation	Trehalose %	Mannitol %	Leucine %	Total Solid Content (mg/mL)	VMD $\pm$ SD (μm)	Span $\pm$ SD
F1 (T80M0-20)	80	0	20	20	4.59 $\pm$ 0.06	1.07 $\pm$ 0.02
F2 (T60M20-20)	60	20	20	20	3.99 $\pm$ 0.02	0.68 $\pm$ 0.04
F3 (T40M40-20)	40	40	20	20	3.69 $\pm$ 0.01	1.61 $\pm$ 0.01
F4 (T80M0-40)	80	0	20	40	4.55 $\pm$ 0.05	1.04 $\pm$ 0.01
F5(T60M20-40)	60	20	20	40	4.64 $\pm$ 0.01	1.01 $\pm$ 0.01
F6 (T40M40-40)	40	40	20	40	4.36 $\pm$ 0.01	1.02 $\pm$ 0.01
F7 (T80M0-60)	80	0	20	60	4.81 $\pm$ 0.03	1.04 $\pm$ 0.01
F8 (T60M20-60)	60	20	20	60	4.55 $\pm$ 0.01	1.01 $\pm$ 0.01
F9 (T40M40-60)	40	40	20	60	4.41 $\pm$ 0.01	1.04 $\pm$ 0.01

VMD: The volume median diameters; SD: standard deviation.

2.3. Phage Powder Preparation

An aliquot of 5 mL of the phage stock was added to 45 mL excipient solution as prepared according to Table 1. The mixtures were spray dried using a Pilotech YC-500 spray dryer (Shanghai Pilotech Instruments and Equipment, Shanghai China) coupled with a high-performance cyclonic separator from Büchi (Buchi Labortechnik AG, Flawil, Switzerland) using an open-loop setting at a drying gas flow rate of 36 m^3/h, a liquid feed rate of 1.8 mL/min and an inlet temperature of 60 °C. The outlet temperature was ~45 °C. The produced powders were collected into scintillation vials and stored in a box with silica gel placed inside a humidity-controlled chamber (RH < 25%) at room temperature until use.

2.4. Particle Morphology

The morphologies of the spray-dried powders were examined using a field emission scanning electron microscope (SEM) (SU-8010, Hitachi, Tokyo, Japan) at 5 kV beam accelerating voltage. The samples were scattered on a carbon tape and sputter coated with 10 nm of gold using a Sputter Coater (Quorum Q150T ES) before imaging.

2.5. Particle Size Distribution

Particle size distributions of the powder formulations were measured by laser diffraction using a Laser Diffraction Particle Size Analyzer LS I3 320 (Beckman Coulter, Miami, FL, USA). Approximately 5 mg of powders were suspended in 7.5 mL of chloroform. The suspended particles were de-aggregated by sonication for five minutes. Immediately after de-aggregation, the suspension was added to the sample compartment dropwise until the optimal obscuration (8–12%) was reached. The stirrer was turned on to minimize aggregation. All measurements were done in triplicate. The size distribution was expressed by the volume median diameter (VMD), and span that defined as the difference in the particle diameters at D_{10} and D_{90} divided by the VMD (D_{10} and D_{90} are defined as the particle diameters at 10% and 90% cumulative volume, respectively).

2.6. Particle Crystallinity

The crystallinity of the produced phage powders and corresponding single excipient powders were examined using an X-ray diffractometer (Smartlab; Rigaku, Japan) under ambient conditions. Samples were spread on glass slides and subjected to Cu Kα radiation at 80 mA and 40 kV. The scattered intensity was collected by a detector for a 2θ range of 5–40° at an angular increment rate of 5° 2θ/min. The data were analyzed using JADE5 software (V.5.0; MaterialsData, Livermore, CA, USA).

2.7. Dynamic Vapor Sorption (DVS)

The moisture sorption profiles of the spray-dried phage powders were analyzed using a DVS instrument (DVS-Intrinsic, Surface Measurement Systems, London, UK). Approximately 5 mg phage powder was placed at RH 0% for vapor desorption for 4 h and the weight was used as the reference mass. The sample was then subjected to a moisture ramping cycle of 0–90% RH at a step increase of 10%. Equilibrium moisture content at each RH was defined at less than dm/dt of 0.02% per minute. The moisture sorption kinetics of the phage powders at 65% RH was also studied by measuring the mass change over a period of 24 h.

2.8. Thermal Analysis

The thermal properties of the phage powders were analyzed by modulated differential scanning calorimetry (mDSC) using DSC 25 equipped with a refrigerated cooling system (TA Instruments, New Castle, DE, USA) and thermogravimetric analysis (TGA) (TGA6, PerkinElmer, Waltham, MA, USA). mDSC measurement was performed on freshly prepared samples using DSC 25 equipped with a refrigerated cooling system. Approximately 4 mg of sample was weighed and sealed in a Tzero aluminum pan with a pinhole in the lid. Sample was equilibrated at −10 °C for 2 min, and then heated to 200 °C at a heating rate of 5 °C/min with modulation of ±1 °C every 60 s. Nitrogen was used as the purge gas at a flow rate of 50 mL/min. For TGA measurement each sample (5 ± 1 mg) was weighed in an alumina crucible and heated from 25 to 400 °C at a rate of 10 °C/min with dynamic nitrogen flow. The experiments were independently conducted twice.

2.9. In Vitro Aerosol Performance

The in vitro aerosol performance of the phage powders were evaluated according to the British Pharmacopoeia (2016) using a multistage liquid impinger (MSLI). For each dispersion, ~10 mg of phage powders were put into a size 3 hydroxypropyl methylcellulose capsule (Capsugel, NSW, Australia) in a humidity controlled chamber (<20% RH). The dispersion was performed using an Osmohaler^{TM} operated at 95 L/min for 2.5 s at room temperature and <35% RH. PBS was used as a rinsing solvent to determine the viable phage deposition profile by plaque assay. The experiment was performed in triplicate. The lower cutoff diameters of the MSLI stages 1–4 at 95 L/min are 10.33, 5.40, 2.46 and 1.35 μm, calculated with the adjustment equations given in Appendix XII C of the British Pharmacopoeia. The recovered rate was determined by the phage titer recovered from all parts (capsule, device, induction port and all the stages of the MSLI) compared with the loaded phage in the powders. The fine particle dose (FPD) of phage/sugar was defined as the phage/sugar recovered from particles with an aerodynamic diameter ≤5.0 μm. The fine particle fraction (FPF) was defined as the FPD with respect to the total recovered dose. To mimic the administration process of phage powder in high-humidity conditions, the capsulated phage powders were incubated in a high-humidity condition (65% RH) for 1 h, followed by the dispersion test described above.

2.10. Quantification of Trehalose by HPLC

The deposition of trehalose at the capsule, inhaler, adaptor and each part of the MSLI was determined using a UPLC system (Model Code CHA D16CHA036G; Waters, Milford, MA, USA) using RI detection. The configuration consisted of an Acquity series of quaternary solvent manager, column manager, RI detector, sample manager-FTN, and Empower® software. An amino acid column (Phenomenex Luna NH_2, 3 μm, 100 Å, 150 × 2 mm) was used. The mobile phase was a mixture of water (30%) and acetonitrile (70%). A volume of 300 μL dispersion sample was mixed with 700 μL acetonitrile before HPLC analysis. The calibration curve for trehalose was linear in the concentration range of 0.05–0.2 mg/mL ($R^2 = 0.999$, $n = 3$).

2.11. Phage Stability in Powder

The concentrations of viable phage in the powder samples immediately after preparation and after storage were determined [32]. Phage powders were first dissolved in PBS to a final concentration of the corresponding total solid content before spray drying. Serial dilutions of the solution samples were performed by adding 20 μL sample to 180 μL PBS. A volume of 150 μL overnight cultured host bacteria was mixed with 4 mL molten soft agar (0.7% agar, 50 °C). The mixture was overlayed onto a solidified NB agar plate made of 1.5% agar (AGAR NO.1, OXOID, Hampshire, UK) and Nutrient Broth (NB, OXOID, Hampshire, UK). Then, 10 μL of diluted phage samples were dropped onto the agar lawn and left to air dry for 30 min, and the plates were incubated overnight at 37 °C. Samples that gave rise to 3–30 pfu were used to determine the phage titer. The phage stability test was performed at 20, 45 days, 2, 3 and 6 months after preparation.

2.12. Statistical Analysis

The analysis of each response of factorial design (stability, FPF and FPF decreased after exposure to the high-humidity condition) was performed in Design Expert software version 12.0.1.0 using Quadratic modeling. One-way analysis of variance (ANOVA) and Fisher pairwise comparison using Minitab were employed to identify any statistically significant differences in production and storage loss, and FPF of phage. A p value of <0.05 was considered statistically significant.

3. Results

3.1. Production Loss AB406 Phage

The viability of AB406 phage immediately after the powder preparation was determined to calculate the production loss (Figure 1). All phage powder formulations noted a titer reduction ranged 0.3–0.5 log. The results were consistent with previous studies evaluating other phages [16,33–35]. ANOVA analysis showed no significant differences between formulations with different compositions and total solid contents. Both trehalose–leucine and trehalose–mannitol–leucine systems could effectively protect AB406 phage from the thermal and dehydration stresses in the spray-drying process.

3.2. Phage and Particle Morphology

Figure 2 shows the SEM images of the spray-dried phage powders. Particles were generally spherical with a wrinkled surface. Significant particle merging was noted for formulations containing no mannitol (F1, F4 and F7) or 20% mannitol (F2, F5, and F8). On the other hand, the addition of a higher portion of mannitol (40%) to the formulations (F3, F6 and F9) could reduce the degree of particle merging. Due to the high-humidity environment in Hong Kong, exposing the produced powders to high humidity during sample collection upon powder production or during sprinkling powders to the carbon tape and golden coating procedure for SEM sample preparation for a short period of time was inevitable. Whether the particle merging was arising from the powder production process or upon the sample preparation for SEM imaging was unclear. Nonetheless, these results were consistent with our previous studies on *Pseudomonas* phage powder [16,17], even though the amount of PBS in the produced *Acinetobacter* phage powders was 10 times higher. From the SEM images, there was no difference noted between formulations prepared from different total solid contents.

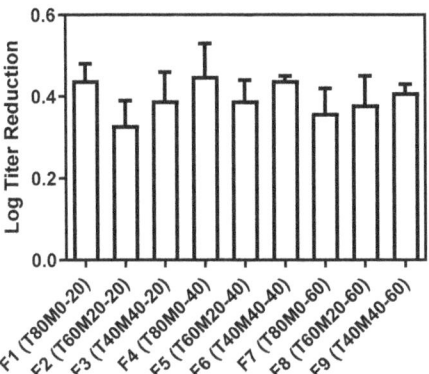

Figure 1. Production loss of AB406 phage in the spray-drying process. Data presented as mean ± standard deviation ($n = 3$).

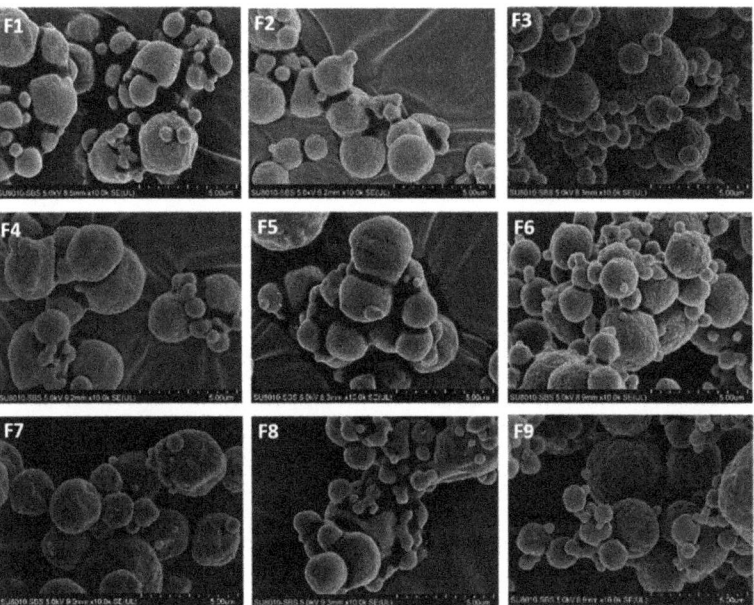

Figure 2. Representative SEM images of F1–F9 (5 μm scale bar).

3.3. Particle Size

The VMD and span of the particles are presented in Table 1. From the result, most particles falling within the inhalable size fraction of less than 5 μm, consistent with the SEM images. With the same total solid content, the formulation with higher mannitol content has a slightly smaller particle size ($p < 0.05$). This is possibly due to the different composition change the surface tension of the liquid feed [36,37], resulting in slightly different droplet sizes and, hence, different particles sizes. With the same excipient composition, the particle size generally increased with increasing total solid content. Although the difference is statistically significant ($p < 0.05$), the variation was very minor due to the small increase in the total solid content.

3.4. Powder Crystallinity

The XRD patterns of fresh phage powders (F1–F3) and spray-dried trehalose, mannitol and leucine are depicted in Figure 3. No significant differences were noted for formulations containing the same composition prepared from various total solid content (Figure S2). From the XRD result, the peak at $2\theta = 6°$ was the primary peak for leucine which is consistent with previous study [38,39]. Except this peak, the peaks at 2θ of 18°, 24°, 29°, 30° and 32° appeared in all formulations with similar intensity, indicating the presence of crystalline leucine. Spray-dried trehalose showed a halo pattern which is a typical XRD profile for amorphous materials, confirming that the spray-dried trehalose is amorphous. The appearance of distinct peaks in the formulations of 40% mannitol are corresponding to the α-form and β-form of mannitol crystals. This was consistent with Kaialy et al. that the XRD profile of α–mannitol specific peaks at 2θ of 10°, 14° and 17° and β–mannitol specific peaks at 2θ of 11°, 15°, 23° and 30° [40].

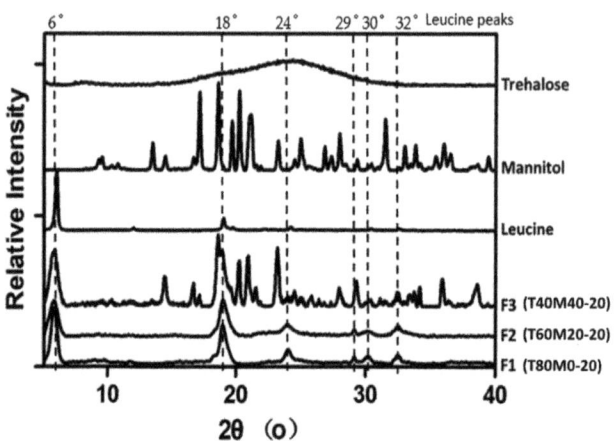

Figure 3. XRD profiles of the spray-dried formulations F1 to F3 and corresponding excipient.

3.5. Residual Moisture Content and Glass Transition Temperature

We next measured the residual moisture content and Tg of the produced powders using TGA and mDSC, respectively (Table 2). The residual moisture content was determined from the TGA profiles (Figure S1) as the mass loss between 25 °C to 100 °C where solvent evaporation occurs. The spray-dried powders had a moisture content of 2–4%, irrespective of the formulation compositions and total solid contents. From the mDSC curves (Figure 4), a glass transition temperature was noted for all nine phage powder formulations and the same excipient compositions resulted in comparable Tg. The Tg of spray-dried phage powders with 80% trehalose and 20% leucine was ~110 °C and it dropped rapidly to ~45 °C and ~15 °C as the trehalose content decreased to 60% and 40%.

3.6. Moisture Sorption

Figure 5A shows the moisture sorption profiles of the phage powders as the RH increased from 0 to 90% at 25 °C. The total solid content did not show a strong influence on the powder moisture sorption ability in low-humidity conditions (≤60% RH) for formulations with the same compositions. Beyond 70% RH, formulations prepared from a lower total solid content tended to have a higher moisture sorption capacity. Formulations containing 80% and 60% trehalose showed the occurrence of recrystallization between 40–60% RH, consistent with our previous study [17], but no recrystallization peak was noted for formulation containing in 40% trehalose, 40% mannitol and 20% leucine. Kinetics of water vapor sorption of F1–F9 under 65% RH at 25 °C were also investigated (Figure 5B). The data revealed that trehalose recrystallization, indicated by the overshoot of change in mass %, took place within 60 min of exposure. The maximum moisture uptake of the spray-dried powders generally increased with decreasing total solid content for formulations with the same composition. With the same total solid content, formulations with 20% mannitol had the highest moisture capacity, agreeing with our previous findings that a small portion of mannitol promotes the recrystallization of trehalose [16,17].

Table 2. Residual moisture content and glass transition temperature of F1–F9.

Formulation	Residual Moisture Content (%)	T_g (°C)
F1 (T80M0-20)	2.93	110.76
F2 (T60M20-20)	1.91	44.82
F3 (T40M40-20)	2.55	15.97
F4 (T80M0-40)	2.57	112.22
F5(T60M20-40)	2.34	45.32
F6 (T40M40-40)	1.77	17.04
F7 (T80M0-60)	3.12	112.95
F8 (T60M20-60)	3.49	45.54
F9 (T40M40-60)	2.77	16.77

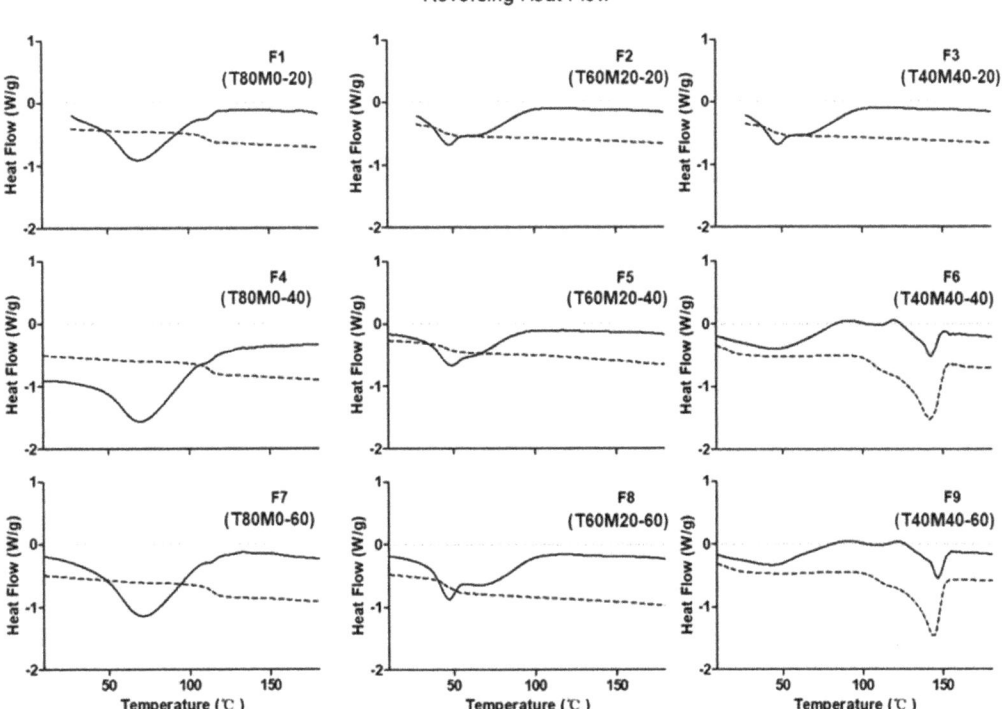

Figure 4. mDSC traces of the spray-dried formulations.

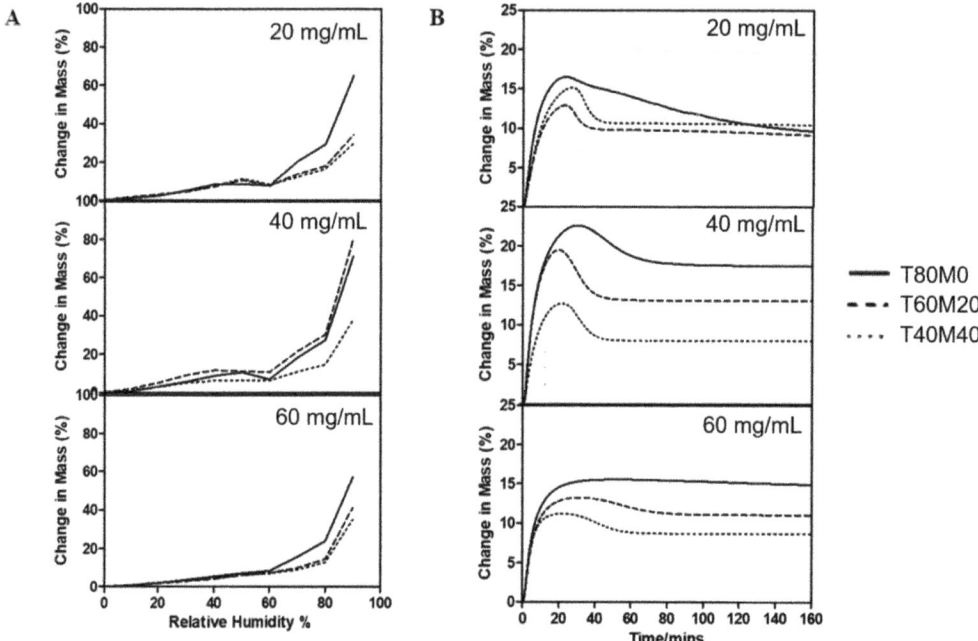

Figure 5. (**A**) DVS traces of F1–F9 as RH increased from 0 to 90% and (**B**) kinetics of water vapor sorption of F1–F9 under 65% RH at 25 °C.

3.7. In Vitro Aerosol Performance and the Effect of High Humidity

The recovery rate and FPF based on the recovered dose of the viable phage and trehalose for F1–F9 after dispersing with an Osmohaler™ at 95 L/min for 2.5 s in the normal (23 °C, <35% RH) and high-humidity conditions (23 °C, after incubating at 65% RH for 1 h) are depicted in Figures 6 and 7, respectively. The deposition profiles of recovered viable phage for all formulations were provided in Figures S3 and S4. As seen in Figures 6A and 7A, the recovery rates of trehalose were in the range of 90–110%, validating the appropriateness of the dispersion experiments. However, the recovery rates of phage for all formulations were <50% for both dispersion conditions, similar to our previous reports [16–18]. Under the normal dispersion condition (minimum exposure to humid air), the aerosol performance of the spray-dried powders were found to be formulation composition and total solid content dependent. Higher FPF was observed in formulations prepared with higher mannitol and lower total solid contents. Among all formulations, F3 gave the higher FPF value of 37% among all formulations studied.

After exposing the phage powders to 65% RH for 1 h, the phage recovery for all formulations dropped around 8% to 10% ($p < 0.05$), with no specific trends on the impacts of formulation composition and total solid content noted. On the other hand, their impacts on the FPF were found to be composition dependent. The extent of FPF reduction in formulations containing trehalose and leucine only (F1, F4 and F7) was the smallest ($p < 0.05$) among the three compositions studied (by ~5%), followed by formulations containing 40% mannitol (F3, F6 and F9, by 15% with $p < 0.01$). A very sharp drop (>30%) occurred for formulations containing in 20% mannitol (F2, F5 and F8, with $p < 0.01$). Overall, both the FPF of trehalose and phage reduced compared with powder dispersed in normal conditions.

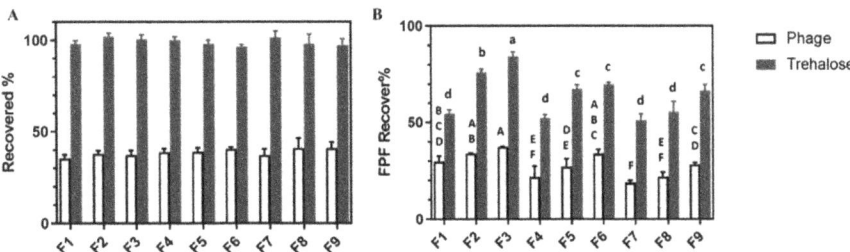

Figure 6. (**A**) The recovered rate and (**B**) the FPF of F1–F9. Data presented as mean ± standard deviation (*n* = 3). Column data marked with different letters indicate significant difference (*p* < 0.05). Uppercase and lowercase letters refer to the comparison of phage and trehalose, respectively.

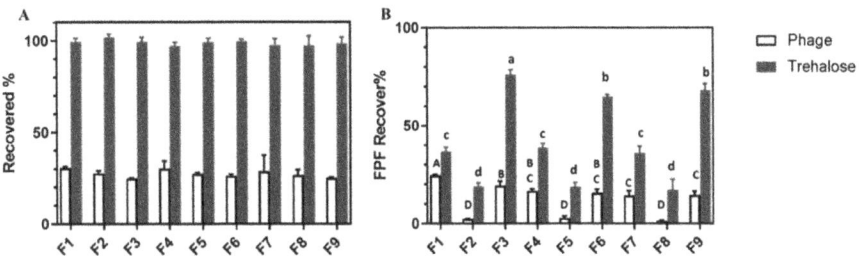

Figure 7. (**A**) The recovered rate and (**B**) the FPF of F1–F9 under 65% RH. Data presented as mean ± standard deviation (*n* = 3). Column data marked with different letters indicate significant difference (*p* < 0.05). Uppercase and lowercase letters refer to the comparison of phage and trehalose, respectively.

3.8. Phage Storage Stability

Since dry powder inhaler products are usually transported, stored and administrated at room temperature, sufficient storage stability of phage powder preparations at room condition is essential. The titer reduction of phage powders after storing at room temperature under desiccation was determined relative to the titer measured in the fresh powder periodically (Figure 8). After a 6-month storage period, a titer loss ranging from 0.5 to 1.8 log was noted. The stabilization of phage in the powder form depended on the formulation compositions as well as the total solid contents. Phages were gradually deactivated with time for formulations containing trehalose (80%) and leucine (20%) only (F1, F4 and F7) regardless of the total solid contents. Their titer reduction upon storage was being more profound compared with formulations containing mannitol (*p* < 0.01). Overall, formulations prepared from the lowest total solid content (20 mg/mL F1–F3) failed to stabilize the incorporated phage as continuous reduction in the phage titer was noted throughout the storage period. These findings were different from our previous observation with *Pseudomonas* phages (PEV2 and PEV40), for which only 1 log titer reduction in 12 month storage [18]. For higher total solid contents, formulations containing 40% trehalose, 40% mannitol and 20% leucine (F6 and F9) provided better storage stability of phage that no-further phage loss after 1 month and <1 log storage loss was noted. Similar findings were reported by Chang et al. that higher total solid content of excipients would minimize the phage titer reduction after spray drying [21].

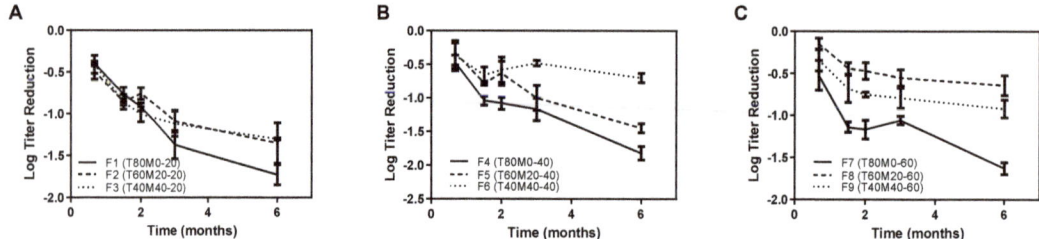

Figure 8. Titer reduction of phage in spray-dried powders after storage at room temperature and RH < 20% relative to titer measured in the fresh powder. (**A**) F1–F3 at a total solid content of 20 mg/mL; (**B**) F4–F6 at a total solid content of 40 mg/mL; and (**C**) F7–F9 at a total solid content of 60 mg/mL.

3.9. Response Surface Methodology Analysis

Response surface methodology (RSM) with a quadratic design model was used to evaluate the relationship between the independent variables (trehalose to mannitol ratio and total solid content) and three selected responses, storage stability, FPF at normal dispersion conditions and FPF reduction after powders incubating in high-humidity conditions. The three-dimensional response surface graphs and corresponding two-dimensional contour plots generated by Design-Expert software are shown in Figure 9. The results indicated that the storage stability and FPF value of phage had linear relationships with the trehalose to mannitol ratio and total solid content. However, a nonlinear relationship between the two independent factors was presented in the FPF reduction of phage.

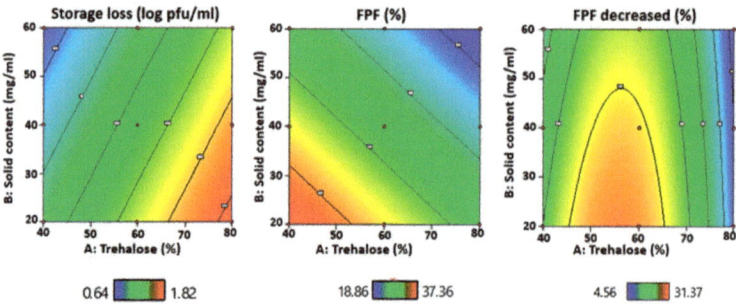

Figure 9. Response surface graphs depicting the influences of the percentage of trehalose and total solid content on the storage stability, FPF of phage and reduction of FPF of phage after incubating in high-humidity conditions.

4. Discussion

Disaccharide sugars were reported to play an important role in stabilizing phage in solid-state formulations with trehalose, sucrose and lactose being the most superior sugars in protecting phage from stresses generated during solidification. Water replacement (replacing water to network with phage via hydrogen bonding to avoid phage protein aggregation) and/or vitrification (immobilizing the phage protein in a glassy matrix) are the two leading hypotheses accounting for their stabilization of proteins/phage in solid-state. Trehalose was chosen for our study because it has a slightly higher glass transition temperature (115 °C) compared with lactose (101 °C) and sucrose (60 °C) [41]. Additionally, more consistent stabilization effects on phage by trehalose were reported in the literature [16–18]. In contrast, discrepancies on the ability of lactose in stabilizing phage in the powder form were reported in the literature. While Chang et al. reported a lactose-leucine binary system could stabilize phage in the powder form [21], Vandenheuvel et al. demonstrated that lactose-only formulations were not able to maintain phage viability [20].

In addition, lactose may cause chemical degradation of proteins via the Maillard reaction which may not be favorable for the long-term storage of phage [42]. Previous reports showing mannitol alone was detrimental to phage [17,43], but the addition of a certain amount of mannitol to the trehalose–leucine system could significantly improve the power properties with less particle merging upon handling and showed no negative impacts on the storage stability of the phage [17]. However, it appeared to have an optimal trehalose-to-mannitol ratio to preserve phage in the powder form. Here, we studied the impacts of this ratio on the stability and aerosol performance of AB406 phage powders. The main reason for adding leucine in dry powder formulations is to improve the dispersibility of the powders, but recent studies showed that a small amount of leucine is needed to improve phage stability in spray-dried powders [21]. The surface-active L-leucine would tend to enrich at the particle surface to minimize the migration of phage to the air–liquid interface during the spray-drying process [39], protecting phage from surface inactivation [44]. In addition, the L-leucine would delay moisture sorption immediately after the powder formed, maintaining the powders in the amorphous form, which is essential for phage stabilization, upon sample collection [21]. Based on previous findings, 20% leucine would be sufficient in ensuring the stability of phage with acceptable dispersibility [21], though it was insufficient to form a continuous shell of crystal leucine on the surface [45]. Similar findings were reported for systems with higher leucine content (up to 40%) [18]. Therefore, we fixed the leucine content to 20% of the total solid content in the present study.

Figure 1 shows minimum titer reduction upon the powder production for all formulations (≤ 0.5 log). The data also agree with our previous findings on *Pseudomonas* phage that a portion up to 40% mannitol in the trehalose-mannitol-leucine systems did not result in more titer loss in spray drying [16,17]. On the other hand, the storage loss of AB406 phage obtained in the present study (Figure 8) were higher than the *Pseudomonas* phage noted in our previous study [18]. It is noteworthy that the mixing ratio of phage suspended in PBS to the excipient solution was 1:9 in the present study, 10 times higher than those used in our previous studies [16–18]. The employed higher phage suspension mixing ratio was originally aimed to increase the phage lung dose for effective treatment. However, the results suggested that a higher amount of residual salt might impair the storage stability of phage. Further investigation is needed to fully understand the effect of salts on the storage stability of phage in powder form.

To stabilize phage during storage in the dried state, it is necessary to remove enough water to immobilize phage inside a non-crystalline glassy sugar matrix. Thus, the glass transition temperature (Tg) is a key parameter for phage stability in the powder form. Recently, Chang et al. investigated the stabilization mechanisms of phages in spray-dried powders [46]. Their results showed that keeping the storage temperatures (Ts) at least ~46 °C below Tg (i.e., Tg–Ts $\geq$ 46 °C) will be essential for phage stabilization. Two factors, the residual moisture content and the incorporation of mannitol, were reported to affect the Tg of trehalose [47] and were investigated. According to Table 2, the residual moisture in all powder formulations were within the optimal range, 3–6%, for phage preservation identified in previous studies [48,49]. Due to the plasticizing effect of water, the Tg of amorphous solid samples were shown to decrease linearly with increasing moisture content [47,50]. However, our results showed that formulations with the same excipient compositions had comparable Tg in spite of their different residual moisture content. The disparity from previous reports might be attributed to the insensitivity of the TGA analysis in differentiating the removal of free water and bound water from the powders in determining the residual moisture. Nonetheless, the TGA analysis confirming there was a low level of water content left in the powders after the spray-drying process. Surprisingly, formulations with 40% trehalose, 40% mannitol and 20% leucine (F3, F6 and F9) had a Tg (~15 °C) lower than the storage temperature (22 °C), but they exhibited superior stabilization effect of the embedded *Acinetobacter* phage after 6 months of storage in low-humidity conditions (<20% RH) (Figure 8). Formulations with the highest trehalose content (F1, F4 and F7) had the storage temperature well below the Tg (Tg–Ts ~90 °C) showing a gradual decrease in phage titer during the storage period. These were different from the greater phage stability in systems with higher Tg as reported in Chang et al. [46]. Cleland et al. reported that high Tg disaccharides might be inefficient in preventing the incorporated proteins from unfolding during dehydration, but adding mannitol to disaccharides (trehalose and sucrose) inhibited aggregation and deamidation during storage to a greater extent than the disaccharide alone systems [51]. This may explain the better storage stability of AB406 in systems with mannitol, despite they have a lower Tg.

Both the size measurements (Table 1) and SEM images (Figure 2) of the produced phage powders showed that most of the particles of all nine formulations were well within the inhalable range. The in vitro aerosol performance of the produced powders, on the basis of the FPF values of sugars ($\geq$50%), also confirmed that they were suitable for pulmonary delivery. Comparing with the sugar excipients, the recovery rate of viable phage was apparently lower even under the normal dispersion condition (Figure 6A). It was likely accounted by the deactivation of phage upon impaction to the inhaler walls during the dispersing process. Apart from the lower recovery of phage, the FPF of phage was also consistently lower than that of the trehalose, but the overall trends in response to the formulation compositions and total solid contents were similar (Figure 6B), suggesting the even distribution of phage within the particles. According to Figure 6B, the FPF value increased with increasing mannitol content. This was likely because the addition of mannitol help minimizing the degree of particle merging upon powder preparation, handling and, hence, dispersion. It might also be accounted by the slightly smaller particle size of the phage powders with higher mannitol content. Similarly, the smaller particle size of the phage powders prepared from the lower total amount of excipients might attributed to their slightly higher FPF. It is worth noting that the FPD of the nine formulations were in the order of 10^6 to 10^7 pfu which were comparable to previous studies on *Pseudomonas* phages [18,21]. The effectiveness of phage powders yielding similar lung dose in treating bacterial lung infection was confirmed in a murine model [22]. Therefore, the promising findings in the *Acinetobacter* phage powders warrant further evaluation on its therapeutic effects in vivo.

The XRD traces confirmed the produced powders were partially amorphous with the crystallinity increase with increasing mannitol content. Amorphous powders are thermodynamically unstable and have a high risk of recrystallization when exposed to moisture, inactivating the embedded phage [21]. To ensure the developed phage powder products are stable in different geographic locations all over the world, powder stability in high-humidity conditions should be considered during formulation development. It is feasible for the final phage product to be manufactured, transported and stored in relatively low-humidity conditions. However, an excellent formulation should also be user friendly for patients and tolerate high-humidity conditions for a reasonable time. To identify an optimal formulation suitable for global distribution, we also investigated the in vitro aerosol performance of phage powders after incubating at 65% RH for 1 h. As shown in DVS profiles (Figure 5), recrystallization takes place at 65% RH within 1 h, the recovery rate of phage and the number of particles able to reach deeper into the lungs (FPF) was expected to decrease after incubating in high-humidity conditions [39], and this was confirmed in Figure 7. As both the FPF of trehalose and phage dropped significantly, the recrystallization of the amorphous content might also lead to the formation of solid bridges between particles [21], making the powders more difficult to dispersed and hence a lower FPF. Overall, the total solid content showed minimum impacts on the FPF of phage, despite the moisture sorption capacity varied. However, the dispersion profiles of phage powders after incubating in high-humidity conditions strongly depend on the formulation compositions. The lung dose of phage powders (both sugars and phage) of formulations with 20% mannitol significantly reduced, while moderate reduction was noted in those contain no or 40% mannitol. These data are largely correlated with the moisture sorption kinetics of the phage powders that formulations with the presence of a small amount of mannitol promote uptake of moisture (Figure 5) and the extent of particle merging noted in the SEM images (Figure 2).

RSM has been a common approach to optimize pharmaceutical formulation [52]. However, the linear relationships noted in the storage loss and FPF in normal dispersion conditions with the studied formulation parameters suggested a higher mannitol content ($\geq$40%) might be beneficial for AB406 phage powder preparation. According to our previous study on *Pseudomonas* phage [17], a mannitol content of 60% would cause significant titer loss compared with formulation with 40% mannitol. Therefore, we postulated the optimal mannitol fraction would lie between 40% to 60%. While further experiments are required to confirm this, F6 had 0.70 log pfu/mL titer loss after a 6-month storage period, a 34% FPF and 18% FPF reduction after incubation at 65% RH for 1 h, and is a promising formulation for further in vivo evaluation.

5. Conclusions

In summary, the influences of formulation composition and total solid content on the physicochemical properties, stability and dispersibility of spray-dried AB406 phage powders were studied. A better powder morphology was observed in the formulation with the higher mannitol percentage (40% mannitol irrespective of the total solid content ranged 20–60 mg/mL). Formulations containing the highest amount of mannitol provided the best storage stability of phage; there was no further phage loss after 1 month, with the higher total solid content resulting in lower storage loss (<1 log). The higher mannitol content was also showed to enhance powder dispersibility. The exposure of phage powders to a high-humidity environment for a short time was found to reduce the phage recovery rate and the FPF due to the recrystallization of amorphous content inactivating the embedded phage. Our results confirmed previous knowledge attained for phage powder preparation could be extended for the preparation of *Acinetobacter* phage with further investigation on the impact of PBS in the final phage powder needed. This is the first report evaluating the impacts of environmental humidity on the dispersion of phage powders, and our findings suggest that this is a factor that may need to be taken into consideration during formulation optimization.

Supplementary Materials: The following are available online at https://www.mdpi.com/article/10.3390/pharmaceutics13081162/s1, Figure S1: TGA profiles of the spray-dried formulations. (A) F1, F4 and F7 at a formulation composition of 80% trehalose, 20% leucine; (B) F2, F5 and F8 at a formulation composition of 60% trehalose, 20% mannitol and 20% leucine; and (C) F3, F6 and F9 at a formulation composition of 40% trehalose, 40% mannitol and 20% leucine, Figure S2: XRD profiles of the spray-dried formulations, Figure S3: The distribution profiles of viable AB406 phage, Figure S4: The distribution profiles of viable AB406 phage under 65% RH.

Author Contributions: Conceptualization, W.Y. and S.S.Y.L.; resources (phage isolation, purification and characterization): Y.L., Y.T.; methodology, W.Y. and B.T.; data curation, W.Y., R.H., X.T. and B.T.; validation, W.Y., R.H., X.T. and B.T.; formal analysis, W.Y. and S.S.Y.L.; data curation, W.Y.; writing—original draft preparation, W.Y.; writing—review and editing, Y.L., Y.T., K.K.W.T. and S.S.Y.L.; supervision, K.K.W.T. and S.S.Y.L. All authors have read and agreed to the published version of the manuscript.

Funding: This research was funded by University Grants Committee Hong Kong, grant number 24300619.

Institutional Review Board Statement: Not applicable.

Informed Consent Statement: Not applicable.

Data Availability Statement: Not applicable.

Acknowledgments: The authors gratefully acknowledge the provision of graduate studentship to W.Y.

Conflicts of Interest: The authors declare no conflict of interest. The authors alone are responsible for the content and writing of this article. The company Livzon Pharmaceutical Group Co., Ltd had no role in the design of the study; in the collection, analyses, or interpretation of data; in the writing of the manuscript, or in the decision to publish the results.

References

1. Gootz, T.D. The global problem of antibiotic resistance. *Crit. Rev. Immunol.* **2010**, *30*, 79–93. [CrossRef]
2. World Health Organization. Global Priority List of Antibiotic-Resistant Bacteria to Guide Research, Discovery, and Development of New Antibiotics. 2017. Available online: https://www.who.int/medicines/publications/global-priority-list-antibiotic-resistant-bacteria/en/ (accessed on 18 February 2020).
3. Czaplewski, L.; Bax, R.; Clokie, M.; Dawson, M.; Fairhead, H.; Fischetti, V.A.; Foster, S.; Gilmore, B.F.; Hancock, R.E.W.; Harper, D.; et al. Alternatives to antibiotics—A pipeline portfolio review. *Lancet Infect. Dis.* **2016**, *16*, 239–251. [CrossRef]
4. Durdu, B.; Kritsotakis, E.I.; Lee, A.C.; Torun, P.; Hakyemez, I.N.; Gultepe, B.; Aslan, T. Temporal trends and patterns in antimicrobial-resistant Gram-negative bacteria implicated in intensive care unit-acquired infections: A cohort-based surveillance study in Istanbul, Turkey. *J. Glob. Antimicrob. Resist.* **2018**, *14*, 190–196. [CrossRef]
5. Falagas, M.E.; Rafailidis, P.I. Attributable mortality of *Acinetobacter baumannii*: No longer a controversial issue. *Crit. Care* **2007**, *11*, 134. [CrossRef] [PubMed]
6. Elizabeth, K.; Jan, B.; Ryszard, M.; Andrzej, G.; Beata, W.-D.; Mzia, K.; Zemphira, A.; Marina, G.; Revaz, A. Clinical phage therapy. In *Phage Therapy: Current Research and Applications*; Caister Academic Press: Norfolk, UK, 2014; Volumes 257–288.
7. Schooley, R.T.; Biswas, B.; Gill, J.J.; Morales, A.C.H.; Lancaster, J.; Lessor, L.; Barr, J.J.; Reed, S.L.; Rohwer, F.; Benler, S.; et al. Development and use of personalized bacteriophage-based therapeutic cocktails to treat a patient with a disseminated resistant acinetobacter baumannii infection. *Antimicrob. Agents Chemother.* **2017**, *61*. [CrossRef] [PubMed]
8. Lavergne, S.; Hamilton, T.; Biswas, B.; Kumaraswamy, M.; Schooley, R.T.; Wooten, D. Phage therapy for a multidrug-resistant acinetobacter baumannii craniectomy site infection. *Open Forum Infect. Dis.* **2018**, *5*, ofy064. [CrossRef]
9. Strathdee, S.A.; Patterson, T.L.; Barker, T. *The Perfect Predator: A Scientist's Race to Save Her Husband from a Deadly Superbug*, 1st ed.; Hachette Books: New York, NY, USA; Boston, MA, USA, 2019.
10. Hua, Y.; Luo, T.; Yang, Y.; Dong, D.; Wang, R.; Wang, Y.; Xu, M.; Guo, X.-K.; Hu, F.; He, P. Phage therapy as a promising new treatment for lung infection caused by carbapenem-resistant *Acinetobacter baumannii* in mice. *Front. Microbiol.* **2018**, *8*, 2659. [CrossRef]
11. Wang, Y.; Mi, Z.; Niu, W.; An, X.; Yuan, X.; Liu, H.; Li, P.; Liu, Y.; Feng, Y.; Huang, Y.; et al. Intranasal treatment with bacteriophage rescues mice from *Acinetobacter baumannii*-mediated pneumonia. *Future Microbiol.* **2016**, *11*, 631–641. [CrossRef]
12. Jeon, J.; Park, J.-H.; Yong, D. Efficacy of bacteriophage treatment against carbapenem-resistant *Acinetobacter baumannii* in Galleria mellonella larvae and a mouse model of acute pneumonia. *BMC Microbiol.* **2019**, *19*, 70. [CrossRef]
13. Cha, K.; Oh, H.K.; Jang, J.Y.; Jo, Y.; Kim, W.K.; Ha, G.U.; Ko, K.S.; Myung, H. Characterization of two novel bacteriophages infecting multidrug-resistant (MDR) *Acinetobacter baumannii* and evaluation of their therapeutic efficacy in vivo. *Front. Microbiol.* **2018**, *9*, 696. [CrossRef]
14. Wienhold, S.-M.; Brack, M.C.; Nouailles, G.; Suttorp, N.W.; Seitz, C.; Ross, A.; Ziehr, H.; Gurtner, C.; Kershaw, O.; Dietert, K.; et al. Witzenrath, intratracheal phage therapy against acinetobacter baumannii lung infection in mice. In *D107. Host Pathogen Interactions*; 2018; A7571.
15. Zhou, Q.; Tang, P.; Leung, S.S.Y.; Chan, J.G.Y.; Chan, H.-K. Emerging inhalation aerosol devices and strategies: Where are we headed? *Adv. Drug Deliv. Rev.* **2014**, *75*, 3–17. [CrossRef]
16. Leung, S.; Parumasivan, T.; Gao, F.G.; Carrigy, N.B.; Vehring, R.; Finlay, W.H.; Morales, S.; Britton, W.J.; Kutter, E.; Chan, H.-K. Production of inhalation phage powders using spray freeze drying and spray drying techniques for treatment of respiratory infections. *Pharm. Res.* **2016**, *33*, 1486–1496. [CrossRef]
17. Leung, S.; Parumasivan, T.; Gao, F.G.; Carter, E.; Carrigy, N.B.; Vehring, R.; Finlay, W.H.; Morales, S.; Britton, W.J.; Kutter, E.; et al. Effects of storage conditions on the stability of spray dried, inhalable bacteriophage powders. *Int. J. Pharm.* **2017**, *521*, 141–149. [CrossRef]
18. Leung, S.; Parumasivan, T.; Nguyen, A.; Gengenbach, T.; Carter, E.; Carrigy, N.B.; Wang, H.; Vehring, R.; Finlay, W.H.; Morales, S.; et al. Effect of storage temperature on the stability of spray dried bacteriophage powders. *Eur. J. Pharm. Biopharm.* **2018**, *127*, 213–222. [CrossRef]
19. Matinkhoo, S.; Lynch, K.H.; Dennis, J.; Finlay, W.H.; Vehring, R. Spray-dried respirable powders containing bacteriophages for the treatment of pulmonary infections. *J. Pharm. Sci.* **2011**, *100*, 5197–5205. [CrossRef]
20. Vandenheuvel, D.; Singh, A.; Vandersteegen, K.; Klumpp, J.; Lavigne, R.; Mooter, G.V.D. Feasibility of spray drying bacteriophages into respirable powders to combat pulmonary bacterial infections. *Eur. J. Pharm. Biopharm.* **2013**, *84*, 578–582. [CrossRef] [PubMed]
21. Chang, R.Y.K.; Wong, J.; Mathai, A.; Morales, S.; Kutter, E.; Britton, W.; Li, J.; Chan, H.-K. Production of highly stable spray dried phage formulations for treatment of Pseudomonas aeruginosa lung infection. *Eur. J. Pharm. Biopharm.* **2017**, *121*, 1–13. [CrossRef] [PubMed]

22. Chang, R.Y.K.; Chen, K.; Wang, J.; Wallin, M.; Britton, W.; Morales, S.; Kutter, E.; Li, J.; Chan, H.-K. Proof-of-principle study in a murine lung infection model of antipseudomonal activity of phage PEV20 in a dry-powder formulation. *Antimicrob. Agents Chemother.* **2018**, *62*, e01714-17. [CrossRef] [PubMed]

23. Vandenheuvel, D.; Meeus, J.; Lavigne, R.; Mooter, G.V.D. Instability of bacteriophages in spray-dried trehalose powders is caused by crystallization of the matrix. *Int. J. Pharm.* **2014**, *472*, 202–205. [CrossRef]

24. STAT 503, PennState Stat. Lesson 9: 3-Level and Mixed-Level Factorials and Fractional Factorials. Available online: https://online.stat.psu.edu/stat503/lesson/9 (accessed on 12 January 2021).

25. Chan, P.K.; Mok, H.; Lee, T.; Chu, I.M.; Lam, W.-Y.; Sung, J.J.Y. Seasonal influenza activity in Hong Kong and its association with meteorological variations. *J. Med. Virol.* **2009**, *81*, 1797–1806. [CrossRef]

26. Brooks, R.T.; Kyker-Snowman, T.D. Forest floor temperature and relative humidity following timber harvesting in southern New England, USA. *For. Ecol. Manag.* **2008**, *254*, 65–73. [CrossRef]

27. Current Results. Average Humidity by US State. Available online: https://www.currentresults.com/Weather/US/annual-average-humidity-by-state.php (accessed on 12 January 2021).

28. Procedures and Protocols. The Actinobacteriophage Database. Available online: https://phagesdb.org/workflow/ (accessed on 14 September 2020).

29. Adriaenssens, E.M.; Lehman, S.M.; Vandersteegen, K.; Vandenheuvel, D.; Philippe, D.L.; Cornelissen, A.; Clokie, M.R.; García, A.J.; De Proft, M.; Maes, M.; et al. CIM® monolithic anion-exchange chromatography as a useful alternative to CsCl gradient purification of bacteriophage particles. *Virology* **2012**, *434*, 265–270. [CrossRef] [PubMed]

30. Zimmer, F.; Souza, A.; Silveira, A.; Santos, M.; Matsushita, M.; Souza, N.; Rodrigues, A. Application of factorial design for optimization of the synthesis of lactulose obtained from whey permeate. *J. Braz. Chem. Soc.* **2017**. [CrossRef]

31. Malcolmson, R.J.; Embleton, J.K. Dry powder formulations for pulmonary delivery. *Pharm. Sci. Technol. Today* **1998**, *1*, 394–398. [CrossRef]

32. Kutter, E.; Sulakvelidze, A. Bacteriophages: Biology and Applications. CRC Press: Boca Raton, FL, USA, 2004.

33. Dini, C.; De Urraza, P. Effect of buffer systems and disaccharides concentration on Podoviridae coliphage stability during freeze drying and storage. *Cryobiology* **2013**, *66*, 339–342. [CrossRef]

34. Merabishvili, M.; Vervaet, C.; Pirnay, J.-P.; De Vos, D.; Verbeken, G.; Mast, J.; Chanishvili, N.; Vaneechoutte, M. Stability of staphylococcus aureus phage ISP after freeze-drying (lyophilization). *PLoS ONE* **2013**, *8*, e68797. [CrossRef]

35. Carrigy, N.; Liang, L.; Wang, H.; Kariuki, S.; Nagel, T.E.; Connerton, I.; Vehring, R. Spray-dried anti-Campylobacter bacteriophage CP30A powder suitable for global distribution without cold chain infrastructure. *Int. J. Pharm.* **2019**, *569*, 118601. [CrossRef] [PubMed]

36. Kulkarni, S.S.; Suryanarayanan, R.; Rinella, J.V.; Bogner, R.H. Mechanisms by which crystalline mannitol improves the reconstitution time of high concentration lyophilized protein formulations. *Eur. J. Pharm. Biopharm.* **2018**, *131*, 70–81. [CrossRef]

37. Mandato, S.; Rondet, E.; Delaplace, G.; Barkouti, A.; Galet, L.; Accart, P.; Ruiz, T.; Cuq, B. Liquids' atomization with two different nozzles: Modeling of the effects of some processing and formulation conditions by dimensional analysis. *Powder Technol.* **2012**, *224*, 323–330. [CrossRef]

38. Sou, T.; Kaminskas, L.; Nguyen, T.-H.; Carlberg, R.; McIntosh, M.P.; Morton, D.A. The effect of amino acid excipients on morphology and solid-state properties of multi-component spray-dried formulations for pulmonary delivery of biomacromolecules. *Eur. J. Pharm. Biopharm.* **2013**, *83*, 234–243. [CrossRef]

39. Li, L.; Sun, S.; Parumasivan, T.; Denman, J.A.; Gengenbach, T.; Tang, P.; Mao, S.; Chan, H.-K. l-Leucine as an excipient against moisture on in vitro aerosolization performances of highly hygroscopic spray-dried powders. *Eur. J. Pharm. Biopharm.* **2016**, *102*, 132–141. [CrossRef] [PubMed]

40. Kaialy, W.; Hussain, T.; Alhalaweh, A.; Nokhodchi, A. Towards a more desirable dry powder inhaler formulation: Large spray-dried mannitol microspheres outperform small microspheres. *Pharm. Res.* **2014**, *31*, 60–76. [CrossRef]

41. Roe, K.D.; Labuza, T.P. Glass transition and crystallization of amorphous trehalose-sucrose mixtures. *Int. J. Food Prop.* **2005**, *8*, 559–574. [CrossRef]

42. Stojanovska, S.; Gruevska, N.; Tomovska, J.; Tasevska, J. Maillard reaction and lactose structural changes during milk processing. *Mail. React. Lact. Struct. Chang. Milk Process.* **2017**, *2*, 139–145.

43. Zhang, Y.; Zhang, H.; Ghosh, D. The stabilizing excipients in dry state therapeutic phage formulations. *AAPS Pharmscitech* **2020**, *21*, 1–14. [CrossRef]

44. Trouwborst, T.; De Jong, J.C.; Winkler, K.C. Mechanism of inactivation in aerosols of bacteriophage T1. *J. Gen. Virol.* **1972**, *15*, 235–242. [CrossRef] [PubMed]

45. Feng, A.; Boraey, M.; Gwin, M.; Finlay, P.; Kuehl, P.; Vehring, R. Mechanistic models facilitate efficient development of leucine containing microparticles for pulmonary drug delivery. *Int. J. Pharm.* **2011**, *409*, 156–163. [CrossRef]

46. Chang, R.Y.K.; Kwok, P.C.L.; Khanal, D.; Morales, S.; Kutter, E.; Li, J.; Chan, H. Inhalable bacteriophage powders: Glass transition temperature and bioactivity stabilization. *Bioeng. Transl. Med.* **2020**, *5*, e10159. [CrossRef]

47. Drake, A.C.; Lee, Y.; Burgess, E.M.; Karlsson, J.O.M.; Eroglu, A.; Higgins, A.Z. Effect of water content on the glass transition temperature of mixtures of sugars, polymers, and penetrating cryoprotectants in physiological buffer. *PLoS ONE* **2018**, *13*, e0190713. [CrossRef]

48. Puapermpoonsiri, U.; Ford, S.; van der Walle, C. Stabilization of bacteriophage during freeze drying. *Int. J. Pharm.* **2010**, *389*, 168–175. [CrossRef]

49. Zhang, Y.; Peng, X.; Zhang, H.; Watts, A.B.; Ghosh, D. Manufacturing and ambient stability of shelf freeze dried bacteriophage powder formulations. *Int. J. Pharm.* **2018**, *542*, 1–7. [CrossRef] [PubMed]

50. Greco, S.; Authelin, J.-R.; Leveder, C.; Segalini, A. A practical method to predict physical stability of amorphous solid dispersions. *Pharm. Res.* **2012**, *29*, 2792–2805. [CrossRef] [PubMed]

51. Cleland, J.L.; Lam, X.; Kendrick, B.; Yang, J.; Yang, T.; Overcashier, D.; Brooks, D.; Hsu, C.; Carpenter, J.F. A specific molar ratio of stabilizer to protein is required for storage stability of a lyophilized monoclonal antibody. *J. Pharm. Sci.* **2001**, *90*, 310–321. [CrossRef]

52. Bezerra, M.A.; Santelli, R.E.; Oliveira, E.P.; Villar, L.S.; Escaleira, L.A. Response surface methodology (RSM) as a tool for optimization in analytical chemistry. *Talanta* **2008**, *76*, 965–977. [CrossRef] [PubMed]

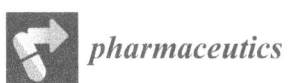

Article

Drug Combination of Ciprofloxacin and Polymyxin B for the Treatment of Multidrug–Resistant *Acinetobacter baumannii* Infections: A Drug Pair Limiting the Development of Resistance

Junwei Wang [1], Marc Stegger [2], Arshnee Moodley [3,4],* and Mingshi Yang [1,5,*]

[1] Department of Pharmacy, Faculty of Health and Medical Sciences, University of Copenhagen, Universitetsparken 2, DK-2100 Copenhagen, Denmark
[2] Department of Bacteria, Parasites and Fungi, Statens Serum Institut, DK-2300 Copenhagen, Denmark
[3] Department of Veterinary and Animal Sciences, University of Copenhagen, DK-1870 Frederiksberg C, Denmark
[4] Animal and Human Health, International Livestock Research Institute, Nairobi 00100, Kenya
[5] Wuya College of Innovation, Shenyang Pharmaceutical University, Wenhua Road No. 103, Shenyang 110016, China
* Correspondence: a.moodley@cgiar.org (A.M.); mingshi.yang@sund.ku.dk (M.Y.)

Abstract: Polymyxins are considered as last–resort antibiotics to treat infections caused by *Acinetobacter baumannii*. However, there are increasing reports of resistance in *A. baumannii* to polymyxins. In this study, inhalable combinational dry powders consisting of ciprofloxacin (CIP) and polymyxin B (PMB) were prepared by spray–drying. The obtained powders were characterized with respect to the particle properties, solid state, in vitro dissolution and in vitro aerosol performance. The antibacterial effect of the combination dry powders against multidrug–resistant *A. baumannii* was assessed in a time–kill study. Mutants from the time–kill study were further investigated by population analysis profiling, minimum inhibitory concentration testing, and genomic comparisons. Inhalable dry powders consisting of CIP, PMB and their combination showed a fine particle fraction above 30%, an index of robust aerosol performance of inhaled dry powder formulations in the literature. The combination of CIP and PMB exhibited a synergistic antibacterial effect against *A. baumannii* and suppressed the development of CIP and PMB resistance. Genome analyses revealed only a few genetic differences of 3–6 SNPs between mutants and the progenitor isolate. This study suggests that inhalable spray–dried powders composed of the combination of CIP and PMB is promising for the treatment of respiratory infections caused by *A. baumannii*, and this combination can enhance the killing efficiency and suppress the development of drug resistance.

Keywords: drug combination; inhalable dry powders; resistance development; synergistic effect

Citation: Wang, J.; Stegger, M.; Moodley, A.; Yang, M. Drug Combination of Ciprofloxacin and Polymyxin B for the Treatment of Multidrug–Resistant *Acinetobacter baumannii* Infections: A Drug Pair Limiting the Development of Resistance. *Pharmaceutics* **2023**, *15*, 720. https://doi.org/10.3390/pharmaceutics15030720

Academic Editors: Michael Yee Tak Chow and Philip Chi Lip Kwok

Received: 27 December 2022
Revised: 10 February 2023
Accepted: 16 February 2023
Published: 21 February 2023

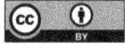
1. Introduction

Respiratory infections are a leading health threat causing millions of deaths worldwide annually [1]. Moreover, the number of respiratory infections caused by multidrug–resistant (MDR) bacteria is growing rapidly, especially those infections caused by *Pseudomonas aeruginosa* [2], *Klebsiella pneumonia* [3] and *Acinetobacter baumannii* [4], and are they associated with high morbidity and mortality [5].

Among those bacterial species, *A. baumannii* should be highlighted as it is extremely difficult to treat and can readily acquire resistance to multiple antibiotics during treatment [6]. In addition, this pathogen usually survives in hospital environment and can cause nosocomial infections, especially in patients in intensive care units (ICUs). Polymyxins such as polymyxin B and polymyxin E (also known as colistin) are considered as the last–resort treatment of *A. baumannii* infections, since other antibiotics are less effective [7]. However, there are increasing reports of unsuccessful polymyxin monotherapy of *A. baumannii* respiratory infections [8], and hence polymyxin resistance is becoming an inevitable therapeutic issue [9–11].

Combination therapy has been shown to contribute to better clinical outcomes than monotherapy, improving the survival of patients suffering from MDR pathogens infections [12–14], especially when a combination exhibits synergistic effect. Drug pairs with synergistic effects can afford an amplified antibacterial effect compared to single used antibiotics, enhancing bacteria kill rate and narrowing the time window of the resistant development [13]. A polymyxin–based combination treatment has been considered as a promising treatment option against MDR *A. baumannii* [15–17]. In a clinical study, a synergistic effect was observed when polymyxin B was combined with levofloxacin, tobramycin and meropenem to treat MDR *A. baumannii* infections [18]. However, the antibacterial effect will also eliminate susceptible bacteria, and antibiotic residues can select for mutants with a reduced susceptibility to the same antibiotics [19,20]. Furthermore, the wide use of drug combinations can also result in cross–resistance or collateral sensitivity [20]. Nevertheless, it is promising that recent studies have shown that cross–resistance can be used to rationally design dosing regimens to avoid resistance development instead of promoting it [21,22]. Therefore, it is important to assess not only the killing efficiency but also the drug resistance development when adopting antibiotic combination therapy [23,24].

The combination of polymyxins and fluoroquinolones has been reported to be effective against MDR *P. aeruginosa* and MDR *A. baumannii* [25,26], but the re–sensitization of the strain by this antibiotic combination has not been reported. In this study, a combination of ciprofloxacin (CIP) and polymyxin B sulfate (PMB) was formulated into inhalable dry powders and tested against *A. baumannii* strain K31. The dry powders were characterized and evaluated with respect to the particle properties, solid state, in vitro aerosol performance, in vitro dissolution and in vitro antibacterial effect. In addition, the antibacterial activity and resistance evolution of the PMB and CIP combination were investigated.

2. Materials and Methods

2.1. Chemicals

United States Pharmacopeia (USP) standard CIP and PMB were purchased from Nanjing Sunlida Biological Technology Co., Ltd. (Nanjing, China). Sodium sulfate and acetonitrile were purchased from Sigma–Aldrich (Copenhagen, Denmark); dialysis bags (Biotech RC Dialysis Tubing) with 20 kD typical molecular weight cut–offs were obtained from Spectrum Laboratories (Compton, CA, USA). E–TEST strips (CIP and PMB) were purchased from bioMérieux SA (Marcy–l'Étoile, France).

2.2. Strains

A. baumannii K31 is a human clinical strain that was isolated in August 2017 from a wound infection (part of the biorepository at Department of Veterinary and Animal Sciences, University of Copenhagen). Minimum inhibitory concentrations (MICs) to aztreonam, CIP, PMB and tobramycin are presented in Table 1.

Table 1. Minimum inhibitory concentrations (MICs) of different antibiotic against *A. baumannii* K31.

Antibiotics	MICs (µg/mL)	MIC Break Points (µg/mL)	
		S≤	R>
Aztreonam	64	N	N
Ciprofloxacin	32	0.25	0.5
Polymyxin B *	1	–	–
Tobramycin	256	4	4

S: susceptible; R: resistant; according to European Committee on Antimicrobial Susceptibility Testing (EUCAST) [27]. N: No breakpoints, and susceptibility testing is not recommended as the bacterial species is a poor target for therapy with this antibiotic (isolates may be reported as R without prior testing). * No breakpoints listed for polymyxin B, but colistin breakpoints are S ≤ 2 and R > 2 (PMB and colistin both belong to polymyxins group).

2.3. Wet Milling

As a hydrophobic compound, ciprofloxacin was prepared by media milling methods to form a homogeneous nanocrystal suspension to be used as feeding solutions [28]. Briefly, 1.0 g of raw ciprofloxacin was dispersed in 20 mL Poloxamer 188 (F68) aqueous solution (0.5%, w/v). Glass beads with two different sizes (1 mm and 2 mm diameter) were mixed as media in the milling process. This mixture was then homogenized for 24 h at room temperature with ~40 mL of milling media by a magnetic stirrer (900 rpm) to prepare nanocrystal suspensions. The micronized particles were collected by centrifugation, washed twice with purified water and dispersed again as feeding solution.

2.4. The Spray–Drying Process

CIP and PMB dry powders were prepared using a Büchi 290 spray drier (BÜCHI Labortechnik; Falwil, Switzerland). The susceptibility profiles (MICs) of antibiotics were important as a preliminary guidance for formulation preparation. In this study, a ratio of 32:1 (CIP/PMB) was determined to be used in the combination dry powder. This ratio was selected based on the MIC value of CIP and PMB. Feeding solutions for each formulation and corresponding composition are listed in Table 2. PMB was dissolved in water or CIP suspension to be prepared as the feeding solutions. The spray–drying conditions were as follows: the inlet and outlet temperature were 100 °C and 46–52 °C respectively; the drying airflow rate was 35 m^3/h; the atomization air flow rate was 700 L/h; the feeding rate of the solution/suspension was 3 mL/min. The spray–dried powders were collected in glass vials and stored in a desiccator at room temperature until further characterization.

Table 2. Feeding solutions for spray–drying.

Dry Powders	Abbreviation	Solid Contents of Feeding Solution	
		PMB Solution (mg/mL)	CIP Suspension (mg/mL)
PMB spray–dried powder	PMB–SD	9.6	–
CIP spray–dried powder	CIP–SD	–	9.8
PMB–CIP co–spray–dried powder	PMB–CIP–SD	0.31	9.8

The size distribution of nanoparticles in CIP suspension was measured by dynamic light scattering, see detailed description in Supplementary Materials.

2.5. Morphology

Samples were fixed on a sticky carbon tape and sputtered with gold by a sputter–coater (Leica EM ACE200, Leica Microsystems GmbH, Wetzlar, Germany). Images were captured at an acceleration voltage of 2.00 kV by scanning electron microscopy (SEM) (Quanta 3D FEG, Thermo Fisher Scientific, Waltham, MA, USA).

2.6. Particle Size

The mean particle sizes of the dry powders were determined by laser diffraction (Malvern Mastersizer 2000, Malvern Instruments, Malvern, Cambridge, UK) equipped with a dry powder feeder unit (Scirrocco 2000 powder feeder, Malvern Instruments Malvern, Cambridge, UK). Dry powder samples were dispersed by air at a pressure of 3 bars. The refractive index was set to 1.520 for the measurement of the samples. The samples were measured in triplicate. The size distributions of the samples are presented via the span, calculated using the following equation:

$$\text{Span} = \frac{\text{Dv}_{90} - \text{Dv}_{10}}{\text{Dv}_{50}} \tag{1}$$

The Dv_{10}, Dv_{50}, and Dv_{90} were also reported, which refer to the volumetric diameter at 10%, 50% and 90% cumulative number, respectively.

2.7. X-ray Powder Diffraction (XRPD)

The XRPD patterns of the powders were collect by an X-ray diffractometer (X'Pert PRO MPD, PANalytical, Almelo, The Netherlands) with a slit detector Ni–filtered CuKα1 source generated at 40 mA and 45 kV. Data were collected from 5° to 38° 2θ, the step width was 0.04° and the scan speed was 5°·min^{-1}. The diffraction patterns of unprocessed raw materials (i.e., CIP, and PMB), physical mixtures of raw materials and spray–dried samples (i.e., CIP–SD, PMB–SD, PMB–CIP–SD) were collected.

2.8. Dynamic Vapor Sorption (DVS)

The water sorption–desorption properties of the samples were described by a VTI–SA$^+$ (TA Instruments, New Castle, DE, USA). Sample preparation began with a drying step then continued with a sorption–desorption cycle. Briefly, approximately 10 mg of powder for each sample was added in a quartz holder, and then exposed in the instrument under 0% relative humidity (RH) at 60 °C for 180 min or until a constant weight (less than 0.001 wt. % change over 5 min) was reached. After drying, samples were cooled down and maintained at 25 °C. The samples were exposed to the following sorption–desorption cycle: 0 to 90% in 10% step size and the same for desorption. Each step's running time was less than 120 min, or until it reached an equilibrated weight (less than 0.001 wt. % change) over 5 min. Data were recorded every 2 min or when a ≥0.0100 wt. % change occurred. Profiles of weight records during the sorption–desorption cycle were collected to present the water sorption–desorption properties of the samples.

2.9. In Vitro Dissolution

Specific amounts (200 mg approximately) of CIP–SD, PMB–SD, PMB–CIP–SD and raw materials (CIP and PMB) were added to dialysis bags and sealed individually. Each dialysis bag was then transferred into 200 mL of dissolution medium (50 mM PBS, pH 7.4). All samples were incubated in a shaking water bath (100 rpm) at 37 °C. At predetermined time points (20 min, 40 min, 1 h, 1.5 h, 2 h, 4 h, 8 h and 24 h), 10 mL of dissolution medium was withdrawn and replaced with fresh medium. Samples were centrifuged first. The concentrations of CIP and PMB were measured using an HPLC (1260 Infinity, Agilent Technologies, Santa Clara, CA, USA) with a reverse–phase column (Agilent C18 150 × 4.6 mm, Agilent Technologies, USA). The mobile phases consisted of a 26% acetonitrile and 74% 30 mM solution of sodium sulfate (pH 2.5, adjusted with phosphoric acid), and the flow rate was 1 mL/min. The samples were detected at 215 nm by a UV detector. Calibration curves were prepared for CIP (1–40 μg/mL, limit of quantification was 50 ng/mL, $r^2 > 0.999$) and PMB (10–100 μg/mL, limit of quantification was 8 μg/mL, $r^2 > 0.999$). The peak areas for polymyxin B1 and B2 were summed for the quantification of PMB. The dissolution rates of the samples were compared via their cumulative dissolution profiles. All samples in the dissolution study were tested in triplicates.

2.10. In Vitro Aerosol Performance

The in vitro aerosol performances of the spray–dried powders were assessed using a Next Generation Impactor (NGI, Copley Scientific, Nottingham, UK). Prior to the tests, the collection plates of NGI were coated with a Tween 20 solution (0.5% (w/v)) to minimize particle bouncing. A low–resistance–type RS01 Monodose dry powder inhaler (Plastiape, Osnago, Italy) was used as the dry powder inhaler device for all tests, and a mouthpiece adapter was used to connect the inhaler to the throat (stainless steel USP induction) of the NGI. About 30 mg of dry powder was put into size 3 hydroxypropyl methylcellulose (HPMC) capsules (Capsugel, Greenwood, SC, USA) for each formulation. One capsule was loaded in the inhaler and emitted in each run at an air flow rate of 90 L/min for 2.6 s. The corresponding pressure drop for the device was adjusted to ~3.9 KPa with the current NGI setting. The powders deposited in the stages of the NGI, the USP throat, the capsule and the inhaler were collected with 1.7% (v/v) acetic acid solution, and the concentrations of CIP and PMB in the samples were determined by HPLC (described in the Section 2.9).

Fine particle fractions (FPF) and emitted dose (ED) were calculated for the evaluation of aerosol performance. The FPFs of the formulations were calculated as the percentage mass of the drug with an aerodynamic diameter smaller than 5 µm of the drug collected from the tests. ED values were defined as the mass percentage of drug recovered from all NGI parts relative to the total drug recovered from the experiments. For each formulation, three independent batches were used for the in vitro aerosol performance evaluation.

2.11. Time–Kill Assay

Overnight bacterial cultures of *A. baumannii* K31 were adjusted to 5×10^5 colony-forming units (CFU)/mL in cation–adjusted Mueller–Hinton broth (200 mL), transferred to glass flasks and incubated for 30 min at 37 °C to reach the early exponential growth phase. Spray–dried powders (CIP–SD, PMB–SD and PMB–CIP–SD) were sealed in a dialysis bag and added to each culture flask at the time point of zero. A sequential combination group was set here to compare with the fixed–dose combination. For this sequential addition, PMB–SD was added at time point zero with other groups, and the CIP–SD was added after sampling at 24 h. The experimental design and treatment groups are described in Table 3. After the antibiotics were added, the flasks were incubated at 37 °C for 48 h. At time intervals of 2 h, 6 h, 12 h, 24 h, 36 h and 48 h, 150 µL of culture was withdrawn from the flasks and serially diluted in saline. The diluted culture was then spotted (20 µL of each dilution) on Mueller–Hinton agar plates. After 24 h incubation, the colonies were counted, and CFU/mL values were calculated for each group. Experiments were performed in duplicate, and data have been presented as the mean value of the two counts. To verify the dissolution influence when using drug powders in the time–kill study, a parallel study was performed by employing the antibiotic solution with the same group setting as that used in the spray–dried powders group (description in Supplementary Results).

Table 3. Group setting and corresponding antibiotic addition plan.

Code	Name	Treatment	Concentration (µg/mL)	
			CIP	PMB
a	Control	no antibiotic	–	–
b	PMB–SD	add PMB–SD at time zero	–	1
c	CIP–SD	add CIP–SD at time zero	32	–
d	PMB–CIP–SD	add PMB–SD and CIP–SD at time zero	32	1
e	PMB–SD–CIP–SD	add PMB–SD at the beginning then add CIP–SD added after 24 h	32	1

Concentrations of CIP and PMB tested corresponded to pure drug formulations.

2.12. Population Analysis Profiling (PAP)

Bacteria from the different treatment groups in the time–kill assay were included in the PAP analysis (Figure 1). Briefly, at time intervals of 24 h and 48 h, bacteria were sampled from each group of the time–kill assay, centrifuged and washed twice, and then spread on a 5% blood agar plate and incubated at 37 °C overnight. After incubation, three colonies from each of the 24 h and 48 h plates were randomly selected, and each strain yielded a lineage that was then used for PAP analysis and confirmatory MIC testing. Antibiotic–free solutions were used as a reference.

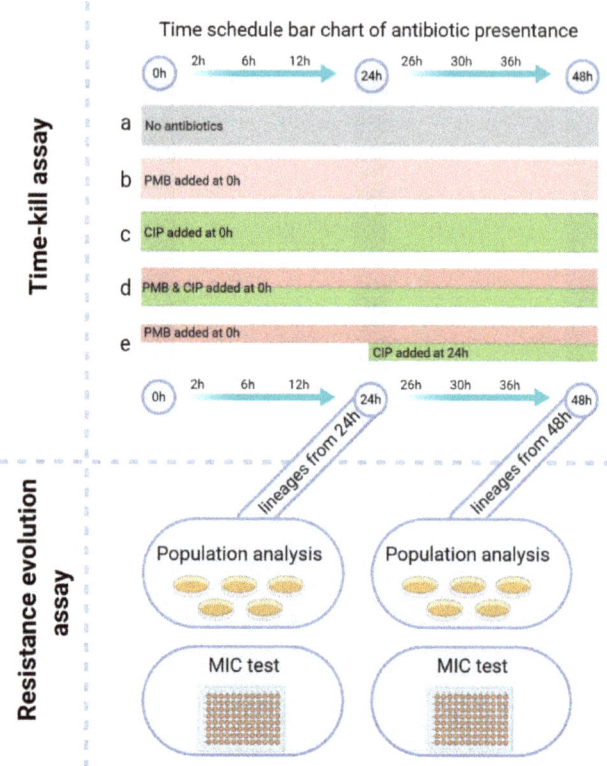

Figure 1. Graphic representation of the in vitro microbiology study. Colored bars in the time schedule represent different addition times and durations of spray–dried antibiotic dry powder application; the group codes correspond to Table 3. Lineages from different time–kill assay (at 24 and 48 h) groups were used for further assaying resistance development.

Each isolate was adjusted to 0.5 MacFarland (10^8 CFU/mL) in 0.85% saline. The starting suspension and serial dilutions (10–1 to1–6 diluted in 0.85% saline) were spotted (20 µL) on Mueller–Hinton agar plates without or with varying concentrations of PMB (0.5, 1, 2, 4, 8, and 16 µg/mL) and CIP (16, 32, 64, 128, 256, and 512 µg/mL). Colonies were counted after 48 h of incubation at 37 °C. PAP values were based on CFU counting and the corresponding drug and drug concentration colonies were counted. The results are grouped with the corresponding group in the time–kill assay (24 h and 48 h).

2.13. MIC Testing

The MICs of all isolates at the start of the PAP experiment were determined by E–TEST for CIP and PMB, performed according to the manufacturer's recommendations (BioMérieux, Marcy–l'Étoile, France). Briefly, each isolate was adjusted to 5×10^8 CFU/mL and spread using a cotton swab on a Mueller–Hinton agar plate. E–test strips were placed on the plates and incubated at 37 °C for 20 h, and the MIC was read where the bacterial growth intersected the test strip. Isolates with MICs below test limits were re–tested by broth microdilution method. Briefly, two–fold serial dilutions from 1 to 512 µg/mL were diluted in Mueller–Hinton broth in a 96–well microtiter plate, and a 0.5 MacFarland standard inoculum (fresh overnight culture) of each group was diluted and transferred into each well to afford a final inoculum of 5×10^5 CFU/mL. All plates were incubated for 20 h at 37 °C, and the MIC value was the concentration at which no bacterial growth was visible in the well. The MICs of the isolates were compared with the original *A. baumannii* K31 (Table 1), and value changes were recorded. The results have been grouped via the corresponding group name in the time–kill assay (24 h and 48 h). For each lineage in the time–kill groups, three isolates were selected, and data have been presented as the mean and standard deviation.

2.14. Genome Sequencing and Analysis

The 48 h lineage values after time–kill study were used for the identification of sequence variations. The lineages derived from solutions were used to avoid the uncertainty of dry powders (Supplementary materials, Table S2). From the original K31 strain, as well as the 48 h lineages of the control, PMB–Sol and CIP–Sol groups, one colony was picked for genome sequencing analysis. For the 48 h lineages of the PMB–CIP–Sol and PMB–Sol–CIP–Sol groups, three colonies were picked for sequencing.

All colonies were then re–cultured overnight in Mueller–Hinton broth at 37 °C. Genomic DNA was extracted using the DNeasy Blood and Tissue kit (Qiagen, Venlo, The Netherlands). The purity and concentration of extracted DNA were assayed using the Nanodrop and Qubit instruments, respectively. The Nextera XT library preparation kit was used to prepare a sequencing library. The prepared library was sequenced on a MiSeq using a paired–end 2×250 bp sequencing strategy, according to standard Illumina protocols (Illumina, San Diego, CA, USA).

To identify sequence variations, the raw sequence data were aligned to an annotated *A. baumannii* 1656–2 reference chromosome (GenBank accession no. CP001921) [29] using NASP v1.2.0 [30] by using BWA–MEM v0.7.12 [31], and the variants were called using GATK [32]. To retain only high–quality variant calling, the respective position was not included when a minimum of 10–depth sequencing was not met, or the nucleotide variant was shown in <90% of the base calls per individual isolates.

2.15. Statistical Analysis

The results are indicated with the appropriate number of replicates (n) and represented as the mean value $\pm$ standard. Statistics were carried out using GraphPad Prism version 8.0 for Windows. *p*-values below 5% ($p < 0.05$) were considered as statistically significant, as determined by analysis of variance (ANOVA) followed by a *t*-test.

3. Results

3.1. Preparation and Characterization of Spray–Dried Powders

Prior to spray–drying, the CIP was wet–milled to nanoparticles of around 362 nm, as measured by dynamic light scattering (description in Supplementary results). Upon spray–drying, the CIP nanoparticles obtained from the wet–milling were transformed to spherical particles, i.e., CIP–SD, in a size range of 1–6 μm (Table 4), measured by laser diffraction. The CIP–SD particles were spherical and composed of fine grains (Figure 2c). The spray–dried PMB (PMB–SD) particles were hollow and wrinkled, in a size range of 0.7–6.4 μm (Table 2). Co–spray–dried samples, i.e., PMB–CIP SD, resembled CIP–SD particles (Figure 2e), and their sizes ranged 0.7–6.4 μm (Table 2).

Table 4. Particle sizes of dry powder formulations.

Sample Name	Diameter (μm)			Span (μm)
	Dv_{10}	Dv_{50}	Dv_{90}	
PMB–SD	1.2 ± 0.1	2.7 ± 0.1	5.7 ± 0.3	1.6 ± 0.1
CIP–SD	0.7 ± 0.1	2.6 ± 0.2	6.4 ± 0.3	2.2 ± 0.1
PMB–CIP SD	0.7 ± 0.1	2.7 ± 0.1	6.3 ± 0.1	2.0 ± 0.1

Dv_{10}, Dv_{50}, and Dv_{90} are volumetric diameters at 10%, 50% and 90% cumulative numbers, respectively. Data shown are representative of triplicate tests (mean $\pm$ SD, n = 3).

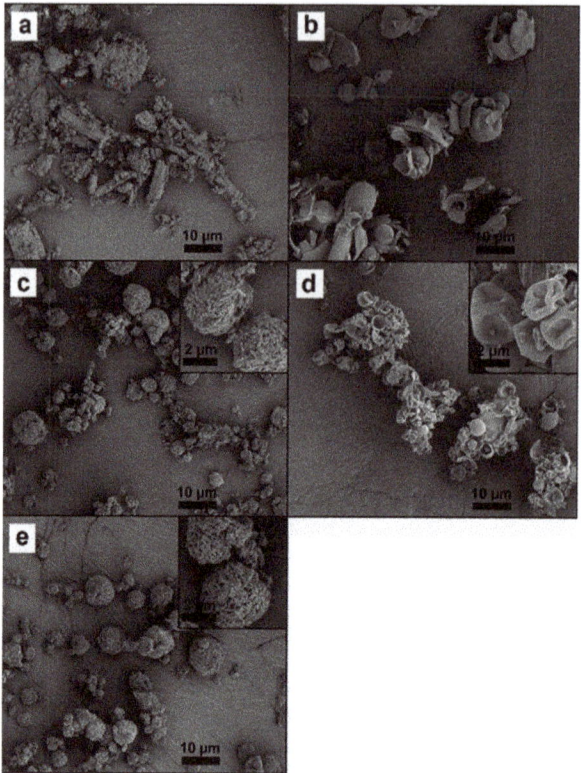

Figure 2. SEM pictures of raw CIP (**a**), raw PMB (**b**), CIP–SD (**c**), PMB–SD (**d**) and PMB–CIP–SD (**e**).

As for the solid states of the different formulations, the PMB remained amorphous after the spray–drying process, whereas the CIP–SD exhibited different crystalline forms from raw CIP (Figure 3). The diffraction patterns of the co–spray–dried PMD–CIP–SD powders resemble those of CIP–SD.

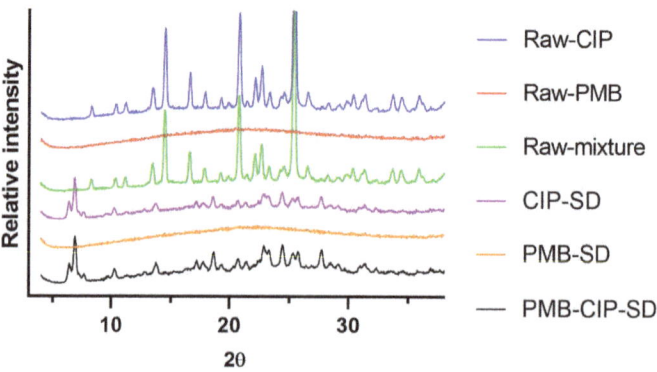

Figure 3. Powder diffraction patterns of raw CIP, raw PMB, physical mixture, CIP–SD, PMB–SD and PMB–CIP–SD.

In the DVS analyses, CIP–SD exhibited a rapid water sorption until 30% RH, followed by a slow water sorption in the range of 30–70% RH, and another burst of rapid water sorption until 90% RH (Figure 4). The CIP–SD underwent a total of 25% (*w*/*w*) of its weight gain up to 90% RH. The removal of water from the CIP–SD seemed to complete with desorption, whereas the desorption exhibited a different profile from the sorption. There was negligible desorption of water from 90% to 50% RH, which was followed by a rapid loss of water from 50% to 40% RH, and from 20% to 10% RH. In contrast, the sorption and desorption profiles of PMB–SD are mostly overlaid, with a total 38% (*w*/*w*) of the weight gain occurring up to 90% RH. The sorption–desorption profiles of PMB–CIP–SD resemble those of CIP–SD.

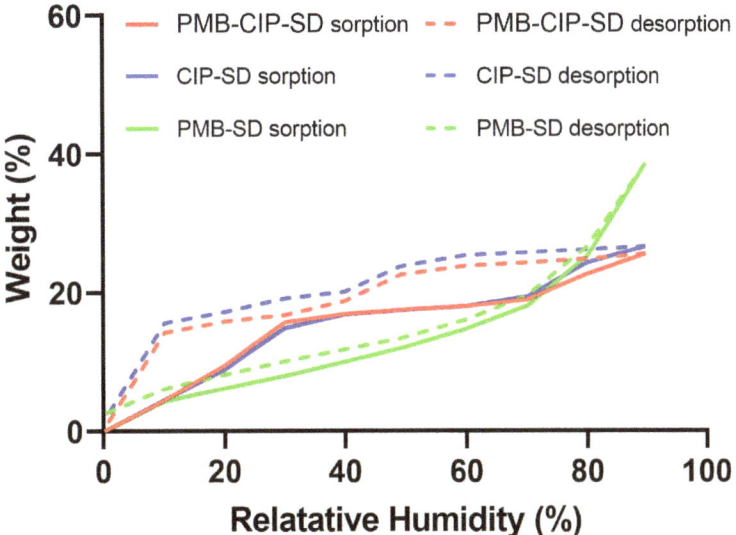

Figure 4. Dynamic vapor sorption isotherm of different formulations. The solid line and dotted line represent the sorption and desorption processes, respectively.

3.2. In Vitro Dissolution and Aerosol Performance of Spray–Dried Powders

The dissolution rates of PMB from different samples, i.e., raw PMB, PMB–SD and PMB–CIP–SD, are similar, and they were all faster than CIP (Figure 5). The dissolution rates of spray–dried CIP samples i.e., CIP–SD and PMB–CIP–SD, were similar, and were faster than that of raw CIP.

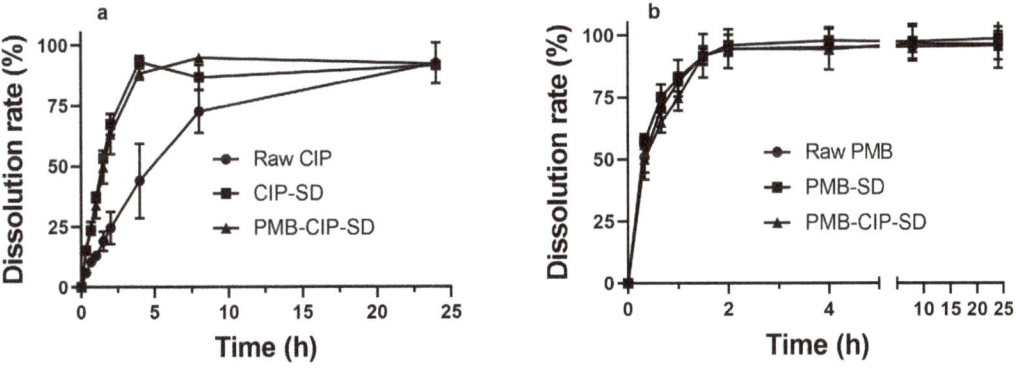

Figure 5. In vitro accumulated dissolution profiles of CIP (**a**) and PMB (**b**) (mean ± SD, n = 3).

All spray–dried powders exhibited relatively high FPF and ED values of over 40% and 70%, respectively (Figure 6). PMB–SD exhibited significantly higher FPF and ED compared to CIP–SD. The FPF and ED values of PMB–CIP SD are similar to those of PMB–SD ($p < 0.05$).

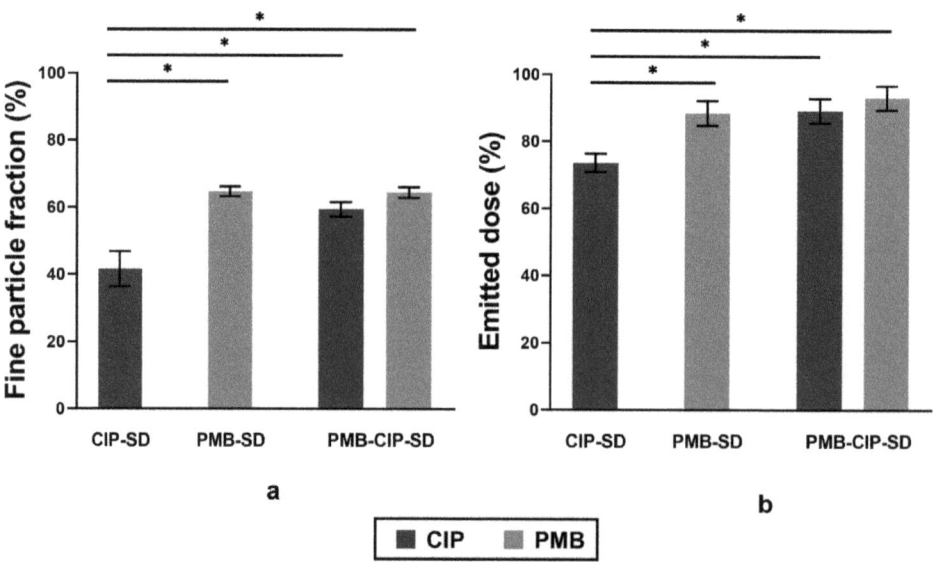

Figure 6. Fine particle fractions (FPF) (**a**) and emitted dose (ED) (**b**) of spray–dried formulations (mean ± SD, n = 3). Significant differences ($p < 0.05$) are indicated with asterisk.

3.3. Time–Kill Assay

The growth of bacteria treated with CIP–SD was inhibited for the first 24 h ($0.7 \log_{10}$ CFU/mL decrease as compared to the control, Figure 7), followed by regrowth from 24 h to 36 h, ultimately reaching a similar $\log_{10}$ CFU/mL to the control (i.e., 14.7 of $\log_{10}$ CFU/mL inoculum increase after 48 h of incubation). PMB–SD exhibited a bacteriostatic effect during the first 6 h, with a $5.6 \log_{10}$ CFU/mL inoculum reduction. A regrowth could be seen after 6 h, but there was apparent inhibition compared to the control and CIP–SD–treated group (Figure 7). PMB–CIP–SD exhibited a similar bacteriostatic activity to the PMB group in the first 6 h, followed by regrowth. It also exhibited a stronger inhibition effect than the PMB group. As for PMB–SD–CIP–SD, a similar killing activity to that of PMB–SD could be observed at 0–24 h. However, the regrowth was slow between 24 and 48 h, and was similar to that of PMB–CIP–SD during the same period. The changes in $\log_{10}$ CFU/mL after 24 and 48 h incubation as compared to the inoculum are listed in Figure 7b. PMB–CIP–SD exhibited the strongest inhibition effect among the samples, followed by PMB–SD–CIP–SD, PMB–SD, and CIP–SD.

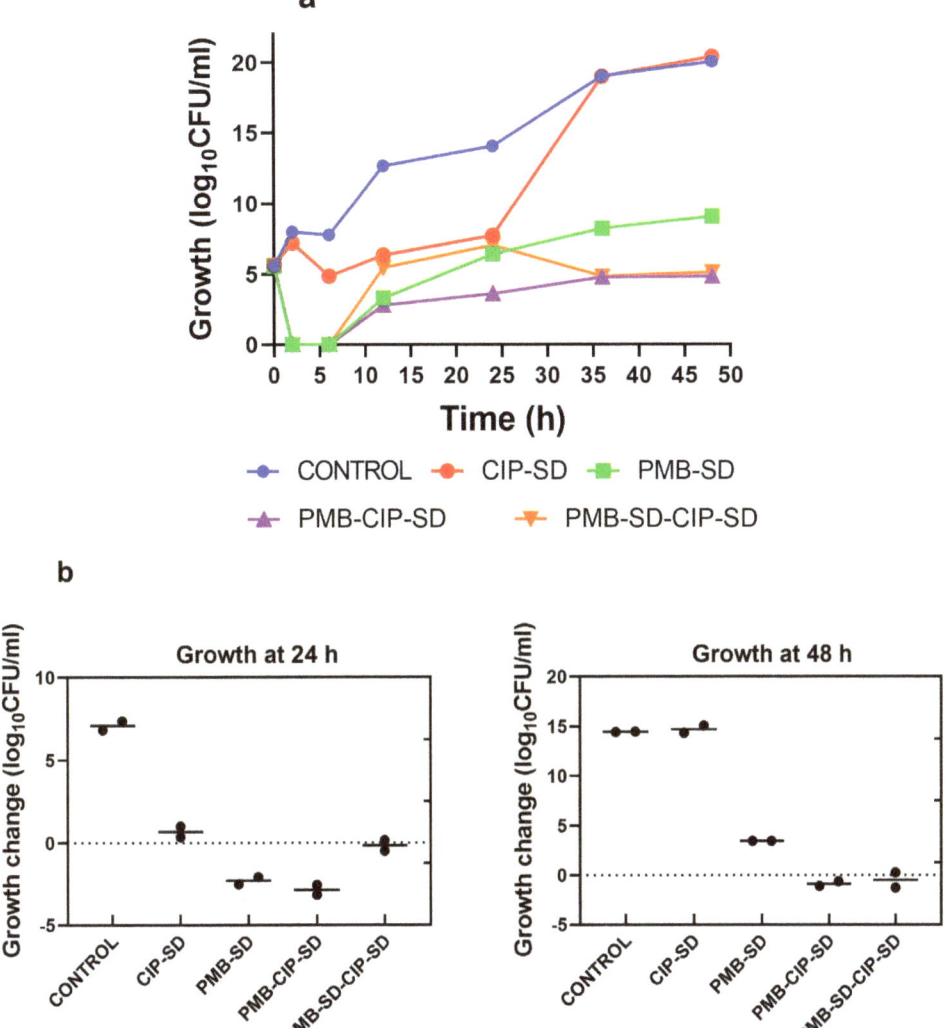

Figure 7. Time–kill assay with *A. baumannii* K31 treated with different formulations (**a**) and a histogram of the change in growth after 24 h and 48 h incubation compared to the inoculum (**b**). Data are presented as the means of two experiments.

3.4. Population Analysis Profile

In the population analysis of PMB using different concentrations, the PMB–SD 24 h and 48 h lineages were shown to be a resistant subpopulation that survived up to 16 µg/mL of PMB (Figure 8a,b). No resistant subpopulations were observed in the CIP–SD lineages (24 h and 48 h). the CIP–SD lineages became susceptible to lower concentrations of PMB compared to the control lineages. As shown in Figure 8a,b, reduced populations of the CIP–SD 24 h lineage and 48 h lineage can be observed at 1 µg/mL and 0.5 µg/mL of PMB, respectively. As for the drug combinations, PMB–CIP–SD was similar to CIP–SD. However, the PMB–SD–CIP–SD 24 h lineage was similar to the PMB–SD 24 h lineage, while the PMB–SD–CIP–SD 48 h lineage was similar to the CIP–SD 48 h lineage.

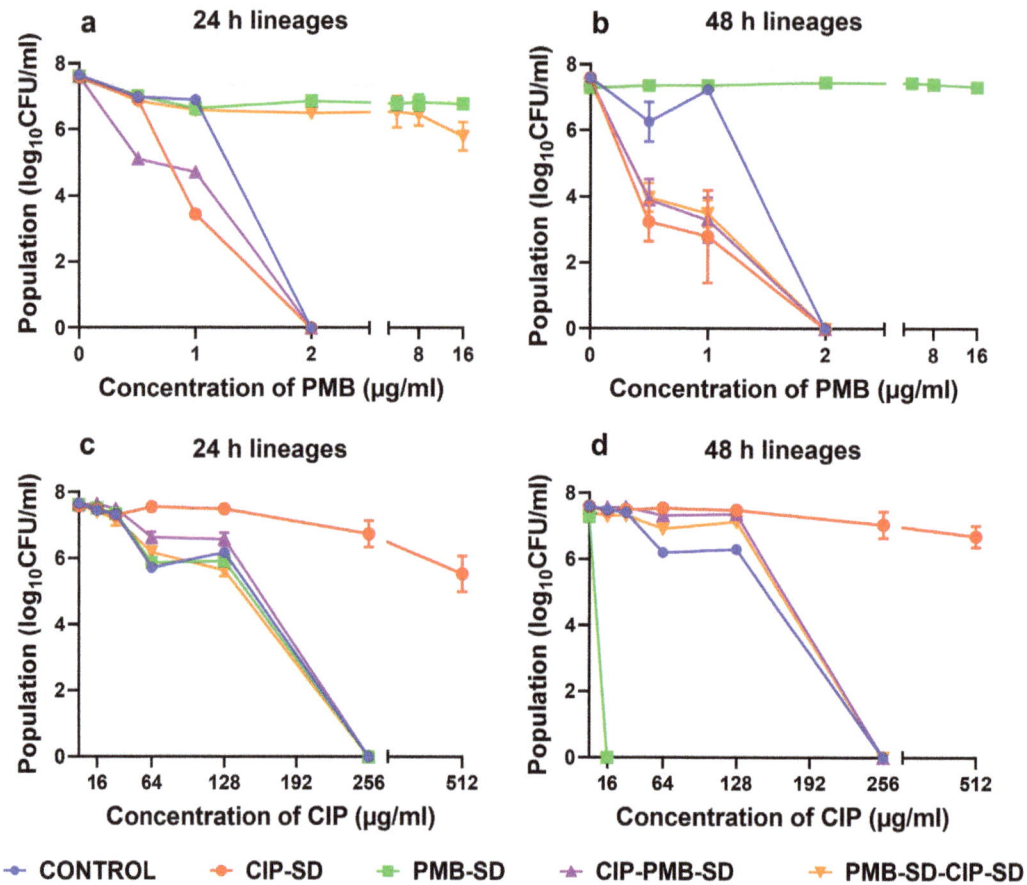

Figure 8. Population analysis profiles of lineages against PMB and CIP (mean ± SEM, n = 3). Lineages were treated with different antibiotics and have been coded by the names in the experimental design of the time–kill assay (Figure 1 and Table 3). (**a**,**c**) The results of lineages (after 24 h treatment in the time–kill assay) against different concentrations of PMB and CIP in the population analysis respectively; (**b**,**d**) the results of lineages (after 48 h treatment in the time–kill assay) against different concentrations of PMB and CIP in the population analyses, respectively.

When the different lineages were exposed to varying concentrations of CIP, the CIP–SD lineages (24 h and 48 h) appeared to survive 512 µg/mL of CIP (Figure 8c,d). The PMB–SD 24 h lineage, PMB–CIP–SD 24 h lineage, PMB–CIP–SD 48 h lineage, PMB–SD–CIP–SD 24 h lineage, and PMB–SD–CIP–SD 48 h lineage were similar to the control lineages, i.e., no growth was seen at 256 µg/mL of CIP. Interestingly, the PMB–SD 48 h lineages were eliminate at 16 µg/mL of CIP (Figure 8d), which is much lower than the value of the control lineages (256 µg/mL).

3.5. Changes in MIC of Lineages

The change in MIC of PMB and CIP in various lineages isolated from the time–kill study are shown in Figure 9a,b, respectively. We observed a prominent increase in the MIC of PMB in the PMB–SD 48 h lineage, contrary to the MIC of the other lineages of PMB (Figure 9a). We also noted an increase in the MIC of CIP against the CIP–SD 24 h lineage and 48 h lineage, as well as a decrease in the CIP MIC for the PMB–SD 48 h lineage (Figure 9b). There was no change in the CIP MIC of other lineages.

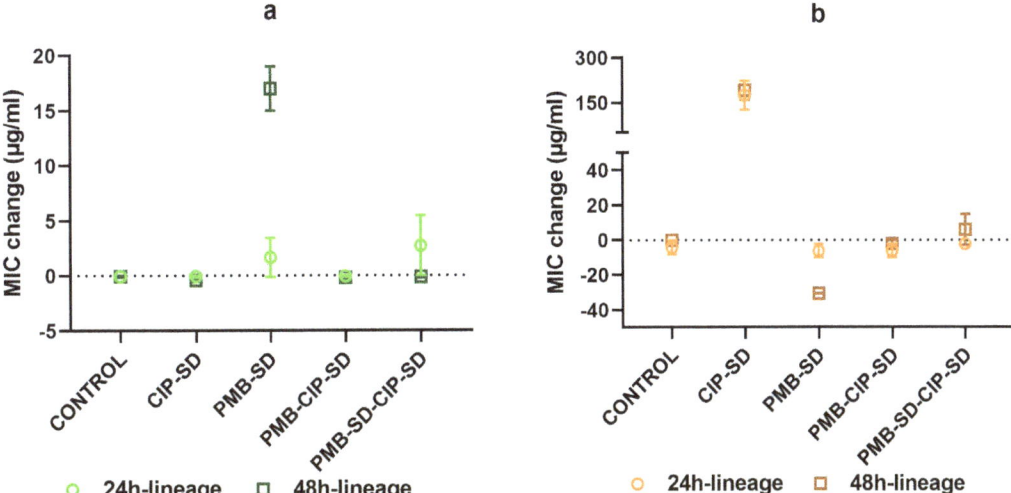

Figure 9. Change in MIC of PMB (**a**) and CIP (**b**) against lineages isolated from time–kill assay (mean ± SEM, n = 4). Lineages are grouped by names in the experimental design of the time–kill assay (Figure 1 and Table 3).

3.6. Genomic Analyses

After purging repetitive and duplicated regions in the reference chromosome, we detected a total of 12 mutations in all sequenced isolates (n = 10) across ~3.2 Mb (80.39%) of the reference genome. All mutations were found in coding regions, with 59% (7/12) being non–synonymous (Supplementary Table S3).

4. Discussion

Spray–drying is a useful technology for preparing inhalable dry powders [33], with possibilities emerging of formulating drug combinations by the co–spray–drying of two or multiple active pharmaceutical ingredients (API) [34,35]. CIP is a poorly water–soluble fluoroquinolone antibiotic, and PMB is a water–soluble antibiotic. To load these two antibiotics with different solubilities, CIP was wet–milled to a homogeneous nano–suspension (Table S1 in Supplementary materials), and then mixed with PMB solution at a designated mass ratio prior to spray drying. The obtained PMB–CIP–SD exhibited a similar size distribution (Table 4) to CIP–SD and PMB–SD. According to the DVS results, CIP–SD showed abrupt sorption from 0 to 30% RH, followed by relatively gentle sorption from 30 to 70%, which indicates that CIP was able to form a hydrate when in contact with water [36]. The XRPD analyses suggest that the raw CIP was an anhydrate, and a CIP 3.7 hydrate was obtained in the spray–dried powders [37,38], i.e., CIP–SD and PMB–CIP–SD. This can be attributed to the interaction between water molecules and the CIP lattice during the wet ball–milling process, resulting in CIP hydrate nanoparticles [37]. This suggests that the conditions of the spray–drying process used in this study did not remove the water bound in the CIP nanoparticles.

There are no differences in the dissolution rates of PMB in different spray–dried powders (i.e., PMB–SD and PMB–CIP–SD). Similar dissolution rates of CIP were also observed in different spray–dried powders (i.e., CIP–SD and PMB–CIP–SD). The dissolution rate of the CIP derived from the spray–dried powders was higher than that of the raw CIP material (Figure 5). One possible reason is that the sizes of CIP in the spray–dried powders were smaller than those in raw CIP materials [39]. In addition, their solid forms were different (Figure 3). It is apparent that the dissolution rates of PMB were faster than those of the CIP from the dry powders in all formulations. This can be attributed to the differences in the intrinsic dissolution rates of PMB and CIP 3.7 hydrate.

In general, all spray–dried powders used in this study are inhalable, since a FPF value above 30% is an index of robust aerosol performance [16]. Notably, PMB–SD possesses a significantly higher respirable fraction compared to CIP–SD (Figure 6), while they have similar geometric particle sizes and size distributions (Table 4). The respirable faction of PMB–CIP–SD was around 60%. The inclusion of PMB in the spray–dried formulations seemed to improve the aerosol performance of CIP formulations. Studies on the spray–drying of PMB are rare, while spray–drying colistin (polymyxin E), its congener, has been more intensively studied. Colistin is known to improve the aerosol performance of co–spray–dried powders by inhibiting the cohesiveness of spray–dried particles [40,41].

As shown in Figure 6, the antibacterial effect of the combination of PMB–CIP–SD against *A. baumannii* K31 is more effective than those of either antibiotic used alone (i.e., CIP–SD and PMB–SD). The reduction in the $\log_{10}$ CFU/mL of PMB–CIP–SD was more than 2-fold at both 24 and 48 h, indicating the combination exerted a synergistic effect [42]. This indicates that the combination of PMB and CIP may be a promising candidate to treat infections caused by resistant *A. baumannii*, owing to their synergistic effects. While antibiotic combinations with synergistic effects eliminate bacteria rapidly, they may also create a window for mutant populations to develop and proliferate, resulting in an increase in resistance development [19,20]. Therefore, in the subsequent experiments, various lineages collected from the time–kill study were investigated by PAP analysis and MIC testing so as to gain further insights into the resistance development and collateral sensitivity of the drug combination.

The lineages collected at 48 h in the time–kill study with individual antibiotics (i.e., CIP–SD or PMB–SD) exhibited resistance. Interestingly, though, the PMB–SD lineages exhibited susceptibility to CIP. The CIP MIC decreased from 32 to 4.7 µg/mL. In addition, as shown in PAP, the resistant subpopulation was reduced in the presence of CIP, which could be considered as indicating collateral sensitivity [43,44].

The lineages treated by the combinations (i.e., PMB–CIP–SD and PMB–SD–CIP–SD) exhibited slower resistance development as compared to strains exposed to the individual antibiotics alone. The similar PAP and unchanged MICs seen in the PMB and CIP were similar to the findings for the control (i.e., bacteria that were not exposed to antibiotics). One possible reason is that the combination rapidly and more effective eradicated the bacteria than the individual antibiotics alone, limiting the time window of regrowth of the resistant mutants [20]. Another reason could be that the presence of PMB induced collateral sensitivity in the CIP. It has been reported that the development of resistance to an antibiotic combination could be limited when the resistance to one antibiotic confers collateral sensitivity to the other antibiotic [22].

The only difference between the two combined formulations, i.e., PMB–CIP–SD and PMB–SD–CIP–SD, is the sequence of the addition of CIP–SD in the time–kill study. The intention of testing PMB–SD–CIP–SD was to investigate whether the sequential use of antibiotics (PMB–SD first, followed by CIP–SD) afforded a better bactericidal effect and the greater inhibition of resistance development than the fixed–dose combination (PMB–CIP–SD). In addition, this will shorten the exposure time of CIP, and can take advantage of the collateral sensitivity of PMB. The results show that even though CIP–SD was added to the bacterial culture 24 h after the treatment of PMB (i.e., PMB–SD–CIP–SD), the antibacterial effects of the two formulations at 48 h were similar (Figures 7–9). The possible reason for this could be that the change in the population with collateral sensitivity (treated with PMB solution) within 24 h was not high enough to induce the antibacterial activity (i.e., time–kill, PAP and MIC). The mutant frequencies were estimated, and 59% of identified mutants were found to be non–synonymous. This suggests that the single–drug–treated lineages collected in this study adapted to the antibiotics (CIP and PMB) without mutation [44].

Pharmaceutics **2023**, *15*, 720

Consequently, the collateral susceptibility observed in this study can be attributed to the pre–adaptation phenomenon, which has been found to be associated with beta–lactamase and efflux pump activities [45,46].

Contemporary antibiotic treatments via the oral route and injection cannot always reach an adequate bacteria–killing effect for chronic respiratory infection [47]. The optimization of the exposure–response relationships of antibiotics is beneficial to the treatment of severe infections in the lung, which can be performed via the pulmonary administration of antibiotics [47]. The pulmonary administration of antibiotics such as tobramycin and colistin was first undertaken using nebulized solutions [48]. Inhaled tobramycin, i.e., TOBI® Podhaler™, was approved first in 2013 by the FDA as an inhaled antibiotic dry powder product, bringing obvious clinical benefits to respiratory infection treatment [49]. The need for dry powder inhalers is increasing rapidly since they are portable and convenient for use [50]. Moreover, the development of new inhaled antibiotic combinations has not stopped. For example, besides the antibiotic pairs that afford synergistic effects [51,52], new combinations, such as antibiotic–biologicals, are also being studied in inhalable dry powder forms [53]. In addition, new delivery systems, such as nanoparticles and liposomes aiming to overcome the mucus/sputum barrier and prolong the drug retention time in the lung of inhaled antibiotics for the treatment of chronic respiratory infection, have been investigated and developed, as these delivery systems could provide additional functionality to the treatment [52,54].

In brief, resistance development is an important factor that should be considered in rational combination designs, and collateral sensitivity/resistance studies may offer more opportunities, and inspire the development of new resistance–limiting combinations.

5. Conclusions

This study demonstrates that inhalable dry powders consisting of CIP and PMB can be readily produced by spray–drying. The fixed–dose combination of CIP and PMB is affordable and more effective against multidrug–resistant *A. baumannii*. In addition, this combination exerts a synergistic effect, and can better suppress the development of resistance as compared to individual antibiotics alone.

Supplementary Materials: The following supporting information can be downloaded at: https://www.mdpi.com/article/10.3390/pharmaceutics15030720/s1, Figure S1: DVS isotherms for PMB–SD, CIP–SD and PMB–CIP–SD; Figure S2: Time–kill assay result of *A. baumannii* K31 treated with different solutions; Figure S3: Population analysis profiles of lineages used against PMB and CIP; Figure S4: Changes in MIC of PMB and CIP against lineages isolated from time–kill assay. Table S1: Particle size of micronized CIP nano–suspension; Table S2: Group setting and corresponding antibiotic supplementation plan; Table S3: Genetic differences between isolates from different experimental groups with the reference of *A. baumannii* 1656–2.

Author Contributions: J.W.: methodology, formal analysis, investigation, writing—original draft. M.S.: data curation, writing—review and editing. A.M.: methodology, formal analysis, supervision, writing—review and editing. M.Y.: conceptualization, funding acquisition, supervision, writing—review and editing. All authors have read and agreed to the published version of the manuscript.

Funding: J.W. was supported by the China Scholarship Council (CSC No: 201609110097). M.Y. was founded by Liaoning Pan Deng Xue Zhe Scholar (No. XLYC2002061), the National Natural Science Foundation of China (No. 82173768), and the Overseas Expertise Introduction Project for Discipline Innovation ("111 Project") (No. D20029).

Institutional Review Board Statement: Not applicable.

Informed Consent Statement: Not applicable.

Data Availability Statement: Data are available on request.

Acknowledgments: We acknowledge the Core Facility for Integrated Microscopy, Faculty of Health and Medical Sciences, University of Copenhagen, for the technical support.

Conflicts of Interest: The authors declare no conflict of interest.

References

1. World Health Organization. The Top 10 Causes of Death. 2018. Available online: http://www.who.int (accessed on 10 February 2020).
2. Trinh, T.D.; Zasowski, E.J.; Claeys, K.C.; Lagnf, A.M.; Kidambi, S.; Davis, S.L.; Rybak, M.J. Multidrug-resistant *Pseudomonas aeruginosa* lower respiratory tract infections in the intensive care unit: Prevalence and risk factors. *Diagn. Microbiol. Infect. Dis.* **2017**, *89*, 61–66. [CrossRef] [PubMed]
3. Bassetti, M.; Righi, E.; Carnelutti, A.; Graziano, E.; Russo, A. Multidrug-resistant *Klebsiella pneumoniae*: Challenges for treatment, prevention and infection control. *Expert Rev. Anti-Infect. Ther.* **2018**, *16*, 749–761. [CrossRef] [PubMed]
4. Ibrahim, S.; Al-Saryi, N.; Al-Kadmy, I.M.S.; Aziz, S.N. Multidrug-resistant *Acinetobacter baumannii* as an emerging concern in hospitals. *Mol. Biol. Rep.* **2021**, *48*, 6987–6998. [CrossRef]
5. Ikuta, K.S.; Swetschinski, L.R.; Aguilar, G.R.; Sharara, F.; Mestrovic, T.; Gray, A.P.; Weaver, N.D.; Wool, E.; Han, C.; Hayoon, A.G.; et al. Global mortality associated with 33 bacterial pathogens in 2019: A systematic analysis for the Global Burden of Disease Study 2019. *Lancet* **2022**, *400*, 2221–2248. [CrossRef] [PubMed]
6. Ayoub Moubareck, C.; Hammoudi Halat, D. Insights into *Acinetobacter baumannii*: A Review of Microbiological, Virulence, and Resistance Traits in a Threatening Nosocomial Pathogen. *Antibiotics* **2020**, *9*, 119. [CrossRef]
7. Yang, Q.; Pogue, J.M.; Li, Z.; Nation, R.L.; Kaye, K.S.; Li, J. Agents of Last Resort: An Update on Polymyxin Resistance. *Infect. Dis. Clin.* **2020**, *34*, 723–750. [CrossRef]
8. Lopez, J.S.; Banerji, U. Combine and conquer: Challenges for targeted therapy combinations in early phase trials. *Nat. Rev. Clin. Oncol.* **2017**, *14*, 57–66. [CrossRef]
9. Cheah, S.-E.; Johnson, M.D.; Zhu, Y.; Tsuji, B.T.; Forrest, A.; Bulitta, J.B.; Boyce, J.D.; Nation, R.L.; Li, J. Polymyxin Resistance in *Acinetobacter baumannii*: Genetic Mutations and Transcriptomic Changes in Response to Clinically Relevant Dosage Regimens. *Sci. Rep.* **2016**, *6*, 26233. [CrossRef]
10. Arroyo, L.A.; Herrera, C.M.; Fernandez, L.; Hankins, J.V.; Trent, M.S.; Hancock, R.E.W. The pmrCAB operon mediates polymyxin resistance in *Acinetobacter baumannii* ATCC 17978 and clinical isolates through phosphoethanolamine modification of lipid A. *Antimicrob. Agents Chemother.* **2011**, *55*, 3743–3751. [CrossRef]
11. Lima, W.G.; de Brito, J.C.M.; Cardoso, B.G.; Cardoso, V.N.; Paiva, M.; De Lima, M.E.; Fernandes, S.O.A. Rate of polymyxin resistance among *Acinetobacter baumannii* recovered from hospitalized patients: A systematic review and meta-analysis. *Eur. J. Clin. Microbiol. Infect. Dis.* **2020**, *39*, 1427–1438. [CrossRef]
12. Moo, C.-L.; Yang, S.-K.; Yusoff, K.; Ajat, M.; Thomas, W.; Abushelaibi, A.; Lim, S.-H.-E.; Lai, K.-S. Mechanisms of Antimicrobial Resistance (AMR) and Alternative Approaches to Overcome AMR. *Curr. Drug Discov. Technol.* **2020**, *17*, 430–447. [CrossRef] [PubMed]
13. Tyers, M.; Wright, G.D. Drug combinations: A strategy to extend the life of antibiotics in the 21st century. *Nat. Rev. Microbiol.* **2019**, *17*, 141–155. [CrossRef] [PubMed]
14. Pulingam, T.; Parumasivam, T.; Gazzali, A.M.; Sulaiman, A.M.; Chee, J.Y.; Lakshmanan, M.; Chin, C.F.; Sudesh, K. Antimicrobial resistance: Prevalence, economic burden, mechanisms of resistance and strategies to overcome. *Eur. J. Pharm. Sci.* **2022**, *170*, 106103. [CrossRef] [PubMed]
15. Wences, M.; Wolf, E.R.; Li, C.; Singh, N.; Bah, N.; Tan, X.; Huang, Y.; Bulman, Z.P. Combatting Planktonic and Biofilm Populations of Carbapenem-Resistant *Acinetobacter baumannii* with Polymyxin-Based Combinations. *Antibiotics* **2022**, *11*, 959. [CrossRef] [PubMed]
16. Lee, S.H.; Teo, J.; Heng, D.; Ng, W.K.; Zhao, Y.; Tan, R.B. Tailored Antibiotic Combination Powders for Inhaled Rotational Antibiotic Therapy. *J. Pharm. Sci.* **2016**, *105*, 1501–1512. [CrossRef]
17. Almangour, T.A.; Garcia, E.; Zhou, Q.; Forrest, A.; Kaye, K.S.; Li, J.; Velkov, T.; Rao, G.G. Polymyxins for the treatment of lower respiratory tract infections: Lessons learned from the integration of clinical pharmacokinetic studies and clinical outcomes. *Int. J. Antimicrob. Agents* **2021**, *57*, 106328. [CrossRef]
18. Sobieszczyk, M.E.; Furuya, E.Y.; Hay, C.M.; Pancholi, P.; Della-Latta, P.; Hammer, S.M.; Kubin, C.J. Combination therapy with polymyxin B for the treatment of multidrug-resistant Gram-negative respiratory tract infections. *J. Antimicrob. Chemother.* **2004**, *54*, 566–569. [CrossRef]
19. Michel, J.-B.; Yeh, P.J.; Chait, R.; Moellering, R.C.; Kishony, R. Drug interactions modulate the potential for evolution of resistance. *Proc. Natl. Acad. Sci. USA* **2008**, *105*, 14918–14923. [CrossRef]
20. Torella, J.P.; Chait, R.; Kishony, R. Optimal Drug Synergy in Antimicrobial Treatments. *PLOS Comput. Biol.* **2010**, *6*, e1000796. [CrossRef]
21. Roemhild, R.; Andersson, D.I. Mechanisms and therapeutic potential of collateral sensitivity to antibiotics. *PLOS Pathog.* **2021**, *17*, e1009172. [CrossRef]
22. Aulin, L.B.S.; Liakopoulos, A.; van der Graaf, P.H.; Rozen, D.E.; van Hasselt, J.G.C. Design principles of collateral sensitivity-based dosing strategies. *Nat. Commun.* **2021**, *12*, 5691. [CrossRef]
23. Szybalski, W.; Bryson, V. Genetic studies on microbial cross resistance to toxic agents I: Cross resistance of *Escherichia coli* to fifteen antibiotics1, 2. *J. Bacteriol.* **1952**, *64*, 489. [CrossRef] [PubMed]

24. Liu, J.; Gefen, O.; Ronin, I.; Bar-Meir, M.; Balaban, N.Q. Effect of tolerance on the evolution of antibiotic resistance under drug combinations. *Science* **2020**, *367*, 200–204. [CrossRef] [PubMed]
25. Lin, Y.-W.; Han, M.-L.; Zhao, J.; Zhu, Y.; Rao, G.; Forrest, A.; Song, J.; Kaye, K.S.; Hertzog, P.; Purcell, A.; et al. Synergistic Combination of Polymyxin B and Enrofloxacin Induced Metabolic Perturbations in Extensive Drug-resistant *Pseudomonas aeruginosa*. *Front. Pharmacol.* **2019**, *10*, 1146. [CrossRef] [PubMed]
26. Buyck, J.M.; Tulkens, P.M.; Van Bambeke, F. Activities of antibiotic combinations against resistant strains of *Pseudomonas aeruginosa* in a model of infected THP-1 monocytes. *Antimicrob. Agents Chemother.* **2015**, *59*, 258–268. [CrossRef] [PubMed]
27. The European Committee on Antimicrobial Susceptibility Testing. Breakpoint Tables for Interpretation of MICs and Zone Diameters. Version 8.1. 2018. Available online: http://www.eucast.org (accessed on 20 November 2019).
28. Wang, J.; Grégoire, N.; Marchand, S.; Kutter, J.P.; Mu, H.; Moodley, A.; Couet, W.; Yang, M. Improved antibacterial efficiency of inhaled thiamphenicol dry powders: Mathematical modelling of in vitro dissolution kinetic and in vitro antibacterial efficacy. *Eur. J. Pharm. Sci.* **2020**, *152*, 105435. [CrossRef] [PubMed]
29. Park, J.Y.; Kim, S.; Kim, S.-M.; Cha, S.H.; Lim, S.-K.; Kim, J. Complete Genome Sequence of Multidrug-Resistant *Acinetobacter baumannii* Strain 1656-2, Which Forms Sturdy Biofilm. *J. Bacteriol.* **2011**, *193*, 6393–6394. [CrossRef] [PubMed]
30. Sahl, J.W.; Lemmer, D.; Travis, J.; Schupp, J.M.; Gillece, J.D.; Aziz, M.; Driebe, E.M.; Drees, K.P.; Hicks, N.D.; Williamson, C.H.D.; et al. NASP: An accurate, rapid method for the identification of SNPs in WGS datasets that supports flexible input and output formats. *Microb. Genom.* **2016**, *2*, e000074. [CrossRef]
31. Durbin, L.R. Fast and accurate short read alignment with Burrows-Wheeler transform. *Bioinformatics* **2009**, *25*, 1754–1760.
32. McKenna, A.; Hanna, M.; Banks, E.; Sivachenko, A.; Cibulskis, K.; Kernytsky, A.; Garimella, K.; Altshuler, D.; Gabriel, S.; Daly, M.; et al. The Genome Analysis Toolkit: A MapReduce framework for analyzing next-generation DNA sequencing data. *Genome Res.* **2010**, *20*, 1297–1303. [CrossRef]
33. Ziaee, A.; Albadarin, A.B.; Padrela, L.; Femmer, T.; O'Reilly, E.; Walker, G. Spray drying of pharmaceuticals and biopharmaceuticals: Critical parameters and experimental process optimization approaches. *Eur. J. Pharm. Sci.* **2019**, *127*, 300–318. [CrossRef]
34. Weers, J.G.; Miller, D.P.; Tarara, T.E. Spray-Dried PulmoSphere™ Formulations for Inhalation Comprising Crystalline Drug Particles. *AAPS PharmSciTech* **2019**, *20*, 103. [CrossRef] [PubMed]
35. Leng, D.; Kissi, E.O.; Löbmann, K.; Thanki, K.; Fattal, E.; Rades, T.; Foged, C.; Yang, M. Design of Inhalable Solid Dosage Forms of Budesonide and Theophylline for Pulmonary Combination Therapy. *AAPS PharmSciTech* **2019**, *20*, 137. [CrossRef] [PubMed]
36. Sheokand, S.; Modi, S.R.; Bansal, A.K. Dynamic Vapor Sorption as a Tool for Characterization and Quantification of Amorphous Content in Predominantly Crystalline Materials. *J. Pharm. Sci.* **2014**, *103*, 3364–3376. [CrossRef]
37. Mafra, L.; Santos, S.M.; Siegel, R.; Alves, I.; Paz, F.A.A.; Dudenko, D.; Spiess, H.W. Packing Interactions in Hydrated and Anhydrous Forms of the Antibiotic Ciprofloxacin: A Solid-State NMR, X-ray Diffraction, and Computer Simulation Study. *J. Am. Chem. Soc.* **2012**, *134*, 71–74. [CrossRef] [PubMed]
38. Paluch, K.J.; McCabe, T.; Müller-Bunz, H.; Corrigan, O.I.; Healy, A.M.; Tajber, L. Formation and Physicochemical Properties of Crystalline and Amorphous Salts with Different Stoichiometries Formed between Ciprofloxacin and Succinic Acid. *Mol. Pharm.* **2013**, *10*, 3640–3654. [CrossRef] [PubMed]
39. Sun, J.; Wang, F.; Sui, Y.; She, Z.; Zhai, W.; Deng, Y. Effect of particle size on solubility, dissolution rate, and oral bioavailability: Evaluation using coenzyme Q_{10} as naked nanocrystals. *Int. J. Nanomed.* **2012**, *7*, 5733–5744. [CrossRef]
40. Mangal, S.; Park, H.; Zeng, L.; Yu, H.H.; Lin, Y.-W.; Velkov, T.; Denman, J.A.; Zemlyanov, D.; Li, J.; Zhou, Q. Composite particle formulations of colistin and meropenem with improved in-vitro bacterial killing and aerosolization for inhalation. *Int. J. Pharm.* **2018**, *548*, 443–453. [CrossRef]
41. Shetty, N.; Ahn, P.; Park, H.; Bhujbal, S.; Zemlyanov, D.; Cavallaro, A.-A.; Mangal, S.; Li, J.; Zhou, Q.T. Improved physical stability and aerosolization of inhalable amorphous ciprofloxacin powder formulations by incorporating synergistic colistin. *Mol. Pharm.* **2018**, *15*, 4004–4020. [CrossRef]
42. Lorian, V. *Antibiotics in Laboratory Medicine*, 5th ed.; Lippincott Williams & Wilkins: Philadelphia, PA, USA, 2005.
43. Lázár, V.; Singh, G.P.; Spohn, R.; Nagy, I.; Horváth, B.; Hrtyan, M.; Busa-Fekete, R.; Bogos, B.; Méhi, O.; Csörgő, B.; et al. Bacterial evolution of antibiotic hypersensitivity. *Mol. Syst. Biol.* **2013**, *9*, 700. [CrossRef]
44. Rodriguez de Evgrafov, M.; Gumpert, H.; Munck, C.; Thomsen, T.T.; Sommer, M.O. Collateral resistance and sensitivity modulate evolution of high-level resistance to drug combination treatment in *Staphylococcus aureus*. *Mol. Biol. Evol.* **2015**, *32*, 1175–1185. [CrossRef]
45. Sánchez-Romero, M.A.; Casadesús, J. Contribution of phenotypic heterogeneity to adaptive antibiotic resistance. *Proc. Natl. Acad. Sci. USA* **2014**, *111*, 355–360. [CrossRef]
46. Dawan, J.; Kim, J.C.; Ahn, J. Insights into collateral susceptibility and collateral resistance in *Acinetobacter baumannii* during antimicrobial adaptation. *Lett. Appl. Microbiol.* **2021**, *73*, 168–175. [CrossRef] [PubMed]
47. Traini, D.; Young, P.M. Delivery of antibiotics to the respiratory tract: An update. *Expert Opin. Drug Deliv.* **2009**, *6*, 897–905. [CrossRef] [PubMed]
48. Nightingale, S.L. Tobramycin Inhalation Product Approved for Use in Cystic Fibrosis Therapy. *JAMA* **1998**, *279*, 645. [CrossRef]
49. Hickey, A.J.; Durham, P.; Dharmadhikari, A.; Nardell, E. Inhaled drug treatment for tuberculosis: Past progress and future prospects. *J. Control. Release* **2016**, *240*, 127–134. [CrossRef]

50. Fiel, S.B.; Roesch, E.A. The use of tobramycin for *Pseudomonas aeruginosa*: A review. *Expert Rev. Respir. Med.* **2022**, *16*, 503–509. [CrossRef] [PubMed]
51. Yu, S.; Wang, S.; Zou, P.; Chai, G.; Lin, Y.-W.; Velkov, T.; Li, J.; Pan, W.; Zhou, Q.T. Inhalable liposomal powder formulations for co-delivery of synergistic ciprofloxacin and colistin against multi-drug resistant gram-negative lung infections. *Int. J. Pharm.* **2020**, *575*, 118915. [CrossRef]
52. Yu, S.; Pu, X.; Ahmed, M.U.; Yu, H.H.; Mutukuri, T.T.; Li, J.; Zhou, Q.T. Spray-freeze-dried inhalable composite microparticles containing nanoparticles of combinational drugs for potential treatment of lung infections caused by *Pseudomonas aeruginosa*. *Int. J. Pharm.* **2021**, *610*, 121160. [CrossRef]
53. Lin, Y.; Quan, D.; Chang, R.Y.K.; Chow, M.Y.; Wang, Y.; Li, M.; Morales, S.; Britton, W.J.; Kutter, E.; Li, J.; et al. Synergistic activity of phage PEV20-ciprofloxacin combination powder formulation—A proof-of-principle study in a *P. aeruginosa* lung infection model. *Eur. J. Pharm. Biopharm.* **2021**, *158*, 166–171. [CrossRef]
54. Chai, G.; Hassan, A.; Meng, T.; Lou, L.; Ma, J.; Simmers, R.; Zhou, L.; Rubin, B.K.; Zhou, Q.; Longest, P.W.; et al. Dry powder aerosol containing muco-inert particles for excipient enhanced growth pulmonary drug delivery. *Nanomed. Nanotechnol. Biol. Med.* **2020**, *29*, 102262. [CrossRef]

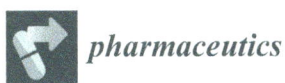 *pharmaceutics*

Review

Optimizing Spray-Dried Porous Particles for High Dose Delivery with a Portable Dry Powder Inhaler

Yoen-Ju Son [1], Danforth P. Miller [2] and Jeffry G. Weers [2,*]

[1] Genentech, South San Francisco, CA 94080, USA; son.yoen-ju@gene.com
[2] Cystetic Medicines, Inc., Burlingame, CA 94010, USA; dmiller@cysteticmedicines.com
* Correspondence: jweers@cysteticmedicines.com; Tel.: +1-650-339-3832

Abstract: This manuscript critically reviews the design and delivery of spray-dried particles for the achievement of high total lung doses (TLD) with a portable dry powder inhaler. We introduce a new metric termed the product density, which is simply the TLD of a drug divided by the volume of the receptacle it is contained within. The product density is given by the product of three terms: the packing density (the mass of powder divided by the volume of the receptacle), the drug loading (the mass of drug divided by the mass of powder), and the aerosol performance (the TLD divided by the mass of drug). This manuscript discusses strategies for maximizing each of these terms. Spray drying at low drying rates with small amounts of a shell-forming excipient (low Peclet number) leads to the formation of higher density particles with high packing densities. This enables ultrahigh TLD (>100 mg of drug) to be achieved from a single receptacle. The emptying of powder from capsules is directly proportional to the mass of powder in the receptacle, requiring an inhaled volume of about 1 L for fill masses between 40 and 50 mg and up to 3.2 L for a fill mass of 150 mg.

Keywords: packing density; product density; small porous particles; corrugated particles

Citation: Son, Y.-J.; Miller, D.P.; Weers, J.G. Optimizing Spray-Dried Porous Particles for High Dose Delivery with a Portable Dry Powder Inhaler. *Pharmaceutics* **2021**, *13*, 1528. https://doi.org/10.3390/pharmaceutics13091528

Academic Editors: Philip Chi Lip Kwok and Michael Yee Tak Chow

Received: 28 July 2021
Accepted: 7 September 2021
Published: 21 September 2021

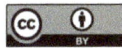
1. Introduction

Traditionally, large doses of inhaled drugs have been administered by jet nebulization. High dose nebulized drugs include Virazole® (ribavirin inhalation solution) for the treatment of respiratory syncytial virus [1,2], Nebupent® (pentamidine inhalation solution) for prophylaxis against *Pneumocystis jiroveci* in immunocompromised AIDS/HIV and organ transplant patients [3,4], and TOBI® (tobramycin inhalation solution) for the treatment of *Pseudomonas aeruginosa* infections in cystic fibrosis (CF) patients [5,6].

Jet nebulizers have limitations that can impact patient adherence [7]. They are bulky, noisy, require a power source, and have a high daily treatment burden. The daily treatment burden considers not only the time to administer the drug but also the time for set-up, disassembly, cleaning, and disinfection of the delivery device. Compliance with cleaning nebulizers is typically poor [8] and this can lead to contamination of the nebulizer with bacteria, possibly increasing the risk of administration of new, more virulent pathogens to at-risk patients during treatment [9]. Aqueous solutions of drugs for inhalation often must be reconstituted from lyophilized powder or stored at refrigerated temperatures to maintain chemical stability of the drug substance. Jet nebulizers also produce high levels of fugitive aerosol.

The higher delivery efficiency of vibrating mesh nebulizers can decrease the daily treatment burden [10,11] but this often requires nebulization of hypertonic solutions that pose greater risk of causing irritation in the lungs [12].

Relative to jet nebulizers, dry powder inhalers enable dramatic decreases in administration time and daily treatment burden. The transition from a nebulized treatment with tobramycin inhalation solution (TOBI®) to tobramycin inhalation powder (TOBI® Podhaler™) led to a reduction in administration time by ~30 min/day [13,14]. This translated into a high preference for the inhaled powder among CF patients [13] with improvements in adherence [15,16] and pharmacoeconomics [16,17]. Portable dry powder inhalers do not require a power source and are easy to carry in a pocket or purse, enabling discreet use outside the home [14].

1.1. High Dose Delivery with Portable Dry Powder Inhalers

Most subjects can empty 40–50 mg of powder from a receptacle in a single inhalation [Sections 4.3 and 4.4]. As the dose increases and powder mass exceeds 100 mg, the options become less satisfactory. This is exemplified by TOBI Podhaler (powder mass = 194 mg) and Bronchitol® (powder mass = 400 mg), which require administration of four and ten capsules twice daily, respectively (Figure 1). There remains a clear unmet need for improving drug delivery with a portable inhaler when the inhaled powder mass exceeds 100 mg.

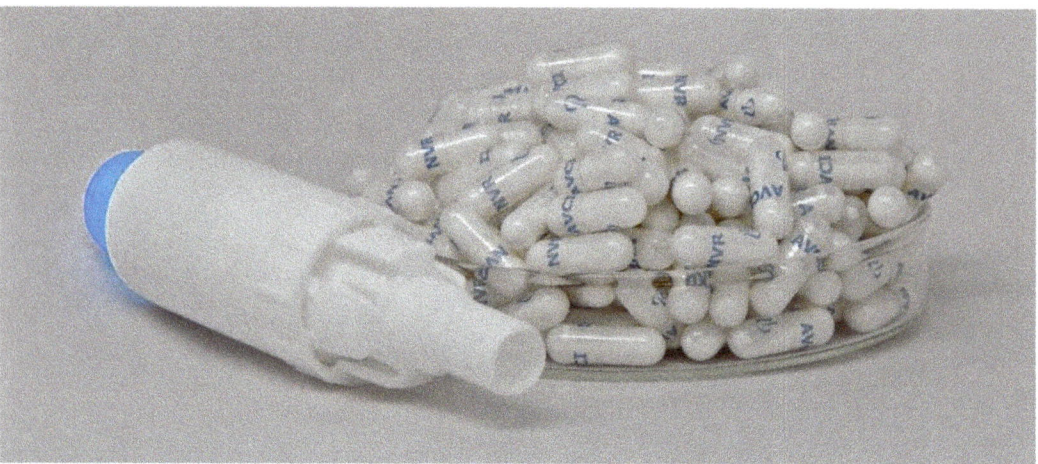

Figure 1. The unit dose Podhaler DPI and a month's supply of 240 capsules.

Indeed, Hickey et al. defined the challenges associated with high dose delivery well: "Effective high dose delivery of inhaled dry powders is a balance of the influence of product performance (drug formulation, metering, and device) and dose delivery (mass on a single breath, number of breaths per dose) with respect to patient adherence to therapy over potentially long periods of treatment." [18].

1.2. Definition of Ranges of Total Lung Dose

Sibum et al. [19] proposed a definition of high powder doses based on the highest mass of drug that can be delivered with standard adhesive mixtures comprising micronized drug and coarse lactose carrier particles (i.e., lactose blends). They suggested that the upper bound for drug loading in lactose blends is 0.1 mg/mg, after which the drug may not be associated with the carrier and the blend may be mechanically unstable with poor dose reproducibility [20]. The maximum fill mass for marketed adhesive mixtures is 25 mg, resulting in a breakpoint at nominal doses $\geq$2.5 mg.

Given that inhalation products have markedly different aerosol performance metrics, we prefer to use the total lung dose (TLD) as the defining metric. Adhesive mixtures comprising a force control agent such as magnesium stearate can achieve a TLD of about 0.5 mg/mg of the nominal dose [21,22]. Hence, the breakpoint between low and high doses would equate to a TLD of ~1 mg. Potent asthma and COPD therapeutics (e.g., inhaled corticosteroids and bronchodilators) have TLD values less than ~0.1 mg, falling well within the low-dose classification (Figure 2). Figure 2 also delineates less potent drugs subdivided into three additional groups: moderate, high, and ultrahigh total lung doses. To put the delivery challenge in perspective, this dose range covers six orders of magnitude.

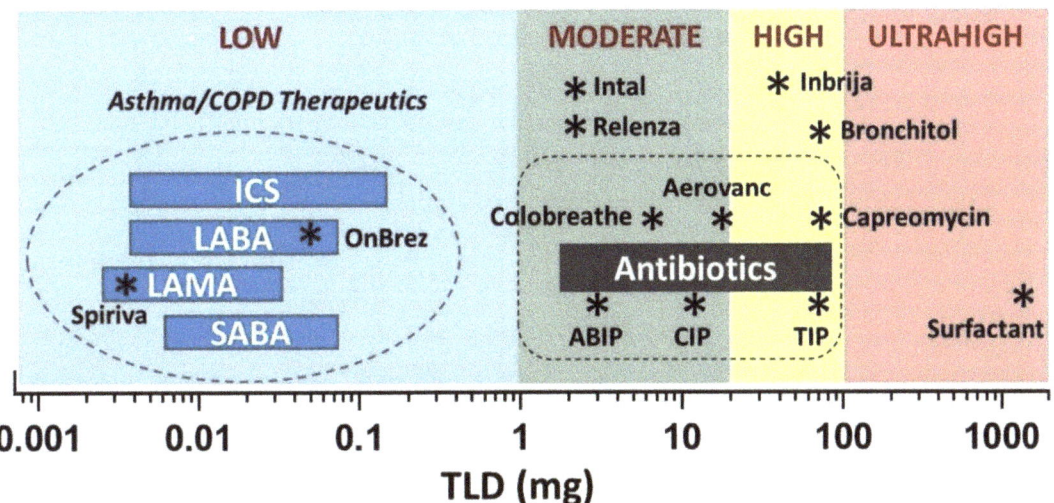

Figure 2. The total lung dose, *TLD* (*) of various inhaled drugs. The *TLD* is divided into low, moderate, high, and ultrahigh dose categories. Abbreviations: ICS, inhaled corticosteroid; LABA, long-acting beta-agonist; LAMA, long-acting muscarinic antagonist; SABA, short-acting beta-agonist; ABIP, amphotericin B inhalation powder (Nektar Therapeutics, San Francisco, CA, USA); CIP, Ciprofloxacin DPI (Bayer, Leverkusen, Germany); TIP, TOBI Podhaler (Novartis, Basel, Switzerland).

As discussed, there is a limit to the mass of powder that can be inhaled in a single inhalation using a capsule-based dry powder inhaler. Porous particle formulations have achieved a *TLD* up to ~20 mg in a single inhalation [23]. We define the range of *TLD* from 1 to 20 mg as moderate doses. For inhaled antibiotics, this group includes Ciprofloxacin DPI, Amphotericin B Inhalation Powder (ABIP), Aerovanc®, and Colobreathe®. The *TLD* range from 20 to 100 mg may require either multiple receptacles and/or multiple inhalations from a large receptacle to deliver the *TLD*. This dose range is defined as high doses and includes products such as TOBI Podhaler (*TLD* ~70 mg), Bronchitol® (*TLD* ~70 mg), and Inbrija® (*TLD* ~40 mg). Finally, *TLD* values above 100 mg are defined as ultrahigh doses. This group currently has no approved products but includes aspirational products such as pulmonary surfactant (*TLD* > 1000 mg, assuming a 20 mg/kg dose to a 60 kg adult).

At some point, the *TLD* can become impractical for delivery with a portable DPI, as it would require an excessive number of receptacles and too many inhalations per receptacle. This practical limit is likely less than 1 g unless a significant innovation in drug delivery is achieved. It is possible that these high doses could be delivered with a powder nebulizer over multiple breaths, but this may encompass many of the challenges associated with liquid nebulizers [24].

The balance of this review is focused on how to maximize the *TLD* that can be delivered from a given sized receptacle for spray-dried powders. To aid in this endeavor, we introduce a new metric termed the 'product density'.

2. Product Density

The product density ($\rho_{product}$) is simply the *TLD* achieved with a portable DPI divided by the volume of the receptable (V_r) that contains the powder. Both terms can be easily measured experimentally. The two most common types of receptacles in non-reservoir-based DPIs are capsules and laminated foil-foil blisters. The receptacle volume of blisters is typically between 0.03 and 0.2 mL, while capsule volumes vary between about 0.2 and 1.0 mL. Some recent DPI designs contain larger volume blisters and use compressed 'pucks' to enable larger fill masses [25–27]. The *TLD* can be determined in vivo by imaging (e.g., gamma scintigraphy) [28] and pharmacokinetic methods [29]. Alternatively, the *TLD* can be estimated in vitro with anatomical throat models (e.g., an Alberta idealized throat, AIT) [30,31]. Estimates can also be made using cascade impactor data but given the dependence of regional deposition on both size and flow rate, it is more appropriate to use a stage grouping (e.g., the stage grouping from stage 3 to the micro-orifice collector (MOC) in a Next Generation Impactor) as opposed to a cutoff size [32,33]. This stage grouping corresponds to particles with an impaction parameter less than ~467 μm^2 L min^{-1} [32]. Unfortunately, the 'type' of aerosol performance data available varies from product to product. When available, priority is given to the use of in vivo imaging and pharmacokinetic results, followed by in vitro anatomical throat data, and then in vitro impactor data. While there may be differences in the in vivo and in vitro measures of *TLD*, we do not believe that these differences materially impact the results and conclusions of the study.

The product density can be subdivided into three terms that capture the essence of key design features of a high dose product (Equation (1)).

$$\rho_{product} = \frac{TLD}{V_r} = \left(\frac{m_{powder}}{V_r} \right) \left(\frac{m_{drug}}{m_{powder}} \right) \left(\frac{TLD}{m_{drug}} \right) \tag{1}$$

The three terms comprise: (1) the mass of powder (m_{powder}) that can be filled into the receptacle volume ('*packing density*'), (2) the mass of drug (m_{drug}) divided by the mass of powder ('*drug loading*'), and (3) the fraction of the drug that is delivered into the lungs ('*aerosol performance*').

2.1. Packing Density

The packing density depends on the characteristics of the powder and the specifics of the filling process. The density of the powder bed depends not only on the particle density but also on how close the particles are able to be packed in the powder bed, which depends on the cohesive forces between particles.

Fine, cohesive powders are typically filled with vacuum drum fillers. These fillers, originally designed during the development of Exubera®, utilize ultrasonic energy to induce powder flow from a trough into a truncated cone-shaped filling cavity located on a rotating cylinder [34–36]. Acoustic energy may also be used to fluidize powder in the trough [36]. Drum fillers enable accurate and precise filling of fine cohesive powders down to fill masses of ~1 mg with an RSD of ≤2% [34]. The loosely compacted pucks are easily broken up during a 'capsule polishing' step where the surface of the capsules is dedusted.

The size of the void space within the receptacle depends on the size and shape of the receptacle and the corresponding size and shape of the puck as well as the number of pucks filled. The volume of the receptacle filled may also be influenced by the free volume needed within the receptacle for effective powder emptying. For example, for blister-based receptacles, powder properties (e.g., physical stability and chemical stability) can be negatively impacted if the powder is touching the lid foil during heat sealing.

2.2. Drug Loading

In the term drug loading, the 'drug' comprises only the active drug substance. It does not include the mass of the counterion in salts (or conformer in cocrystals), the mass in a drug that is not part of the active agent (e.g., in a prodrug), or the mass associated with excipients and residual process aids. For high dose delivery, it is highly desirable to maximize the drug loading in the formulation. With that said, the use of excipients is often necessary and, as we will show, critical for optimizing high dose delivery (Section 4).

2.3. Aerosol Performance

Aerosol performance depends on the nature of the formulation and the delivery device, and how the two components work in concert to optimize drug delivery to the target site within the lungs.

2.4. Optimization of Product Density

Taken together, the three terms encompass all aspects of the formulation, manufacturing process, and product performance, hence the term 'product density'. Attempts to improve one term may negatively impact another. For example, in some formulations, increasing powder compression during filling to increase the packing density may diminish aerosol performance. Drug delivery with neat formulations to increase drug loading may also reduce aerosol performance or increase dosing variability. Indeed, the constraints imposed for high dose delivery are unique for each drug being considered and the development of the drug product often becomes an optimization exercise. There is no single right answer and there are typically multiple approaches to arrive at an acceptable drug product, especially for drugs that require a moderate *TLD*.

3. Product Densities in Inhaled Drug Products

The product density metrics for the drug products pictured in Figure 2 are presented in Table 1.

Table 1. Product density metrics for various late-stage and marketed products.

Drug Product	Packing Density (mg/mL)	Drug Loading (mg/mg)	Aerosol Performance (mg/mg)	Product Density (mg/mL)
Spiriva® HandiHaler®	18.3	0.003	0.20	0.012
Onbrez® Breezhaler®	83.3	0.006	0.34	0.17
Intal® Spinhaler®	54.1	0.91	0.11	5.4
Relenza®	125.0	0.20	0.23	5.8
Colobreathe®	391.9	0.44	0.12	20.7
TOBI® Podhaler™	131.1	0.58	0.63	47.1
Ciprofloxacin DPI	135.1	0.65	0.53	46.5
ABIP	27.0	0.50	0.70	9.5
Capreomycin DPI	100.0	0.69	0.30	20.7
Aerovanc®	100.0	0.83	0.50	41.5
Bronchitol®	133.3	1.0	0.18	23.3
Inbrija®	52.6	0.84	0.50	22.1

3.1. Low Dose Products

As discussed, drugs for asthma and COPD are highly potent with *TLD*s less than ~0.1 mg (Figure 2). Table 1 includes product density metrics for two COPD drug products comprising adhesive mixtures: Spiriva® HandiHaler® (Boehringer Ingelheim, Ingelheim am Rhein, Germany) [37,38] and Onbrez® Breezhaler® (Novartis) [22,39]. The drugs in these products are bronchodilators: tiotropium bromide, a muscarinic receptor antagonist, and indacaterol maleate, a beta-agonist. Owing to the low nominal doses required, the drug loadings in these formulations are very low (0.003 and 0.006 mg/mg, respectively). The fill masses and resulting packing densities are also low (18.3 and 83.3 mg/mL, respectively), as are the *TLD* values (0.20 and 0.34 mg/mg, respectively). These metrics result in product densities for Spiriva and Onbrez of 0.012 and 0.17 mg/mL, respectively.

The magnitude of the flow rate dependence for these formulations was assessed using the Q_{index} [40]. The Q_{index} is the percent difference in *TLD* between pressure drops of 1 and 6 kPa, normalized by the higher of the two values. Formulations with Q_{index} values <15% are defined as having low flow rate dependence, between 15 and 45% medium flow rate dependence, and >45% high flow rate dependence [40]. The Q_{index} values for Spiriva HandiHaler and Onbrez Breezhaler were −25.0 and −31.0%, respectively, indicative of medium flow rate dependence [40]. A medium flow rate dependence is characteristic of lactose blends [40].

3.2. Intal® (Cromolyn Sodium Inhalation Powder)

Cromolyn sodium (also known as sodium cromoglycate) is a bronchodilator developed from the plant extract Khellin. At the time it was developed, Intal (Fisons, Loughborough, UK) was considered to be a high dose product, delivering 20 mg of micronized cromolyn sodium to asthma patients from a size 2 capsule with the Spinhaler® DPI (packing density = 54.1 mg/mL). The drug loading is quite high (0.91 mg/mg) owing to formulation as the disodium salt (i.e., without excipients). The TLD varies between 0.055 and 0.17 mg/mg with variations in inspiratory flow rate (mean = 0.113 mg/mg) [41], leading to a product density of ~5.4 mg/mL. On average, the TLD/capsule is about 2 mg. The Q_{index} for Intal is +73.7%, indicative of a high flow rate dependence [40].

3.3. Relenza® (Zanamivir Inhalation Powder)

Relenza (GSK) is a dry powder formulation of the antiviral zanamivir, used for the treatment of influenza. The drug product comprises an adhesive mixture of 5 mg of micronized drug blended with 20 mg of coarse lactose carrier particles (drug loading: 0.2 mg/mg) [42]. Twenty-five milligrams of the formulated powder was filled into laminated foil blisters (V_r ~ 0.16 mL) for a packing density of 125.0 mg/mL. A dose consists of administration of the contents of two blisters (total powder dose = 50 mg). The TLD of 0.23 mg/mg was determined with an anatomical throat model [43], resulting in a product density of 5.8 mg/mL. The TLD/blister is ~1.2 mg or ~2.4 mg/dose.

3.4. Colobreathe® (Colistimethate Powder for Inhalation)

Colobreathe (Forest Laboratories) is approved in Europe for the treatment of chronic *Pseudomonas aeruginosa* infections in cystic fibrosis (CF) patients [44,45]. Colobreathe delivers an emitted dose of 125 mg of neat colistimethate sodium from the Turbospin® dry powder inhaler twice daily [44,45]. The packing density is high (391.9 mg/mL) as the entire 145 mg powder dose is loaded into a single size 2 hard gelatin capsule. Colistimethate sodium is a prodrug of colistin that is intended to improve the biocompatibility of the cyclic peptide [46]. Colistin is first derivatized with methanesulfonic acid, and then converted into the sodium salt [46]. This results in a drug loading of the active colistin drug substance of ~0.44 mg/mg [46]. The aerosol performance of Colobreathe is poor compared to the spray-dried formulations, detailed below, with a total lung dose determined by gamma scintigraphy of 0.12 mg/mg [47]. These factors contribute to a product density of just 20.7 mg/mL. If colistimethate is treated as a neat drug (i.e., not as a prodrug), the product density increases to 46.1 mg/mL, comparable to the small porous particles detailed below. The in vitro TLD of neat colistimethate powder measured in the idealized Alberta throat model with CF patient inspiratory flow profiles, is highly dependent on flow rate ($Q_{index} = -45.8\%$). The low TLD is also expected to lead to significant variability in TLD associated with differences in the anatomical features of the oropharynx among patients [48,49].

3.5. TOBI® Podhaler™ (Tobramycin Inhalation Powder)

TOBI Podhaler (Novartis) is also administered to CF patients as a maintenance treatment for chronic *P. aeruginosa* infections in the airways [13,14,16]. The drug product was developed as a life cycle extension to the nebulized TOBI® drug product, significantly decreasing the burden of treatment while also improving patient convenience [13,14,16]. TOBI Podhaler is prepared using the solution-based PulmoSphere™ manufacturing process [14,50] wherein tobramycin sulfate is dissolved in the continuous phase of a perfluorooctyl bromide-in-water emulsion [14,50]. During drying, the evaporating liquid in the emulsion droplets leaves behind nanopores in the dried particles.

On a dry basis, the spray-dried drug product comprises 85% tobramycin sulfate and 15% excipients (2:1 molar ratio of distearoylphosphatidylcholine (DSPC):calcium chloride) [51]. When expressed in terms of tobramycin content and including residual solvents, the drug loading is 0.58 mg/mg with ~20% of the mass in the composition taken up by the sulfate counterion. The small porous particles have a median geometric size of about 3 μm. The drug product is filled into a size 2 HPMC capsule with a 48.5 mg fill mass yielding a packing density of 131.1 mg/mL. The nominal dose of 112 mg (28 mg per capsule) is administered in four capsules with the Podhaler dry powder inhaler twice daily, for a daily dose of 224 mg/day. The emitted dose is greater than 90% with about 63% of the nominal dose delivered into the lungs [52]. This results in a product density of 47.1 mg/mL and a TLD/capsule of 17.6 mg. The TLD in TOBI Podhaler is independent of inspiratory flow rate over the range of breathing profiles typically achieved by CF patients (Q_{index} = +0.3%) [40,52].

3.6. Ciprofloxacin DPI (Ciprofloxacin Powder for Inhalation)

Ciprofloxacin is a broad-spectrum antibiotic with activity against both Gram-positive and Gram-negative bacteria. Ciprofloxacin DPI (Bayer) was developed for the treatment of chronic infections in CF and non-CF bronchiectasis patients [53,54]. Ciprofloxacin DPI is prepared by the suspension based PulmoSphere manufacturing process, using the poorly soluble zwitterionic form of the drug at neutral pH [50,54]. This process results in small porous particles of micronized crystalline drug particles coated with porous shell comprising a 2:1 molar ratio of DSPC:CaCl$_2$. Formulation of the neutral form of the drug provides for dissolution-limited delivery in the lungs, enhancing the pharmacokinetic/pharmacodynamic metrics (e.g., the AUC/MIC ratio) and efficacy of the drug in the lungs [54]. The drug loading in the spray-dried drug product is 0.65 mg/mg. Using a drum filler, 50 mg of the powder is loaded into size 2 HPMC capsules, giving a packing density of 135.1 mg/mL. The nominal dose of the drug product is 32.5 mg, with delivery from a single capsule twice daily (65 mg daily dose). The aerosol performance as determined by gamma scintigraphy is about 0.53 mg/mg [55]. These results provide a product density of 46.5 mg/mL and a TLD/capsule of 17.2 mg. Moreover, as per TOBI Podhaler, the Q_{index} is low (Q_{index} = −12.2%) [54].

3.7. Amphotericin B Inhalation Powder (ABIP)

Amphotericin B inhalation powder (Nektar Therapeutics) was developed for prophylaxis of immunocompromised patients against the development of invasive fungal infections [56–58]. The drug product completed end-of-Phase 2 meetings with health authorities, but the program was discontinued after the pulmonary business unit of Nektar was sold to Novartis. The suspension based PulmoSphere formulation comprised 50% w/w crystalline amphotericin B with the remainder being the PulmoSphere excipients (i.e., a 2:1 mol:mol ratio of DSPC:CaCl$_2$) [56]. The drug is administered with a loading dose followed by weekly maintenance doses [58]. Given the relatively low maintenance dose (5 or 10 mg), the fill mass occupies only a small percentage of the size 2 capsule volume. As a result, the packing density is just 27.0 mg/mL. The aerosol performance of ABIP is independent of flow rate and inhaled volume with an emitted dose of 96 ± 3%, an MMAD of 2.3 μm, an FPF$_{S3-F}$ of 83% of the nominal dose, and a Q_{index} of just +1.3% [56]. The TLD is about 0.7 mg/mg. This results in a product density of about 9.5 mg/mL, and a TLD/capsule of about 3.5 mg.

3.8. Capreomycin Inhalation Powder

Capreomycin is an antibiotic that is commonly used in the treatment of tuberculosis in combination with other antibiotics. Core-shell particles of capreomycin sulfate (~87% capreomycin) were prepared by spray drying the drug with leucine as a shell-forming excipient [59,60]. On a dry basis, the drug product contained 16.7% w/w leucine. The spray-dried powder had a water content of 5.3% w/w, resulting in a drug loading of ~0.69 mg/mg. Thirty milligrams of powder was filled into size 3 capsules (packing density = 100.0 mg/mL) and the contents of up to 12 capsules (total powder dose of 360 mg) were administered to healthy adult subjects [60]. The MMAD of capreomycin inhalation powder was 4.74 μm. The FPF_{S2-F} was 50% of the nominal dose and the FPF_{S4-F} was 10% of the nominal dose. Splitting the difference yields an FPF_{S3-F} of about 30% of the nominal dose. Overall, this results in a packing density of 20.7 mg/mL and a TLD/capsule of 6.2 mg. The TLD for the full 12 capsules was about 74.5 mg, i.e., comparable to that of the TOBI Podhaler.

3.9. Aerovanc® (Vancomycin Inhalation Powder)

Aerovanc (Savara Pharmaceuticals) is intended to treat Gram-positive infections (e.g., methicillin-resistant *Staphylococcus aureus*, MRSA) in CF patients. The small porous particles were manufactured by spray drying a solution-based liquid feed that contained 83% vancomycin and 17% excipients [61–63]. The core-shell particles contained vancomycin in the core of the particle with a shell of leucine. Thirty milligrams of Aerovanc was filled into size 3 HPMC capsules providing a packing density of 100.0 mg/mL [61]. Aerosol delivery into the lungs and systemic circulation was about 0.50 mg/mg [61,62]. Overall, these features resulted in a product density comparable to the other small porous particle formulations, i.e., 41.5 mg/mL and a TLD/capsule of 12.5 mg.

3.10. Bronchitol® (Mannitol Inhalation Powder)

Bronchitol (mannitol inhalation powder) improves mucociliary clearance in CF patients [64–66]. The 400 mg nominal dose of mannitol is subdivided into ten size 3 capsules (V_r = 0.30 mL), each containing 40 mg of the powder formulation (packing density = 133.3 mg/mL). The drug product is administered twice daily for an 800 mg daily nominal dose. Bronchitol is manufactured by spray drying a solution of neat mannitol (drug loading = 1.0 mg/mg) to produce fine crystalline drug particles. The aerosol performance of spray-dried mannitol with a variant of the RS01 dry powder inhaler (Osmohaler™, R = 0.036 $kPa^{0.5}$ L^{-1} min) was determined by SPECT imaging in nine healthy subjects [66]. The measured TLD was 0.175 mg/mg [66]. This leads to a product density of 23.3 mg/mL and a TLD/capsule of 7.0 mg. The TLD per dose is ~70 mg. The treatment burden is high with Bronchitol with the need for patients to load and inhale the contents of twenty capsules daily.

As with the other neat drug formulations (i.e., Intal and Colobreathe), the flow rate dependence is high. The flow rate dependence of inhaled mannitol was assessed with the lower resistance version of the Osmohaler (R = 0.021 $kPa^{0.5}$ L^{-1} min) used for bronchoprovocation testing. The TLD decreased from 0.199 mg/mg at a flow rate of 67 L min^{-1} to 0.098 mg/mg at a mean flow rate of 121 L min^{-1}, corresponding to a high Q_{index} of −52.0% [66].

3.11. Inbrija® (Levodopa Inhalation Powder)

Inbrija (Acorda Therapeutics) is prescribed to Parkinson's patients during their "off-period" when symptoms are high and plasma dopamine levels are low [67]. Pulmonary administration enables rapid increases in plasma dopamine. The drug product on a dry basis comprises 90% w/w levodopa with the remaining 10% w/w being a mixture of dipalmitoylphosphatidylcholine (DPPC) and sodium chloride [25,68–70]. The spray-dried drug product also contains residual moisture. Inbrija is manufactured as large porous particles (ARCUS™ technology) as first described by Edwards et al. [71]. The median geometric diameter of the corrugated particles is about 6 to 8 μm [70]. The large size necessitates that the particle density be low to make the particles respirable. Indeed, the poured bulk density of the large porous particles is about 0.02 to 0.05 g/cm^3 [70]. Hence, the volume of powder that must be inhaled is large. About 50 mg of powder containing 42 mg of levodopa is filled into size 00 HPMC capsules (V_r = 0.95 cm^3), resulting in a packing density of about 52.6 mg/mL and a drug loading of 0.84 mg/mg. Despite the large volume of powder, emptying of the capsule typically requires only a single inhalation by the patient.

Patients with Parkinson's disease take the drug on demand up to five times daily for a maximum daily nominal dose of 420 mg (two capsules per dose) [25]. The drug is administered with the Inbrija dry powder inhaler, a capsule-based inhaler derived from the Turbospin aerosol engine and adapted to use a size 00 capsule. The in vitro emitted dose is about 86% with approximately 50% of the drug delivered into the lungs (i.e., aerosol performance ~ 0.5 mg/mg) [23,70]. This leads to a product density of about 22.1 mg/mL and a TLD/capsule of 21.0 mg.

4. Increasing TLD and Product Density in Spray Dried Powders

The discussion that follows is not intended to be an exhaustive review of manuscripts related to high dose delivery of inhaled therapeutics.

Here, we use specific examples to illustrate trends in the field and their impact on the TLD and product density. For a more comprehensive review of the literature, readers should consult the recent themed issue edited by Das, Stewart, and Tucker [72], which contains numerous reviews of interest [19,73–79], as well as other recent reviews dedicated to high dose delivery [80–82].

4.1. Why Not Just Formulate Neat Drug?

As suggested, there is currently a limit to the mass of powder that can be administered in a single inhalation. Hence, there is a strong desire to maximize the TLD/m_{powder}. This ratio is simply the product of the last two terms in the product density (Equation (1)). Stated another way, there is a desire to increase the drug loading (i.e., minimize or eliminate excipients including counterions and coformers) and to maximize aerosol performance in these high dose formulations. One group has gone so far as to suggest that the improvements in aerosol performance observed with spray-dried particles in Table 1 (TLD~40–70% of the nominal dose) can be duplicated through improvements in device design and that "designing and developing more powerful DPIs seems a better solution for improving dispersion" [19]. It remains to be seen whether this can be realized with more cohesive powders sans excipients and whether this will compromise the consistency of dose delivery (e.g., via increases in flow rate dependence and variability associated with oropharyngeal filtering of particles, as was observed with the neat Intal, Bronchitol, and Colobreathe formulations) [40,66]. The product density metrics for these examples are presented in Table 2.

Table 2. Product densities from selected research studies.

Drug Product	Packing Density (mg/mL)	Drug Loading (mg/mg)	Aerosol Performance (mg/mg)	Product Density (mg/mL)
Clofazimine RS01 [83]	66.7	1.0	0.45	30.0
Tobra Form I RS00 [84]	83.3	0.95	0.53	41.9
Tobra Form 2 RS00 [84]	83.3	1.0	0.34	28.4
TobraPS RS01 [85,86]	176.5	0.91	0.65	104.4
Tobra Cyclops [87,88]	85.7	0.95	0.34	27.7
Levodopa Cyclops [89,90]	85.7	0.98	0.24	20.2
Ciprofloxacin FB-DPI [91]	192.3	0.30	0.67	38.7
Levofloxacin iSPERSE [92]	133.3	0.51	0.40	48.0
TSLP Fab T-326 [93,94]	405.4	0.50	0.73	148.1
Levofloxacin T-326 [93]	405.4	0.80	0.69	223.8
FDC R/K RS00 [95]	66.7	1.0	0.61	40.7

It is worth noting that formulating neat crystalline drugs with a high true density does not necessarily translate into a high packing density or tapped density [96]. Indeed, the tapped densities achieved with neat crystalline drug powders, especially particles of respirable size, are often similar to what is observed with spray-dried particles. This is due to a low packing density resulting from significant porosity in the powder bed.

4.1.1. Neat Jet-Milled Clofazimine

Clofazimine is used in combination with rifampicin and dapsone in the treatment of leprosy. There is growing evidence that the drug may also have activity in the treatment of non-tuberculosis mycobacterial infections [97].

Brunaugh et al. [83] assessed the aerosol performance of neat jet-milled clofazimine powder (drug loading: 1.0 mg/mg) administered with the low resistance RS01 DPI (Table 2). The milling process resulted in a median particle diameter by laser diffraction of 1.8 μm. Twenty milligrams of the powder was loaded into a size 3 capsule for a packing density of 66.7 mg/mL. The aerodynamic particle size distributions were determined on a Next Generation Impactor at pressure drops of 1 and 4 kPa, corresponding to flow rates of 47 and 93 L min^{-1}, respectively. The fine particle dose on stages 3 to MOC (i.e., FPD$_{S3-F}$) were approximately 9.5 and 8.5 mg, respectively, suggesting that throat deposition increases at the very high flow rates achieved with the low resistance device. The Q_{index} shows a medium flow rate dependence with a value of −17.6%. For the purposes of the product density calculation, the mean of the two FPD$_{S3-F}$ values was used, i.e., 9.0 mg. This corresponds to an estimated *TLD* of 0.45 mg/mg. Overall, the product density was ~30.0 mg/mL, or about 50% lower than the small porous particle formulations in Table 1.

The *TLD*/capsule of ~9.0 mg sits comfortably in the moderate dose region where many technology solutions exist. The advantage of jet milling is that the process is simple and product development is also simplified by the absence of excipient. The process depends critically on the ability to effectively mill the drug to respirable sizes and the interparticle cohesive forces in the resulting agglomerated drug particles. As such, this process is not universal for all drugs. The use of shell-forming excipients was introduced, in part, to control the surface properties independent of the nature of the drug substance.

4.1.2. Tobramycin Base Formulation—1

A number of studies have been conducted with inhaled tobramycin. These studies are motivated by the desire to reduce the daily treatment burden by increasing the product density. As discussed, approximately 20% of the mass in the TOBI Podhaler spray-dried particles is from the sulfuric acid used to make the sulfate salt. As such, formulation as the free base has the potential to significantly increase the drug loading in tobramycin formulations.

Pilcer et al. [84] utilized gamma scintigraphy to determine the *TLD* for two high drug loading tobramycin free base formulations in nine patients with CF. Tobra Form 1 comprised lipid-coated crystals of tobramycin manufactured by spray drying a suspension of tobramycin base in isopropanol with 5% dissolved lipids (3:1 w:w ratio of cholesterol to Phospholipon). Tobra Form 2 was simply neat micronized tobramycin free base. Twenty-five milligrams of each powder was filled into size 3 capsules (packing density = 83.3 mg/mL). The capsules were loaded into an RS00 DPI. The *TLD*s for Tobra Form 1 and Tobra Form 2 were 0.53 and 0.34 mg/mg, respectively. The interpatient variability in the *TLD* increased from 19% for Tobra Form 1 to 36% for Tobra Form 2, consistent with previous studies where interpatient variability in the *TLD* decreased with increases in *TLD* [48,49].

This example illustrates the potential for suspension-based spray drying to deliver lipid-coated crystals with good aerosol performance with use of just 5% *w/w* lipid as a shell former. It also further illustrates the challenges associated with neat drug formulations, both from aerosol performance and variability in dose delivery perspectives.

4.1.3. Tobramycin Base Formulation—2

Buttini et al. [85,86] combined a solution of tobramycin base in water with an alcoholic solution of sodium stearate to form a 1% w/v liquid feed. The liquid feed was then spray dried to form amorphous particles of tobramycin base coated with just 1% w/w sodium stearate (TobraPS). Accounting for residual water in the formulation, the drug loading was 0.91 mg/mg. The dry powder was loaded into different sized capsules ranging from size 3 to size 0. The capsules were loaded into variants of the RS01 DPI modified to actuate and deliver the different sized capsules. The data for the size 0 capsule are presented in Table 2.

One hundred twenty milligrams of TobraPS powder was loaded into a size 0 capsule (packing density = 176.5 mg/mL). The aerosol performance of the lipid-coated particles was comparable or slightly better than TOBI Podhaler. Owing to the use of tobramycin base and increases in packing density, TobraPS achieved a significantly greater product density (104.4 mg/mL) compared to TOBI Podhaler (47.1 mg/mL). This, coupled with the use of a larger sized receptacle, enabled TobraPS to achieve a comparable TLD to TOBI Podhaler (~70 mg) by administration of TobraPS from a single size 0 capsule. As shown in Sections 4.3 and 4.4, this fill mass can be emptied by most CF patients in two or three inhalations. Overall, this approach decreases the number of capsules from four to one and the total number of inhalations from eight to two or three, a notable improvement.

4.1.4. Tobramycin Base Formulation—3

Hoppentocht et al. [87,88] spray dried neat tobramycin base from water to form an amorphous powder. The residual water content in the drug product was not disclosed. For the purposes of this estimate of product density, the drug loading is assumed to be 0.95 mg/mg. Thirty milligrams of amorphous tobramycin powder was loaded into the Cyclops single-dose cartridge (SDC) in the single-use disposable DPI. Although not specified, it is assumed that the study was run with the standard SDC that has a 0.35 mL volume. This results in a packing density of about 85.7 mg/mL.

Single ascending doses of 30, 60, 120, and 240 mg (requiring 1–8 devices) were administered to eight adult patients with non-CF bronchiectasis (age range from 57 to 73 years). Local tolerability and systemic pharmacokinetics were assessed. The aerosol performance of Tobra Cyclops was estimated from the systemic bioavailability in comparison with the systemic bioavailability results observed for TOBI Podhaler in CF patients in a Phase 1 clinical study [98]. This estimate assumes that the pulmonary bioavailability of tobramycin is ~100% of the TLD. According to early work on the development of an inhaled biopharmaceutical classification system (iBCS), drugs that are not permeability or dissolution limited typically have pulmonary bioavailabilities approaching 100% [99]. Indeed, the high pulmonary bioavailability of inhaled tobramycin was demonstrated in pharmacokinetic studies by Li and Byron [100]. In the Phase 1 study with TOBI Podhaler, a 112 mg dose was found to be equivalent to a 300 mg dose of TOBI. The dose-normalized AUC_{0-12h}/mg was 0.041 h mg/L. The corresponding dose-normalized AUC_{0-12h}/mg values for Tobra Cyclops were 0.013 (30 mg), 0.017 (60 mg), 0.019 (120 mg), and 0.022 h mg/L (240 mg). For the two higher doses, the relative bioavailability of Tobra Cyclops is about half that observed for TOBI Podhaler. The TLD for TOBI Podhaler was determined in the Alberta idealized throat model (0.63 mg/mg) [52]. This leads to an estimate of the aerosol performance of 0.34 mg/mg and a product density of 27.7 mg/mL for Tobra Cyclops. The TLD/device is ~9.7 mg.

4.1.5. Levodopa Formulation Co-Milled with Force Control Agent

Another manufacturing option is to co-mill the drug substance with a force-control agent (FCA) such as magnesium stearate, leucine, or a phospholipid under high-shear mixing processes such as mechanofusion [101,102].

In this example, Luinstra et al. [89,90] co-milled levodopa with 2% w/w leucine. Thirty milligrams of the coated drug particles was loaded into the Cyclops single-use disposable DPI (packing density = 85.7 mg/mL) and the systemic pharmacokinetics (i.e., the target for CNS delivery) and tolerability of inhaled levodopa was assessed in eight patients with Parkinson's disease. The aerosol performance was calculated from the systemic bioavailability of inhaled levodopa from the Cyclops DPI relative to results published for Inbrija and an oral SINEMET 25–100 tablet. SINEMET 25–100 has an oral bioavailability of 71% for levodopa at steady state [23,103,104]. Based on the bioavailability relative to the oral control, Inbrija has a TLD of about 0.46 mg/mg. This is consistent with aerosol performance metrics for Inbrija which suggest a TLD of about 0.50 mg/mg [69,70]. The dose normalized bioavailability of the 30 mg dose of inhaled levodopa from the Cyclops device is about 1.9 times lower than that of Inbrija, suggesting a TLD of about 0.24 mg/mg. This results in a product density of ~20.2 mg/mL and a moderate TLD of ~7 mg/device.

4.1.6. Fixed Dose Combinations

Several groups have explored the development of fixed dose combinations of two or more drugs [95,105–108]. In many of these studies the more hydrophobic drug is used as a shell-forming material with the more hydrophilic/hygroscopic drug present in the core of the spray dried core-shell particles [95,107]. The shell-forming drug helps to improve the physical stability, chemical stability, and aerosol performance of the drug that is less stable to changes in RH. For antibiotics, the two drugs may also work synergistically to lower the dose needed for effective bacterial killing, thereby decreasing the TLD/mg powder [105,106,108].

For example, Momin et al. [95] studied a fixed dose combination of 60% kanamycin/ 40% rifampicin spray-dried from a 70/30 % v/v mixture of ethanol/water with no added excipients (drug loading = 1.0 mg/mg) (designated as FDC R/K RS00 in Table 2). Twenty milligrams of the powder was filled into a size 3 capsule (packing density = 66.7 mg/mL) and the powder was administered with the RS00 DPI at a flow rate of 100 L/min and an inhaled volume of 4 L. Surprisingly, the FPF_{S3-F} differed for the two drugs, with about 0.68 mg/mg of the shell-forming rifampicin and 0.54 mg/mg of the kanamycin deposited on S3-F. The average of the two values was used for the aerosol performance, i.e., 0.61 mg/mg. This resulted in a product density of 40.7 mg/mL and a TLD/capsule of ~12.2 mg (Table 2).

4.1.7. Excipients

Overall, the results presented above suggest that there are options to significantly improve the drug loading in high dose formulations. It is clear that, as the dose increases, a conscious attempt should be made to minimize the percentage of excipients in the formulation. All of the examples presented provide options for moderate TLD delivery. Spray-dried formulations containing small amounts of shell-forming excipients achieve better aerosol performance and improved dose consistency relative to neat drug particles.

While minimizing excipients and process aids is important for high dose formulations, there are many reasons to add excipients beyond improving aerosol performance. Salts are often preferred because of their improved solubility, purity, and crytallizability relative to neutral forms. For labile drug substances, excipients can be used to improve the physical and chemical stability of the drug substance. We add excipients to improve the tolerability and safety of the drug product. We add excipients to improve efficacy by controlling pharmacokinetic/pharmacodynamic metrics. We add excipients to improve the consistency of dosing by reducing variability associated with oropharyngeal filtering of particles, variability associated with inspiratory flow rate, and variability associated with coformulation effects in fixed dose combinations. In addition, yes, we add excipients to reduce interparticle cohesive forces, thereby enabling improvements in aerosol performance, packing density, and targeting within the respiratory tract.

To put this in perspective, let us consider the formulations comprising tobramycin base detailed above. From a regulatory perspective, TOBI Podhaler was filed as a 505(b)(2) NDA, with nebulized TOBI as the reference listed drug (RLD). As such, key features of the drug product (e.g., use of the sulfate salt of the drug substance) were maintained. This allowed the development of TOBI Podhaler to leverage the extensive systemic and pulmonary safety established by TOBI in both nonclinical and clinical studies. This further enabled TOBI Podhaler to go straight from a Phase 1 single ascending dose study in CF patients to Phase 3. The TOBI Podhaler dose for Phase 3 was selected based on its equivalence to TOBI in terms of systemic drug levels [98].

Tobramycin is an aminoglycoside antibiotic containing three glycosidic rings and five primary amine groups. TOBI was formulated at pH 6.0 by the addition of sulfuric acid to tobramycin base to provide a stable formulation. This avoided the use of preservatives and antioxidants (e.g., phenol and sodium bisulfite) which had been demonstrated to contribute to bronchospasm when inhaled by CF patients [6,109]. One challenge with the use of tobramycin base is the high pH of the drug in water (pH~10). The multiple amine groups, high dose, and twice daily administration provides the potential for significant buffering capacity (i.e., raising concerns about altering the physiologic pH in the lungs). The TOBI Inhalation Solution monograph suggests that nebulized liquids can be safely administered below pH 8.7 [6]. While long-term safety studies have been conducted with TOBI and TOBI Podhaler with the sulfate salt, the long-term safety of tobramycin base has yet to be established and, as such, needs to be kept in mind for future life cycle product designs.

The physicochemical stability of the formulated drug product is critical to the development and registration of dry powder inhalation products. This is especially important for amorphous materials which tend to have lower physical and chemical stability. While tobramycin base can be crystallized, salts of tobramycin cannot [51]. As is expected, the stability of the amorphous phase is significantly greater for the salt forms of tobramycin with the sulfate salt having a much higher glass transition temperature than the hydrochloride salt or the free base (at 11.3% RH, the T_g values are 105, 72, and 63 °C, respectively) [51,110]. At 43% RH, the T_g of tobramycin base is equivalent to a storage temperature of 25 °C. Amorphous tobramycin base presents additional physical stability challenges, crystallizing at RH values > 53% RH [51,87].

In TOBI Podhaler, the high T_g of tobramycin sulfate and high gel to liquid crystal phase transition temperature of the phospholipid acyl chains in the spray-dried drug product enables room temperature stability (physical, chemical, and aerosol) over a period of three years [14,110]. Maintaining long-term stability requires a delicate balance of physical form, formulation/process, and packaging. The general rule of thumb is that for long-term stability the T_g of the amorphous phase should be at least 50 °C above the storage temperature [111]. For tobramycin base, the low T_g suggests that room temperature stability may be challenging, even when using laminated foil blisters with very low water permeability. This can possibly be mitigated through refrigerated storage with very tight packaging. Peelable blisters such as those used in single-use disposable DPIs may not provide a sufficient moisture barrier to maintain long-term stability of amorphous tobramycin base. Shell formers such as leucine, trileucine, and sodium stearate may be added to reduce the instantaneous drop in aerosol performance when inhalers are operated at high RH [112–116]. They may also slow changes in physical form and drug content on storage.

We raise these points to reinforce the concept that there are many reasons that formulators add excipients (including counterions) to formulations and that these considerations need to be kept in mind during formulation development.

4.2. Why Not Take the Air Out?

While significant attention has been paid to maximizing drug loading and aerosol performance in high dose products, comparatively little time has been invested in maximizing the packing density of particles in the receptacle. As discussed, the packing density depends not only on the particle density, but also on the void spaces between particles and details around the filling process.

For porous particles, the aerodynamic diameter, d_a, is related to the geometric diameter of the particles (d_g) and the particle density (ρ_p) by Equation (2):

$$d_a = d_g \sqrt{\rho_p} \tag{2}$$

To achieve an equivalent aerodynamic diameter with larger sized particles, the particle density must be decreased. Given that this relationship is proportional to the square root of particle density, marked reductions in particle density are necessary for modest increases in particle size. This is readily apparent for the spray-dried formulations in Table 1. Small porous particles with d_g = 1–4 μm (e.g., TOBI Podhaler, Ciprofloxacin DPI, Aerovanc) achieve higher packing densities and product densities than large porous particles with d_g = 6–8 μm (e.g., Inbrija) owing, in part, to their greater particle densities (Table 1). The question is whether the particle density can be increased further by reducing particle corrugation or porosity while still maintaining acceptable powder flow and aerosol performance.

4.2.1. Small Dense Particles

Pulmatrix, Inc. developed the iSPERSE™ technology to address this question [92,117]. iSPERSE particles comprise fine spray-dried particles (d_g < 5.0 μm) with a tapped density > 0.4 g cm^{-3}. The increased tapped density relative to many lower density porous particle formulations is due, in part, to the incorporation of high-density inorganic salts in the particles. Unfortunately, little data have been published demonstrating the capability of the technology.

In one study, Manzanedo et al. [92] studied iSPERSE powders comprising 75–90% levofloxacin with the remainder being a 1:2 w:w mixture of leucine and sodium chloride. For this estimate, we will use the higher drug loading of 0.9 mg/mg. A fill mass of 40 mg in a size 3 capsule was administered with the RS01 DPI (packing density = 133.3 mg/mL). The FPD$_{S2-F}$ was presented and varied between 0.39 and 0.62 mg/mg (mean = 0.51 mg/mg). Obviously, the FPD$_{S3-F}$ will be less than this—let us assume 0.4 mg/mg. This yields an approximate product density of 48.0 mg/mL which is comparable to the values for small porous particle formulations (e.g., TOBI Podhaler, Ciprofloxacin DPI, Aerovanc) listed in Table 1. They claim to be able to fill up to 100 mg in a size 3 capsule (packing density = 333 mg/mL) but provide no data to support this assertion [92].

4.2.2. Coated Crystals

Another path to increasing the particle density is via spray drying of suspension-based liquid feeds comprising crystalline drug particles [53,54,56,84]. In this process, the crystalline particles are typically coated with a layer of shell-forming excipient. Numerous examples of coated crystals are provided in this review, including Ciprofloxacin DPI [53,54], ABIP [56], and Tobra Form 1 [84]. Given that the drug makes up the bulk of the spray-dried particle and most crystalline drugs have true densities >1 g/cm^3, the particle density of particles prepared from suspension-based liquid feeds is expected to be higher. The fill mass of crystalline Ciprofloxacin DPI is 50 mg (packing density = 135.1 mg/mL). During dose-ranging studies, higher doses of the drug were studied but produced no added clinical benefit [118]. Nonetheless, fill masses up to 75 mg were developed in support of these studies (packing density = 202.7 mg/mL). This led to an increase in product density to ~69.8 mg/mL. A recent review by Weers et al. [56] provides considerations for spray drying suspension-based liquid feeds. This includes formulation and engineering solutions that enable maintenance of drug crystallinity irrespective of the physicochemical properties of the drug, including its aqueous solubility [56].

4.2.3. Modifications of Packing Density

So far, the discussion has focused on modifications of particle density. Let us now turn attention to the packing of the particles in the powder bed. For gravitationally stable coarse particles (d_g > 100 μm), close packing within the powder bed is achieved with spherical particles [119–121]. Any decreases in sphericity increase bed porosity and reduce the packing density [119]. As particles become finer, increases in interparticle cohesive forces begin to negatively impact close packing of particles [119]. In this scenario it may be necessary to reduce cohesive forces via changes in particle morphology. These changes not only improve particle fluidization and dispersion, but they also enable close packing within the powder bed.

The impact of variations in surface corrugation on the packing density of fine cohesive powders comprising an antibody fragment (Fab) was studied by Son et al. [93,94].

The degree of surface corrugation is controlled through variations in the feedstock composition (e.g., solids loading, concentration of shell former) and by variations in the rate of drying. This can be described conceptually in the context of the Peclet number, a dimensionless number that describes the interplay of diffusion and evaporation in an atomized droplet during spray drying, viz [122–126]:

$$Pe = \frac{\kappa}{D} = \frac{\text{evaporation rate}}{\text{diffusion rate}} \tag{3}$$

When an atomized droplet is dried slowly, the solutes within the liquid droplet have time to diffuse throughout the shrinking droplet. This leads to the formation of fine, higher density particles with a smooth particle morphology (i.e., no surface roughness). In contrast, if an atomized droplet is dried quickly relative to the diffusion rates of the solutes, the slow-diffusing solutes become enriched on the surfaces of the drying droplets, leading to low-density particles. Components with low solubility or high surface activity are concentrated at the interface of the receding droplet. The resulting particles are often hollow. Depending on the material properties of the shell, the particle may collapse upon drying to form a lower density corrugated morphology akin to a 'wrinkled raisin'. By varying the Peclet number it is possible to control the degree of surface corrugation.

The process conditions and micromeritic properties of three of the anti-TSLP Fab formulations studied by Son et al. [93,94] are summarized in Table 3. Scanning electron microscopy images of the particles are presented in Figure 3.

Table 3. Process conditions and micromeritic properties of three formulations comprising 50% w/w of an anti-human thymic stromal lymphopoietin (TSLP) antibody fragment (CSJ117) [93,94]. Adapted with permission from Virginia Commonwealth University and Respiratory Drug Delivery, 2020.

Anti-TSLP Fab (CSJ117)	Lot A7	Lot A1	Lot A13
Morphology	Smooth spheres	Dimpled spheres	Corrugated particles
Trileucine (% w/w)	0	2.5	15
Solids Loading	1.0	1.0	1.0
Drying conditions [a]	Fast	Slow	Fast
$\times 50$ (μm) [b]	1.19	1.43	1.36
$\times 90$ (μm) [b]	1.87	2.39	2.94
SSA (m^2/g) [b]	6.35	6.01	14.90
Bulk density (g/cm^3)	0.21	0.29	0.10
Tapped density (g/cm^3)	0.34	0.57	0.15
Puck density (g/cm^3)	0.38	0.64	0.28
Compressibility (inh)	10.5	10.9	46.4

[a] Slow drying conditions: feed rate = 2.5 mL/min; outlet temperature = 55 °C; airflow rate = 300 L/min. Fast drying conditions: feed rate = 5.0 mL/min; outlet temperature = 70 °C; airflow rate = 600 L/min. [b] $\times 50$: 50% of the particles in the volume distribution have a primary particle size less than the $\times 50$; $\times 90$: 90% of the particles in the volume distribution have a primary particle size less than the $\times 90$; SSA: specific surface area.

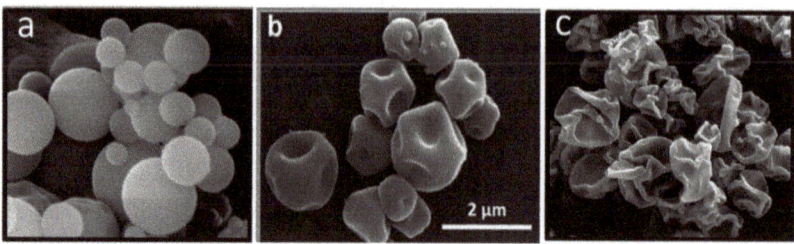

Figure 3. Scanning electron microscopy images of anti-TSLP Fab (CSJ117) particles spray dried with increasing Peclet numbers: (**a**) smooth spheres with 0% trileucine (Lot A7), (**b**) dimpled spheres with 2.5% trileucine (Lot A1), (**c**) corrugated spheres with 15% trileucine (Lot A13) [93].

A modified compressibility index listed in Table 3 was defined to reflect parameters important for inhaled drug products comprising fine drug particles. Instead of using the poured bulk density and tapped density in the calculation, the inhaled compressibility index uses the tapped density and the puck density. The puck density is the bulk density measured under the compression used to form pucks during drum filling. While the standard (Carr's) compressibility index and Hausner ratios provide information on the flowability of the bulk powder, these values are not reflective of the ability to fill these particles with high accuracy and precision on drum fillers, nor are they predictive of the resulting aerosol properties. The inhaled compressibility index provides a better metric to assess the impact of the degree of powder compression on filling and its resultant influence on aerosol performance [93,94]. Compressibility index values on the order of 10 indicate low degrees of powder compression on filling while values on the order of 40 indicate a high level of compression.

In the absence of a shell-forming excipient such as trileucine, the spray-dried antibody forms smooth spheres (Figure 3a). Unfortunately, a high coordination number and packing density is not achievable with particles of this size; cohesive forces between the particles leads to particle bridging and large void spaces within the powder bed, even on compression to form a puck during drum filling (Figure 4). The puck density following compression of the spherical particles during filling was just 0.38 g/cm^3.

The addition of 15% trileucine as a shell former and rapid drying conditions lead to significant increases in particle corrugation and specific surface area (SSA) for the core-shell powder formulation (Figure 3c). From the standpoint of packing density, the increased corrugation leads to a low particle density as the asperities on the particle surfaces prevent close packing. As a result, the puck density for the powder bed is just 0.28 g/cm^3 (Table 3). This low puck density occurred despite the high compressibility index of this powder, i.e., the tapped density is significantly lower.

Introducing a small amount of corrugation within the particles (e.g., dimpling) by processing at a low Peclet number is sufficient to reduce the interparticle cohesive forces and improve packing within the powder bed (Figure 3b). For example, a powder with only 2.5% w/w trileucine manufactured using 'slow' drying conditions was able to pack more effectively, with a puck density of 0.64 g/cm^3 (Table 3).

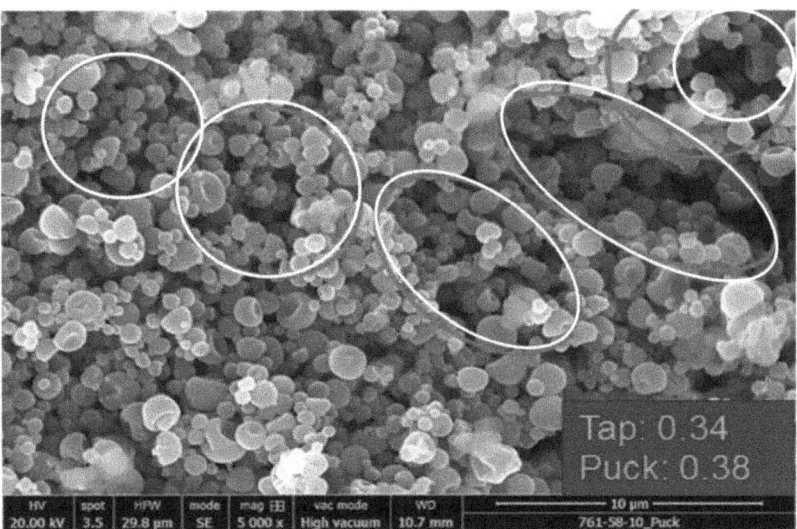

Figure 4. Scanning electron micrograph image of compressed spherical anti-TSLP Fab particles (Lot A7) showing large voids in powder bed [93].

To be suitable for high dose powder delivery, a powder with an improved packing density must also empty and disperse effectively from the capsule during patient inspiration. The low compressibility index observed for the dimpled spheres suggests that the filling process may have an insignificant impact on powder dispersion [93,94]. For a 150 mg fill mass in a size 2 capsule (packing density = 405.4 mg/mL), the emitted dose of the dimpled particles was 83% after the first inhalation and 88% after the second inhalation [93,94]. The TLD was 0.69 mg/mg after the first inhalation, increasing to 0.83 mg/mg of the emitted dose after the second inhalation (2 L volume of air per actuation) [93,94]. This equates to a TLD of 110 mg of the dry powder and 55 mg of anti-TLSP Fab from a single size 2 capsule. The low Peclet Fab particles have a product density of 148.1 mg/mL (Table 2), which is about three-fold higher than is achieved by the small porous particle formulations presented in Table 1. A dramatic increase in product density occurs despite the formulation containing 50% excipients. The excipients include glass formers (trehalose, mannitol) and a buffer (histidine) to stabilize the antibody physically and chemically in an amorphous solid (glass), thereby enabling room temperature stability of the formulated drug product. A levofloxacin formulation spray dried at low Peclet numbers with a higher drug loading pushed the envelope even further, achieving a product density of 223.8 mg/mL (Table 2) [93].

The significant increases in packing density and product density achieved with these low Peclet number formulations enable delivery of high and ultrahigh TLD from a single capsule. While most studies to date have been conducted with DPIs utilizing size 3 and size 2 capsules, the design of two DPIs have been modified to incorporate larger sized capsules. Acorda Therapeutics modified the Turbospin device to increase the capsule size from size 2 to size 00 for the Inbrija drug product [25]. This markedly increased the receptacle volume from 0.37 to 0.95 mL. Similarly, the design of the RS01 DPI has been modified to incorporate size 2 and size 0 capsules from the original size 3 capsules [26,86]. The aerosol engines driving powder dispersion in these devices remain the same.

Figure 5 displays the TLD as a function of the packing density for various sized capsules. For the products detailed in Table 1, the product densities are less than 50 mg/mL and they typically utilize size 2 and size 3 capsules. As such, it is clear from Figure 5 how the TLD/capsule is limited to about 20 mg. The impact of increasing product density and capsule size on the TLD/capsule is readily apparent. Ultrahigh TLD greater than 100 mg can be achieved at high product densities in size 0 and size 00 capsules for product densities greater than 160 and 110 mg/mL, respectively.

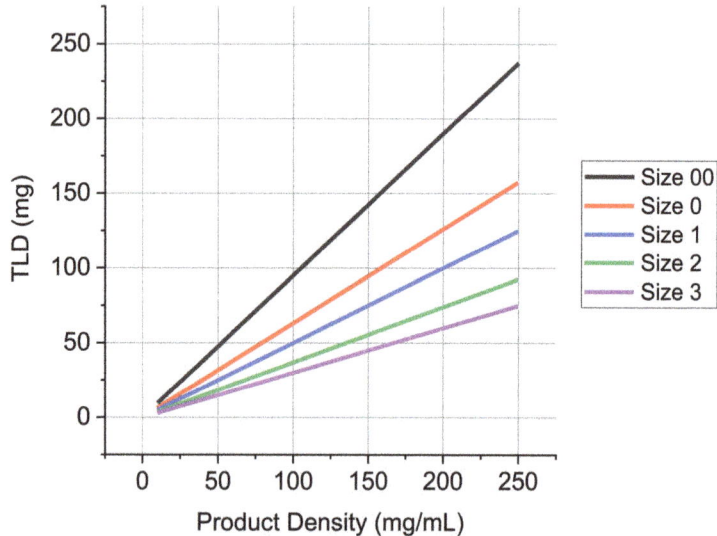

Figure 5. TLD as a function of the product density for various sized capsules.

To put the product densities observed with low Peclet number formulations in perspective, the TLD for the ten administered capsules in Bronchitol is about 70 mg. In principle this could be accomplished by the inhalation of the contents of a single size 2 or size 0 capsule. Similarly, a product density of 200 mg/mL with tobramycin would allow for the administration of the current 70 mg TLD from a single size 2 capsule versus the four capsules in the current drug product.

Moving to a single larger-sized capsule to administer the full dose may not only reduce the daily treatment burden, administration time, and potential for capsule handling errors, it may also reduce the cost of goods (capsules, packaging), improve the shelf life (less moisture uptake in a larger dose), and reduce environmental impact (less packaging). Many patients, especially elderly patients, or those with neuropathy, may also find handling larger sized capsules to be easier.

Increasing the product density may also have important implications for blister-based multidose DPIs, potentially extending the range of TLD that can be achieved in this class of inhalers to 5–10 mg. This may enable less potent actives such as immunoglobulins, hormones, and kinase inhibitors to be delivered in a multi-dose DPI (MD-DPI) alone or in combination with potent asthma/COPD therapeutics.

4.3. Capsule Emptying

One concern with high dose delivery using passive DPIs is whether a patient's inspiratory effort is sufficient to effectively fluidize and disperse the powder, and whether the inhaled volume of air is sufficient to empty powder from the capsule.

The inhaled volume required to empty the powder contents from a capsule was determined by laser photometry [127,128]. The laser photometer generates a laser light sheet that intersects the flow path of the emitted aerosol immediately downstream of the inhaler mouthpiece (Figure 6A). The obscuration of the laser sheet caused by the emitted aerosol bolus is detected by a photodetector. The photodetector's response is linear with obscuration and Beer's Law is used to convert the response into a relative aerosol concentration. It is relative in the sense that it is not corrected for differences in scattering intensity that result from the presence of different sized particles in the laser light path over the period of powder emptying. The signal intensity is observed as a voltage pulse whose width corresponds to the duration of the aerosol emission process. Simulated inspiratory flow profiles are generated using a custom breath simulator. The breath simulator is equipped with a computer controlled proportional solenoid valve. When the system is connected to a vacuum source, the valve opening can be varied in a controlled manner to mimic a patient's inspiratory flow profile.

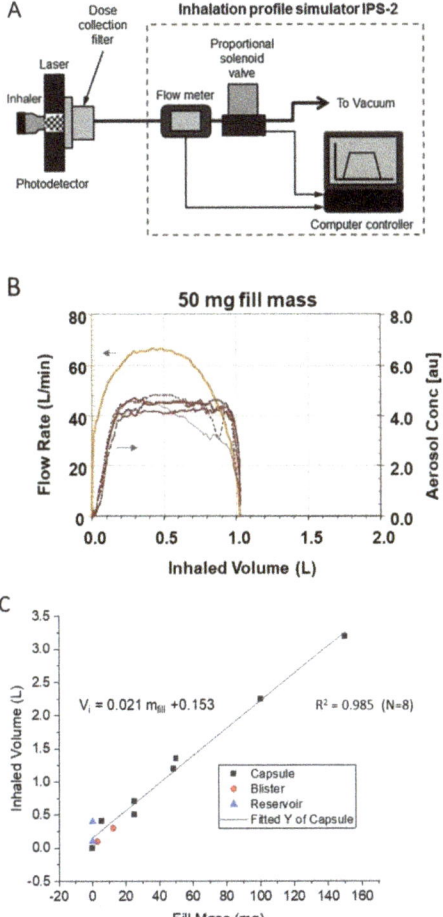

Figure 6. (**A**) Diagram of laser photometer system utilized to determine inhaled volume required to empty powder from a DPI [127,128]. The diagram was reproduced from [127] with permission from Elsevier, 2016; (**B**) Plot of a representative inspiratory flow profile and corresponding powder emptying profile for TOBI Podhaler using the laser photometer system; (**C**) Plot of the inhaled volume required to empty a fill mass for various inhaled products. DPIs included in the plot are: Asmanex® Twisthaler®, Pulmicort® Flexhaler®, Spiriva HandiHaler, Advair® Diskus®, Onbrez Breezhaler, indacaterol Simoon™, vardenafil AOS®, Cipro T-326, TOBI Podhaler, CSJ117 T-326 [93,127,128]. It should be noted that the curve is dominated by capsule DPIs except at low fill masses.

Figure 6B illustrates the typical output for the laser photometer with a simulated inspiratory flow profile for a CF patient with the Podhaler device (Vi ~1.1 L and PIF ~66 L/min), along with the emptying profiles for four capsules containing 50 mg of tobramycin inhalation powder. For this inspiratory flow profile, the bulk of the powder is emptied with a single inhalation.

As the packing density increases within the same sized capsule, the inhaled volume needed to empty the powder increases in proportion to the mass of powder in the capsule (i.e., it is largely independent of the volume of powder) (Figure 6C).

For low dose asthma/COPD therapeutics, the inhaled volume required to empty the powder from reservoirs, blisters, and capsules is $\leq$0.7 L, with the upper end of the range being defined by capsule based DPIs with a 25 mg fill mass of lactose (Figure 6C). For the ~50 mg of powder in TOBI Podhaler, the required inhaled volume increases to about 1.1 to 1.2 L. The 150 mg fill mass for the anti-TSLP Fab in a size 2 capsule requires 3.3 L of inhaled volume to empty. For the 145 mg fill mass in Colobreathe, the predicted inhaled volume is ~3.2 L, while a 400 mg fill mass (e.g., Bronchitol) would require a minimum inhaled volume of 8.6 L to empty. The inhaled volume that subjects can achieve with portable dry powder inhalers depends on many factors, some of which are detailed in the examples below.

4.4. Inhaled Volumes of Patients

Azouz et al. [129] studied inspiratory flow profiles in 88 asthma and COPD patients. The mean inhaled volumes (Vi) were 1.10 L for pediatric asthma patients with an age of 8.8 $\pm$ 3.1 years, 1.62 L for adult asthma patients with a mean age of 48.7 $\pm$ 16.0 years, and 1.63 L for adult COPD patients with a mean age of 66.0 $\pm$ 9.6 years. Decreases in Vi were observed with increases in device resistance. Given that the Vi required for emptying asthma/COPD DPIs is $\leq$0.7 L, only a single inhalation would be needed, even for most pediatric patients. This is consistent with clinical practice.

Tiddens et al. [130] studied the inspiratory flow profiles of 96 patients with CF while inhaling through a test device containing a series of flow resistors. When inhaling against a resistance of 0.024 $kPa^{0.5}$ L^{-1} min, 73% of children aged 6–10 years could achieve a Vi of 1.0 L. This decreased to 30% for a Vi of 1.5 L, and only 3% could reach a Vi of 2.0 L. For children with CF between the ages of 11–18 years, 92% could achieve a Vi of 1.0 L, decreasing to 62% of patients for a Vi of 1.5 L, and 33% for a Vi of 2.0 L. For adults older than age 18, 97% of patients could achieve a Vi of 1.0 L, 77% a Vi of 1.5 L, and 51% a Vi of 2.0 L. A small trend towards decreased Vi with increasing device resistance was observed. A marked decrease in Vi was noted with decreases in FEV_1. Although most patients can achieve the ~1.2 L inhaled volume needed to empty a TOBI Podhaler capsule in a single inhalation, some cannot. To ensure that all patients receive their dose, the TOBI Podhaler instructions for use (IFU) call for two inhalations and subsequent inspection of the capsule to ensure that the dose is emptied. For Colobreathe (145 mg fill mass), 3–4 inhalations are needed by most patients to generate the 3.2 L of inhaled volume needed to empty the capsule. For the 120 mg fill mass of TobraPS, the Vi required to empty the powder from the size 0 capsule is about 2.7 L (i.e., 2–3 inhalations for most patients). Given that CF patients find that inhaling the contents of four capsules with two inhalations per capsule to be significantly more convenient and preferred relative to 15–20 min of jet nebulization, it is likely that 2–3 inhalations from a single capsule over a period of 1–2 min will not be a significant barrier to patient adherence. Nonetheless, factors that influence adherence with high dose powder delivery deserve more attention.

Haynes et al. [52] reported the inspiratory flow profiles of 38 patients with CF ranging in age from 6 to 71 years with the TOBI Podhaler device. Across all patients, inhaled volumes ranged from 0.6 to 3.1 L. For patients in the age groups 6–10, 11–18, and >18 years, the mean Vi values were 1.2, 1.6, and 2.1 L, respectively. Ten inhalation profiles that spanned the range of peak inspiratory flow (PIF) and Vi were selected for assessment of the TLD with the Alberta idealized throat model. As per the IFU, two inhalations were taken per capsule. The measured TLD was found to be independent of PIF and Vi over the range of simulated inhalation profiles, indicating that two inhalations are sufficient to achieve effective dose delivery to the lungs in most CF patients.

Luinstra et al. [89] assessed the inspiratory flow profiles of 13 adult patients with Parkinson's disease with a test inhaler with resistance values varying from 0.037 to 0.061 kPa$^{0.5}$ L^{-1} min. Inhaled volumes ranged from 1.2 to 3.5 L, with mean Vi increasing from about 1.8 to about 2.4 L as the device resistance decreased. It may be surprising to learn that in the Inbrija drug product, the large volume of low-density powder is emptied from the size 00 capsule in a single inhalation. The fill mass in Inbrija is 50 mg, suggesting that an inhaled volume of ~1.2 L should be sufficient to empty the capsule (Figure 6C). As described by Luinstra et al. [89], all the patients in their study achieved a $Vi \geq 1.2$ L. Hence, the concerns expressed about using low density porous particles for 'high dose delivery', especially for moderate TLDs in the range from 1 to 20 mg, are unfounded [19]. Even the high 42 mg TLD requires only two inhalations from two capsules.

Sahay et al. [131] studied the inspiratory flow profiles of 35 adult patients with pulmonary arterial hypertension (PAH) using variants of the RS01 DPI that had resistance values between 0.017 and 0.051 kPa$^{0.5}$ L^{-1} min. Mean Vi values increased from 1.7 to 1.9 L as the resistance of the device decreased. With the higher resistance DPI, the mean Vi decreased from 1.8 to 1.2 L when FEV$_1$ values were decreased from >60% predicted to <50% predicted. Adult patients with PAH have lower inhaled volumes than adults with asthma, COPD, CF, or Parkinson's disease, due in part to most PAH patients being female [131].

In summary, the inhaled volume that subjects achieve depends on many factors including their sex, age, the nature of their disease, the severity of their disease, and the inspiratory flow profile they achieve through the device. Most subjects inhale at only 40–80% of their maximum inspiratory pressure when using DPIs [132]. The effort that patients provide may also have an impact on their inhaled volume. The inhaled volume that subjects achieve is also dependent on the resistance of the DPI being utilized. For spray-dried formulations with minimal flow rate dependence, it may be advantageous to use a lower resistance DPI for high and ultrahigh dose delivery to minimize the number of inhalations required to empty the capsule. Achieving high dose delivery with a minimal number of inhalations is especially challenging in CF given the low Vi of many children.

5. Novel Devices for High Dose Delivery

At the top of the design considerations for a novel high dose DPI are the dose, treatment regimen, and intended patient population (sex, age, disease). The nature of the device may change significantly depending on whether the required TLD is moderate, high, or ultrahigh. The inhaled volume of women and children may be significantly lower than those of adult men, affecting the number of inhalations needed to empty a dose.

The device design must also consider the nature of the formulation. Will the powder be crystalline or amorphous? How will the dose be packaged? How will the dose be prepared for inhalation? How will the patient interact with the device? Additional questions to ponder are detailed below.

Is the intent to develop a single-use disposable device that can be emptied in a single inhalation or is the intent to develop a unit-dose device that accommodates a large receptacle with an ultrahigh powder dose that is emptied over multiple inhalations? For single-use disposable DPIs [133,134], the device is used once and then discarded. They are the preferred device when the drug product is administered just a few times (e.g., vaccines [135] or inhaled oxytocin for the prevention of post-partum hemorrhage [136]), when the dosing regimen calls for less frequent dosing (e.g., once weekly as in ABIP), or when the patient is immunocompromised and there is concern about the risk of infection when reusing the device. It has been suggested that single-use devices may also be preferred for amorphous powder formulations as accumulation of residual amorphous powder in the device can negatively impact device performance at elevated RH. For two marketed amorphous drug products (i.e., TOBI Podhaler and Exubera), this issue is effectively mitigated via modifications to the device and by shortening the device use life (or in the case of Exubera the transjector use life) to one week [34,137].

While single-use disposable DPIs may be suitable for the delivery of moderate doses in a single inhalation, questions remain regarding their utility in high dose chronic applications that may require many devices per day. To be successful in high dose delivery, the TLD/receptacle would need to be much greater than can be achieved with unit dose capsule DPIs with size 2 or 3 capsules. Otherwise, one is simply swapping a capsule for a device, which makes little sense.

For a device with a large volume receptacle, the critical question is, from a human-factors perspective, how many inhalations are reasonable before patients become nonadherent? Inhaling multiple times off the same receptacle may also lead to a more central deposition in the lungs as there will be no 'chase' air at the end of the inhalation to drive the powder peripherally. Is this acceptable for your drug product? Can the design help to minimize the inhaled volume needed to deliver the dose without negatively impacting powder dispersion and tolerability?

What will be the optimal device resistance be? As the device resistance increases, the inhaled volume that subjects achieve will tend to decrease. This can negatively impact the number of inhalations required to empty a large-volume receptacle. Alternatively, low resistance devices where subjects inhale at about 100 L/min may lead to increases in throat deposition for some formulations, thereby reducing aerosol performance and increasing variability.

With this as background, let us explore some of the new high dose device options. Comprehensive reviews of this topic are available [78].

5.1. Twincer® and Cyclops® DPIs

The Twincer and Cyclops are single-use disposable DPIs that use air classifiers to increase inertial forces acting on the powder to aid in powder dispersion [19,87,138]. The Cyclops DPI is about the size of a ~0.5 cm stack of credit cards. Powder formulations also include coarse lactose 'sweeper' crystals to increase the emitted dose by removing powder adhered to the walls of the device. The crystals are retained in the device and not inhaled by the subject. The intent with these devices is to maximize the TLD/mg powder by administering neat drug or formulations with minimal amounts of excipient and delivering these formulations with high efficiency to the lungs.

Both devices use a pre-loaded single-use cartridge with a peelable lidding foil. Delivery is simple and intuitive. After the foil strip is removed, the user inhales once, holds their breath for 5–10 s, and then discards the used device. Consistent with unit dose DPIs that employ a size 2 capsule, most subjects can empty and disperse up to ~50 mg fill mass from a standard single-dose cartridge (0.35 mL) in a single inhalation.

The inhaled volume required to empty approximately 50 mg of powder from a standard single-dose cartridge (0.35 mL) depends on the nature of the material and the flow rate/pressure drop attained by the inhalation maneuver. For the aminoglycoside amikacin, the complete dose is dispersed in about 1.0 L of inhaled volume at 6 and 4 kPa, and with about 1.5 L at a 2 kPa pressure drop [139]. These results are comparable to the ~1.2 L of inhaled volume required to empty a capsule of comparable volume in TOBI Podhaler.

For a 55 mg fill mass of isoniazid in the standard single dose cartridge (SDC), the drug emptied with a lower Vi of 0.23 to 0.33 L [140]. A larger (0.52 mL) SDC is also available. Sibum et al. [139] were able to achieve a fill mass of 150 mg of isoniazid by hand filling the entire SDC volume with drum-filled pucks (packing density = 288.5 mg/mL). The inhaled volume required to empty the powder was 0.38 to 0.43 L, significantly less than is reported to date for capsule inhalers.

Based on non-compendial laser diffraction testing in the absence of a throat, it was claimed that these devices achieve high fine particle fractions and low throat deposition in vivo [87,89]. Pharmacokinetic studies with tobramycin in bronchiectasis patients [88] and levodopa in Parkinson's patients [90] suggest that lung delivery may be significantly less than suggested by these in vitro measurements. The dose-normalized systemic C_{max} and AUC values observed with the Cyclops-based products are approximately two-fold lower than is observed with TOBI Podhaler and Inbrija (Section 4.1). These results suggest that lung delivery from the Cyclops is on the order of 25–35% of the nominal dose, which is consistent with the marketed Novolizer® and Genuair® DPIs that incorporate air classifier technologies [140,141]. Hence, while the Cyclops device is suitable for moderate dose delivery, it may have limited potential for chronic high dose delivery unless significant improvements in aerosol performance are achieved.

To put this in perspective, achieving equivalent delivery of levodopa as the Inbrija drug product (i.e., a TLD of 40 mg up to five times daily) with the clinical 30 mg Cyclops device would require approximately 900 devices/month ((6 devices/dose)(up to 5 doses/day)(30 days/month)) (Table 1, Table 2). For a 0.5 cm device thickness, this equates to a stack of devices 4.5 m high. Of course, the performance of the drug/device combination product could be optimized to decrease the number of required devices. However, even if the device delivered the entire 40 mg TLD in one inhalation from a single device, up to 150 devices would still be required per month. In our opinion, this type of chronic multidose/day high TLD product is not a practical application for the Cyclops technology. Additional work is needed to see if spray-dried formulations with high packing densities may enable significant increases in the dose loaded into a cartridge, in line with the isoniazid data pointed out above.

5.2. Orbital® DPI

In contrast, the Orbital multi-breath DPI contains a large-volume cylindrical puck that has been demonstrated to encapsulate up to 400 mg of powder [27,142]. As such, it represents a step change in the mass of powder present in the receptacle compared to capsule based DPIs, providing a potential device solution for ultrahigh dose delivery.

To date, in vitro emptying studies have been conducted using an inhaled volume of 4 L. For mannitol-containing formulations, the emptying was independent of the fill mass, demonstrating a curious emptying profile where each inhalation decreases the mass of powder within the puck by about half, enabling emitted doses greater than 90% in about four 'shots'.

In another study, Zhu et al. [142] demonstrated that emptying of tobramycin powder from the puck could be controlled by varying the diameter and number of holes in the puck. They selected a geometry that enabled a comparable dose of tobramycin to TOBI Podhaler to be delivered in four shots without the need to use multiple capsules (Vi = 16 L). The challenge with these emptying studies is that the 4 L inhaled volume is significantly larger than what CF patients can achieve (Section 4.4). Additional work is needed to better understand the hole size and number of holes required for optimal emptying with realistic inhaled volumes. The optimal emptying rate must also consider its impact on tolerability and powder dispersion. High emptying rates may lead to incomplete powder dispersion. This is true not only for the Orbital device, but for all large-volume receptacles, including the FB-DPI dosing sphere, and large volume capsules.

5.3. FB-DPI

The team at Virginia Commonwealth University have developed several novel DPIs including a fluidized bed high dose DPI (FB-DPI) [91]. In an early iteration of the device, drug product is loaded into a large-volume dosing sphere with a 10 mm inner diameter and four 0.5 mm holes. This equates to a receptacle volume of ~0.52 mL. The dosing sphere is placed within a bed of about sixty 4.76 mm PTFE mixing beads. When air is drawn through the device, the mixing beads fluidize, facilitating emptying and dispersion of powder from the dosing sphere. The powder then passes through a grid to provide secondary dispersion on the way to the patient. The FB-DPI is currently used in conjunction with VCU's highly efficient excipient enhanced growth (EEG) formulation technologies [143]. In one study, Farkas et al. [91] loaded 100 mg of a ciprofloxacin EEG formulation containing mannitol, leucine, and poloxamer 188 into the dosing sphere (drug loading = ~0.30 mg/mg, packing density = 192.3 mg/mL) (Table 2). To assess aerosol performance, the flow rate was set at 60 L/min (4 kPa pressure drop), the inhaled volume at 4 L, and four inhalations were taken (*Vi* = 16 L). This resulted in an emitted dose of 71.4% and an $FPF_{<5 \ \mu m}$ of 93.3% of the emitted dose. Given the flow rate, this is also a close approximation of FPF_{S3-F}. This leads to aerosol performance of 0.67 mg/mg and a product density of 38.7 mg/mL. The *TLD* of ciprofloxacin was about 20 mg/dosing sphere. This is comparable to what was achieved with Ciprofloxacin DPI from a size 2 capsule with an inhaled volume of 1.3 L (Table 1).

6. Maximizing Safety and Tolerability at High Doses

Irritation or inflammation in the respiratory tract following pulmonary administration of inhaled therapeutics and excipients can cause treatment-emergent adverse events including bronchospasm, dyspnea, oropharyngeal pain, hoarseness, voice alteration, dysgeusia, wheezing, and cough. Adverse events are an important consideration in the development of inhaled therapeutics as they can result in poor adherence, discontinuation, and, ultimately, failure of treatment. Post-inhalation cough is the most reported adverse event for high dose delivery. Two recent reviews provide significant detail on post-inhalation cough with therapeutic aerosols [12,144].

Increases in the mass of drug and excipient deposited on epithelial lining fluid (ELF) can increase irritation and inflammation, irrespective of whether the drug is administered as a dry powder or a liquid aerosol. Nonetheless, there remains a bias that inhaled powders are inherently less tolerable than nebulized liquids.

Delivery of high doses of dry powder to the respiratory tract does not necessarily result in a direct irritant effect on the respiratory epithelium [12]. The nature of the material deposited in ELF matters. For example, lactose blends contain between about 12.5 and 25 mg of lactose. Most of the lactose is deposited near cough receptors in the upper respiratory tract. Yet this material does not cause airway irritation. Instead, drug or excipient materials that change osmolality, pH, or ion composition of ELF may activate release of leukotrienes and prostaglandins and cause local inflammation [12,144]. The magnitude of the effect may be potentiated by pulmonary disease and underlying inflammation in the lungs, especially for drugs with tussive potential.

Lung irritation, including cough, is impacted by the nature of the formulation. Cough may be elevated for salt forms of drugs with pK_a values less than 7.0 due to disproportionation of the salt in the ELF to form the free base and corresponding acid [12]. This can also occur with acidic drugs, disproportionating to the acid and corresponding base. The lower the pK_a of the acid used to make the salt, the greater the proton ion concentration on the epithelium, and the greater the irritant effect. The impact of salt disproportion may be mitigated by using a neutral form of the drug, through the use of a cocrystal or by forming salts from acids with higher pK_a values [12]. This was demonstrated with inhaled bronchodilator, indacaterol, where a switch from the maleate salt (pK_a = 1.85) to the acetate salt (pK_a = 4.75) significantly reduced the incidence of post-inhalation cough [12,145,146].

There is also a dose-dependent increase in airway irritation that is related to changes in osmolality via administration of ionizable species (e.g., salts) to ELF (Figure 7).

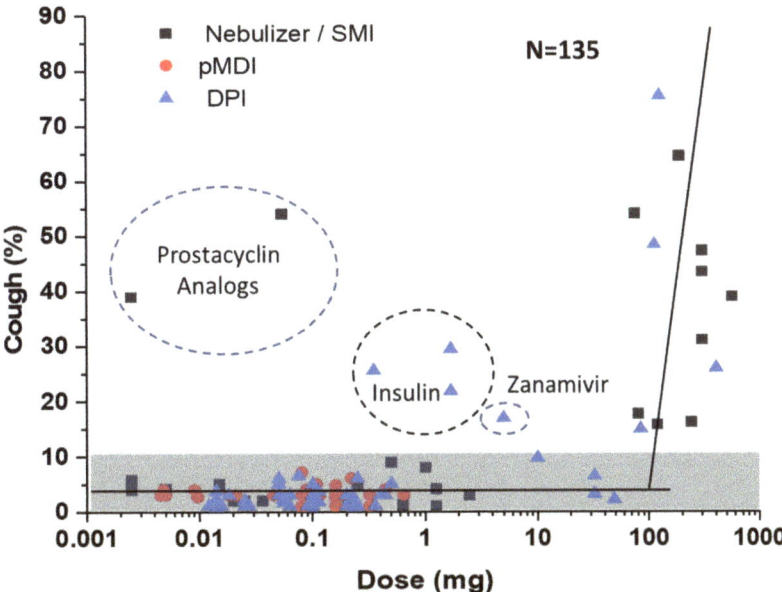

Figure 7. Impact of increases in nominal dose on the incidence of post-inhalation cough. The results are also presented with respect to the various delivery systems (square: nebulizers and soft mist inhalers (SMIs); circle: pressurized metered dose inhalers (pMDIs); triangle: dry powder inhalers (DPIs)). Reproduced with permission from [12]. Copyright Elsevier, 2020.

Post-inhalation cough increases markedly when the nominal dose of ionizable drugs exceeds about 10 mg [12]. For example, tobramycin contains five primary amine groups that can be protonated. When deposited in ELF, tobramycin sulfate produces a high osmolality in the vicinity of dissolving particles [12]. This is potentiated by the fact that cough receptors are enriched at bifurcations and other points where aerosols tend to accumulate [147]. In inhaled tobramycin, post-inhalation cough is generally mild to moderate in intensity and decreases with use. The intensity of the cough may be reduced by inhaling at lower flow rates. The cough threshold is lower in pediatrics than in adults.

In contrast to the high degree of cough observed with tobramycin sulfate, inhalation of the zwitterionic form of ciprofloxacin at neutral pH, at a comparable powder mass and with the same excipients, leads to minimal cough and airway irritation [12,54]. This is presumably due to the low osmolality of the poorly soluble neutral form of the drug in ELF [12,54]. Airway irritation can be mitigated by utilizing neutral forms of drugs, cocrystals instead of salts, and poorly soluble excipients [12]. For inhaled antibiotics, utilizing the poorly soluble neutral form of a molecule may have further utility due to its slow clearance from the lungs. This provides improved pulmonary targeting leading to improved pharmacokinetic/pharmacodynamic metrics (e.g., the ratio of AUC/MIC) and bacterial killing efficiency [54,148,149].

One concern with the use of poorly soluble drugs and excipients is that the presence of undissolved particulate matter in the lungs may result in adverse lung changes through a process of macrophage recruitment and stimulation with secondary lung damage and fibrosis [150]. However, there are examples from Table 1 where poorly soluble drug particles that are slowly cleared have no significant adverse effects in long-term nonclinical toxicology studies (e.g., ABIP, Ciprofloxacin DPI), and in long-term Phase 3 clinical studies [151,152]. Clearly, more studies are needed to better understand the link between slow particle clearance and adverse effects.

7. Conclusions

- Emptying of powder from capsules is highly dependent on the fill mass and less so on the fill volume. Most subjects can inhale approximately 40–50 mg of powder from a capsule in a single inhalation (requires ~1 L of inhaled volume).

- To date, the highest TLD/receptacle that can be emptied in a single inhalation for a marketed product is ~20 mg. This was achieved with Inbrija, a low density large porous particle formulation. This defines the upper limit for moderate TLDs (moderate TLD range is from 1 to 20 mg).

- For efficient high dose delivery (TLD = 20–100 mg), it is advantageous to maximize the TLD/m_{powder}. Maximizing dose delivery within this mass of powder requires achieving as high a TLD as possible with as little excipient as possible. The best spray-drying options to achieve this goal are: (1) lipid coated crystals prepared by spray drying suspension-based liquid feeds with ≤5% lipid excipient, and (2) core-shell particles prepared by spray drying a solution of drug and ≤5% of a shell forming excipient (e.g., trileucine) at low Peclet numbers.

- The mass of powder loaded into a given sized receptacle can be increased via increases in the packing density. This can be achieved to a high degree with the low Peclet core-shell particles noted above.

- For high dose delivery, target TLD values can be achieved from a single larger sized capsule with multiple inhalations needed to empty the capsule. The required inhaled volume is proportional to the mass of powder in the capsule. A 150 mg fill mass requires about 3.25 L of inhaled volume to empty (i.e., approximately three inhalations or less for most subjects). This enables a TLD of 80–100 mg from a single size 2 capsule.

- Ultrahigh doses (TLD > 100 mg) require large receptacles (e.g., size 0 or size 00 capsules) or novel DPIs (e.g., the large volume cylindrical puck in the Orbital DPI or the dosing sphere in the FB-DPI).

- It is critical to better understand how the size and number of holes in larger sized receptacles impact powder emptying. Further, it is critical that these emptying studies be conducted with realistic patient breathing profiles, as opposed to the standard 4 L inhaled volumes typically used in aerosol testing.

- Evidence established to date suggests that high doses of neat drug particles (sans excipient) have significantly decreased aerosol performance and poor dose consistency. The addition of small amounts of shell forming excipient is necessary to improve aerosol performance, packing density, dose consistency, and, ultimately, product density.

- The inhalation of large doses of powder does not lead to increases in local irritation in the lungs. It depends on the nature of the powder inhaled.

- While significant progress has been made in increasing the dose of powder that can be delivered from a portable DPI, we have limited understanding of the practical limits of high dose powder delivery both from a tolerability perspective, but also from a patient adherence perspective. How many inhalations are practical and at what point is a liquid nebulizer or possibly a powder nebulizer a better solution?

- Overall, ultrahigh doses of drug (>100 mg) can be deposited in the lungs with a portable DPI in three to four inhalations when using a device with a receptacle volume greater than 0.6 mL and spray-dried porous particles with a high packing density greater than 150 mg/mL.

Author Contributions: Y.-J.S., D.P.M. and J.G.W. equally contributed to writing of this review. Y.-J.S., D.P.M. and J.G.W. have read and agreed to the published version of the manuscript.

Funding: This research received no external funding.

Conflicts of Interest: Y.S. is an employee of Genentech, while D.M. and J.W. are employees of cystetic Medicines, Inc. Genentech and cystetic Medicines had no role in the collection, analyses, and interpretation of the data, or in the writing of the review. The decision to publish the results received formal approval from the Genentech publication approval committee. The authors are inventors on a patent application directed to results presented in this review (U.S. Patent Application 2021/0069106A1, assigned to Novartis AG). J.W. is also an inventor of the PulmoSphere technology which was used to formulate several drug products discussed in this review (e.g., TOBI Podhaler, Amphotericin B Inhalation Powder, and Ciprofloxacin DPI).

References

1. Walsh, B.K.; Betit, P.; Fink, J.B.; Pereira, L.M.; Arnold, J. Characterization of ribavirin aerosol with small particle aerosol generator and vibrating mesh micropump aerosol technologies. *Respir. Care* **2016**, *61*, 577–585. [CrossRef]
2. Newth, C.J.; Clark, A.R. In vitro performance of the small particle aerosol generator (Spag-2). *Pediatr. Pulmonol.* **1989**, *7*, 183–188. [CrossRef]
3. Smaldone, G.C.; Fuhrer, J.; Steigbigel, R.T.; McPeck, M. Factors determining pulmonary deposition of aerosolized pentamidine in patients with human immunodeficiency virus infection. *Am. Rev. Respir. Dis.* **1991**, *143*, 727–737. [CrossRef]
4. Conte, J.E., Jr.; Golden, J.A. Concentrations of aerosolized pentamidine in bronchoalveolar lavage, systemic absorption, and excretion. *Antimicrob. Agents Chemother.* **1988**, *32*, 1490–1493. [CrossRef]
5. Ramsey, B.W.; Pepe, M.S.; Quan, J.M.; Otto, K.L.; Montgomery, A.B.; Williams-Warren, J.; Vasiljev, K.M.; Borowitz, D.; Bowman, C.M.; Marshall, B.C.; et al. Intermittent administration of inhaled tobramycin in patients with cystic fibrosis. Cystic fibrosis inhaled tobramycin study group. *N. Engl. J. Med.* **1999**, *340*, 23–30. [CrossRef] [PubMed]
6. Godden, D.J.; Borland, C.; Lowry, R.; Higenbottam, T.W. Chemical specificity of coughing in man. *Clin. Sci.* **1986**, *70*, 301–306. [CrossRef] [PubMed]
7. Briesacher, B.A.; Quittner, A.L.; Saiman, L.; Sacco, P.; Fouayzi, H.; Quittell, L.M. Adherence with tobramycin inhaled solution and health care utilization. *BMC Pulm. Med.* **2011**, *11*, 5. [CrossRef] [PubMed]
8. Blau, H.; Mussaffi, H.; Mei Zahav, M.; Prais, D.; Livne, M.; Czitron, B.M.; Cohen, H.A. Microbial contamination of nebulizers in the home treatment of cystic fibrosis. *Child Care Health Dev.* **2007**, *33*, 491–495. [CrossRef]
9. Rottier, B.L.; van Erp, C.J.; Sluyter, T.S.; Heijerman, H.G.; Frijlink, H.W.; Boer, A.H. Changes in performance of the PARI eFlow rapid and PARI LC plus during 6 months use by CF patients. *J. Aerosol Med. Pulm. Drug Deliv.* **2009**, *22*, 263–269. [CrossRef]
10. Dhand, R. Nebulizer that use a vibrating mesh or plate with multiple apertures to generate aerosol. *Respir. Care* **2002**, *47*, 1406–1416. [PubMed]
11. Weers, J. Inhaled antimicrobial therapy—Barriers to effective treatment. *Adv. Drug Deliv. Rev.* **2015**, *85*, 24–43. [CrossRef]
12. Sahakijpijarn, S.; Smyth, H.D.C.; Miller, D.P.; Weers, J.G. Post-inhalation cough with therapeutic aerosols: Formulation considerations. *Adv. Drug Deliv. Rev.* **2020**, *165–166*, 127–141. [CrossRef] [PubMed]
13. Konstan, M.W.; Flume, P.A.; Kappler, M.; Chiron, R.; Higgins, M.; Brockhaus, F.; Zhang, J.; Angyalosi, G.; He, E.; Geller, D.E. Safety, efficacy and convenience of tobramycin inhalation powder in cystic fibrosis patients: The EAGER trial. *J. Cyst. Fibros.* **2011**, *10*, 54–61. [CrossRef]
14. Geller, D.E.; Weers, J.; Heuerding, S. Development of an inhaled dry-powder formulation of tobramycin using PulmoSphere™ technology. *J. Aerosol Med. Pulm. Drug Deliv.* **2011**, *24*, 175–182. [CrossRef]
15. Somayaji, R.; Parkins, M.D. Tobramycin inhalation powder: An efficient and efficacious therapy for the treatment of *Pseudomonas aeruginosa* infection in cystic fibrosis. *Ther. Deliv.* **2015**, *6*, 121–137. [CrossRef] [PubMed]
16. Hamed, K.; Debonnett, L. Tobramycin inhalation powder for the treatment of pulmonary *Pseudomonas aeruginosa* infection in patients with cystic fibrosis: A review based on clinical evidence. *Ther. Adv. Respir. Dis.* **2017**, *11*, 193–209. [CrossRef]
17. Panguluri, S.; Gunda, P.; Debonnett, L.; Hamed, K. Economic evaluation of tobramycin inhalation powder for the treatment of chronic pulmonary pseudomonas aeruginosa infection in patients with cystic fibrosis. *Clin. Drug Investig.* **2017**, *37*, 795–805. [CrossRef] [PubMed]
18. Hickey, A.J.; Stewart, I.E.; Jones, A. Why we need to deliver large amounts of powder to the lungs and the concurrent challenges. *Drug Deliv. Lungs* **2019**, *30*, 1–4.
19. Sibum, I.; Hagedoorn, P.; de Boer, A.H.; Frijlink, H.W.; Grasmeijer, F. Challenges for pulmonary delivery of high powder doses. *Int. J. Pharm.* **2018**, *548*, 325–336. [CrossRef] [PubMed]
20. Grasmeijer, F.; Hagedoorn, P.; Frijlink, H.W.; de Boer, A.H. Drug content effects on the dispersion performance of adhesive mixtures for inhalation. *PLoS ONE* **2013**, *8*, e71339.
21. Jetzer, M.W.; Schneider, M.; Morrical, B.D.; Imanidis, G. Investigations on the mechanism of magnesium stearate to modify aerosol performance in dry powder inhaled formulations. *J. Pharm. Sci.* **2018**, *107*, 984–998. [CrossRef]
22. Weers, J.G.; Clark, A.R.; Rao, N.; Ung, K.; Haynes, A.; Khindri, S.K.; Perry, S.A.; Machineni, S.; Colthorpe, P. In vitro-in vivo correlations observed with indacaterol-based formulations delivered with the Breezhaler®. *J. Aerosol Med. Pulm. Drug Deliv.* **2015**, *28*, 268–280. [CrossRef] [PubMed]
23. FDA. *Clinical Pharmacology and Biopharmaceutics Review(s)*; Application Number: 209184Orig1s000; FDA: Silver Spring, MD, USA, 2018.

24. Ruppert, C.; Kuchenbuch, T.; Schmidt, S.; Markart, P.; Gessler, T.; Schmehl, T.; Seeger, W.; Günther, A. Dry powder nebulization of a recombinant surfactant protein c-based surfactant for treatment of acute respiratory distress syndrome. *Crit. Care* **2007**, *11*, 208. [CrossRef]
25. Acorda Therapeutics. Inbrija®(Levodopa Inhalation Powder): US Prescribing Information. 2018. Available online: https://www.inbrija.com/ (accessed on 25 July 2021).
26. Parumasivam, T.; Leung, S.S.; Tang, P.; Mauro, C.; Britton, W.; Chan, H.K. The delivery of high-dose dry powder antibiotics by a low-cost generic inhaler. *AAPS J.* **2017**, *19*, 191–202. [CrossRef]
27. Young, P.M.; Crapper, J.; Philips, G.; Sharma, K.; Chan, H.K.; Traini, D. Overcoming dose limitations using the Orbital® multi-breath dry powder inhaler. *J. Aerosol Med. Pulm. Drug Deliv.* **2014**, *27*, 138–147. [CrossRef]
28. Conway, J. Lung imaging—Two dimensional gamma scintigraphy, SPECT, CT and PET. *Adv. Drug Deliv. Rev.* **2012**, *64*, 357–368. [CrossRef] [PubMed]
29. Newman, S.; Steed, K.; Hooper, G.; Källén, A.; Borgström, L. Comparison of gamma scintigraphy and a pharmacokinetic technique for assessing pulmonary deposition of terbutaline sulphate delivered by pressurized metered dose inhaler. *Pharm. Res.* **1995**, *12*, 231–236. [CrossRef] [PubMed]
30. Ruzycki, C.A.; Martin, A.R.; Finlay, W.H. An exploration of factors affecting in vitro deposition of pharmaceutical aerosols in the Alberta Idealized Throat. *J. Aerosol Med. Pulm. Drug Deliv.* **2019**, *32*, 405–417. [CrossRef] [PubMed]
31. Byron, P.R.; Weers, J.G.; Clark, A.R.; Sandell, D.; Mitchell, J.P. Achieving deposition equivalence: The state of the art. In Proceedings of the Respiratory Drug Delivery Europe 2017, Nice, France, 25–28 April 2017; Volume 1, pp. 101–111.
32. Weers, J. Regional deposition of particles within the respiratory tract should be linked to impaction parameter, not aerodynamic size. *J. Aerosol Med. Pulm. Drug Deliv.* **2018**, *31*, 116–118. [CrossRef] [PubMed]
33. Weers, J.G.; Rao, N.; Kadrichu, N. Is aerodynamic diameter a good metric for understanding regional deposition? In Proceedings of the Respiratory Drug Delivery Europe 2019, Lisbon, Portugal, 7–10 May 2019; Volume 1, pp. 59–66.
34. Stevenson, C.L.; Bennett, D.B. Development of the Exubera® insulin pulmonary delivery system. In *Mucosal Delivery of Biopharmaceuticals: Biology, Challenges and Strategies*; Das Neves, J., Sarmento, B., Eds.; Springer: Boston, MA, USA, 2014; pp. 461–481.
35. Parks, D.J.; Rocchio, M.J.; Naydo, K.; Wightman, D.E.; Smith, A.E. Powder Filling Systems, Apparatus, and Methods. U.S. Patent US5826633A, 27 October 1998.
36. Stout, G.; Pham, X.; Rocchio, M.J.; Naydo, K.A.; Parks, D.J.; Reich, P. Powder Filling Apparatus and Methods of Their Use. U.S. Patent US6182712, 6 February 2001.
37. Chodosh, S.; Flanders, J.S.; Kesten, S.; Serby, C.W.; Hochrainer, D.; Witek, T.J., Jr. Effective delivery of particles with the handihaler dry powder inhalation system over a range of chronic obstructive pulmonary disease severity. *J. Aerosol Med. Pulm. Drug Deliv.* **2001**, *14*, 309–315. [CrossRef]
38. Brand, P.; Meyer, T.; Weuthen, T.; Timmer, W.; Berkel, E.; Wallenstein, G.; Scheuch, G. Lung deposition of radiolabeled tiotropium in healthy subjects and patients with chronic obstructive pulmonary disease. *J. Clin. Pharmacol.* **2007**, *47*, 1335–1341. [CrossRef]
39. Abadelah, M.; Chrystyn, H.; Larhrib, H. Use of inspiratory profiles from patients with chronic obstructive pulmonary disease (COPD) to investigate drug delivery uniformity and aerodynamic dose emission of indacaterol from a capsule based dry powder inhaler. *Eur. J. Pharm. Sci.* **2019**, *134*, 138–144. [CrossRef]
40. Weers, J.; Clark, A. The impact of inspiratory flow rate on drug delivery to the lungs with dry powder inhalers. *Pharm. Res.* **2017**, *34*, 507–528. [CrossRef] [PubMed]
41. Newman, S.P.; Hollingworth, A.; Clark, A.R. Effect of different modes of inhalation on drug delivery from a dry powder inhaler. *Int. J. Pharm.* **1994**, *102*, 127–132. [CrossRef]
42. MacConnachie, A.M. Zanamivir (Relenza)—A new treatment for influenza. *Inten. Crit. Care Nurs.* **1999**, *15*, 369–370. [CrossRef]
43. Delvadia, R.; Hindle, M.; Longest, P.W.; Byron, P.R. In vitro tests for aerosol deposition ii: Ivivcs for different dry powder inhalers in normal adults. *J. Aerosol Med. Pulm. Drug Deliv.* **2013**, *26*, 138–144. [CrossRef]
44. Schuster, A.; Haliburn, C.; Döring, G.; Goldman, M.H. Safety, efficacy and convenience of colistimethate sodium dry powder for inhalation (Colobreathe DPI) in patients with cystic fibrosis: A randomised study. *Thorax* **2013**, *68*, 344–350. [CrossRef]
45. Schwarz, C. Colobreathe® for the treatment of cystic fibrosis-associated pulmonary infections. *Pulm. Ther.* **2015**, *1*, 19–30. [CrossRef]
46. Bergen, P.J.; Li, J.; Rayner, C.R.; Nation, R.L. Colistin methanesulfonate is an inactive prodrug of colistin against *Pseudomonas aeruginosa*. *Antimicrob. Agents Chemother.* **2006**, *50*, 1953–1958. [CrossRef] [PubMed]
47. Su, S.; Riccobene, T.; Scott, C. Lung deposition of inhaled colistimethate sodium in cystic fibrosis patients. *Eur. Respir. J.* **2014**, *44*, P1975.
48. Borgström, L.; Olsson, B.; Thorsson, L. Degree of throat deposition can explain the variability in lung deposition of inhaled drugs. *J. Aerosol Med. Pulm. Drug Deliv.* **2006**, *19*, 473–483. [CrossRef]
49. Cipolla, D.; Chan, H.K.; Schuster, J.; Farina, D. Personalizing aerosol medicine: Development of delivery systems tailored to the individual. *Ther. Deliv.* **2010**, *1*, 667–682. [CrossRef]
50. Weers, J.; Tarara, T. The PulmoSphere™ platform for pulmonary drug delivery. *Ther. Deliv.* **2014**, *5*, 277–295. [CrossRef] [PubMed]

51. Miller, D.P.; Tan, T.; Tarara, T.E.; Nakamura, J.; Malcolmson, R.J.; Weers, J.G. Physical characterization of tobramycin inhalation powder: I. Rational design of a stable engineered-particle formulation for delivery to the lungs. *Mol. Pharm.* **2015**, *12*, 2582–2593. [CrossRef] [PubMed]

52. Haynes, A.; Geller, D.; Weers, J.; Ament, B.; Pavkov, R.; Malcolmson, R.; Debonnett, L.; Mastoridis, P.; Yadao, A.; Heuerding, S. Inhalation of tobramycin using simulated cystic fibrosis patient profiles. *Pediatr. Pulmonol.* **2016**, *51*, 1159–1167. [CrossRef] [PubMed]

53. McShane, P.J.; Weers, J.G.; Tarara, T.E.; Haynes, A.; Durbha, P.; Miller, D.P.; Mundry, T.; Operschall, E.; Elborn, J.S. Ciprofloxacin dry powder for inhalation (Ciprofloxacin DPI): Technical design and features of an efficient drug-device combination. *Pulm. Pharmacol. Ther.* **2018**, *50*, 72–79. [CrossRef]

54. Weers, J. Comparison of phospholipid-based particles for sustained release of ciprofloxacin following pulmonary administration to bronchiectasis patients. *Pulm. Ther.* **2019**, *5*, 127–150. [CrossRef]

55. Stass, H.; Nagelschmitz, J.; Kappeler, D.; Sommerer, K.; Kietzig, C.; Weimann, B. Ciprofloxacin dry powder for inhalation in patients with non-cystic fibrosis bronchiectasis or chronic obstructive pulmonary disease, and in healthy volunteers. *J. Aerosol Med. Pulm. Drug Deliv.* **2017**, *30*, 53–63. [CrossRef] [PubMed]

56. Weers, J.G.; Miller, D.P.; Tarara, T.E. Spray-dried PulmoSphere™ formulations for inhalation comprising crystalline drug particles. *AAPS PharmSciTech* **2019**, *20*, 103. [CrossRef]

57. Lee, J.D.; Kugler, A.R.; Lori, S.K.; Eldon, M.A. Amphotericin B inhalation powder (ABIP) is well tolerated with low systemic amphotericin B exposure in healthy subjects. In Proceedings of the 2nd Conference of Advances Against Aspergillosis, Athens, Greece, 22–25 February 2006; pp. 214–215.

58. Kugler, A.R.; Lee, J.D.; Samford, L.K.; Sahner, D. Clinical pharmacokinetics (pk) following multiple doses of amphotericin b inhalation powder (ABIP). In Proceedings of the Conference of Focus on Fungal Infections, San Diego, CA, USA, 17 April 2007; pp. 225–226.

59. Fiegel, J.; Garcia-Contreras, L.; Thomas, M.; VerBerkmoes, J.; Elbert, K.; Hickey, A.; Edwards, D. Preparation and in vivo evaluation of a dry powder for inhalation of capreomycin. *Pharm. Res.* **2008**, *25*, 805–811. [CrossRef]

60. Dharmadhikari, A.S.; Kabadi, M.; Gerety, B.; Hickey, A.J.; Fourie, P.B.; Nardell, E. Phase i, single-dose, dose-escalating study of inhaled dry powder capreomycin: A new approach to therapy of drug-resistant tuberculosis. *Antimicrob. Agents Chemother.* **2013**, *57*, 2613–2619. [CrossRef] [PubMed]

61. Lord, J.; Jouhikainen, J.T.; Snyder, H.E.; Soni, P.; Kuo, M.-C. Dry Powder Vancomycin Compositions and Associated Methods. U.S. Patent US10561608, 18 February 2020.

62. Lord, J. In Aerovanc™: A novel dry powder inhaler for the treatment of methicillin-resistant staphylococcus aureus infection in cystic fibrosis patients. In Proceedings of the Respiratory Drug Delivery, Fajardo, Puerto Rico, 4–8 May 2014; pp. 563–567.

63. Waterer, G.; Lord, J.; Hofmann, T.; Jouhikainen, T. Phase I, dose-escalating study of the safety and pharmacokinetics of inhaled dry-powder vancomycin (Aerovanc) in volunteers and patients with cystic fibrosis: A new approach to therapy for methicillin-resistant staphylococcus aureus. *Antimicrob. Agents Chemother.* **2020**, *64*, 3. [CrossRef] [PubMed]

64. Hurt, K.; Bilton, D. Inhaled mannitol for the treatment of cystic fibrosis. *Exp. Rev. Respir. Med.* **2012**, *6*, 19–26. [CrossRef]

65. Jaques, A.; Daviskas, E.; Turton, J.A.; McKay, K.; Cooper, P.; Stirling, R.G.; Robertson, C.F.; Bye, P.T.P.; LeSouëf, P.N.; Shadbolt, B.; et al. Inhaled mannitol improves lung function in cystic fibrosis. *Chest* **2008**, *133*, 1388–1396. [CrossRef]

66. Yang, M.Y.; Verschuer, J.; Shi, Y.; Song, Y.; Katsifis, A.; Eberl, S.; Wong, K.; Brannan, J.D.; Cai, W.; Finlay, W.H.; et al. The effect of device resistance and inhalation flow rate on the lung deposition of orally inhaled mannitol dry powder. *Int. J. Pharm.* **2016**, *513*, 294–301. [CrossRef]

67. Farbman, E.S.; Waters, C.H.; LeWitt, P.A.; Rudzińska, M.; Klingler, M.; Lee, A.; Qian, J.; Oh, C.; Hauser, R.A. A 12-month, dose-level blinded safety and efficacy study of levodopa inhalation powder (CVT-301, Inbrija) in patients with Parkinson's disease. *Parkinson's Relat. Disord.* **2020**, *81*, 144–150. [CrossRef] [PubMed]

68. LeWitt, P.A.; Pahwa, R.; Sedkov, A.; Corbin, A.; Batycky, R.; Murck, H. Pulmonary safety and tolerability of inhaled levodopa (CVT-301) administered to patients with Parkinson's disease. *J. Aerosol Med. Pulm. Drug Deliv.* **2018**, *31*, 155–161. [CrossRef] [PubMed]

69. Lipp, M.M.; Batycky, R.; Moore, J.; Leinonen, M.; Freed, M.I. Preclinical and clinical assessment of inhaled levodopa for off episodes in Parkinson's disease. *Sci. Transl. Med.* **2016**, *8*, 360–366. [CrossRef] [PubMed]

70. Batycky, R.P.; Lipp, M.M.; Kamerkar, A.; Penachio, E.D.; Kee, K.D. Capsules Containing High Doses of Levodopa for Pulmonary Use. U.S. Patent US8685442B1, 1 April 2014.

71. Edwards, D.A.; Hanes, J.; Caponetti, G.; Hrkach, J.; Ben-Jebria, A.; Eskew, M.L.; Mintzes, J.; Deaver, D.; Lotan, N.; Langer, R. Large porous particles for pulmonary drug delivery. *Science* **1997**, *276*, 1868–1871. [CrossRef] [PubMed]

72. Das, S.C.; Stewart, P.J.; Tucker, I.G. The respiratory delivery of high dose dry powders. *Int. J. Pharm.* **2018**, *550*, 486–487. [CrossRef]

73. Brunaugh, A.D.; Smyth, H.D.C. Formulation techniques for high dose dry powders. *Int. J. Pharm.* **2018**, *547*, 489–498. [PubMed]

74. Scherließ, R.; Etschmann, C. DPI formulations for high dose applications—Challenges and opportunities. *Int. J. Pharm.* **2018**, *548*, 49–53. [CrossRef]

75. Ranjan, R.; Srivastava, A.; Bharti, R.; Ray, L.; Singh, J.; Misra, A. Preparation and optimization of a dry powder for inhalation of second-line anti-tuberculosis drugs. *Int. J. Pharm.* **2018**, *547*, 150–157. [CrossRef] [PubMed]

76. Kukut Hatipoglu, M.; Hickey, A.J.; Garcia-Contreras, L. Pharmacokinetics and pharmacodynamics of high doses of inhaled dry powder drugs. *Int. J. Pharm.* **2018**, *549*, 306–316. [CrossRef]
77. D'Angelo, I.; Conte, C.; La Rotonda, M.I.; Miro, A.; Quaglia, F.; Ungaro, F. Improving the efficacy of inhaled drugs in cystic fibrosis: Challenges and emerging drug delivery strategies. *Adv. Drug Deliv. Rev.* **2014**, *75*, 92–111. [CrossRef] [PubMed]
78. Momin, M.A.M.; Tucker, I.G.; Das, S.C. High dose dry powder inhalers to overcome the challenges of tuberculosis treatment. *Int. J. Pharm.* **2018**, *550*, 398–417. [CrossRef]
79. Yeung, S.; Traini, D.; Lewis, D.; Young, P.M. Dosing challenges in respiratory therapies. *Int. J. Pharm.* **2018**, *548*, 659–671. [CrossRef] [PubMed]
80. Lau, M.; Young, P.M.; Traini, D. A review of co-milling techniques for the production of high dose dry powder inhaler formulation. *Drug Dev. Ind. Pharm.* **2017**, *43*, 1229–1238. [CrossRef]
81. Velkov, T.; Abdul Rahim, N.; Zhou, Q.T.; Chan, H.K.; Li, J. Inhaled anti-infective chemotherapy for respiratory tract infections: Successes, challenges and the road ahead. *Adv. Drug Deliv. Rev.* **2015**, *85*, 65–82. [CrossRef]
82. Traini, D.; Young, P.M. Delivery of antibiotics to the respiratory tract: An update. *Exp. Opin. Drug Deliv.* **2009**, *6*, 897–905. [CrossRef]
83. Brunaugh, A.D.; Jan, S.U.; Ferrati, S.; Smyth, H.D.C. Excipient-free pulmonary delivery and macrophage targeting of clofazimine via air jet micronization. *Mol. Pharm.* **2017**, *14*, 4019–4031. [CrossRef]
84. Pilcer, G.; Vanderbist, F.; Amighi, K. Spray-dried carrier-free dry powder tobramycin formulations with improved dispersion properties. *J. Pharm. Sci.* **2009**, *98*, 1463–1475. [CrossRef]
85. Parlati, C.; Colombo, P.; Buttini, F.; Young, P.M.; Adi, H.; Ammit, A.J.; Traini, D. Pulmonary spray dried powders of tobramycin containing sodium stearate to improve aerosolization efficiency. *Pharm. Res.* **2009**, *26*, 1084–1092. [CrossRef] [PubMed]
86. Buttini, F.; Balducci, A.G.; Colombo, G.; Sonvico, F.; Montanari, S.; Pisi, G.; Rossi, A.; Colombo, P.; Bettini, R. Dose administration maneuvers and patient care in tobramycin dry powder inhalation therapy. *Int. J. Pharm.* **2018**, *548*, 182–191. [CrossRef] [PubMed]
87. Hoppentocht, M.; Akkerman, O.W.; Hagedoorn, P.; Frijlink, H.W.; de Boer, A.H. The Cyclops for pulmonary delivery of aminoglycosides; a new member of the Twincer™ family. *Eur. J. Pharm. Biopharm.* **2015**, *90*, 8–15. [CrossRef]
88. Hoppentocht, M.; Akkerman, O.W.; Hagedoorn, P.; Alffenaar, J.W.; van der Werf, T.S.; Kerstjens, H.A.; Frijlink, H.W.; de Boer, A.H. Tolerability and pharmacokinetic evaluation of inhaled dry powder tobramycin free base in non-cystic fibrosis bronchiectasis patients. *PLoS ONE* **2016**, *11*, e0149768. [CrossRef] [PubMed]
89. Luinstra, M.; Rutgers, A.W.; Dijkstra, H.; Grasmeijer, F.; Hagedoorn, P.; Vogelzang, J.M.; Frijlink, H.W.; de Boer, A.H. Can patients with Parkinson's disease use dry powder inhalers during off periods? *PLoS ONE* **2015**, *10*, e0132714. [CrossRef] [PubMed]
90. Luinstra, M.; Rutgers, W.; van Laar, T.; Grasmeijer, F.; Begeman, A.; Isufi, V.; Steenhuis, L.; Hagedoorn, P.; de Boer, A.; Frijlink, H.W. Pharmacokinetics and tolerability of inhaled levodopa from a new dry-powder inhaler in patients with parkinson's disease. *Ther. Adv. Chronic Dis.* **2019**, *10*, 1–10. [CrossRef] [PubMed]
91. Farkas, D.R.; Hindle, M.; Longest, P.W. Characterization of a new high-dose dry powder inhaler (DPI) based on a fluidized bed design. *Ann. Biomed. Eng.* **2015**, *43*, 2804–2815. [CrossRef]
92. Manzanedo, D.; Brande, M.; Kramer, S.R.; Yee, L.W.; DeHaan, W.H.; Clarke, R.W.; Lipp, M.M.; Sung, J.C. Formulation characterization of a novel levofloxacin pulmonary dry powder drug delivery technology. In Proceedings of the Respiratory Drug Delivery 2012, Phoenix, AZ, USA, 13–17 May 2012; pp. 713–716.
93. Son, Y.-J.; Huang, D.; Miller, D.; Weers, J.G. High dose delivery of inhaled therapeutics. U.S. Patent Application No. 16/963678, 11 March 2021.
94. Weers, J.G.; Miller, D. Increased packing density of fine particles in spray-dried formulations. In Proceedings of the Respiratory Drug Delivery 2020, Palm Springs, CA, USA, 26–30 April 2020; pp. 455–458.
95. Momin, M.A.M.; Tucker, I.G.; Doyle, C.S.; Denman, J.A.; Sinha, S.; Das, S.C. Co-spray drying of hygroscopic kanamycin with the hydrophobic drug rifampicin to improve the aerosolization of kanamycin powder for treating respiratory infections. *Int. J. Pharm.* **2018**, *541*, 26–36. [CrossRef]
96. Hancock, B.C.; Colvin, J.T.; Mullarney, M.P.; Zinchuk, A.V. The relative densities of pharmaceutical powders, blends, dry granulations, and immediate release tablets. *Pharm. Technol.* **2003**, *27*, 64–80.
97. Banaschewski, B.; Verma, D.; Pennings, L.J.; Zimmerman, M.; Ye, Q.; Gadawa, J.; Dartois, V.; Ordway, D.; van Ingen, J.; Ufer, S.; et al. Clofazimine inhalation suspension for the aerosol treatment of pulmonary nontuberculous mycobacterial infections. *J. Cyst. Fibros.* **2019**, *18*, 714–720. [CrossRef]
98. Geller, D.E.; Konstan, M.W.; Smith, J.; Noonberg, S.B.; Conrad, C. Novel tobramycin inhalation powder in cystic fibrosis subjects: Pharmacokinetics and safety. *Pediatr. Pulmonol.* **2007**, *42*, 307–313. [CrossRef] [PubMed]
99. Hastedt, J.E.; Bäckman, P.; Clark, A.R.; Doub, W.; Hickey, A.; Hochhaus, G.; Kuehl, P.J.; Lehr, C.-M.; Mauser, P.; McConville, J.; et al. Scope and relevance of a pulmonary biopharmaceutical classification system aaps/fda/usp workshop March 16–17, 2015 in Baltimore, MD. *AAPS Open* **2016**, *2*, 1. [CrossRef]
100. Li, M.; Byron, P.R. Tobramycin disposition in the rat lung following airway administration. *J. Pharmacol. Exp. Ther.* **2013**, *347*, 318–324. [CrossRef]
101. Begat, P.; Morton, D.A.; Shur, J.; Kippax, P.; Staniforth, J.N.; Price, R. The role of force control agents in high-dose dry powder inhaler formulations. *J. Pharm. Sci.* **2009**, *98*, 2770–2783. [CrossRef]

102. Lau, M.; Young, P.M.; Traini, D. Co-milled api-lactose systems for inhalation therapy: Impact of magnesium stearate on physico-chemical stability and aerosolization performance. *Drug Dev. Indust. Pharm.* **2017**, *43*, 980–988. [CrossRef]
103. Yeh, K.C.; August, T.F.; Bush, D.F.; Lasseter, K.C.; Musson, D.G.; Schwartz, S.; Smith, M.E.; Titus, D.C. Pharmacokinetics and bioavailability of SINEMET CR: A summary of human studies. *Neurology* **1989**, *39*, 25–38. [PubMed]
104. Safirstein, B.E.; Ellenbogen, A.; Zhao, P.; Henney, H.R., 3rd; Kegler-Ebo, D.M.; Oh, C. Pharmacokinetics of inhaled levodopa administered with oral carbidopa in the fed state in patients with Parkinson's disease. *Clin. Ther.* **2020**, *42*, 1034–1046. [CrossRef] [PubMed]
105. Adi, H.; Young, P.M.; Chan, H.K.; Stewart, P.; Agus, H.; Traini, D. Co-spray dried antibiotics for dry powder lung delivery. *J. Pharm. Sci.* **2008**, *97*, 3356–3366. [CrossRef] [PubMed]
106. Pilcer, G.; Rosière, R.; Traina, K.; Sebti, T.; Vanderbist, F.; Amighi, K. New co-spray-dried tobramycin nanoparticles-clarithromycin inhaled powder systems for lung infection therapy in cystic fibrosis patients. *J. Pharm. Sci.* **2013**, *102*, 1836–1846. [CrossRef]
107. Shetty, N.; Ahn, P.; Park, H.; Bhujbal, S.; Zemlyanov, D.; Cavallaro, A.; Mangal, S.; Li, J.; Zhou, Q.T. Improved physical stability and aerosolization of inhalable amorphous ciprofloxacin powder formulations by incorporating synergistic colistin. *Mol. Pharm.* **2018**, *15*, 4004–4020. [CrossRef]
108. Brunaugh, A.D.; Sharma, S.; Smyth, H. Inhaled fixed-dose combination powders for the treatment of respiratory infections. *Exp. Opin. Drug Deliv.* **2021**, *18*, 1–15. [CrossRef] [PubMed]
109. Nikolaizik, W.H.; Jenni-Galović, V.; Schöni, M.H. Bronchial constriction after nebulized tobramycin preparations and saline in patients with cystic fibrosis. *Eur. J. Pediatr.* **1996**, *155*, 608–611. [CrossRef] [PubMed]
110. Miller, D.P.; Tan, T.; Nakamura, J.; Malcolmson, R.J.; Tarara, T.E.; Weers, J.G. Physical characterization of tobramycin inhalation powder: II. State diagram of an amorphous engineered particle formulation. *Mol. Pharm.* **2017**, *14*, 1950–1960. [CrossRef] [PubMed]
111. Hancock, B.C.; Shamblin, S.L.; Zografi, G. Molecular mobility of amorphous pharmaceutical solids below their glass transition temperatures. *Pharm. Res.* **1995**, *12*, 799–806. [CrossRef]
112. Hickey, A.J.; Gonda, I.; Irwin, W.J.; Fildes, F.J. Effect of hydrophobic coating on the behavior of a hygroscopic aerosol powder in an environment of controlled temperature and relative humidity. *J. Pharm. Sci.* **1990**, *79*, 1009–1014. [CrossRef]
113. Wang, Z.; Wang, H.; Vehring, R. Leucine enhances the dispersibility of trehalose-containing spray-dried powders on exposure to a high-humidity environment. *Int. J. Pharm.* **2021**, *601*, 120561. [CrossRef] [PubMed]
114. Yu, J.; Romeo, M.C.; Cavallaro, A.A.; Chan, H.K. Protective effect of sodium stearate on the moisture-induced deterioration of hygroscopic spray-dried powders. *Int. J. Pharm.* **2018**, *541*, 11–18. [CrossRef]
115. Shetty, N.; Park, H.; Zemlyanov, D.; Mangal, S.; Bhujbal, S.; Zhou, Q.T. Influence of excipients on physical and aerosolization stability of spray dried high-dose powder formulations for inhalation. *Int. J. Pharm.* **2018**, *544*, 222–234. [CrossRef]
116. Lechuga-Ballesteros, D.; Charan, C.; Stults, C.L.; Stevenson, C.L.; Miller, D.P.; Vehring, R.; Tep, V.; Kuo, M.C. Trileucine improves aerosol performance and stability of spray-dried powders for inhalation. *J. Pharm. Sci.* **2008**, *97*, 287–302. [CrossRef] [PubMed]
117. Lawlor, C.P.; Tauber, M.K.; Brogan, J.T.; Zhu, L.; Currie, D.F.; Trautman, B.G.; Sung, J.C. Levofloxacin dry powders engineered for efficient pulmonary delivery and stability. In Proceedings of the Respiratory Drug Delivery, Fajardo, Puerto Rico, 4–8 May 2014; Volume 2, pp. 549–552.
118. Stass, H.; Delesen, H.; Nagelschmitz, J.; Staab, D. Safety and pharmacokinetics of ciprofloxacin dry powder for inhalation in cystic fibrosis: A Phase I, randomized, single-dose, dose-escalation study. *J. Aerosol Med. Pulm. Drug Deliv.* **2015**, *28*, 106–115. [CrossRef] [PubMed]
119. Yu, A.B.; Zou, R.P. Prediction of the porosity of particle mixtures. *KONA* **1998**, *16*, 68–81. [CrossRef]
120. Yang, R.Y.; Zou, R.P.; Yu, A.B. Effect of material properties on the packing of fine particles. *J. Appl. Phys.* **2003**, *94*, 3025–3034. [CrossRef]
121. Xiang, J. The effect of air on the packing structure of fine particles. *Powder Technol.* **2009**, *191*, 280–293. [CrossRef]
122. Vehring, R. Pharmaceutical particle engineering via spray drying. *Pharm. Res.* **2008**, *25*, 999–1022. [CrossRef]
123. Ordoubadi, M.; Gregson, F.K.A.; Wang, H.; Nicholas, M.; Gracin, S.; Lechuga-Ballesteros, D.; Reid, J.P.; Finlay, W.H.; Vehring, R. On the particle formation of leucine in spray drying of inhalable microparticles. *Int. J. Pharm.* **2021**, *592*, 120102. [CrossRef]
124. Lechanteur, A.; Evrard, B. Influence of composition and spray-drying process parameters on carrier-free DPI properties and behaviors in the lung: A review. *Pharmaceutics* **2020**, *12*, 55. [CrossRef]
125. Weers, J.G.; Miller, D.P. Formulation design of dry powders for inhalation. *J. Pharm. Sci.* **2015**, *104*, 3259–3288. [CrossRef]
126. Boraey, M.A.; Vehring, R. Diffusion controlled formation of microparticles. *J. Aerosol Sci.* **2014**, *67*, 131–143. [CrossRef]
127. Ung, K.T.; Chan, H.K. Effects of ramp-up of inspired airflow on in vitro aerosol dose delivery performance for certain dry powder inhalers. *Eur. J. Pharm. Sci.* **2016**, *84*, 46–54. [CrossRef] [PubMed]
128. Ung, K.T.; Rao, N.; Weers, J.G.; Clark, A.R.; Chan, H.-K. In vitro assessment of dose delivery performance of dry powders for inhalation. *Aerosol Sci. Technol.* **2014**, *48*, 1099–1110. [CrossRef]
129. Azouz, W.; Chetcuti, P.; Hosker, H.S.; Saralaya, D.; Stephenson, J.; Chrystyn, H. The inhalation characteristics of patients when they use different dry powder inhalers. *J. Aerosol Med. Pulm. Drug Deliv.* **2015**, *28*, 35–42. [CrossRef]
130. Tiddens, H.A.; Geller, D.E.; Challoner, P.; Speirs, R.J.; Kesser, K.C.; Overbeek, S.E.; Humble, D.; Shrewsbury, S.B.; Standaert, T.A. Effect of dry powder inhaler resistance on the inspiratory flow rates and volumes of cystic fibrosis patients of six years and older. *J. Aerosol Med.* **2006**, *19*, 456–465. [CrossRef] [PubMed]

131. Sahay, S.; Holy, R.; Lyons, S.; Parsley, E.; Maurer, M.; Weers, J. Impact of human behavior on inspiratory flow profiles in patients with pulmonary arterial hypertension using AOS™ dry powder inhaler device. *Pulm. Circ.* **2021**, *11*, 2045894020985345. [CrossRef] [PubMed]
132. Clark, A.R. The role of inspiratory pressures in determining the flow rates though dry powder inhalers; a review. *Curr. Pharm. Design* **2015**, *21*, 3974–3983. [CrossRef]
133. De Boer, A.H.; Hagedoorn, P. The role of disposable inhalers in pulmonary drug delivery. *Exp. Opin. Drug Deliv.* **2015**, *12*, 143–157. [CrossRef]
134. Friebel, C.; Steckel, H. Single-use disposable dry powder inhalers for pulmonary drug delivery. *Exp. Opin. Drug Deliv.* **2010**, *7*, 1359–1372. [CrossRef]
135. Gomez, M.; McCollum, J.; Wang, H.; Ordoubadi, M.; Jar, C.; Carrigy, N.B.; Barona, D.; Tetreau, I.; Archer, M.; Gerhardt, A.; et al. Development of a formulation platform for a spray-dried, inhalable tuberculosis vaccine candidate. *Int. J. Pharm.* **2021**, *593*, 120121. [CrossRef] [PubMed]
136. Prankerd, R.J.; Nguyen, T.H.; Ibrahim, J.P.; Bischof, R.J.; Nassta, G.C.; Olerile, L.D.; Russell, A.S.; Meiser, F.; Parkington, H.C.; Coleman, H.A.; et al. Pulmonary delivery of an ultra-fine oxytocin dry powder formulation: Potential for treatment of postpartum haemorrhage in developing countries. *PLoS ONE* **2013**, *8*, e82965. [CrossRef]
137. Maltz, D.; Paboojian, S.J. In Device engineering insights into Tobi podhaler: A development case study of high efficiency powder delivery to cystic fibrosis patients. In Proceedings of the Respiratory Drug Delivery Europe 2011, Berlin, Germany, 3–6 May 2011; pp. 55–66.
138. De Boer, A.H.; Hagedoorn, P.; Westerman, E.M.; Le Brun, P.P.; Heijerman, H.G.; Frijlink, H.W. Design and in vitro performance testing of multiple air classifier technology in a new disposable inhaler concept (Twincer) for high powder doses. *Eur. J. Pharm. Sci.* **2006**, *28*, 171–178. [CrossRef] [PubMed]
139. Sibum, I.; Hagedoorn, P.; Botterman, C.O.; Frijlink, H.W.; Grasmeijer, F. Automated filling equipment allows increase in the maximum dose to be filled in the Cyclops® high dose dry powder inhalation device while maintaining dispersibility. *Pharmaceutics* **2020**, *12*, 645. [CrossRef]
140. Newman, S.P.; Hirst, P.H.; Pitcairn, G.R. Scintigraphic evaluation of lung deposition with a novel inhaler device. *Curr. Opin. Pulm. Med.* **2001**, *7*, S12–S14.
141. Newman, S.P.; Sutton, D.J.; Segarra, R.; Lamarca, R.; de Miquel, G. Lung deposition of aclidinium bromide from Genuair, a multidose dry powder inhaler. *Respiration* **2009**, *78*, 322–328. [CrossRef] [PubMed]
142. Zhu, B.; Padroni, M.; Colombo, G.; Phillips, G.; Crapper, J.; Young, P.M.; Traini, D. The development of a single-use, capsule-free multi-breath tobramycin dry powder inhaler for the treatment of cystic fibrosis. *Int. J. Pharm.* **2016**, *514*, 392–398. [CrossRef] [PubMed]
143. Son, Y.-J.; Longest, P.W.; Tian, G.; Hindle, M. Evaluation and modification of commercial dry powder inhalers for the aerosolization of a submicrometer excipient enhanced growth (EEG) formulation. *Eur. J. Pharm. Sci.* **2013**, *49*, 390–399. [CrossRef]
144. Chang, R.Y.K.; Kwok, P.C.L.; Ghassabian, S.; Brannan, J.D.; Koskela, H.O.; Chan, H.-K. Cough as an adverse effect on inhalation pharmaceutical products. *Br. J. Pharmacol.* **2020**, *177*, 4096–4112. [CrossRef] [PubMed]
145. Tolerability of Indacaterol Salts (Maleate, Xinafoate and Acetate) in Comparison to Placebo in Patients with Mild to Moderate Persistent Asthma. Novartis. Available online: https://clinicaltrials.gov/ct2/show/NCT00624702 (accessed on 25 July 2021).
146. Beeh, K.M.; Kirsten, A.M.; Tanase, A.M.; Richard, A.; Cao, W.; Hederer, B.; Beier, J.; Kornmann, O.; van Zyl-Smit, R.N. Indacaterol acetate/mometasone furoate provides sustained improvements in lung function compared with salmeterol xinafoate/fluticasone propionate in patients with moderate-to-very-severe COPD: Results from a Phase II randomized, double-blind 12-week study. *Int. J. Chron. Obstuct. Pulmon. Dis.* **2018**, *13*, 3923–3936. [CrossRef]
147. Canning, B.J.; Chang, A.B.; Bolser, D.C.; Smith, J.A.; Mazzone, S.B.; McGarvey, L. Anatomy and neurophysiology of cough: Chest guideline and expert panel report. *Chest* **2014**, *146*, 1633–1648. [CrossRef]
148. Wong, J.P.; Yang, H.; Blasetti, K.L.; Schnell, G.; Conley, J.; Schofield, L.N. Liposome delivery of ciprofloxacin against intracellular *Francisella tularensis* infection. *J. Control. Release* **2003**, *92*, 265–273. [CrossRef]
149. Dalhoff, A. Pharmacokinetics and pharmacodynamics of aerosolized antibacterial agents in chronically infected cystic fibrosis patients. *Clin. Microbiol. Rev.* **2014**, *27*, 753–782. [CrossRef] [PubMed]
150. Jones, R.M.; Neef, N. Interpretation and prediction of inhaled drug particle accumulation in the lung and its associated toxicity. *Xenobiotica* **2012**, *42*, 86–93. [CrossRef] [PubMed]
151. De Soyza, A.; Aksamit, T.; Bandel, T.J.; Criollo, M.; Elborn, J.S.; Operschall, E.; Polverino, E.; Roth, K.; Winthrop, K.L.; Wilson, R. Respire 1: A Phase III placebo-controlled randomised trial of ciprofloxacin dry powder for inhalation in non-cystic fibrosis bronchiectasis. *Eur. Respir. J.* **2018**, *51*, 1702052. [CrossRef] [PubMed]
152. Aksamit, T.; De Soyza, A.; Bandel, T.J.; Criollo, M.; Elborn, J.S.; Operschall, E.; Polverino, E.; Roth, K.; Winthrop, K.L.; Wilson, R. Respire 2: A Phase III placebo-controlled randomised trial of ciprofloxacin dry powder for inhalation in non-cystic fibrosis bronchiectasis. *Eur. Respir. J.* **2018**, *51*, 1702053. [CrossRef] [PubMed]

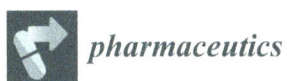

Review

Inhaled Antifungal Agents for Treatment and Prophylaxis of Bronchopulmonary Invasive Mold Infections

Kévin Brunet [1,2,3,*,†], Jean-Philippe Martellosio [1,2,4,†], Frédéric Tewes [1,2], Sandrine Marchand [1,2,5] and Blandine Rammaert [1,2,4,*]

1   Institut National de la Santé et de la Recherche Médicale, INSERM U1070, Pôle Biologie Santé, 1 rue Georges Bonnet, 86022 Poitiers, France; jean-philippe.martellosio@chu-poitiers.fr (J.-P.M.); frederic.tewes@univ-poitiers.fr (F.T.); sandrine.marchand@univ-poitiers.fr (S.M.)
2   Faculté de Médecine et Pharmacie, Université de Poitiers, 6 rue de la Milétrie, 86073 Poitiers, France
3   Laboratoire de Mycologie-Parasitologie, Centre Hospitalier Universitaire de Poitiers, 2 rue de la Milétrie, 86021 Poitiers, France
4   Service de Maladies Infectieuses et Tropicales, Centre Hospitalier Universitaire de Poitiers, 2 rue de la Milétrie, 86021 Poitiers, France
5   Laboratoire de Pharmacologie-Toxicologie, Centre Hospitalier Universitaire de Poitiers, 2 rue de la Milétrie, 86021 Poitiers, France
*   Correspondence: kevin.brunet@univ-poitiers.fr (K.B.); blandine.rammaert.paltrie@univ-poitiers.fr (B.R.)
†   These authors contributed equally to this work.

Abstract: Pulmonary mold infections are life-threatening diseases with high morbi-mortalities. Treatment is based on systemic antifungal agents belonging to the families of polyenes (amphotericin B) and triazoles. Despite this treatment, mortality remains high and the doses of systemic antifungals cannot be increased as they often lead to toxicity. The pulmonary aerosolization of antifungal agents can theoretically increase their concentration at the infectious site, which could improve their efficacy while limiting their systemic exposure and toxicity. However, clinical experience is poor and thus inhaled agent utilization remains unclear in term of indications, drugs, and devices. This comprehensive literature review aims to describe the pharmacokinetic behavior and the efficacy of inhaled antifungal drugs as prophylaxes and curative treatments both in animal models and humans.

Keywords: antifungal drugs; aerosol; invasive fungal disease; animal model; antifungal prophylaxis

Citation: Brunet, K.; Martellosio, J.-P.; Tewes, F.; Marchand, S.; Rammaert, B. Inhaled Antifungal Agents for Treatment and Prophylaxis of Bronchopulmonary Invasive Mold Infections. *Pharmaceutics* **2022**, *14*, 641. https://doi.org/10.3390/pharmaceutics14030641

Academic Editors: Philip Chi Lip Kwok and Michael Yee Tak Chow

Received: 1 February 2022
Accepted: 9 March 2022
Published: 14 March 2022

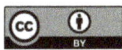

1. Introduction

Bronchopulmonary invasive mold infections (IMI) are a major cause of mortality in immunocompromised patients such as transplant recipients and hematological patients with high-risk neutropenia [1,2]. Three main systemic antifungal classes are used to treat invasive fungal diseases. Systemic triazoles (posaconazole, itraconazole, voriconazole, isavuconazole) and polyenes (amphotericin B (AmB)) are the classes of choice for prophylaxis and treatment, but they suffer from drug-drug interactions and toxicity, while echinocandins are poorly active against molds [3].

Aerosols are an interesting route of administration, theoretically limiting systemic toxicity while ensuring high concentrations at the site of infection [4]. However, due to their physiochemical properties and pharmacokinetic characteristics, some antifungal agents are not good candidates for nebulization and should preferably be delivered intravenously. For example, AmB, which has a high molecular weight and a low permeability across biological membranes, is attractive for delivery by nebulization. Triazoles, which have a high permeability across the respiratory barrier, are less attractive to inhale as a solution, since a low residence time in the lungs is obtained. Molecules with a high respiratory barrier permeability need to be delivered as solid particles with a slow dissolution/release rate, or as advanced formulations that can control permeability to increase their residence time in the lungs after inhalation [5].

Although in some cases inhaled antifungals may be appropriate, clinical experience is still poor and leads to difficulties in their use by physicians. Indeed, the associated indications, materials used for nebulization, and suitable regimens remain unclear. In an effort to facilitate the use of inhaled antifungals, we performed a comprehensive review of their use as prophylaxes and curative treatments of pulmonary IMI in animal models and clinical cases.

2. Materials and Methods

Using PubMed Medline, we searched for articles in English and French that included at least one of the following groups: animal model, rat, mouse, and human. The search query used the following list of keywords: fungi, aerosol, antifungal drug, nebulized, aerosolized, aerosol, inhaled, fluconazole, flucytosine, 5-fluorocytosine, micafungin, caspofungin, echinocandin, isavuconazole, itraconazole, voriconazole, posaconazole, and amphotericin B. Articles of interest cited by the articles found were also reviewed. We included articles published from 1950. Only invasive mold infections were included in the analysis; data from the treatment of chronic or allergic bronchopulmonary aspergillosis (ABPA), fungal colonization, and severe asthma with fungal sensitization (SAFS) were excluded. Infections due to *Pneumocystis jirovecii*, yeasts, and dimorphic fungi were excluded. This search was updated on 31 December 2021.

3. Results

3.1. Selection Criteria for Choosing an Inhaler for Pulmonary Administration of Antifungals

Based on the dosing capacity of each existing technology, only dry powder inhalers (DPIs) and nebulizers are capable of delivering the high dose (usually more than 10 mg) needed to treat pulmonary fungal infections. Nebulizers can deliver several hundred milligrams of a drug to the lungs depending on the drug solubility and the tolerability of long nebulization times [6]. They can be used to deliver solutions or suspensions such as liposomal suspensions of AmB. The efficacy of nebulized antifungals to treat lung infections depends on the total amount of drug reaching the lungs and where the droplets deposit in the lungs. As IMIs are generally spread throughout the lungs, it is important to obtain sufficiently high antifungal agent concentrations all over the pulmonary tree. Liquid droplet deposition in the lungs is controlled by three main factors: airway geometry, aerodynamic particle size, and inhaled flow rate. The aerodynamic size distribution of the droplets emitted by the nebulizer is usually described by the mass median aerodynamic diameter (MMAD) and the geometric standard deviation (GSD). The MMAD refers to the diameter of the droplets above and below which 50% of the mass of drug is contained. The GSD indicates the magnitude of dispersity from the MMAD value. In general, aerosols with an MMAD between 1 and 5 μm are considered respirable [7]. These droplets are large enough to avoid elimination during exhalation and small enough to avoid deposition in the oropharynx [8–10]. More precisely, particles with an MMAD between 2 and 5 μm impact the upper or central airways, while particles with an MMAD of 1–2-μm deposit in the respiratory alveolar zone or peripheral airways [10,11]. Thus, the MMAD is an important parameter when choosing a nebulizer, as it allows estimation of where in the lungs the aerosol should deposit.

There are different types of nebulizers (jet nebulizers, high-frequency nebulizers often termed ultrasonic nebulizers such as vibrating mesh nebulizers, and colliding liquid jet nebulizers), which have different aerosol generation mechanisms and allow different aerosol output rates [12]. The most common nebulizers found in hospitals to treat spontaneously breathing patients are jet nebulizers, and they have been the most used in studies reporting the inhalation of antifungals [12,13]. These nebulizers use compressed air or oxygen to generate a polydispersed aerosol, with only about 5% of the aerosol being respirable, the remainder being returned to the reservoir containing the solution/suspension. In some cases, helium/oxygen (heliox) mixtures are used to reduce the resistance of the patient's airway and, hypothetically, deliver more aerosol to obstructed airways [12]. The patient inhales the aerosol while tidal breathing from a reservoir through a mouthpiece or face mask. Hence, no specific inhalation maneuver is required. During mechanical ventilation, nebulizers can be connected to the inspiratory limb of the ventilator circuit, and the antifungal can be administered continuously or only during inspiration. In these cases, ultrasonic vibrating mesh nebulizers are attractive. They do not require compressed gas but use a high-frequency vibrating membrane filled with micrometer-sized holes to produce droplets. There is virtually no additional gas flow output from the nebulizer to interfere with ventilator operation [12].

Among the most commonly used jet nebulizers, there is a change in MMAD from 6.8 μm to 2.5 μm in standard use [14]. For example, Roth et al. tested three different jet nebulizers loaded with an AmB solution at 10 mg/mL, with droplets with an MMAD between 2 and 3 μm: Respirgard II® (Marquest Inc., Englewood, CO, USA), Cirrus® (Intersurgical, Wokingham, United Kingdom), and Pari IS-2® (Pari-Werk, Starnberg, Germany) [15]. Jet nebulizers seem to generate particles of optimal MMAD compared to ultrasonic nebulizers. Beyer et al. demonstrated that various jet nebulizers generate AmB-loaded droplets with an MMAD of 3 to 5 μm, whereas aerosols generated by ultrasonic nebulizers contained larger droplets (MMAD > 5 μm) [8].

Besides the MMAD, other parameters such as the fine particle fraction (FPF) and the respirable delivered dose (RDD) can influence the choice of nebulizer. The FPF is the percentage of the aerosol with an MMAD between 1 and 5 μm that deposits in the lungs. For commonly used jet nebulizers, the FPF can vary from 80% to less than 40% depending on the jet nebulizer used [14]. Additionally, pulmonary doses of antifungals reaching the lungs may vary by a factor of two when comparing different nebulizers [12,16]. The RDD is calculated by multiplying the total aerosol output by the FPF, and represents the amount (mg) of respirable aerosol deposited in the lungs. When administering high doses of an aerosol, as with antifungal agents, optimizing the nebulization time may be essential to improving patient adherence to treatment. At first glance, we might consider increasing the output rate of the nebulizer to reduce the nebulization time. However, increasing the nebulizer output rate also increases the MMAD of the droplets and reduces the FPF, thereby reducing the rate of deposition of respirable aerosol [14]. For jet nebulizers, the general recommended drug solution volume is 4 to 6 mL, at a flow rate of 8 L/min [10]. In this condition, the administration lasts 10 to 20 min in clinical studies [4,17,18]. Among jet nebulizers, the breath-enhanced nebulizer system allows better drug delivery than the standard system [10].

Aerosol therapy with DPIs has gained attention in the last decade, mainly due to their ability to deliver large doses (up to 10 mg) of a drug quickly (in one puff), and due to the increased chemical stability of active molecules in a dry powder form compared to solutions. Therefore, most antibiotics approved for pulmonary inhalation are now available or under development in a dry powder form [19]. Because of the increased efficacy of aerosolized antibiotic delivery by DPIs compared to nebulizers, a much lower total dose (two to six times) is required with DPIs to achieve similar lung exposure [19]. DPIs are actuated and driven by the patient's inspiratory flow and a powerful, deep inhalation by the DPI is required to disaggregate the powder formulation into respirable particles as efficiently as possible in order to ensure that the drug is delivered to the lungs. Therefore, powder engineering is mandatory to achieve effective aerosolization, and the off-label tests that have been used clinically to nebulize antifungal molecules from solutions intended for IV administration cannot be performed with antifungal powders which are not intended for inhalation. This has limited the clinical data available on the DPI of antifungal agents.

Highlights (criteria for choosing an inhaler):

- Dry powder inhalers (DPIs) and nebulizers are used to deliver antifungal agents;
- Solutions or suspensions of antifungal agents can be nebulized with nebulizers while DPIs are used to nebulize powder;
- Jet nebulizers seem to generate optimal particles compared to other nebulizers;

- Jet nebulizers use compressed gas to generate polydispersed aerosols which are inhaled by the patient through a mouthpiece or face mask. Nebulizers can be connected to the inspiratory limb of the ventilator circuit during mechanical ventilation;
- Mesh nebulizers are also widely used during mechanical ventilation.

3.2. Amphotericin B

Amphotericin B (AmB) is a broad-spectrum antifungal agent from the polyene family [20]. Several pharmaceutical forms of AmB exist: the historic deoxycholate formulation (AmBd), and various formulations using lipid compounds developed with the aim of limiting the nephrotoxicity of AmB. Three lipid formulations are approved by the United States Food and Drug Administration (FDA, Silver Spring, MD, USA) and the European Medicines Agency (EMA, Amsterdam, the Netherlands), and are commercially available in several countries: liposomal AmB (L-AmB), amphotericin B lipid complex (ABLC), and amphotericin B colloidal dispersion (ABCD). The antifungal effects of AmB in the lung are dose- and concentration-dependent [21,22], although AmB pulmonary diffusion is low when administered systemically [23]. Given its relatively high molecular weight (924 g/mol) and low-lipophilic properties represented by a LogD of -2.8 at pH 7.4 [23], AmB should have a long residence time in the lungs after nebulization. AmB is thus a good candidate for inhalation and was administered to humans by nebulization of various liquid formulations [24]. However, most of the clinical studies were performed using liquid AmB formulations designed for parenteral administration that have been repurposed for nebulization and used off-label to treat lower airway infections; additionally, the optimal drug dosing often remains undefined. New formulations of AmB have been recently developed for administration by DPI but in vivo studies have not been performed on these formulations [25,26].

The pharmacodynamics of L-AmB is poorly understood due to its complex pharmacokinetics [27,28]. Indeed, several measurements can be conducted: total AmB, protein bound drug, liposome associated drug, and freely circulating drug. Classically, total concentrations of AmB in both plasma and tissues are measured; however, only free AmB will be active. Consequently, the pharmacokinetic data obtained from L-AmB inhalation are difficult to analyze. The pharmacokinetics of AmBd is better understood due to the absence of liposomes. In this context, most authors refer to the minimal inhibitory concentration (MIC) to assess the efficacy of AmB in the alveolar compartments, although this is questionable due to the dose- and concentration-dependent behavior of AmB [29].

3.2.1. Pharmacokinetics

In Animal Models

The pharmacokinetics of nebulized AmBd (n-AmBd) have been assessed in a non-infected rat model and compared to those of intraperitoneal (IP) injections [30]. Non-immunosuppressed rats were exposed to n-AmBd by jet nebulizer (air flow 8 L/min; drug solution 0.3 L/min). AmBd was efficiently delivered to the lungs while limiting accumulation in other organs. After n-AmBd nebulization of 1.6 mg/kg, concentrations were undetectable (<0.1 µg/g) in the serum, spleen, liver, kidney, and brain. Elimination from the lungs was progressive with a half-time elimination of 4.8 days after 3.2 mg/kg of n-AmBd. The maximal dose tolerated through nebulization by rats without toxicity was 60 mg/kg as determined by microscopic organ examination and animal behavior. n-AmBd pharmacokinetics have also been evaluated in a sheep model [31]. AmBd has been nebulized in animals using an ultrasonic nebulizer connected to an endotracheal tube. The drug concentration was measured in the bronchoalveolar fluid (BALF). However, the authors did not calculate the epithelial lining fluid (ELF) concentration. The peak concentration was achieved after 0.5 h in the BALF, and a slow decrease in the concentration was observed over 24 h. The peak concentrations were identical with two different doses: 5 mg and 30 mg, showing that the peak concentration of AmB in the bronchi was not directly proportional to the dose, while the area under the curve in BALF was superior with the higher dose. These data indicate that n-AmBd may reduce the systemic toxicity due to its very low systemic passage and high concentration in the lungs. Moreover, its long half-life allows several days of interval between administrations [8,32]. The distribution in the organs of nebulized L-AmB (n-L-AmB) was studied in male BALB/c 30 g mice [33]. After 1 h of nebulization of different formulations of L-AmB (8.56 to 20.03 mg of AmB) with a nose-only Collison nebulizer, L-AmB was not detected in serum at any point in time.

To find the best candidate formulation for nebulization, various formulations of AmB have been tested in similar models with divergent results. Several authors have shown that the distribution between different formulations is similar. The aerosol delivery of AmBd and L-AmB have been compared in vivo in rats [34]. The authors demonstrated that both formulations were well delivered in lungs with low systemic exposure. Both formulations led to physicochemical characteristics suitable for nebulization with the same delivered dose. In addition, liposomes are physically stable enough to be nebulized. In another naive rat model, four nebulized commercial formulations of AmB (AmBd, L-AmB, ABLC, and ABCD) were compared [35]. The distribution in the lungs after nebulization was identical whatever the formulation, and AmB was detectable after six weeks in lungs, but undetectable in serum. On the other hand, other studies have shown that L-AmB or ABLC were better candidates for nebulization with higher lung retention than AmBd. In a murine model comparing n-AmBd and n-L-AmB, the drug concentration in the lungs was 8.6 times higher with n-L-AmB [36]. In a rat model of invasive pulmonary aspergillosis, the concentration of nebulized ABLC (n-ABLC) was higher and more prolonged than that of n-AmBd in the lungs one day and seven days after treatment [37]. Moreover, n-L-AmB had no effect on surfactant function, while n-AmBd inhibited its activity [38,39]. Deoxycholic acid alone inhibited surfactant surface activity and perturbed lipid organization. Therefore, the authors proposed L-AmB as a better formulation for nebulization [39].

New formulations of AmB were developed to be used through nebulization. For example, AmB liposomes coated with alveolar macrophage-specific ligands led to a high lung concentration and a low plasma concentration in rats [40,41]. Another formulation of n-AmB using sodium deoxycholate sulfate was tested in rats [42]. Compared to n-AmBd, this formulation was less toxic for the organs, as assessed by histopathology, and provided the highest lung and plasma concentrations. Other authors have developed polymeric and lipid nanoparticles of AmB via a spray-drying technique using hydroxypropylmethycellulose and stearylamine with oleic acid [43]. This technique led to alveolar drug delivery for a long period (30–35 h).

In Human

In lung transplant recipients, IMIs are responsible for tracheobronchitis, bronchial anastomosis necrosis, pneumonia, and disseminated infections [44]. *Aspergillus* spp. are the most frequent fungi retrieved from the lungs of these patients. Antifungal drugs are used as prophylaxis after transplantation, and the regular control of transplant anastomosis is performed through bronchoscopy. It is thus easier to implement clinical studies using broncho-alveolar lavage (BAL) in this particular population. AmBd concentrations were measured in the bronchial secretion aspirate and BAL fluid (BALF) of 39 lung transplant recipients up to 24 h after one nebulization of 6 mg/d of AmBd, for a minimum of seven days [45]. The mean concentration in BALF was 11 µg/mL. The drug concentration in the ELF was calculated assuming that 1% of the recovered BALF corresponded to the volume of ELF. The concentration of AmB necessary to prevent *Aspergillus* is not known but the MIC of most of *Aspergillus* species is above 1 µg/mL. However, in the most proximal zone where bronchial anastomosis is located, this concentration is achieved only during the initial hours after nebulization. The proposed dosing regimen to better prevent *Aspergillus* infection of the bronchial anastomosis is thus 6 mg every 8 h during the early weeks post-transplantation [4].

Nebulized lipid formulations of AmB offer higher concentrations [23], a longer half-life, and a longer persistence in the BALF than n-AmBd, enhancing lung penetration [9]. L-AmB reaches different lung compartments after nebulization. The highest concentration was found in the alveolar compartment (24.5 ± 3.1% of total AmB introduced in the nebulizer), followed by the bronchial compartment (11.6 ± 1.3%) [46]. In two different studies in lung transplant patients, the administration of nebulized ABLC 1 mg/kg/day or L-AmB 25 mg/day resulted in high enough AmB concentrations in the ELF or BALF for *Aspergillus* spp. prophylaxis up to 7 to 14 days after the last inhaled dose [47,48]. In another study, technetium-labelled ABLC was administered using an AeroEclipse (Amherst, NY, USA) nebulizer in 12 lung transplant recipients. About 17 to 20% of the dose was deposited in the lungs. The evaluation of the size of the nebulized particles revealed a similar size to that of the *Aspergillus* conidia, and therefore, suggested a similar distribution in the tracheobronchial tract [16]. AmB concentrations of 0.50 ± 0.31 μg/mL were obtained in the ELF of eight lung transplant recipients in the 30 to 60 min following completion of the nebulization of 30 mg AmBd (5 mg/mL in 15–20 min). These concentrations are equal to the MIC of most *Aspergillus* species (i.e., 0.5 mg/L) [1].

Numerous studies have demonstrated no evidence of significant systemic absorption after nebulization (undetectable concentrations < 0.2 μg/mL at peak 1 h), under various dosing regimens (n-AmBd 6 mg/day to 10 mg/8 h; n-L-AmB 25 mg three times a week to 40 mg/day; n-ABLC 50 mg twice a week to 1 mg/kg/day) and various drug concentrations and nebulizers [8,45,47–53]. Only one study found therapeutic serum levels (2 μg/mL) in three out of five patients treated with n-AmBd at 20 mg b.i.d [54]. AmBd was detectable in serum (<1 μg/mL) after 10 mg b.i.d. of n-AmBd [52]. None of the four patients who received n-L-AmB at 20 mg b.i.d had detectable serum levels. In comparison, steady-state peak plasma concentrations of AmB are typically between 1.2 and 2.4 mg/mL following intravenous AmBd at 0.5–1 mg/kg, and between 7 and 12 mg/mL following intravenous L-AmB at 1 mg/kg [52]. Consequently, n-AmB led to high lung concentrations with no or very low systemic absorption. Lipid formulations seem more interesting due to their higher concentration in lungs and longer half-life, which is presumed to result in better adherence to treatment and less contamination of the nebulizer [17]. It is feasible to administer nebulized lipid formulations of AmB every one or two weeks rather than once daily for AmBd, which is more convenient for the patient. However, due to insufficient data concerning AmB concentrations at the bronchial anastomosis site in lung transplant recipients, it has been suggested that a higher frequency of administration is maintained until the suture is healed [48]. Lipid formulations are usually easier to administer as they are already in solution and do not foam, in contrast to n-AmBd [15]. Moreover, it has been shown during in vitro studies that AmBd inhibits bovine surfactant functions [38,39], whereas Monforte et al. revealed that n-L-AmB induced no changes in the lipid content of human pulmonary surfactant [55]. Albeit lower than with other systemic drugs, the cost for prophylaxis with n-L-AmB is about six fold that for a six-month n-AmBd treatment [17]. The main drawbacks of n-AmB are its unreliable distribution in the native lung in single-lung transplant recipients, who remain at risk for IMIs, due to a predominant distribution in the transplant [45], and the fact that it does not prevent extra-pulmonary infections such as candidemia.

Highlights (nebulized AmB pharmacokinetics):
- Nebulized AmB is well delivered in the bronchial and alveolar compartments with concentrations in the ELF or BALF above most fungal MICs;
- There is no or very weak systemic absorption;
- Lipid formulations have a higher concentration and a longer half-life in the BALF and do not alter surfactant functions; however, they are more expensive.

3.2.2. Efficacy of n-AmB for Curative Treatment of IMI

Animal Models

To evaluate the efficacy of n-AmB, invasive pulmonary aspergillosis (IPA) models are the most studied. n-AmBd was tested on male Sprague Dawley rats (125–150 g) [56]. Rats were immunosuppressed with 100 mg of cortisone (three times per week, subcutaneously) and intratracheally inoculated with 10^6 spores of *A. fumigatus*. One nebulization (air chamber with air flow 8 L/min; drug solution 0.3 L/min; exposure time 15 min/4.5 mL AmB; dose 1.6 mg/kg) two days after infection delayed death but did not improve survival. Comparable results were observed with one nebulization started 24 h after inoculation and continued daily for six days [56]. In the same model, combinations of one dose of n-AmBd at 1.6 mg/kg two days before inoculation with itraconazole (ITZ), SCH39304, or placebo were studied [57]. n-AmBd combined with ITZ or SCH39304 significantly improved survival at day 24 compared to n-AmBd combined with placebo.

In another study, the four commercially available formulations of AmB (AmBd, L-AmB, ABLC, and ABCD) were nebulized and compared in naive and infected rat aspergillosis model [35]. All AmB formulations were effective in prolonging survival when treatment was started 16 h after intratracheal fungal inoculation. Two studies have compared n-L-AmB and n-AmBd for IPA treatment in rats [39,58]. The two formulations prolonged rat survival. Both forms are more effective than systemic treatment, but n-L-AmB was more effective than n-AmBd to increase survival [58].

Combining n-AmB and systemic antifungal drugs could optimize IPA treatment. Results from rat aspergillosis models are, however, contradictory. One study have shown that n-L-AmB combined with systemic L-AmB did not improve survival but prevented dissemination [58]. Others have shown that n-L-AmB combined with systemic AmB (AmBd or L-AmB) is superior to either treatment alone [59]. Finally, n-L-AmB was tested in combination with intraperitoneal micafungin [60]. In total, 10 mg of n-L-AmB alone was effective to improve survival and decrease fungal burden. A combination with intraperitoneal micafungin at 1 mg/kg/day was more effective. Other formulations used for nebulization such as non-ionic surfactant vesicles containing AmB [61] or AmB polymethacrylic acid nanoparticle [62] showed good results during in vivo models. These formulations were also effective in prophylaxis.

Clinical Studies

Twenty-two publications, mostly case reports and case series, gathering 100 patients have reported the use of n-AmB as an adjunctive treatment for IMIs (see Supplementary Materials, Table S1) [18,63–84]. Curative nebulized treatment has been used in two forms of aspergillosis, tracheobronchial (TBA) and invasive pulmonary aspergillosis (IPA), mainly in lung cancer patients or lung transplant recipients.

n-AmBd has been used in 34 patients (Supplementary Metarials, Table S1). Different dosing regimens have been used, mostly 12.5 mg once or twice daily in recent studies, in combination with systemic anti-mold drugs and/or interventional bronchoscopic treatment and/or topical instillation of AmB [64–71]. Cure rates ranged between 36% and 67% in the two largest series [66,67]. The position of nebulization as a first line or salvage therapy was not described. Three previously described case reports involved pulmonary mucormycosis [72–75,79]. n-AmBd dosage varied from 6 mg t.i.d to 30 mg twice a week in combination with systemic AmB +/− topical instillation of AmBd +/− interventional bronchoscopic treatment or surgical treatment. All three patients were eventually cured.

Nebulized lipid formulations have been reported in a total of 67 patients (Supplementary Table S1). Peghin et al. reported a series of 22 lung transplant recipients with invasive aspergillosis (15 IPA, 7 ulcerative TBA) treated with n-L-AmB and a systemic mold-active drug. The global cure rate was 55% [18]. Safdar and Rodriguez reported a series of 32 immunosuppressed patients with various IMIs treated with n-ABLC 50 mg once or twice daily combined with various systemic antifungal agents. The global cure rate was 50% [79]. Various pulmonary IMIs including infections due to *Mucorales*, *Scedosporium* spp., *Hormographiella aspergillata*, *Fusarium* spp. and *Microascus* have been successfully treated using n-ABLC (25 to 100 mg once daily) [75,80,82] or n-L-AmB 25 mg three times a week [63,81], in combination with systemic antifungal agents and/or interventional bronchoscopic treatment and/or topical instillation of AmB. A unique publication reported the use of successful monotherapy with n-ABLC 50 mg/d in a case of IPA [77].

Curative Treatment Guidelines

The Infectious Disease Society of America (IDSA), the Infectious Disease Community of Practice (IDCOP), and The International Society for Heart and Lung Transplantation (ISHLT) have each issued recommendations for the use of adjunctive n-AmB in the curative treatment of IMIs [85–87] (Table 1).

Table 1. Guidelines for the use of nebulized AmB in treatment for invasive mold infections in lung transplant recipients.

Ref	Type of IFD	n-AmB	Evidence
Patterson, 2016 [86]	TBA in lung transplants associated with anastomotic endobronchial ischemia or ischemic reperfusion injury due to airway ischemia	Adjunctive inhaled AmB is recommended in association with a systemic antimold antifungal (strong recommendation; moderate-quality evidence).	"No consistent evidence"
Husain, 2016 [87]	TBA	n-AmB alone is not recommended as a primary treatment of TBA (C-III). Although it has been proposed as an adjunctive therapy in an endobronchial prothesis infection, more evidence is needed.	Morales, 2009 [80]
	IPA	Addition of n-AmB to a standard regimen of treatment is not routinely recommended (C-III). However, the authors also declare that n-AmB could be used in combination with voriconazole/other systemic antifungal drugs, depending on the severity of IFD, or possibly in situations in which large cavitary lesions might render the penetration of systemic agents difficult.	Additional evidence would be helpful
Husain, 2019 [85]	TBA associated with anastomotic endo-bronchial ischemia, or ischemic reperfusion injury due to airway ischemia associated with lung transplant	Inhaled AmB (in conjunction with systemic antifungal therapy) may be used (weak; low).	

Highlights (nebulized AmB in curative treatment):

- Adjunctive therapy with n-AmB has been used for pulmonary IMIs in combination with systemic drugs, but its efficacy as a primary and/or salvage therapy has not been elucidated in randomized studies;
- n-AmBd and n-L-AmB have been not compared, but animal models suggest that n-L-AmB is more efficient than n-AmBd;
- n-AmB is only recommended in association with systemic antifungal agents in TBA in lung transplants associated with anastomotic endobronchial ischemia or ischemic reperfusion injury due to airway ischemia with low evidence.

3.2.3. Efficacy of n-AmB for Prophylaxis of IMI

Animal Models

n-AmB prophylaxis have been studied in animal models of aspergillosis, on rats [35,37,56,88,89], mice [36], and guinea pigs [90]. The only study assessing n-AmB for mucormycosis prophylaxis showed negative results with n-L-AmB [91].

n-L-AmB (0.8 mg/kg) administered two hours before challenge led to 100% survival at day eight in an aspergillosis rat model [88]. In another rat model (10^5 *Aspergillus* spores intratracheally, discontinued corticoid immunosuppression), prophylaxis with n-AmBd administered at 1.6 mg/kg two days before inoculation decreased mortality to 11% compared to 93.8% with placebo at three weeks [89]. In the rat model previously described in the curative section [56], nebulization administered two days before inoculation delayed mortality and dramatically reduced *Aspergillus* colony forming units in the lungs.

Some authors have used new formulations of AmB such as inhalation of AmB dry powder with success in a guinea pig model of aspergillosis [90]. A single inhaled dose of dry powder at 0.05, 0.5, 4, or 10 mg/kg was administered 24 h prior to infection. This treatment improved survival and decreased the fungal burden. n-AmBd and n-L-AmB seem to be as effective regardless of the time of administration (1, 2, or 3 days) before inoculation when compared to corticoid immunosuppressed mice intranasally inoculated with *Aspergillus* spores [36]. Comparisons of the four commercialized formulations give contradictory results. They have been equally effective for survival when administered one week before inoculation in an aspergillosis rat model [35]. When prophylaxis was started six weeks before challenge, only n-L-AmB was effective, probably due to the longer half-life of L-AmB compared to other formulations. In another model, n-ABLC was more effective than n-AmBd to prolong survival [37]. A meta-analysis of n-AmB as a prophylactic for IPA on immunosuppressed animal was performed in 2015 [92]. A meta-analysis concluded that n-AmB was effective for prophylaxis in IPA with no significant variation between lipid formulations of AmB and AmBd. Moreover, they found no more adverse events (AEs) in the n-AmBd group.

Clinical Studies in Hematology

Most of the available studies are related to primary prophylaxis. Data on n-AmB as secondary prophylaxis for IPA in immunosuppressed patients are scarce [78].

Non-randomized studies have shown a decrease in IPA incidence rates with n-AmBd prophylaxis in high-risk hematological patients, i.e., acute myeloid leukemia (AML) and myelodysplastic syndrome (SMD) undergoing intensive chemotherapy, or autologous and allogenic stem cell transplantation (SCT) [50,93–96] (Supplementary Table S2). However, these studies lacked a control group or statistical comparison, or failed to reach significance. A prospective study of 102 patients undergoing allogenic SCT demonstrated significantly less possible/probable/proven IMI when patients received adequate n-AmBd prophylaxis (15 mg b.i.d., $\geq$7 days) compared with inadequate n-AmBd prophylaxis (<7 days) (2.4% vs. 18.8% at day 120, $p < 0.05$) [97]. In a retrospective cohort of 354 allogenic SCT patients receiving n-AmBd 25 mg/d as prophylaxis, the five-year incidence rate of probable or proven IA was 2.5% [98]. This is significantly lower than the 6.6% of a historical control cohort without antifungal prophylaxis. In comparison, the rate of proven and probable invasive fungal disease in AML/SMD patients undergoing induction chemotherapy was reduced from 8% to 2%, and the rate of IPA from 7% to 1% with posaconazole prophylaxis in a randomized controlled trial [99].

The only two randomized trials assessing the efficacy of n-AmBd (10 mg b.i.d.) compared to a control group in high-risk neutropenic patients did not show significant differences in the possible/probable/proven IPA incidence [100,101].

Three comparative studies assessed the efficacy of nebulized lipid formulations of AmB for prophylaxis in high-risk hematological patients (Supplementary Table S3). Two prospective studies compared prophylaxis with n-L-AmB 12.5 mg twice a week + fluconazole 400 mg/day to a historical control group treated with fluconazole 400 mg/day only [102,103]. Hullard-Pulstinger et al. found a non-significant decrease in probable/proven IA in the n-L-AmB group compared to a control group (2.1% vs. 3.8%), but few events occurred [103]. Chong et al. showed a significant decrease in probable/proven IA in the n-L-AmB group compared to the historical control group (9.5% vs. 23.4%, $p = 0.006$) [102].

One randomized double-blind controlled study evaluated the incidence rate of probable/proven IPA in 271 high-risk neutropenic patients: 139 patients received prophylactic n-L-AmB 12.5 mg twice weekly + fluconazole until neutrophil recovery > 300/mm^3, 132 patients received nebulized placebo + fluconazole. This trial showed a significant decrease in probable/proven IPA in the n-L-AmB group (4.3% vs. 13.6%, OR 0.26, 95% CI [0.09–0.72]) [2]. A meta-analysis from 2015 showed a lower incidence of IPA among patients who underwent n-AmBd or n-L-AmB prophylaxis (OR 0.42, 95% CI [0.22–0.79], $p = 0.007$) [92].

Clinical Studies in Lung Transplant Recipients

Due to the lack of randomized studies, surveys of antifungal prophylaxis strategy in lung transplant centers worldwide and in the US have been published between 2006 and 2015 [104–108]. These studies showed great variations between centers, with an increasing use of n-AmB. In each of these surveys, most centers used universal antifungal prophylaxis. n-AmB was the most used antifungal agent, alone or in combination with oral voriconazole or itraconazole. Prophylaxis is most often initiated during the 24 h post-transplantation [104] and the duration varies from three to six months to life-long.

Non-comparative studies have shown a low incidence rate of IA < 5% with either n-AmBd or nebulized lipid formulations of AmB alone, or in association with systemic antifungal prophylaxis [18,53,109–116] (Supplementary Tables S4 and S5). The use of n-AmBd resulted in a significant decrease in IA incidence in several prospective and retrospective studies, in comparison with historical controls without antifungal prophylaxis [4,117–120].

Two studies comparing n-AmBd and n-L-AmB showed no significant differences in the incidence rates of IA [17,52] (Supplementary Table S6). A randomized double-blind trial compared the incidence rate of IFI during the first two months post-transplantation in 100 patients receiving prophylactic n-AmBd 25 mg or n-ABLC 50 mg for four days then weekly for seven weeks. Doses were doubled in mechanically ventilated patients. There was no significant difference in the incidence of IMI between the two groups, 14.3% vs. 11.8%, respectively [121]. In conclusion, the three comparative studies showed no significant differences in terms of efficacy between n-L-AmB and n-AmBd for IFI prophylaxis, even though IMI incidence rate was lower with n-L-AmB prophylaxis in all three studies [17,52,121].

Mechanically Ventilated COVID-19 Patients

Since patients hospitalized in critical care are at high risk for IPA, Van Ackerbroeck et al. have tested antifungal prophylaxis with n-AmBL [122]. Authors have shown that inhaled liposomal amphotericin-B (under a twice-weekly prophylactic regimen of 12.5 mg) reduced the incidence of COVID-19-associated pulmonary aspergillosis in mechanically ventilated COVID-19 patients (RR 0.15, 95% CI [0.05–0.48]).

Prophylaxis Guidelines

Several groups (European Society of Clinical Microbiology and Infectious Disease (ESCMID), IDCOP, ISHLT, and IDSA) have proposed guidelines for indications, dosing regimens, and the duration of n-AmB antifungal prophylaxis in hematological patients (Table 2) or transplant recipients (Table 3).

Table 2. Guidelines for prophylactic use of nebulized AmB in hematological patients.

Ref	Criteria	n-AmBd	n-L-AmB
Mellinghoff, 2018 [123]	Neutrophils < 500/mm^3, >7 days. (AlloSCT and ALL excluded)	Recommendation against its use (D-I)	Recommended B-II (second choice after posaconazole) 12.5 mg × 2/week in combination with fluconazole 400 mg/day
Patterson, 2016 [86]	Prolonged neutropenia (induction/reinduction therapy for AL, and alloSCT recipients following conditioning or during treatment of GVHD)	n-AmB may be considered (weak recommendation; low-quality evidence) AmB lipid formulations are generally better tolerated than AmBd	
Ullman, 2018 [124]	Prolonged and profound neutropenia	Not mentioned	Recommended B-I (second choice after posaconazole) 12.5 mg × 2/week in combination with fluconazole 400 mg/day
	AlloSCT recipients until neutrophil recovery	Not mentioned	Recommended B-II (ex-aqueous first choice with posaconazole) 12.5 mg × 2/week in combination with fluconazole 400 mg/day

Table 2. *Cont.*

Ref	Criteria	n-AmBd	n-L-AmB
Maertens, 2018 [125]	Induction AML/MDS	Recommendation against its use (A-I)	Recommended B-I (second choice after posaconazole) 10 mg × 2/week in combination with fluconazole 400 mg/day
	AlloSCT with high-risk mold infection		Not recommended if low incidence of mold infections (<5%), recommended B-II (third choice) if high incidence of mold infections (>5%) 10 mg × 2/week in combination with fluconazole 400 mg/day

AlloSCT: allogeneic stem cell transplantation; ALL: acute lymphoblastic leukemia; AML: acute myeloid leukemia; MDS: myelodysplastic syndrome; AmB: amphotericin B; n-AmB: nebulized AmB; AmBd: deoxycholate AmB; L-AmB: liposomal AmB.

Table 3. Guidelines for prophylactic use of nebulized AmB in lung transplant recipients.

Ref	Criteria	n-AmBd	n-AmB Lipid Formulation
Husain, 2016 [87]	Lung transplant recipients	n-AmB ± fluconazole or an echinocandin should be used in the first 2–4 weeks post-transplantation (B-I)	
Patterson, 2016 [86]	Lung transplant recipients	n-AmB may be considered (weak recommendation; low-quality evidence) AmB lipid formulations are generally better tolerated than AmBd	
Ullman, 2018 [124]	Lung transplant recipients	B-II 25 mg/day for 4 days, followed by 25 mg/week for 7 weeks	Recommended A-I (first choice) More AEs with AmBd but similar efficacy; various possible protocols: ABLC 50 mg/d for 4 d, then 50 mg/w for 7 w. ABLC 50 mg/day for 2 w., then 1×/w for 10 w. L-AmB 25 mg × 3/w. (day 1–60) post SOT, then 1×/w. (day 60–180)
	Heart transplant recipients	n-AmB universal prophylaxis is recommended in second choice (C-I). First choice is targeted prophylaxis with echinocandins	
Husain and Camargo, 2019 [85]	Lung transplant recipients	AmBd 20 mg × 3/d or 25 mg/d (weak; low)	ABLC 50 mg 1×/2d for 2 w., then 1×/w for 13 w. (week; low) L-AmB 25 mg × 3/w. for 2 months, then 1×/w. for 6 m., then 2×/m. thereafter (weak; low)
	Heart transplant recipients	Not cited Targeted prophylaxis with itraconazole or voriconazole or echinocandins is recommended in patients at risk	

AmB: amphotericin B; n-AmB: nebulized AmB; AmBd: deoxycholate AmB; L-AmB: liposomal AmB; SOT: solid organ transplantation; AEs: adverse events.

Highlights (nebulized AmB in prophylaxis):

- Several authors have shown the high efficacy of n-AmBd or n-L-AmBL alone or in combination with systemic drugs to prevent IPA in lung transplant recipients;
- In hematological patients with high-risk neutropenia, n-L-AmB has been associated with a decrease in probable/proven IPA incidence while the results with n-AmBd were discordant;
- In lung transplant recipients, n-AmBd or nebulized lipid formulations of AmB could be used in first or second intention;
- In hematological patients with high-risk neutropenia, n-L-AmB is recommended in second intention after posaconazole.

3.2.4. Tolerance

No systemic adverse events (AEs) have been observed, especially no change in creatinine levels with either n-AmBd or n-L-AmB. Some mild and transient AEs are common with both formulations (cough, dysgeusia, nausea) with great rate differences between studies (see Supplementary Tables S2–S5), since they are dose-dependent [51]. n-AmBd AEs range from 0% to 100% of patients [4,17,49–52,54,94–98,100,112,119,121,126,127]. Several studies have reported an incidence of 30–40% [4,17,52,119,121] or even 50–100% of AEs [51,97,100,127]. AEs are less frequent with nebulized lipid formulations, ranging from 0% to 36.5% of patients [2,17,18,52,53,102,103,109,112,121,128] in all studies but one [129] (i.e., coughing in 74% of patients), with no severe AE. Bronchospasm and wheezing have also been reported with n-AmBd, n-L-AmB, and n-ABLC [4,17,18,51,52,54,97,121]. These AEs are rare and easily managed with salbutamol inhalation before the procedure or by halving the drug concentration [18,98]. A decline in pulmonary function has been reported in about 5% of patients (between 0 and 32%) in most studies with nebulized lipid formulations of AmB [48,53,121,128,129] and in 10.6 to 50.0% with n-AmBd [121,126]. This reversible AE has been reported both in neutropenic and lung transplant patients. Thus, local and irritative AEs of n-AmB clearly outweigh the systemic AEs observed when AmB is administered intravenously.

Treatment-limiting AEs range from 0 to 33% with n-AmBd, [17,51,97,98,100,126], and are close to 0% when using salbutamol premedication [98]. They most often range between 0 and 6% with nebulized lipid formulations [17,18,52,53,109,121,128], except in two studies that reported discontinuation rates of 42.7% [103] and 45% [2], mainly due to discomfort in the first study and patients' weakness and technical problem in the second.

Three studies have compared n-AmBd and nebulized lipid formulations of AmB for prophylaxis in lung transplant patients. n-AmBd is associated with more AEs than lipid formulations and seems to result in more treatment discontinuations. Two non-randomized studies have shown no significant differences in the incidence of AEs and treatment-limiting AEs between n-AmBd and n-L-AmB [17,52] (see Supplementary Table S6). There is only one randomized trial comparing the tolerance of n-AmBd and lipid formulations [121]. In this study, 100 lung transplant patients were randomized to receive antifungal prophylaxis with either n-AmBd or n-ABLC for seven weeks. There were more patients who experienced at least one AE in the AmBd group than in the ABLC group (42% vs. 28%): cough (10.6% vs. 2.1%), dyspnea (19.9% vs. 2.1%), nausea (8.5% vs. 2.1%), wheezing (6.4% vs. 4.2%), dysgeusia (10.6% vs. 7.7%), and bronchospasm (25% vs. 20.4%). The decline in pulmonary function (decline of FEV1 > 20%) was similar in the two groups (10.6% vs. 11.1%). Patients who received n-AmBd were more likely to experience AEs (OR = 2.16, 95% CI [1.10–4.24], p = 0.02). Treatment-limiting AEs were higher in the AmBd group (12.2% vs. 5.9%), although this finding did not reach significance due to a lack of power [121]. A meta-analysis of these three prospective studies in lung-transplant recipients was unable to compare the AEs of n-AmBd and nebulized lipid formulations due to non-uniform reporting of the data [130]. In terms of treatment-limiting AEs, meta-analysis showed a 4% rate with nebulized lipid formulations vs. 8% for n-AmBd not reaching significance (HR 0.57, 95% CI [0.22–1.50]).

Highlights (nebulized AmB tolerance):

- Global tolerance of n-AmB is good with no or very few systemic AEs;
- Mild and transient AEs are common with both formulations (cough, dysgeusia, nausea);
- Bronchospasm and wheezing are rare and easily managed with salbutamol inhalation or by halving drug concentration;
- Decline in pulmonary function is rare but has been reported in about 5% of patients;
- AEs are less frequent with lipid formulations.

3.3. Triazoles

3.3.1. Voriconazole

Voriconazole (VRZ) is a relatively lipophilic molecule with a LogD = 1.8 at pH 7.4, with an ELF/plasma ratio between 6 and 11 when administered by a systemic route in humans [23]. Several studies have investigated the aerodynamic properties of nebulized voriconazole (n-VRZ) using commercially available solutions concentrated at 6.25 to 10 mg/mL. The MMAD was 2.4 to 2.98 μm and the FPF was 71.7–93.0% [131–134]. These results suggested an appropriate distribution of the nebulized droplets into the distal zones of the lung but a rapid systemic absorption.

The pharmacokinetics of n-VRZ was investigated in non-infected racing pigeons [135]. After nebulization for 15 min at 10 mg/mL of an intravenous commercially available solution, the authors showed a low concentration in the lungs with no detection after one hour and a fast decrease in plasma. A non-commercial aqueous solution of VRZ solubilized with sulfobutyl ether-beta-cyclodextrin was nebulized in mice [136]. High concentrations were observed in the lungs and plasma within 30 min. The ratio of lung/plasma concentration was 1.4 after a single inhaled dose and 2.9 after multiple doses. A rapid distribution from lung to blood was observed. In another model, chronically inhaled voriconazole was well tolerated in a rat model [133].

A rapid distribution of n-VRZ from lungs to plasma was also observed in humans. Therapeutic drug levels in human lung tissues occurred 30 min after inhalation of a solution at 10 mg/mL, and maximal pulmonary concentrations were 1.4 times higher than plasma concentrations [133,134]. In a study including six patients, n-VRZ was rapidly absorbed into systemic circulation with detectable serum concentrations 15 min after nebulization of 40 mg. Median plasma concentrations were 100 times lower twelve hours after the last nebulization in the inhalation group, who received 40 mg b.i.d for two days, compared to the oral group (400 mg b.i.d at day 1, 200 mg b.i.d at day 2) (8 vs. 1224 ng/mL, $p < 0.0001$) [137]. There was a non-significant trend towards a higher median ELF/plasma concentration ratio in the inhalation group (21, 95% CI [6–63]) compared to the oral group (8, 95% CI [3–20]; $p = 0.2$).

Different formulations have been tested to try to retain VRZ in the lungs, such as nanoparticles [138], dry powder insufflation of crystalline and amorphous VRZ formulations [139], polylactic-co-glycolic acid (PGLA) nanoparticles [140], chitosan-coated PGLA nanoparticles [141], and inhalable dry powder by spray freeze drying [142]. These formulations showed good aerosol properties with efficient lung deposition and higher concentrations in the lungs than intravenous VRZ. These formulations led to clinically relevant concentrations in plasma but with variable systemic absorption.

n-VRZ has solely been studied for curative treatment in humans and not for prophylaxis. One mouse model of IPA showed that aqueous solutions of VRZ solubilized with sulfobutyl ether-beta-cyclodextrin improved survival when administered as prophylaxis and were more efficient than IP injection of AmB [134]. In humans, four case reports have been reported thus far using n-VRZ as an adjunctive treatment of IMI (see Supplementary Table S7). Two publications involving three lung transplant recipients and one immunosuppressed patient with IPA showed clinical and/or radiological cure or improvement with n-VRZ 40 mg administered one to three times daily, alone or as adjunctive treatment [131,132]. n-VRZ 40 mg once or twice daily has also been used as an adjunctive treatment for *Scedosporium apiospermum* and *Microascus* sp. invasive infections with good results [82,143].

Highlights (voriconazole):

- Nebulized voriconazole is well delivered in lungs but leads to rapid systemic absorption;
- The ELF/plasma concentration ratio is not significantly different between nebulized and oral voriconazole.

3.3.2. Itraconazole

Itraconazole (ITZ) is a highly lipophilic molecule with a ratio of 3:1 in lung tissue versus plasma when administered systemically [144]. Due to this lipophilic characteristic, it must be solubilized to be aerosolized [145].

Nanoparticles of ITZ were synthetized with different technologies: evaporative precipitation of aqueous solution (EPAS), spray freezing into liquid (SFL), and ultra-rapid freezing (URF) [146]. These formulations allow ITZ to rapidly dissolve. Lung deposition was similar between EPAS and SFL, with high lung concentrations [147]. The amorphous nanoparticles produced by SFL showed higher concentrations in the lungs and serum than oral solutions [148]. The aerosolization of amorphous ITZ produced by SFL has no pro-inflammatory effect nor tissue toxicity [149]. A nanostructured ITZ solid solution was developed by URF technology [150]. This formulation led to high lung deposition but high systemic concentration. The efficacy of these formulations was assessed in experimental models. The EPAS and SFL of ITZ both achieved high lung concentrations with reduced systemic exposure in a murine model of IPA [151]. These forms of ITZ were more effective in prophylaxis for *A. flavus* aspergillosis than oral suspension or placebo. SFL showed better results than EPAS in survival studies. Aerosolized nanostructured formulations of ITZ produced by SFL were tested in aspergillosis prophylaxis models and compared with ITZ by oral gavage [152]. The aerosolized formulation was used two days before inoculation and continued for seven days post-inoculation. This treatment was more effective than ITZ by oral gavage for improved survival, and histopathological examination of lung biopsies displayed less lesions. The pulmonary delivery of an ITZ cyclodextrin solubilized solution was compared with colloidal dispersion of an ITZ nanoparticle formulation synthetized by URF [153]. These two formulations had the same lung deposition with deep lung delivery and the same pharmacokinetic profile. ITZ cyclodextrin solubilized solution had, however, a more rapid systemic distribution [153]. The authors also compared the bioavailability of amorphous ITZ nanoparticles synthetized by URF versus crystalline ITZ nanoparticles produced by wet milling [154]. Although both formulations allowed similar deep lung delivery due to compatible aerodynamic diameters, amorphous nanoparticles of ITZ showed a higher systemic bioavailability.

Using a wet-milling process with organic milling beads, a stable nanosuspension of ITZ at 20% was synthetized [155]. Nebulization of this suspension led to a high and long-lasting lung concentration with a minimal systemic exposure in rats. A single dose of 22.5 mg/kg led to 25.4 h of half-life. These nanosuspensions were tested in Japanese quail [156]. This formulation permitted high lung concentrations with a low systemic exposure in young quail. Moreover, a nanosuspension of ITZ at 10% or 4% was effective for aspergillosis treatment in this model [157]. Treatment was once daily for 30 min, starting 2 h after inoculation for six days, which increased survival and was well tolerated.

More recently, some authors synthetized ITZ-loaded nanostructured lipid carriers for pulmonary treatment of IPA in falcons [158]. This formulation can be easily nebulized and effectively penetrated the respiratory tract.

Several authors have evaluated the endotracheal insufflator device for the administration of dry powder and have shown that it can be used in preclinical trials [159]. This material was used to test three ITZ dry powders for inhalation [160]. ITZ was prepared by spray-drying a mannitol solution in which ITZ was dispersed or solubilized. The concentrations of ITZ in lungs were high for two of the formulations but with high systemic bioavailabilities. Micronized cocrystal powders, micronized using the jet-milling system with succinic acid (SA) or l-tartaric acid (TA), and amorphous spray-dried formulations of ITZ were also evaluated [161]. Micronized cocrystals are promising formulations for enhancing the pulmonary absorption of poorly soluble compounds.

Finally, the relationship between the in vitro dissolution of ITZ powder and its fate in vivo was assessed [162]. The authors showed that the dissolution of ITZ in the lungs may be increased to avoid local irritation and rapid elimination by macrophages. However, high dissolution led to a fast systemic absorption and a lower lung retention.

Highlights (itraconazole):

- Nebulized itraconazole is well delivered in lungs but leads to rapid systemic absorption;
- Advanced formulations are in development to control the permeability and/or the release rate in pulmonary compartments.

3.3.3. Other Triazoles

The aerodynamic properties of nebulized molecules of IV posaconazole solutions have been characterized. With an MMAD of 3.0 to 3.4 μm and a FPF of 78–79% for solutions concentrated at 6 to 12 mg/mL, an appropriate distribution in the lungs is suggested [132]. Although posaconazole is a lipophilic molecule with a LogD of 2.15 at pH 7.4, it is not a good candidate for nebulization. Nebulized posaconazole has not been tested to treat IMIs.

A new triazole drug, named PC945 (opelconazole), was developed to optimize topical treatment with tissue retention and physicochemical properties adapted to inhalation [163,164]. Opelconazole inhalation resulted in high local concentrations, prolonged lung retention, slow absorption from the lung, and low plasma concentrations [165]. Intranasal PC945 showed an increased survival in a murine model of IPA. This compound was able to decrease the fungal load and in vivo biomarkers of aspergillosis in the BAL and serum and showed superiority to voriconazole and posaconazole [166]. Moreover, the drug acted synergistically with commonly used triazoles (posaconazole, VRZ, ITZ) [167]. Phase I and IIa were recently performed and showed only mild-to-moderate AEs in 29 subjects. Opelconazole was used in a compassionate program on nine patients and positive clinical results were observed in eight [164]. Since opelconazole was poorly absorbed, the drug should not be used alone in disseminated forms of IMI but could represent a new option of great value in combination with systemic treatment or in prophylaxis.

Another new triazole drug, PC1244, showed efficacy against IPA when administered intranasally [168]. This compound showed better activity than VRZ and posaconazole against azole-resistant *Aspergillus* [169].

Highlights (other triazoles):

- As with other triazoles, posaconazole nebulization leads to rapid systemic absorption;
- New triazole antifungal agents showed efficacy in nebulization in IPA animal models.

3.4. Other Antifungal Agents

Among other antifungal agents, imidazoles (ketoconazole, miconazole, prochloraz) are not used as aerosolized agents since they lead to histamine release and airway constriction [170].

Since echinocandins are poorly effective against molds, few studies have been performed on this topic. However, pharmacokinetic data have shown that caspofungin is well delivered to the lungs with higher maximal concentrations and AUC compared to IV routes [171]. Several authors have developed new formulations of caspofungin to improve alveolar concentrations [172]. Inhaled micafungin was used for the treatment of two *Scopulariospsis/Microascus* infections and led to high ELF concentrations with low plasmatic passage and was well tolerated [173].

Pneumocandin L-693,989, an experimental echinocandin, administered at 5 mg/kg 2 h before inoculation was effective in improving survival in a rat model of IPA [88]. In another rat model of IPA, an aerosol of hamycin at 0.68 mg/kg administered two days before infection delayed mortality compared to the control group [174]. Administered as a curative treatment, at the same dosage of 0.68 mg/kg 24 h after inoculation daily for six days, nebulized hamycin was effective.

The pharmacokinetics of nebulized terbinafine was assessed in Hispaniolan Amazon parrots. The time above MIC remained low in the study conditions [175]. The lack of efficacy of this drug as prophylaxis was demonstrated in an aspergillosis rat model nebulized with terbinafine at 1.6 mg/kg two days before inoculation [176].

New drugs, some belonging to new families, are actually under development. These new drugs include fosmanogepix (a novel Gwt1 enzyme inhibitor), ibrexafungerp (a first-in-class triterpenoid), and olorofim (a novel dihydroorotate dehydrogenase enzyme inhibitor) [164]. The use of these drugs by nebulized routes should be evaluated to bring new families of inhaled drugs.

3.5. Perspectives/Recommendations for Future Research

- Perform prospective randomized studies to evidence the efficacy of n-AmB in the prophylaxis and curative treatment of IMIs, especially in particular settings such as severe or refractory infections, or large cavitary lesions;
- Perform prospective randomized studies to compare the efficacy and tolerance of lipid formulations of AmB and AmBd;
- Continue the development of opelconazole;
- Test new antifungal agents (fosmanogepix, ibrexafungerp, olorofim) by nebulized route;
- Evaluate n-AmB on emerging IMIs such as mucormycosis.

4. Conclusions

Animal models and clinical data have shown that AmB presents adequate physico-chemical characteristics for nebulization compared to other antifungal drugs which need appropriate formulations to be retained in the lungs. n-AmB leads to high alveolar concentrations and no or very low systemic passage. Most animal studies have proposed lipid forms of AmB as the best candidates for nebulization due to better lung penetration, a higher half-life, and the improvement of survival. The choice of nebulizer is crucial in humans; jet nebulizers seem to generate more optimal particles compared to ultrasonic nebulizers. Combining systemic treatments for nebulization could prevent fungal dissemination. n-AmB was thus tested as an adjunctive therapy, as a primary and salvage therapy for refractory pulmonary IMIs in patients. Although the results seem to favor increased efficacy, no randomized controlled prospective studies have elucidated the impact of n-AmB on survival. In prophylaxis, several authors showed a high efficacy of n-AmB to prevent IA. In hematological patients with high-risk neutropenia, even if data are scarce, n-L-AmB showed a decrease in probable/proven IPA incidence. Global tolerance of n-AmB is good, with no or very few systemic AEs, bronchospasm, and wheezing being less frequent with lipid formulations.

Prospective randomized studies are mandatory to evidence the efficacy of n-AmB in prophylaxis and curative treatments. To recommend n-AmB outside of salvage therapy or prophylaxis in lung transplant recipients is complex due to the lack of evidence. Moreover, most data come from IPA. It would be interesting to evaluate the effect of n-AmB on emerging IMIs such as mucormycosis. Prospective randomized studies would also be useful to compare the efficacy and tolerance of lipid formulations of AmB and AmBd. Finally, the development of opelconazole must be continued. Indeed, it could represent a new option in the treatment of IMIs by nebulized routes.

Supplementary Materials: The following are available online at https://www.mdpi.com/article/10.3390/pharmaceutics14030641/s1, Table S1: Nebulized AmB used as curative treatment for invasive mold infections, Table S2: Nebulized AmBd as prophylaxis in hematological patients, Table S3: Nebulized lipid formulations of AmB (L-AmB or ABLC) as prophylaxis in hematological patients, Table S4: Nebulized AmBd as prophylaxis in lung transplant recipients, Table S5: Nebulized AmB lipid formulations as prophylaxis in lung transplant recipients, Table S6: Comparative studies of nebulized AmBd prophylaxis and nebulized lipid formulations of AmB prophylaxis, Table S7: Studies of n-voriconazole used as curative treatment for invasive mold.

Author Contributions: Conceptualization, J.-P.M., K.B., and B.R.; methodology, J.-P.M., K.B., and B.R.; investigation, J.-P.M., K.B., and F.T.; writing—original draft preparation, J.-P.M., K.B., F.T., and B.R.; writing—review and editing, F.T., B.R., and S.M.; supervision, B.R. and S.M.; project administration, B.R. and S.M. All authors have read and agreed to the published version of the manuscript.

Funding: This research received no external funding.

Institutional Review Board Statement: Not applicable.

Informed Consent Statement: Not applicable.

Conflicts of Interest: Kevin Brunet received travel grants from Gilead, MSD, and Pfizer, and speaker's fees from Gilead; Blandine Rammaert received travel grants from Pfizer and MSD, and speaker's fees from MSD, Gilead, Astellas, and Iqone; Jean-Philippe Martellosio received a travel grant from Pfizer.

References

1. Marra, F.; Partovi, N.; Wasan, K.M.; Kwong, E.H.; Ensom, M.H.H.; Cassidy, S.M.; Fradet, G.; Levy, R.D. Amphotericin B Disposition after Aerosol Inhalation in Lung Transplant Recipients. *Ann. Pharmacother.* **2002**, *36*, 46–51. [CrossRef] [PubMed]
2. Rijnders, B.J.; Cornelissen, J.J.; Slobbe, L.; Becker, M.J.; Doorduijn, J.K.; Hop, W.C.J.; Ruijgrok, E.J.; Löwenberg, B.; Vulto, A.; Lugtenburg, P.J.; et al. Aerosolized Liposomal Amphotericin B for the Prevention of Invasive Pulmonary Aspergillosis during Prolonged Neutropenia: A Randomized, Placebo-Controlled Trial. *Clin. Infect. Dis.* **2008**, *46*, 1401–1408. [CrossRef] [PubMed]
3. Van Daele, R.; Spriet, I.; Wauters, J.; Maertens, J.; Mercier, T.; Van Hecke, S.; Brüggemann, R. Antifungal Drugs: What Brings the Future? *Med. Mycol.* **2019**, *57*, S328–S343. [CrossRef] [PubMed]
4. Monforte, V.; Roman, A.; Gavalda, J.; Bravo, C.; Tenorio, L.; Ferrer, A.; Maestre, J.; Morell, F. Nebulized Amphotericin B Prophylaxis for Aspergillus Infection in Lung Transplantation: Study of Risk Factors. *J. Heart Lung Transplant.* **2001**, *20*, 1274–1281. [CrossRef]
5. Brillault, J.; Tewes, F. Control of the Lung Residence Time of Highly Permeable Molecules after Nebulization: Example of the Fluoroquinolones. *Pharmaceutics* **2020**, *12*, E387. [CrossRef] [PubMed]
6. Hastedt, J.E.; Bäckman, P.; Clark, A.R.; Doub, W.; Hickey, A.; Hochhaus, G.; Kuehl, P.J.; Lehr, C.-M.; Mauser, P.; McConville, J.; et al. Scope and Relevance of a Pulmonary Biopharmaceutical Classification System AAPS/FDA/USP Workshop March 16–17th, 2015 in Baltimore, MD. *AAPS Open* **2016**, *2*, 1. [CrossRef]
7. Rubin, B.K.; Williams, R.W. Emerging Aerosol Drug Delivery Strategies: From Bench to Clinic. *Adv. Drug Deliv. Rev.* **2014**, *75*, 141–148. [CrossRef]
8. Beyer, J.; Schwartz, S.; Barzen, G.; Risse, G.; Dullenkopf, K.; Weyer, C.; Siegert, W. Use of Amphotericin B Aerosols for the Prevention of Pulmonary Aspergillosis. *Infection* **1994**, *22*, 143–148. [CrossRef] [PubMed]
9. Solé, A. Invasive Fungal Infections in Lung Transplantation: Role of Aerosolised Amphotericin B. *Int. J. Antimicrob. Agents* **2008**, *32* (Suppl. 2), S161–S165. [CrossRef]
10. Le, J.; Schiller, D.S. Aerosolized Delivery of Antifungal Agents. *Curr. Fungal Infect. Rep.* **2010**, *4*, 96–102. [CrossRef]
11. Sangwan, S.; Condos, R.; Smaldone, G.C. Lung Deposition and Respirable Mass during Wet Nebulization. *J. Aerosol Med.* **2003**, *16*, 379–386. [CrossRef]
12. Martin, A.R.; Finlay, W.H. Nebulizers for Drug Delivery to the Lungs. *Expert Opin. Drug Deliv.* **2015**, *12*, 889–900. [CrossRef] [PubMed]
13. Quon, B.S.; Goss, C.H.; Ramsey, B.W. Inhaled Antibiotics for Lower Airway Infections. *Ann. Am. Thorac Soc.* **2014**, *11*, 425–434. [CrossRef] [PubMed]
14. Adorni, G.; Seifert, G.; Buttini, F.; Colombo, G.; Stecanella, L.A.; Krämer, I.; Rossi, A. Aerosolization Performance of Jet Nebulizers and Biopharmaceutical Aspects. *Pharmaceutics* **2019**, *11*, 406. [CrossRef] [PubMed]
15. Roth, C.; Gebhart, J.; Just-Nübling, G.; von Eisenhart-Rothe, B.; Beinhauer-Reeb, I. Characterization of Amphotericin B Aerosols for Inhalation Treatment of Pulmonary Aspergillosis. *Infection* **1996**, *24*, 354–360. [CrossRef]
16. Corcoran, T.E.; Venkataramanan, R.; Mihelc, K.M.; Marcinkowski, A.L.; Ou, J.; McCook, B.M.; Weber, L.; Carey, M.-E.; Paterson, D.L.; Pilewski, J.M.; et al. Aerosol Deposition of Lipid Complex Amphotericin-B (Abelcet) in Lung Transplant Recipients. *Am. J. Transplant.* **2006**, *6*, 2765–2773. [CrossRef] [PubMed]
17. Monforte, V.; Ussetti, P.; Gavaldà, J.; Bravo, C.; Laporta, R.; Len, O.; García-Gallo, C.L.; Tenorio, L.; Solé, J.; Román, A. Feasibility, Tolerability, and Outcomes of Nebulized Liposomal Amphotericin B for Aspergillus Infection Prevention in Lung Transplantation. *J. Heart Lung Transplant.* **2010**, *29*, 523–530. [CrossRef]
18. Peghin, M.; Monforte, V.; Martin-Gomez, M.-T.; Ruiz-Camps, I.; Berastegui, C.; Saez, B.; Riera, J.; Ussetti, P.; Solé, J.; Gavaldá, J.; et al. 10 Years of Prophylaxis with Nebulized Liposomal Amphotericin B and the Changing Epidemiology of *Aspergillus* spp. Infection in Lung Transplantation. *Transpl. Int.* **2016**, *29*, 51–62. [CrossRef]
19. Kukut Hatipoglu, M.; Hickey, A.J.; Garcia-Contreras, L. Pharmacokinetics and Pharmacodynamics of High Doses of Inhaled Dry Powder Drugs. *Int. J. Pharm.* **2018**, *549*, 306–316. [CrossRef]
20. Adler-Moore, J.P.; Gangneux, J.-P.; Pappas, P.G. Comparison between Liposomal Formulations of Amphotericin B. *Med. Mycol.* **2016**, *54*, 223–231. [CrossRef]
21. Andes, D.; Stamsted, T.; Conklin, R. Pharmacodynamics of Amphotericin B in a Neutropenic-Mouse Disseminated-Candidiasis Model. *Antimicrob. Agents Chemother.* **2001**, *45*, 922–926. [CrossRef]
22. Wiederhold, N.P.; Tam, V.H.; Chi, J.; Prince, R.A.; Kontoyiannis, D.P.; Lewis, R.E. Pharmacodynamic Activity of Amphotericin B Deoxycholate Is Associated with Peak Plasma Concentrations in a Neutropenic Murine Model of Invasive Pulmonary Aspergillosis. *Antimicrob. Agents Chemother.* **2006**, *50*, 469–473. [CrossRef]
23. Felton, T.; Troke, P.F.; Hope, W.W. Tissue Penetration of Antifungal Agents. *Clin. Microbiol. Rev.* **2014**, *27*, 68–88. [CrossRef] [PubMed]

24. Diot, P.; Rivoire, B.; Le Pape, A.; Lemarie, E.; Dire, D.; Furet, Y.; Breteau, M.; Smaldone, G.C. Deposition of Amphotericin B Aerosols in Pulmonary Aspergilloma. *Eur. Respir. J.* **1995**, *8*, 1263–1268. [CrossRef] [PubMed]
25. Mehrabani Yeganeh, E.; Bagheri, H.; Mahjub, R. Preparation, Statistical Optimization and In-Vitro Characterization of a Dry Powder Inhaler (DPI) Containing Solid Lipid Nanoparticles Encapsulating Amphotericin B: Ion Paired Complexes with Distearoyl Phosphatidylglycerol. *Iran J. Pharm. Res.* **2020**, *19*, 45–62. [CrossRef] [PubMed]
26. Gomez, A.I.; Acosta, M.F.; Muralidharan, P.; Yuan, J.X.-J.; Black, S.M.; Hayes, D.; Mansour, H.M. Advanced Spray Dried Proliposomes of Amphotericin B Lung Surfactant-Mimic Phospholipid Microparticles/Nanoparticles as Dry Powder Inhalers for Targeted Pulmonary Drug Delivery. *Pulm. Pharmacol. Ther.* **2020**, *64*, 101975. [CrossRef]
27. Siopi, M.; Mouton, J.W.; Pournaras, S.; Meletiadis, J. In Vitro and In Vivo Exposure-Effect Relationship of Liposomal Amphotericin B against Aspergillus Fumigatus. *Antimicrob. Agents Chemother.* **2019**, *63*, e02673-18. [CrossRef]
28. Stone, N.R.; Bicanic, T.; Salim, R.; Hope, W. Liposomal Amphotericin B (AmBisome®): A Review of the Pharmacokinetics, Pharmacodynamics, Clinical Experience and Future Directions. *Drugs* **2016**, *76*, 485–500. [CrossRef]
29. Groll, A.H.; Rijnders, B.J.A.; Walsh, T.J.; Adler-Moore, J.; Lewis, R.E.; Brüggemann, R.J.M. Clinical Pharmacokinetics, Pharmacodynamics, Safety and Efficacy of Liposomal Amphotericin B. *Clin. Infect. Dis.* **2019**, *68*, S260–S274. [CrossRef]
30. Niki, Y.; Bernard, E.M.; Schmitt, H.J.; Tong, W.P.; Edwards, F.F.; Armstrong, D. Pharmacokinetics of Aerosol Amphotericin B in Rats. *Antimicrob. Agents Chemother.* **1990**, *34*, 29–32. [CrossRef]
31. Koizumi, T.; Kubo, K.; Kaneki, T.; Hanaoka, M.; Hayano, T.; Miyahara, T.; Okada, K.; Fujimoto, K.; Yamamoto, H.; Kobayashi, T.; et al. Pharmacokinetic Evaluation of Amphotericin B in Lung Tissue: Lung Lymph Distribution after Intravenous Injection and Airspace Distribution after Aerosolization and Inhalation of Amphotericin B. *Antimicrob. Agents Chemother.* **1998**, *42*, 1597–1600. [CrossRef] [PubMed]
32. Schmitt, H.J. New Methods of Delivery of Amphotericin B. *Clin. Infect. Dis.* **1993**, *17* (Suppl. 2), S501–S506. [CrossRef]
33. Lambros, M.P.; Bourne, D.W.; Abbas, S.A.; Johnson, D.L. Disposition of Aerosolized Liposomal Amphotericin B. *J. Pharm. Sci.* **1997**, *86*, 1066–1069. [CrossRef] [PubMed]
34. Ruijgrok, E.J.; Vulto, A.G.; Van Etten, E.W. Aerosol Delivery of Amphotericin B Desoxycholate (Fungizone) and Liposomal Amphotericin B (AmBisome): Aerosol Characteristics and in-Vivo Amphotericin B Deposition in Rats. *J. Pharm. Pharmacol.* **2000**, *52*, 619–627. [CrossRef] [PubMed]
35. Ruijgrok, E.J.; Fens, M.H.A.; Bakker-Woudenberg, I.A.J.M.; van Etten, E.W.M.; Vulto, A.G. Nebulization of Four Commercially Available Amphotericin B Formulations in Persistently Granulocytopenic Rats with Invasive Pulmonary Aspergillosis: Evidence for Long-Term Biological Activity. *J. Pharm. Pharmacol.* **2005**, *57*, 1289–1295. [CrossRef] [PubMed]
36. Allen, S.D.; Sorensen, K.N.; Nejdl, M.J.; Durrant, C.; Proffit, R.T. Prophylactic Efficacy of Aerosolized Liposomal (AmBisome) and Non-Liposomal (Fungizone) Amphotericin B in Murine Pulmonary Aspergillosis. *J. Antimicrob. Chemother.* **1994**, *34*, 1001–1013. [CrossRef] [PubMed]
37. Cicogna, C.E.; White, M.H.; Bernard, E.M.; Ishimura, T.; Sun, M.; Tong, W.P.; Armstrong, D. Efficacy of Prophylactic Aerosol Amphotericin B Lipid Complex in a Rat Model of Pulmonary Aspergillosis. *Antimicrob. Agents Chemother.* **1997**, *41*, 259–261. [CrossRef]
38. Griese, M.; Schams, A.; Lohmeier, K.P. Amphotericin B and Pulmonary Surfactant. *Eur. J. Med. Res.* **1998**, *3*, 383–386.
39. Ruijgrok, E.J.; Vulto, A.G.; Van Etten, E.W. Efficacy of Aerosolized Amphotericin B Desoxycholate and Liposomal Amphotericin B in the Treatment of Invasive Pulmonary Aspergillosis in Severely Immunocompromised Rats. *J. Antimicrob. Chemother.* **2001**, *48*, 89–95. [CrossRef]
40. Vyas, S.P.; Quraishi, S.; Gupta, S.; Jaganathan, K.S. Aerosolized Liposome-Based Delivery of Amphotericin B to Alveolar Macrophages. *Int. J. Pharm.* **2005**, *296*, 12–25. [CrossRef]
41. Vyas, S.P.; Khatri, K.; Goyal, A.K. Functionalized Nanocarrier(s) to Image and Target Fungi Infected Immune Cells. *Med. Mycol.* **2009**, *47* (Suppl. 1), S362–S368. [CrossRef]
42. Usman, F.; Nopparat, J.; Javed, I.; Srichana, T. Biodistribution and Histopathology Studies of Amphotericin B Sodium Deoxycholate Sulfate Formulation Following Intratracheal Instillation in Rat Models. *Drug. Deliv. Transl. Res.* **2019**, *10*, 59–69. [CrossRef]
43. Mathpal, D.; Garg, T.; Rath, G.; Goyal, A.K. Development and Characterization of Spray Dried Microparticles for Pulmonary Delivery of Antifungal Drug. *Curr. Drug Deliv.* **2015**, *12*, 464–471. [CrossRef] [PubMed]
44. Doligalski, C.T.; Benedict, K.; Cleveland, A.A.; Park, B.; Derado, G.; Pappas, P.G.; Baddley, J.W.; Zaas, D.W.; Harris, M.T.; Alexander, B.D. Epidemiology of Invasive Mold Infections in Lung Transplant Recipients. *Am. J. Transplant.* **2014**, *14*, 1328–1333. [CrossRef]
45. Monforte, V.; Roman, A.; Gavaldá, J.; López, R.; Pou, L.; Simó, M.; Aguadé, S.; Soriano, B.; Bravo, C.; Morell, F. Nebulized Amphotericin B Concentration and Distribution in the Respiratory Tract of Lung-Transplanted Patients. *Transplantation* **2003**, *75*, 1571–1574. [CrossRef] [PubMed]
46. Fauvel, M.; Farrugia, C.; Tsapis, N.; Gueutin, C.; Cabaret, O.; Bories, C.; Bretagne, S.; Barratt, G. Aerosolized Liposomal Amphotericin B: Prediction of Lung Deposition, in Vitro Uptake and Cytotoxicity. *Int. J. Pharm.* **2012**, *436*, 106–110. [CrossRef]
47. Husain, S.; Capitano, B.; Corcoran, T.; Studer, S.M.; Crespo, M.; Johnson, B.; Pilewski, J.M.; Shutt, K.; Pakstis, D.L.; Zhang, S.; et al. Intrapulmonary Disposition of Amphotericin B After Aerosolized Delivery of Amphotericin B Lipid Complex (Abelcet; ABLC) in Lung Transplant Recipients. *Transplantation* **2010**, *90*, 1215–1219. [CrossRef] [PubMed]

48. Monforte, V.; Ussetti, P.; López, R.; Gavaldà, J.; Bravo, C.; de Pablo, A.; Pou, L.; Pahissa, A.; Morell, F.; Román, A. Nebulized Liposomal Amphotericin B Prophylaxis for Aspergillus Infection in Lung Transplantation: Pharmacokinetics and Safety. *J. Heart Lung Transplant.* **2009**, *28*, 170–175. [CrossRef] [PubMed]
49. Heinemann, V.; Scholz, P.; Vehling, U.; Wachholz, K.; Jehn, U. Inhalation of Amphotericin B for Prophylaxis of Invasive Fungal Infections During Intensive Leukemia Therapy. In *Acute Leukemias IV.*; Büchner, T., Hiddemann, W., Wörmann, B., Schellong, G., Ritter, J., Eds.; Springer: Berlin/Heidelberg, Germany, 1994; Volume 36, pp. 762–764. ISBN 978-3-642-78352-4.
50. Beyer, J.; Barzen, G.; Risse, G.; Weyer, C.; Miksits, K.; Dullenkopf, K.; Huhn, D.; Siegert, W. Aerosol Amphotericin B for Prevention of Invasive Pulmonary Aspergillosis. *Antimicrob. Agents Chemother.* **1993**, *37*, 1367–1369. [CrossRef]
51. Erjavec, Z.; Woolthuis, G.M.; de Vries-Hospers, H.G.; Sluiter, W.J.; Daenen, S.M.; de Pauw, B.; Halie, M.R. Tolerance and Efficacy of Amphotericin B Inhalations for Prevention of Invasive Pulmonary Aspergillosis in Haematological Patients. *Eur. J. Clin. Microbiol. Infect. Dis.* **1997**, *16*, 364–368. [CrossRef]
52. Lowry, C.M.; Marty, F.M.; Vargas, S.O.; Lee, J.T.; Fiumara, K.; Deykin, A.; Baden, L.R. Safety of Aerosolized Liposomal versus Deoxycholate Amphotericin B Formulations for Prevention of Invasive Fungal Infections Following Lung Transplantation: A Retrospective Study. *Transpl. Infect. Dis.* **2007**, *9*, 121–125. [CrossRef]
53. Palmer, S.M.; Drew, R.H.; Whitehouse, J.D.; Tapson, V.F.; Davis, R.D.; McConnell, R.R.; Kanj, S.S.; Perfect, J.R. Safety of Aerosolized Amphotericin B Lipid Complex in Lung Transplant Recipients. *Transplantation* **2001**, *72*, 545–548. [CrossRef] [PubMed]
54. Myers, S.E.; Devine, S.M.; Topper, R.L.; Ondrey, M.; Chandler, C.; O'Toole, K.; Williams, S.F.; Larson, R.A.; Geller, R.B. A Pilot Study of Prophylactic Aerosolized Amphotericin B in Patients at Risk for Prolonged Neutropenia. *Leuk. Lymphoma* **1992**, *8*, 229–233. [CrossRef] [PubMed]
55. Monforte, V.; López-Sánchez, A.; Zurbano, F.; Ussetti, P.; Solé, A.; Casals, C.; Cifrian, J.; de Pablos, A.; Bravo, C.; Román, A. Prophylaxis with Nebulized Liposomal Amphotericin B for Aspergillus Infection in Lung Transplant Patients Does Not Cause Changes in the Lipid Content of Pulmonary Surfactant. *J. Heart Lung Transplant.* **2013**, *32*, 313–319. [CrossRef] [PubMed]
56. Schmitt, H.J.; Bernard, E.M.; Häuser, M.; Armstrong, D. Aerosol Amphotericin B Is Effective for Prophylaxis and Therapy in a Rat Model of Pulmonary Aspergillosis. *Antimicrob. Agents Chemother.* **1988**, *32*, 1676–1679. [CrossRef]
57. Schmitt, H.J.; Bernard, E.M.; Edwards, F.F.; Armstrong, D. Combination Therapy in a Model of Pulmonary Aspergillosis. *Mycoses* **1991**, *34*, 281–285. [CrossRef]
58. Gavaldà, J.; Martín, M.-T.; López, P.; Gomis, X.; Ramírez, J.-L.; Rodríguez, D.; Len, O.; Puigfel, Y.; Ruíz, I.; Pahissa, A. Efficacy of Nebulized Liposomal Amphotericin B in Treatment of Experimental Pulmonary Aspergillosis. *Antimicrob. Agents Chemother.* **2005**, *49*, 3028–3030. [CrossRef]
59. Ruijgrok, E.J.; Fens, M.H.A.M.; Bakker-Woudenberg, I.A.J.M.; van Etten, E.W.M.; Vulto, A.G. Nebulized Amphotericin B Combined with Intravenous Amphotericin B in Rats with Severe Invasive Pulmonary Aspergillosis. *Antimicrob. Agents Chemother.* **2006**, *50*, 1852–1854. [CrossRef]
60. Takazono, T.; Izumikawa, K.; Mihara, T.; Kosai, K.; Saijo, T.; Imamura, Y.; Miyazaki, T.; Seki, M.; Kakeya, H.; Yamamoto, Y.; et al. Efficacy of Combination Antifungal Therapy with Intraperitoneally Administered Micafungin and Aerosolized Liposomal Amphotericin B against Murine Invasive Pulmonary Aspergillosis. *Antimicrob. Agents Chemother.* **2009**, *53*, 3508–3510. [CrossRef]
61. Alsaadi, M.; Italia, J.L.; Mullen, A.B.; Ravi Kumar, M.N.V.; Candlish, A.A.; Williams, R.a.M.; Shaw, C.D.; Al Gawhari, F.; Coombs, G.H.; Wiese, M.; et al. The Efficacy of Aerosol Treatment with Non-Ionic Surfactant Vesicles Containing Amphotericin B in Rodent Models of Leishmaniasis and Pulmonary Aspergillosis Infection. *J. Control Release* **2012**, *160*, 685–691. [CrossRef]
62. Shirkhani, K.; Teo, I.; Armstrong-James, D.; Shaunak, S. Nebulised Amphotericin B-Polymethacrylic Acid Nanoparticle Prophylaxis Prevents Invasive Aspergillosis. *Nanomedicine* **2015**, *11*, 1217–1226. [CrossRef] [PubMed]
63. Godet, C.; Cateau, E.; Rammaert, B.; Grosset, M.; Le Moal, G.; Béraud, G.; Martellosio, J.P.; Iriart, X.; Cadranel, J.; Roblot, F. Nebulized Liposomal Amphotericin B for Treatment of Pulmonary Infection Caused by Hormographiella Aspergillata: Case Report and Literature Review. *Mycopathologia* **2017**, *182*, 709–713. [CrossRef] [PubMed]
64. Birsan, T.; Taghavi, S.; Klepetko, W. Treatment of Aspergillus-Related Ulcerative Tracheobronchitis in Lung Transplant Recipients. *J. Heart Lung Transplant.* **1998**, *17*, 437–438. [PubMed]
65. Zhou, Q.-Y.; Yang, W.-J.; Zhao, X.-Q. Pulmonary Aspergillosis Treated with Inhaled Amphotericin B. *Int. J. Infect. Dis.* **2017**, *54*, 92–94. [CrossRef] [PubMed]
66. Huang, H.; Li, Q.; Huang, Y.; Bai, C.; Wu, N.; Wang, Q.; Yao, X.; Chen, B. Pseudomembranous Necrotizing Tracheobronchial Aspergillosis: An Analysis of 16 Cases. *Chin. Med. J.* **2012**, *125*, 1236–1241. [PubMed]
67. Wu, N.; Huang, Y.; Li, Q.; Bai, C.; Huang, H.-D.; Yao, X.-P. Isolated Invasive Aspergillus Tracheobronchitis: A Clinical Study of 19 Cases. *Clin. Microbiol. Infect.* **2010**, *16*, 689–695. [CrossRef] [PubMed]
68. Dal Conte, I.; Riva, G.; Obert, R.; Lucchini, A.; Bechis, G.; De Rosa, G.; Gioannini, P. Tracheobronchial Aspergillosis in a Patient with AIDS Treated with Aerosolized Amphotericin B Combined with Itraconazole. *Mycoses* **1996**, *39*, 371–374. [CrossRef]
69. Boots, R.J.; Paterson, D.L.; Allworth, A.M.; Faoagali, J.L. Successful Treatment of Post-Influenza Pseudomembranous Necrotising Bronchial Aspergillosis with Liposomal Amphotericin, Inhaled Amphotericin B, Gamma Interferon and GM-CSF. *Thorax* **1999**, *54*, 1047–1049. [CrossRef]
70. Rodenhuis, S.; Beaumont, F.; Kauffman, H.F.; Sluiter, H.J. Invasive Pulmonary Aspergillosis in a Non-Immunosuppressed Patient: Successful Management with Systemic Amphotericin and Flucytosine and Inhaled Amphotericin. *Thorax* **1984**, *39*, 78–79. [CrossRef]

71. Boettcher, H.; Bewig, B.; Hirt, S.W.; Möller, F.; Cremer, J. Topical Amphotericin B Application in Severe Bronchial Aspergillosis after Lung Transplantation: Report of Experiences in 3 Cases. *J. Heart Lung Transplant.* **2000**, *19*, 1224–1227. [CrossRef]

72. Furco, A.; Mouchet, B.; Carbonnelle, M.; Vallerand, H. Pulmonary mucormycosis: Benefit of aerosol amphotericin B? *Rev. Mal. Respir.* **2001**, *18*, 309–313.

73. Alfageme, I.; Reina, A.; Gallego, J.; Reyes, N.; Torres, A. Endobronchial Instillations of Amphotericin B: Complementary Treatment for Pulmonary Mucormycosis. *J. Bronchology Interv. Pulmonol.* **2009**, *16*, 214–215. [CrossRef] [PubMed]

74. McGuire, F.R.; Grinnan, D.C.; Robbins, M. Mucormycosis of the Bronchial Anastomosis: A Case of Successful Medical Treatment and Historic Review. *J. Heart Lung Transplant.* **2007**, *26*, 857–861. [CrossRef] [PubMed]

75. Safdar, A.; O'Brien, S.; Kouri, I.F. Efficacy and Feasibility of Aerosolized Amphotericin B Lipid Complex Therapy in Caspofungin Breakthrough Pulmonary Zygomycosis. *Bone Marrow Transplant.* **2004**, *34*, 467–468. [CrossRef] [PubMed]

76. Castagnola, E.; Moresco, L.; Cappelli, B.; Cuzzubbo, D.; Moroni, C.; Lanino, E.; Faraci, M. Nebulized Liposomal Amphotericin B and Combined Systemic Antifungal Therapy for the Treatment of Severe Pulmonary Aspergillosis after Allogeneic Hematopoietic Stem Cell Transplant for a Fatal Mitochondrial Disorder. *J. Chemother.* **2007**, *19*, 339–342. [CrossRef] [PubMed]

77. Canetti, D.; Cazzadori, A.; Adami, I.; Lifrieri, F.; Cristino, S.; Concia, E. Aerosolized Amphotericin B Lipid Complex and Invasive Pulmonary Aspergillosis: A Case Report. *Infez. Med.* **2015**, *23*, 44–47.

78. Venanzi, E.; Martín-Dávila, P.; López, J.; Maiz, L.; de la Pedrosa, E.G.-G.; Gioia, F.; Escudero, R.; Filigheddu, E.; Moreno, S.; Fortún, J. Aerosolized Lipid Amphotericin B for Complementary Therapy and/or Secondary Prophylaxis in Patients with Invasive Pulmonary Aspergillosis: A Single-Center Experience. *Mycopathologia* **2019**, *184*, 239–250. [CrossRef]

79. Safdar, A.; Rodriguez, G.H. Aerosolized Amphotericin B Lipid Complex as Adjunctive Treatment for Fungal Lung Infection in Patients with Cancer-Related Immunosuppression and Recipients of Hematopoietic Stem Cell Transplantation. *Pharmacotherapy* **2013**, *33*, 1035–1043. [CrossRef]

80. Morales, P.; Galán, G.; Sanmartín, E.; Monte, E.; Tarrazona, V.; Santos, M. Intrabronchial Instillation of Amphotericin B Lipid Complex: A Case Report. *Transplant. Proc.* **2009**, *41*, 2223–2224. [CrossRef]

81. Al Yazidi, L.S.; Huynh, J.; Britton, P.N.; Morrissey, C.O.; Lai, T.; Westall, G.P.; Selvadurai, H.; Kesson, A. Endobronchial Fusariosis in a Child Following Bilateral Lung Transplant. *Med. Mycol. Case. Rep.* **2019**, *23*, 77–80. [CrossRef]

82. Taton, O.; Bernier, B.; Etienne, I.; Bondue, B.; Lecomte, S.; Knoop, C.; Jacob, F.; Montesinos, I. Necrotizing Microascus Tracheo-bronchitis in a Bilateral Lung Transplant Recipient. *Transpl. Infect. Dis.* **2018**, *20*, e12806. [CrossRef]

83. Trujillo, H.; Fernández-Ruiz, M.; Gutiérrez, E.; Sevillano, Á.; Caravaca-Fontán, F.; Morales, E.; López-Medrano, F.; Aguado, J.M.; Praga, M.; Andrés, A. Invasive Pulmonary Aspergillosis Associated with COVID-19 in a Kidney Transplant Recipient. *Transpl. Infect. Dis.* **2021**, *23*, e13501. [CrossRef]

84. Liu, Q.; Kong, L.; Hua, L.; Xu, S. Pulmonary Microascus Cirrosus Infection in an Immunocompetent Patient with Bronchiectasis: A Case Report. *Respir. Med. Case Rep.* **2021**, *34*, 101484. [CrossRef]

85. Husain, S.; Camargo, J.F. Invasive Aspergillosis in Solid-Organ Transplant Recipients: Guidelines from the American Society of Transplantation Infectious Diseases Community of Practice. *Clin. Transplant.* **2019**, *33*, e13544. [CrossRef] [PubMed]

86. Patterson, T.F.; Thompson, G.R.; Denning, D.W.; Fishman, J.A.; Hadley, S.; Herbrecht, R.; Kontoyiannis, D.P.; Marr, K.A.; Morrison, V.A.; Nguyen, M.H.; et al. Practice Guidelines for the Diagnosis and Management of Aspergillosis: 2016 Update by the Infectious Diseases Society of America. *Clin. Infect. Dis.* **2016**, *63*, e1–e60. [CrossRef]

87. Husain, S.; Sole, A.; Alexander, B.D.; Aslam, S.; Avery, R.; Benden, C.; Billaud, E.M.; Chambers, D.; Danziger-Isakov, L.; Fedson, S.; et al. The 2015 International Society for Heart and Lung Transplantation Guidelines for the Management of Fungal Infections in Mechanical Circulatory Support and Cardiothoracic Organ Transplant Recipients: Executive Summary. *J. Heart Lung Transplant.* **2016**, *35*, 261–282. [CrossRef] [PubMed]

88. Kurtz, M.B.; Bernard, E.M.; Edwards, F.F.; Marrinan, J.A.; Dropinski, J.; Douglas, C.M.; Armstrong, D. Aerosol and Parenteral Pneumocandins Are Effective in a Rat Model of Pulmonary Aspergillosis. *Antimicrob. Agents Chemother.* **1995**, *39*, 1784–1789. [CrossRef]

89. Niki, Y.; Bernard, E.M.; Edwards, F.F.; Schmitt, H.J.; Yu, B.; Armstrong, D. Model of Recurrent Pulmonary Aspergillosis in Rats. *J. Clin. Microbiol.* **1991**, *29*, 1317–1322. [CrossRef] [PubMed]

90. Kirkpatrick, W.R.; Najvar, L.K.; Vallor, A.C.; Wiederhold, N.P.; Bocanegra, R.; Pfeiffer, J.; Perkins, K.; Kugler, A.R.; Sweeney, T.D.; Patterson, T.F. Prophylactic Efficacy of Single Dose Pulmonary Administration of Amphotericin B Inhalation Powder in a Guinea Pig Model of Invasive Pulmonary Aspergillosis. *J. Antimicrob. Chemother.* **2012**, *67*, 970–976. [CrossRef]

91. Mihara, T.; Kakeya, H.; Izumikawa, K.; Obata, Y.; Nishino, T.; Takazono, T.; Kosai, K.; Morinaga, Y.; Kurihara, S.; Nakamura, S.; et al. Efficacy of Aerosolized Liposomal Amphotericin B against Murine Invasive Pulmonary Mucormycosis. *J. Infect. Chemother.* **2014**, *20*, 104–108. [CrossRef]

92. Xia, D.; Sun, W.-K.; Tan, M.-M.; Zhang, M.; Ding, Y.; Liu, Z.-C.; Su, X.; Shi, Y. Aerosolized Amphotericin B as Prophylaxis for Invasive Pulmonary Aspergillosis: A Meta-Analysis. *Int. J. Infect. Dis.* **2015**, *30*, 78–84. [CrossRef]

93. Conneally, E.; Cafferkey, M.T.; Daly, P.A.; Keane, C.T.; McCann, S.R. Nebulized Amphotericin B as Prophylaxis against Invasive Aspergillosis in Granulocytopenic Patients. *Bone Marrow Transplant.* **1990**, *5*, 403–406.

94. De Laurenzi, A.; Matteocci, A.; Lanti, A.; Pescador, L.; Blandino, F.; Papetti, C. Amphotericin B Prophylaxis against Invasive Fungal Infections in Neutropenic Patients: A Single Center Experience from 1980 to 1995. *Infection* **1996**, *24*, 361–366. [CrossRef] [PubMed]

95. Hertenstein, B.; Kern, W.V.; Schmeiser, T.; Stefanic, M.; Bunjes, D.; Wiesneth, M.; Novotny, J.; Heimpel, H.; Arnold, R. Low Incidence of Invasive Fungal Infections after Bone Marrow Transplantation in Patients Receiving Amphotericin B Inhalations during Neutropenia. *Ann. Hematol.* **1994**, *68*, 21–26. [CrossRef] [PubMed]

96. Jeffery, G.M.; Beard, M.E.; Ikram, R.B.; Chua, J.; Allen, J.R.; Heaton, D.C.; Hart, D.N.; Schousboe, M.I. Intranasal Amphotericin B Reduces the Frequency of Invasive Aspergillosis in Neutropenic Patients. *Am. J. Med.* **1991**, *90*, 685–692. [CrossRef]

97. Morello, E.; Pagani, L.; Coser, P.; Cavattoni, I.; Cortelazzo, S.; Casini, M.; Billio, A.; Rossi, G. Addition of Aerosolized Deoxycholate Amphotericin B to Systemic Prophylaxis to Prevent Airways Invasive Fungal Infections in Allogeneic Hematopoietic SCT: A Single-Center Retrospective Study. *Bone Marrow Transplant.* **2011**, *46*, 132–136. [CrossRef]

98. Nihtinen, A.; Anttila, V.-J.; Ruutu, T.; Juvonen, E.; Volin, L. Low Incidence of Invasive Aspergillosis in Allogeneic Stem Cell Transplant Recipients Receiving Amphotericin B Inhalation Prophylaxis. *Transpl. Infect. Dis.* **2012**, *14*, 24–32. [CrossRef]

99. Cornely, O.A.; Maertens, J.; Winston, D.J.; Perfect, J.; Ullmann, A.J.; Walsh, T.J.; Helfgott, D.; Holowiecki, J.; Stockelberg, D.; Goh, Y.-T.; et al. Posaconazole vs. Fluconazole or Itraconazole Prophylaxis in Patients with Neutropenia. *N. Engl. J. Med.* **2007**, *356*, 348–359. [CrossRef]

100. Behre, G.F.; Schwartz, S.; Lenz, K.; Ludwig, W.-D.; Wandt, H.; Schilling, E.; Heinemann, V.; Link, H.; Trittin, A.; Boenisch, O.; et al. Aerosol Amphotericin B Inhalations for Prevention of Invasive Pulmonary Aspergillosis in Neutropenic Cancer Patients. *Ann. Hematol.* **1995**, *71*, 287–291. [CrossRef]

101. Schwartz, S.; Behre, G.; Heinemann, V.; Wandt, H.; Schilling, E.; Arning, M.; Trittin, A.; Kern, W.V.; Boenisch, O.; Bosse, D.; et al. Aerosolized Amphotericin B Inhalations as Prophylaxis of Invasive Aspergillus Infections during Prolonged Neutropenia: Results of a Prospective Randomized Multicenter Trial. *Blood* **1999**, *93*, 3654–3661. [PubMed]

102. Chong, G.-L.M.; Broekman, F.; Polinder, S.; Doorduijn, J.K.; Lugtenburg, P.J.; Verbon, A.; Cornelissen, J.J.; Rijnders, B.J.A. Aerosolised Liposomal Amphotericin B to Prevent Aspergillosis in Acute Myeloid Leukaemia: Efficacy and Cost Effectiveness in Real-Life. *Int. J. Antimicrob. Agents* **2015**, *46*, 82–87. [CrossRef]

103. Hullard-Pulstinger, A.; Holler, E.; Hahn, J.; Andreesen, R.; Krause, S.W. Prophylactic Application of Nebulized Liposomal Amphotericin B in Hematologic Patients with Neutropenia. *Onkologie* **2011**, *34*, 254–258. [CrossRef]

104. Dummer, J.S.; Lazariashvili, N.; Barnes, J.; Ninan, M.; Milstone, A.P. A Survey of Anti-Fungal Management in Lung Transplantation. *J. Heart Lung Transplant.* **2004**, *23*, 1376–1381. [CrossRef]

105. He, S.Y.; Makhzoumi, Z.H.; Singer, J.P.; Chin-Hong, P.V.; Arron, S.T. Practice Variation in Aspergillus Prophylaxis and Treatment among Lung Transplant Centers: A National Survey. *Transpl. Infect. Dis.* **2015**, *17*, 14–20. [CrossRef]

106. Husain, S.; Zaldonis, D.; Kusne, S.; Kwak, E.J.; Paterson, D.L.; McCurry, K.R. Variation in Antifungal Prophylaxis Strategies in Lung Transplantation. *Transpl. Infect. Dis.* **2006**, *8*, 213–218. [CrossRef] [PubMed]

107. Mead, L.; Danziger-Isakov, L.A.; Michaels, M.G.; Goldfarb, S.; Glanville, A.R.; Benden, C. International Pediatric Lung Transplant Collaborative (IPLTC) Antifungal Prophylaxis in Pediatric Lung Transplantation: An International Multicenter Survey. *Pediatr. Transplant.* **2014**, *18*, 393–397. [CrossRef] [PubMed]

108. Neoh, C.F.; Snell, G.I.; Kotsimbos, T.; Levvey, B.; Morrissey, C.O.; Slavin, M.A.; Stewart, K.; Kong, D.C.M. Antifungal Prophylaxis in Lung Transplantation–a World-Wide Survey. *Am. J. Transplant.* **2011**, *11*, 361–366. [CrossRef]

109. Borro, J.M.; Solé, A.; de la Torre, M.; Pastor, A.; Fernandez, R.; Saura, A.; Delgado, M.; Monte, E.; Gonzalez, D. Efficiency and Safety of Inhaled Amphotericin B Lipid Complex (Abelcet) in the Prophylaxis of Invasive Fungal Infections Following Lung Transplantation. *Transplant. Proc.* **2008**, *40*, 3090–3093. [CrossRef]

110. Cadena, J.; Levine, D.J.; Angel, L.F.; Maxwell, P.R.; Brady, R.; Sanchez, J.F.; Michalek, J.E.; Levine, S.M.; Restrepo, M.I. Antifungal Prophylaxis with Voriconazole or Itraconazole in Lung Transplant Recipients: Hepatotoxicity and Effectiveness. *Am. J. Transplant.* **2009**, *9*, 2085–2091. [CrossRef]

111. Eriksson, M.; Lemström, K.; Suojaranta-Ylinen, R.; Martelius, T.; Harjula, A.; Sipponen, J.; Halme, M.; Piilonen, A.; Salmenkivi, K.; Anttila, V.J.; et al. Control of Early Aspergillus Mortality after Lung Transplantation: Outcome and Risk Factors. *Transplant. Proc.* **2010**, *42*, 4459–4464. [CrossRef] [PubMed]

112. Koo, S.; Kubiak, D.W.; Issa, N.C.; Dietzek, A.; Boukedes, S.; Camp, P.C.; Goldberg, H.J.; Baden, L.R.; Fuhlbrigge, A.L.; Marty, F.M. A Targeted Peritransplant Antifungal Strategy for the Prevention of Invasive Fungal Disease after Lung Transplantation: A Sequential Cohort Analysis. *Transplantation* **2012**, *94*, 281–286. [CrossRef] [PubMed]

113. Samanta, P.; Clancy, C.J.; Marini, R.V.; Rivosecchi, R.M.; McCreary, E.K.; Shields, R.K.; Falcione, B.A.; Viehman, A.; Sacha, L.; Kwak, E.J.; et al. Isavuconazole Is as Effective as and Better Tolerated Than Voriconazole for Antifungal Prophylaxis in Lung Transplant Recipients. *Clin. Infect. Dis.* **2021**, *73*, 416–426. [CrossRef] [PubMed]

114. Ibáñez-Martínez, E.; Solé, A.; Cañada-Martínez, A.; Muñoz-Núñez, C.F.; Pastor, A.; Montull, B.; Falomir-Salcedo, P.; Valentín, A.; López-Hontangas, J.L.; Pemán, J. Invasive Scedosporiosis in Lung Transplant Recipients: A Nine-Year Retrospective Study in a Tertiary Care Hospital. *Rev. Iberoam. Micol.* **2021**, *38*, 184–187. [CrossRef]

115. Baker, A.W.; Maziarz, E.K.; Arnold, C.J.; Johnson, M.D.; Workman, A.D.; Reynolds, J.M.; Perfect, J.R.; Alexander, B.D. Invasive Fungal Infection After Lung Transplantation: Epidemiology in the Setting of Antifungal Prophylaxis. *Clin. Infect. Dis.* **2020**, *70*, 30–39. [CrossRef]

116. Alissa, D.; AlMaghrabi, R.; Nizami, I.; Saleh, A.; Al Shamrani, A.; Alangari, N.; Al Begami, N.; Al Muraybidh, R.; Bin Huwaimel, S.; Korayem, G.B. Nebulized Amphotericin B Dosing Regimen for Aspergillus Prevention After Lung Transplant. *Exp. Clin. Transplant.* **2021**, *19*, 58–63. [CrossRef]

117. Calvo, V.; Borro, J.M.; Morales, P.; Morcillo, A.; Vicente, R.; Tarrazona, V.; París, F. Antifungal Prophylaxis during the Early Postoperative Period of Lung Transplantation. Valencia Lung Transplant Group. *Chest* **1999**, *115*, 1301–1304. [CrossRef]
118. Minari, A.; Husni, R.; Avery, R.K.; Longworth, D.L.; DeCamp, M.; Bertin, M.; Schilz, R.; Smedira, N.; Haug, M.T.; Mehta, A.; et al. The Incidence of Invasive Aspergillosis among Solid Organ Transplant Recipients and Implications for Prophylaxis in Lung Transplants. *Transpl. Infect. Dis.* **2002**, *4*, 195–200. [CrossRef]
119. Reichenspurner, H.; Gamberg, P.; Nitschke, M.; Valantine, H.; Hunt, S.; Oyer, P.E.; Reitz, B.A. Significant Reduction in the Number of Fungal Infections after Lung-, Heart-Lung, and Heart Transplantation Using Aerosolized Amphotericin B Prophylaxis. *Transplant. Proc.* **1997**, *29*, 627–628. [CrossRef]
120. Linder, K.A.; Kauffman, C.A.; Patel, T.S.; Fitzgerald, L.J.; Richards, B.J.; Miceli, M.H. Evaluation of Targeted versus Universal Prophylaxis for the Prevention of Invasive Fungal Infections Following Lung Transplantation. *Transpl. Infect. Dis.* **2021**, *23*, e13448. [CrossRef] [PubMed]
121. Drew, R.H.; Dodds Ashley, E.; Benjamin, D.K.; Duane Davis, R.; Palmer, S.M.; Perfect, J.R. Comparative Safety of Amphotericin B Lipid Complex and Amphotericin B Deoxycholate as Aerosolized Antifungal Prophylaxis in Lung-Transplant Recipients. *Transplantation* **2004**, *77*, 232–237. [CrossRef]
122. Van Ackerbroeck, S.; Rutsaert, L.; Roelant, E.; Dillen, K.; Wauters, J.; Van Regenmortel, N. Inhaled Liposomal Amphotericin-B as a Prophylactic Treatment for COVID-19-Associated Pulmonary Aspergillosis/Aspergillus Tracheobronchitis. *Crit. Care* **2021**, *25*, 298. [CrossRef] [PubMed]
123. Mellinghoff, S.C.; Panse, J.; Alakel, N.; Behre, G.; Buchheidt, D.; Christopeit, M.; Hasenkamp, J.; Kiehl, M.; Koldehoff, M.; Krause, S.W.; et al. Primary Prophylaxis of Invasive Fungal Infections in Patients with Haematological Malignancies: 2017 Update of the Recommendations of the Infectious Diseases Working Party (AGIHO) of the German Society for Haematology and Medical Oncology (DGHO). *Ann. Hematol.* **2018**, *97*, 197–207. [CrossRef]
124. Ullmann, A.J.; Aguado, J.M.; Arikan-Akdagli, S.; Denning, D.W.; Groll, A.H.; Lagrou, K.; Lass-Flörl, C.; Lewis, R.E.; Munoz, P.; Verweij, P.E.; et al. Diagnosis and Management of Aspergillus Diseases: Executive Summary of the 2017 ESCMID-ECMM-ERS Guideline. *Clin. Microbiol. Infect.* **2018**, *24* (Suppl. 1), e1–e38. [CrossRef] [PubMed]
125. Maertens, J.A.; Girmenia, C.; Brüggemann, R.J.; Duarte, R.F.; Kibbler, C.C.; Ljungman, P.; Racil, Z.; Ribaud, P.; Slavin, M.A.; Cornely, O.A.; et al. European Guidelines for Primary Antifungal Prophylaxis in Adult Haematology Patients: Summary of the Updated Recommendations from the European Conference on Infections in Leukaemia. *J. Antimicrob. Chemother.* **2018**, *73*, 3221–3230. [CrossRef] [PubMed]
126. Dubois, J.; Bartter, T.; Gryn, J.; Pratter, M.R. The Physiologic Effects of Inhaled Amphotericin B. *Chest* **1995**, *108*, 750–753. [CrossRef]
127. Gryn, J.; Goldberg, J.; Johnson, E.; Siegel, J.; Inzerillo, J. The Toxicity of Daily Inhaled Amphotericin B. *Am. J. Clin. Oncol.* **1993**, *16*, 43–46. [CrossRef] [PubMed]
128. Alexander, B.D.; Dodds Ashley, E.S.; Addison, R.M.; Alspaugh, J.A.; Chao, N.J.; Perfect, J.R. Non-Comparative Evaluation of the Safety of Aerosolized Amphotericin B Lipid Complex in Patients Undergoing Allogeneic Hematopoietic Stem Cell Transplantation. *Transpl. Infect. Dis.* **2006**, *8*, 13–20. [CrossRef] [PubMed]
129. Slobbe, L.; Boersma, E.; Rijnders, B.J.A. Tolerability of Prophylactic Aerosolized Liposomal Amphotericin-B and Impact on Pulmonary Function: Data from a Randomized Placebo-Controlled Trial. *Pulm. Pharmacol. Ther.* **2008**, *21*, 855–859. [CrossRef]
130. Bhaskaran, A.; Mumtaz, K.; Husain, S. Anti-Aspergillus Prophylaxis in Lung Transplantation: A Systematic Review and Meta-Analysis. *Curr. Infect. Dis. Rep.* **2013**, *15*, 514–525. [CrossRef]
131. Hilberg, O.; Andersen, C.U.; Henning, O.; Lundby, T.; Mortensen, J.; Bendstrup, E. Remarkably Efficient Inhaled Antifungal Monotherapy for Invasive Pulmonary Aspergillosis. *Eur. Respir. J.* **2012**, *40*, 271–273. [CrossRef]
132. Thanukrishnan, H.; Corcoran, T.E.; Iasella, C.J.; Moore, C.A.; Nero, J.A.; Morrell, M.R.; McDyer, J.F.; Hussain, S.; Nguyen, M.H.; Venkataramanan, R.; et al. Aerosolization of Second-Generation Triazoles: In Vitro Evaluation and Application in Therapy of Invasive Airway Aspergillosis. *Transplantation* **2019**, *103*, 2608–2613. [CrossRef] [PubMed]
133. Tolman, J.A.; Nelson, N.A.; Bosselmann, S.; Peters, J.I.; Coalson, J.J.; Wiederhold, N.P.; Williams, R.O. Dose Tolerability of Chronically Inhaled Voriconazole Solution in Rodents. *Int. J. Pharm.* **2009**, *379*, 25–31. [CrossRef] [PubMed]
134. Tolman, J.A.; Wiederhold, N.P.; McConville, J.T.; Najvar, L.K.; Bocanegra, R.; Peters, J.I.; Coalson, J.J.; Graybill, J.R.; Patterson, T.F.; Williams, R.O. Inhaled Voriconazole for Prevention of Invasive Pulmonary Aspergillosis. *Antimicrob. Agents Chemother.* **2009**, *53*, 2613–2615. [CrossRef] [PubMed]
135. Beernaert, L.A.; Baert, K.; Marin, P.; Chiers, K.; De Backer, P.; Pasmans, F.; Martel, A. Designing Voriconazole Treatment for Racing Pigeons: Balancing between Hepatic Enzyme Auto Induction and Toxicity. *Med. Mycol.* **2009**, *47*, 276–285. [CrossRef] [PubMed]
136. Tolman, J.A.; Nelson, N.A.; Son, Y.J.; Bosselmann, S.; Wiederhold, N.P.; Peters, J.I.; McConville, J.T.; Williams, R.O. Characterization and Pharmacokinetic Analysis of Aerosolized Aqueous Voriconazole Solution. *Eur. J. Pharm. Biopharm.* **2009**, *72*, 199–205. [CrossRef]
137. Andersen, C.U.; Sønderskov, L.D.; Bendstrup, E.; Voldby, N.; Cass, L.; Ayrton, J.; Hilberg, O. Voriconazole Concentrations in Plasma and Epithelial Lining Fluid after Inhalation and Oral Treatment. *Basic Clin. Pharmacol. Toxicol.* **2017**, *121*, 430–434. [CrossRef]
138. Sinha, B.; Mukherjee, B.; Pattnaik, G. Poly-Lactide-Co-Glycolide Nanoparticles Containing Voriconazole for Pulmonary Delivery: In Vitro and in Vivo Study. *Nanomedicine* **2013**, *9*, 94–104. [CrossRef]

139. Beinborn, N.A.; Du, J.; Wiederhold, N.P.; Smyth, H.D.C.; Williams, R.O. Dry Powder Insufflation of Crystalline and Amorphous Voriconazole Formulations Produced by Thin Film Freezing to Mice. *Eur. J. Pharm. Biopharm.* **2012**, *81*, 600–608. [CrossRef]
140. Das, P.J.; Paul, P.; Mukherjee, B.; Mazumder, B.; Mondal, L.; Baishya, R.; Debnath, M.C.; Dey, K.S. Pulmonary Delivery of Voriconazole Loaded Nanoparticles Providing a Prolonged Drug Level in Lungs: A Promise for Treating Fungal Infection. *Mol. Pharm.* **2015**, *12*, 2651–2664. [CrossRef]
141. Paul, P.; Sengupta, S.; Mukherjee, B.; Shaw, T.K.; Gaonkar, R.H.; Debnath, M.C. Chitosan-Coated Nanoparticles Enhanced Lung Pharmacokinetic Profile of Voriconazole upon Pulmonary Delivery in Mice. *Nanomedicine* **2018**, *13*, 501–520. [CrossRef]
142. Liao, Q.; Yip, L.; Chow, M.Y.T.; Chow, S.F.; Chan, H.-K.; Kwok, P.C.L.; Lam, J.K.W. Porous and Highly Dispersible Voriconazole Dry Powders Produced by Spray Freeze Drying for Pulmonary Delivery with Efficient Lung Deposition. *Int. J. Pharm.* **2019**, *560*, 144–154. [CrossRef] [PubMed]
143. Holle, J.; Leichsenring, M.; Meissner, P.E. Nebulized Voriconazole in Infections with Scedosporium Apiospermum–Case Report and Review of the Literature. *J. Cyst. Fibros.* **2014**, *13*, 400–402. [CrossRef] [PubMed]
144. Prentice, A.G.; Glasmacher, A. Making Sense of Itraconazole Pharmacokinetics. *J. Antimicrob. Chemother.* **2005**, *56* (Suppl. 1), i17–i22. [CrossRef]
145. Purvis, T.; Vaughn, J.M.; Rogers, T.L.; Chen, X.; Overhoff, K.A.; Sinswat, P.; Hu, J.; McConville, J.T.; Johnston, K.P.; Williams, R.O. Cryogenic Liquids, Nanoparticles, and Microencapsulation. *Int. J. Pharm.* **2006**, *324*, 43–50. [CrossRef] [PubMed]
146. Yang, W.; Wiederhold, N.P.; Williams, R.O. Drug Delivery Strategies for Improved Azole Antifungal Action. *Expert Opin. Drug Deliv.* **2008**, *5*, 1199–1216. [CrossRef]
147. McConville, J.T.; Overhoff, K.A.; Sinswat, P.; Vaughn, J.M.; Frei, B.L.; Burgess, D.S.; Talbert, R.L.; Peters, J.I.; Johnston, K.P.; Williams, R.O. Targeted High Lung Concentrations of Itraconazole Using Nebulized Dispersions in a Murine Model. *Pharm. Res.* **2006**, *23*, 901–911. [CrossRef] [PubMed]
148. Vaughn, J.M.; McConville, J.T.; Burgess, D.; Peters, J.I.; Johnston, K.P.; Talbert, R.L.; Williams, R.O. Single Dose and Multiple Dose Studies of Itraconazole Nanoparticles. *Eur. J. Pharm. Biopharm.* **2006**, *63*, 95–102. [CrossRef]
149. Vaughn, J.M.; Wiederhold, N.P.; McConville, J.T.; Coalson, J.J.; Talbert, R.L.; Burgess, D.S.; Johnston, K.P.; Williams, R.O.; Peters, J.I. Murine Airway Histology and Intracellular Uptake of Inhaled Amorphous Itraconazole. *Int. J. Pharm.* **2007**, *338*, 219–224. [CrossRef]
150. Yang, W.; Tam, J.; Miller, D.A.; Zhou, J.; McConville, J.T.; Johnston, K.P.; Williams, R.O. High Bioavailability from Nebulized Itraconazole Nanoparticle Dispersions with Biocompatible Stabilizers. *Int. J. Pharm.* **2008**, *361*, 177–188. [CrossRef]
151. Hoeben, B.J.; Burgess, D.S.; McConville, J.T.; Najvar, L.K.; Talbert, R.L.; Peters, J.I.; Wiederhold, N.P.; Frei, B.L.; Graybill, J.R.; Bocanegra, R.; et al. In Vivo Efficacy of Aerosolized Nanostructured Itraconazole Formulations for Prevention of Invasive Pulmonary Aspergillosis. *Antimicrob. Agents Chemother.* **2006**, *50*, 1552–1554. [CrossRef]
152. Alvarez, C.A.; Wiederhold, N.P.; McConville, J.T.; Peters, J.I.; Najvar, L.K.; Graybill, J.R.; Coalson, J.J.; Talbert, R.L.; Burgess, D.S.; Bocanegra, R.; et al. Aerosolized Nanostructured Itraconazole as Prophylaxis against Invasive Pulmonary Aspergillosis. *J. Infect.* **2007**, *55*, 68–74. [CrossRef] [PubMed]
153. Yang, W.; Chow, K.T.; Lang, B.; Wiederhold, N.P.; Johnston, K.P.; Williams, R.O. In Vitro Characterization and Pharmacokinetics in Mice Following Pulmonary Delivery of Itraconazole as Cyclodextrin Solubilized Solution. *Eur. J. Pharm. Sci.* **2010**, *39*, 336–347. [CrossRef] [PubMed]
154. Yang, W.; Johnston, K.P.; Williams, R.O. Comparison of Bioavailability of Amorphous versus Crystalline Itraconazole Nanoparticles via Pulmonary Administration in Rats. *Eur. J. Pharm. Biopharm.* **2010**, *75*, 33–41. [CrossRef] [PubMed]
155. Rundfeldt, C.; Steckel, H.; Scherliess, H.; Wyska, E.; Wlaź, P. Inhalable Highly Concentrated Itraconazole Nanosuspension for the Treatment of Bronchopulmonary Aspergillosis. *Eur. J. Pharm. Biopharm.* **2013**, *83*, 44–53. [CrossRef] [PubMed]
156. Rundfeldt, C.; Wyska, E.; Steckel, H.; Witkowski, A.; Jeżewska-Witkowska, G.; Wlaź, P. A Model for Treating Avian Aspergillosis: Serum and Lung Tissue Kinetics for Japanese Quail (Coturnix Japonica) Following Single and Multiple Aerosol Exposures of a Nanoparticulate Itraconazole Suspension. *Med. Mycol.* **2013**, *51*, 800–810. [CrossRef] [PubMed]
157. Wlaź, P.; Knaga, S.; Kasperek, K.; Wlaź, A.; Poleszak, E.; Jeżewska-Witkowska, G.; Winiarczyk, S.; Wyska, E.; Heinekamp, T.; Rundfeldt, C. Activity and Safety of Inhaled Itraconazole Nanosuspension in a Model Pulmonary Aspergillus Fumigatus Infection in Inoculated Young Quails. *Mycopathologia* **2015**, *180*, 35–42. [CrossRef]
158. Pardeike, J.; Weber, S.; Zarfl, H.P.; Pagitz, M.; Zimmer, A. Itraconazole-Loaded Nanostructured Lipid Carriers (NLC) for Pulmonary Treatment of Aspergillosis in Falcons. *Eur. J. Pharm. Biopharm.* **2016**, *108*, 269–276. [CrossRef]
159. Duret, C.; Wauthoz, N.; Merlos, R.; Goole, J.; Maris, C.; Roland, I.; Sebti, T.; Vanderbist, F.; Amighi, K. In Vitro and in Vivo Evaluation of a Dry Powder Endotracheal Insufflator Device for Use in Dose-Dependent Preclinical Studies in Mice. *Eur. J. Pharm. Biopharm.* **2012**, *81*, 627–634. [CrossRef]
160. Duret, C.; Merlos, R.; Wauthoz, N.; Sebti, T.; Vanderbist, F.; Amighi, K. Pharmacokinetic Evaluation in Mice of Amorphous Itraconazole-Based Dry Powder Formulations for Inhalation with High Bioavailability and Extended Lung Retention. *Eur. J. Pharm. Biopharm.* **2014**, *86*, 46–54. [CrossRef]
161. Karashima, M.; Sano, N.; Yamamoto, S.; Arai, Y.; Yamamoto, K.; Amano, N.; Ikeda, Y. Enhanced Pulmonary Absorption of Poorly Soluble Itraconazole by Micronized Cocrystal Dry Powder Formulations. *Eur. J. Pharm. Biopharm.* **2017**, *115*, 65–72. [CrossRef]

162. Huang, Z.; Lin, L.; McGoverin, C.; Liu, H.; Wang, L.; Zhou, Q.T.; Lu, M.; Wu, C. Dry Powder Inhaler Formulations of Poorly Water-Soluble Itraconazole: A Balance between in-Vitro Dissolution and in-Vivo Distribution Is Necessary. *Int. J. Pharm.* **2018**, *551*, 103–110. [CrossRef] [PubMed]
163. Colley, T.; Alanio, A.; Kelly, S.L.; Sehra, G.; Kizawa, Y.; Warrilow, A.G.S.; Parker, J.E.; Kelly, D.E.; Kimura, G.; Anderson-Dring, L.; et al. In Vitro and In Vivo Antifungal Profile of a Novel and Long-Acting Inhaled Azole, PC945, on Aspergillus Fumigatus Infection. *Antimicrob. Agents Chemother.* **2017**, *61*, e02280-16. [CrossRef] [PubMed]
164. Hoenigl, M.; Sprute, R.; Egger, M.; Arastehfar, A.; Cornely, O.A.; Krause, R.; Lass-Flörl, C.; Prattes, J.; Spec, A.; Thompson, G.R.; et al. The Antifungal Pipeline: Fosmanogepix, Ibrexafungerp, Olorofim, Opelconazole, and Rezafungin. *Drugs* **2021**, *81*, 1703–1729. [CrossRef] [PubMed]
165. Cass, L.; Murray, A.; Davis, A.; Woodward, K.; Albayaty, M.; Ito, K.; Strong, P.; Ayrton, J.; Brindley, C.; Prosser, J.; et al. Safety and Nonclinical and Clinical Pharmacokinetics of PC945, a Novel Inhaled Triazole Antifungal Agent. *Pharmacol. Res. Perspect.* **2021**, *9*, e00690. [CrossRef] [PubMed]
166. Kimura, G.; Nakaoki, T.; Colley, T.; Rapeport, G.; Strong, P.; Ito, K.; Kizawa, Y. In Vivo Biomarker Analysis of the Effects of Intranasally Dosed PC945, a Novel Antifungal Triazole, on Aspergillus Fumigatus Infection in Immunocompromised Mice. *Antimicrob. Agents Chemother.* **2017**, *61*, e00124-17. [CrossRef]
167. Colley, T.; Sehra, G.; Daly, L.; Kimura, G.; Nakaoki, T.; Nishimoto, Y.; Kizawa, Y.; Strong, P.; Rapeport, G.; Ito, K. Antifungal Synergy of a Topical Triazole, PC945, with a Systemic Triazole against Respiratory Aspergillus Fumigatus Infection. *Sci. Rep.* **2019**, *9*, 9482. [CrossRef]
168. Colley, T.; Sehra, G.; Chowdhary, A.; Alanio, A.; Kelly, S.L.; Kizawa, Y.; Armstrong-James, D.; Fisher, M.C.; Warrilow, A.G.S.; Parker, J.E.; et al. In Vitro and In Vivo Efficacy of a Novel and Long-Acting Fungicidal Azole, PC1244, on Aspergillus Fumigatus Infection. *Antimicrob. Agents Chemother.* **2018**, *62*, e01941-17. [CrossRef]
169. Colley, T.; Sharma, C.; Alanio, A.; Kimura, G.; Daly, L.; Nakaoki, T.; Nishimoto, Y.; Bretagne, S.; Kizawa, Y.; Strong, P.; et al. Anti-Fungal Activity of a Novel Triazole, PC1244, against Emerging Azole-Resistant Aspergillus Fumigatus and Other Species of Aspergillus. *J. Antimicrob. Chemother.* **2019**, *74*, 2950–2958. [CrossRef]
170. Gietzen, K.; Penka, L.; Eisenburger, R. Imidazole Fungicides Provoke Histamine Release from Mast Cells and Induce Airway Contraction. *Exp. Toxicol. Pathol.* **1996**, *48*, 529–531. [CrossRef]
171. Yu, I.G.; O'Brien, S.E.; Ryckman, D.M. Pharmacokinetic and Pharmacodynamic Comparison of Intravenous and Inhaled Caspofungin. *J. Aerosol. Med. Pulm. Drug Deliv.* **2021**, *34*, 197–203. [CrossRef]
172. Yu, I.G.; Ryckman, D.M. Assessment and Development of the Antifungal Agent Caspofungin for Aerosolized Pulmonary Delivery. *Pharmaceutics* **2021**, *13*, 504. [CrossRef] [PubMed]
173. Los-Arcos, I.; Berastegui, C.; Martín-Gómez, M.T.; Grau, S.; Campany-Herrero, D.; Deu, M.; Sacanell, J.; Campillo, N.; Bravo, C.; Len, O. Nebulized Micafungin Treatment for Scopulariopsis/Microascus Tracheobronchitis in Lung Transplant Recipients. *Antimicrob. Agents Chemother.* **2021**, *65*, e02174-20. [CrossRef] [PubMed]
174. Dhuley, J.N. Aerosol Hamycin Is Effective for Prophylaxis and Therapy in a Rat Model of Pulmonary Aspergillosis. *Rocz. Akad. Med. Bialymst.* **2001**, *46*, 317–325. [PubMed]
175. Emery, L.C.; Cox, S.K.; Souza, M.J. Pharmacokinetics of Nebulized Terbinafine in Hispaniolan Amazon Parrots (Amazona Ventralis). *J. Avian. Med. Surg.* **2012**, *26*, 161–166. [CrossRef]
176. Schmitt, H.J.; Andrade, J.; Edwards, F.; Niki, Y.; Bernard, E.; Armstrong, D. Inactivity of Terbinafine in a Rat Model of Pulmonary Aspergillosis. *Eur. J. Clin. Microbiol. Infect. Dis.* **1990**, *9*, 832–835. [CrossRef] [PubMed]

MDPI

St. Alban-Anlage 66

4052 Basel

Switzerland

www.mdpi.com

Pharmaceutics Editorial Office

E-mail: pharmaceutics@mdpi.com

www.mdpi.com/journal/pharmaceutics

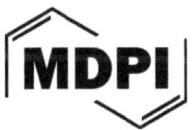

www.ingramcontent.com/pod-product-compliance
Lightning Source LLC
LaVergne TN
LVHW070503100526
83820ZLV00014B/1777